The Handbook of Wellness Medicine

AF148874

The Handbook of Wellness Medicine

Edited by

Waguih William IsHak

Professor and Clinical Chief of Psychiatry, Cedars-Sinai Medical Center and Clinical Professor of Psychiatry, David Geffen School of Medicine, University of California Los Angeles (UCLA), Los Angeles, California, USA

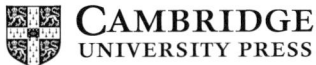
CAMBRIDGE
UNIVERSITY PRESS

CAMBRIDGE
UNIVERSITY PRESS

University Printing House, Cambridge CB2 8BS, United Kingdom

One Liberty Plaza, 20th Floor, New York, NY 10006, USA

477 Williamstown Road, Port Melbourne, VIC 3207, Australia

314–321, 3rd Floor, Plot 3, Splendor Forum, Jasola District Centre,
New Delhi – 110025, India

79 Anson Road, #06–04/06, Singapore 079906

Cambridge University Press is part of the University of Cambridge.

It furthers the University's mission by disseminating knowledge in the pursuit of
education, learning, and research at the highest international levels of excellence.

www.cambridge.org
Information on this title: www.cambridge.org/9781108722056
DOI: 10.1017/9781108650182

© Cambridge University Press 2020

This publication is in copyright. Subject to statutory exception
and to the provisions of relevant collective licensing agreements,
no reproduction of any part may take place without the written
permission of Cambridge University Press.

First published 2020

Printed in the United Kingdom by TJ International Ltd, Padstow Cornwall

A catalogue record for this publication is available from the British Library.

ISBN 978-1-108-72205-6 Paperback

Cambridge University Press has no responsibility for the persistence or accuracy of
URLs for external or third-party internet websites referred to in this publication
and does not guarantee that any content on such websites is, or will remain,
accurate or appropriate.

....

Every effort has been made in preparing this book to provide accurate and up-to-date information that
is in accord with accepted standards and practice at the time of publication. Although case histories are
drawn from actual cases, every effort has been made to disguise the identities of the individuals involved.
Nevertheless, the authors, editors, and publishers can make no warranties that the information
contained herein is totally free from error, not least because clinical standards are constantly changing
through research and regulation. The authors, editors, and publishers therefore disclaim all liability for
direct or consequential damages resulting from the use of material contained in this book. Readers are
strongly advised to pay careful attention to information provided by the manufacturer of any drugs or
equipment that they plan to use.

To my love Asbasia (Hanan) Mikhail-IsHak, MD, FACEP, our sons William and Michael, our parents William Makram IsHak, MD, Nawara Yacoub Dawoud-IsHak, MD, Mr. Aboelkhair Mikhail and Mrs. Aziza Mikhail, and our siblings Rafik William IsHak, MD, FRCS, Albert Mikhail, MD, and Mrs. Lamia Maalouf. For their inspiration, encouragement, and love.

Contents

List of Contributors   *page* xi

Part I Approach to Wellness

Part I aims at introducing the concept of wellness by detailing the definitions, screening/assessment/measurement methods, and the formulation of wellness plans.

1   **Defining Wellness**   1
Waguih William IsHak, Amy Mann, Vicki Manoukian, Sarin Pakhdikian, Monika Chaudhry, Angela Liu, and Ryan Bart

2   **Screening and Assessment Methods for Wellness**   13
Jared M. Greenberg, Enrico G. Castillo, Waguih William IsHak, and Kenneth Wells

3   **The Biopsychosocial Assessment**   23
Lubna Somjee and Sabrina A. Esbitt

4   **Wellness Measurement**   37
Timothy P. Melchert

5   **The Wellness Treatment Plan**   45
Dilani M. Perera and Jeffry Moe

Part II From Illness to Wellness by Organ Systems/Disorders

Part II aims at detailing wellness plans for patients with major illnesses categorized by organ system/disorders. Scientific evidence for specific wellness interventions in each disease state is presented.

6   **The Concept of Wellness in Psychiatric and Substance-Use Disorders**   57
A. George Awad

7   **Neurological and Neurosurgical Disorders and Wellness**   66
Kevin Ding and Isaac Yang

8   **Cardiovascular and Pulmonary Wellness**   79
Waguih William IsHak and Nathalie Herrera

9   **Gastrointestinal System and Wellness**   87
Lori A. Robbins and Edward J. Feldman

10   **Wellness and the Genito-Urinary System**   98
Karyn S. Eilber and Una J. Lee

11   **Reproductive System: Pregnancy and Postpartum Wellness**   116
Dotun Ogunyemi

12   **Allergic, Infectious, and Immunological Processes**   135
Ossama Riaz, Sylvester Orimaye, Thabit Al-Khateeb, Patrick Sodeke, Adeola Awujoola, and Karl Goodkin

13   **Wellness in Endocrine and Metabolic Disorders**   160
Steven Clevenger, Lidia Eskander, Tiffany Lin, and Waguih William IsHak

Part III Special Populations and Special Topics

Part III aims at detailing what assessment methods and interventions could be utilized to improve wellness in each of the specific populations or settings, using scientific evidence.

14 **Wellness Interventions in Patients Living with Chronic Medical Conditions** 177
Alexander J. Steiner, Leslie Aguilar-Hernandez, Demetria R. Pizano, Julieta Dascal, and Waguih William IsHak

15 **Wellness in Older Individuals** 188
Allison M. Mays, Elizabeth Whiteman, and Sonja Rosen

16 **Wellness in Children and Adolescents** 199
Cassidy Zanko and Margaret L. Stuber

17 **Wellness in Pain Disorders** 209
Charles Louy, Chona Sweet, Gabriel Pollock, Catherine de Zagon, Zara Louy, Jeanne M. Weiss, and Dermot P. Maher

18 **Wellness in Cancer and Neoplastic Diseases** 225
Luma Bashmi and Waguih William IsHak

19 **Wellness in Terminal Illness** 237
Monika Chaudhry, Alex Gordon, Emile Tadros, Carrian Sun, Gabriel Tobia, and Waguih William IsHak

20 **Wellness Interventions in the Workplace** 248
Robert A. Chernoff

21 **Wellness Interventions for Physicians and Healthcare Professionals** 258
Matthew Goldenberg and Itai Danovitch

Part IV Wellness Interventions

Part IV aims at describing in detail each intervention, including the scientific evidence behind it and its practical application.

22 **Nutrition** 271
James Lundy

23 **Nutraceuticals and Wellness** 292
Dax Volle and Katrina DeBonis

24 **Pharmaceuticals and Alternatives for Wellness** 302
Thomas Parisi, Blaire Heath, Raymond Wen, and Waguih William IsHak

25 **Exercise, Dance, Tai Chi, Pilates, and Alexander Technique** 315
Ziya Altug

26 **Sleep, Rest, and Relaxation in Improving Wellness** 324
Ashley Ngor and Waguih William IsHak

27 **Sex, Intimacy, and Well-Being** 332
Kailee Marin, Gabriel Tobia, Atef Bakhoum, Lancer Naghdechi, Samuel Korouri, and Waguih William IsHak

28 **Mindfulness, Meditation, and Yoga** 345
Kayse Budd

29 **Forgiveness, Gratitude, and Spirituality** 357
Sindhu A. Idicula, Natasha Thrower, and James Lomax

30 **Positive Neuropsychology, Cognitive Rehabilitation, and Neuroenhancement** 365
Patricia A. Pimental, John B. O'Hara, Jennifer M. Christopher, and Anna M. Ciampanelli

31 **Acupuncture, Herbs, and Ayurvedic Medicine** 378
Lucy Postolov and Suzanne Gilberg-Lenz

32 **The Role of Aesthetics in Wellness** 394
Asbasia A. Mikhail and Ashley Ngor

33 **Massage, Humor, and Music** 403
Soo Liang Ooi and Sok Cheon Pak

34 **Nature and Pets** 413
Vinathe Sharma-Brymer, Katherine Dashper, and Eric Brymer

35 **Circadian Rhythm in the Digital Age** 423
Mona Ezzat-Velinov and Mimi Guarneri

36 **The Arts in Health Settings: Inspirational, Educational, and Therapeutic Approaches to Wellness** 435
Amy Bucciarelli, Gail K. Ellison, Eleanor K. Sommer, and Heather Spooner

37 **Engaging the Five Senses: Taste, Smell, See, Listen, and Touch** 448
Vladimir Bokarius

38 **Emotional Intelligence and Its Role in Sustaining Fulfillment in Life** 463
Harry C. Sax and Bruce L. Gewertz

39 **Psychotherapy and Positive Psychology** 474
Andrea Svicher and Eva-Lotta Brakemeier

40 **Resilience and Wellness** 484
Nathalie Herrera and Waguih William IsHak

41 **Developing Purpose, Meaning, and Achievements** 494
Jennice Vilhauer

42 **Healing and Wellness** 504
Paul Dieppe, Sarah Goldingay, and Sara L. Warber

43 **Connection, Compassion, and Community** 515
Rebecca Hedrick and Kristina Jones

44 **Wellness Interventions for Chronicity and Disability** 525
Anna Klimowicz, Lorne Schussel, and Waguih William IsHak

Part V Wellness through Optimization of Work, Love, and Play

Part V aims at integrating the above knowledge in terms of utilizing time to practically apply the interventions into one's life aspects to maintain wellness.

45 **Work, Love, Play, and Joie de Vivre** 535
Nicole Van Groningen, Waguih William IsHak, Shaina Ganjian, Michael Ong, and Wendelin Slusser

46 **Well-Being and Work–Life Balance: Cultural, Positive Psychology, and Practical Perspectives** 545
Michael Bolton, Ingrid Lobben, Tom Pruzinsky, and Theodore A. Stern

47 **Family Relations, Friendships, and Love** 553
Shelby Alsup, Elli Weisbaum, Talya Vogel, and Daniel J. Siegel

48 **The Role of Leisure, Recreation, and Play in Health and Well-Being** 565
Laura L. Payne and Jaesung An

49 **Wellness and Whole-Person Care** 573
Tom A. Hutchinson and Nora Hutchinson

50 **The Personalized Wellness Life Plan** 582
Waguih William IsHak, Ryan Bart, Yasmine Gohar, Natalie Lorea, Lidia Eskander, Tiffany Chang, Samantha Cohen, Katerina Furman, Piyush Peter Nayyar, and Katrina DeBonis

Appendix I: Wellness Measures 598
Waguih William IsHak

Appendix II: Wellness Apps and Devices 605
Brennan Spiegel, Jonathan A. Almendárez, Samuel Korouri, Angela Liu, and Waguih William IsHak

Index 623

Contributors

Leslie Aguilar-Hernandez, BA candidate
Department of Psychiatry and
Behavioral Neurosciences, Cedars-Sinai
Medical Center, Los Angeles,
California, USA

Thabit Al-Khateeb, MD
Department of Psychiatry and Behavioral
Sciences, James H. Quillen College of
Medicine, East Tennessee State University,
Johnson City, TN, USA

Jonathan A. Almendárez, BA
Department of Psychiatry, Cedars-Sinai
Medical Center, Los Angeles, CA, USA

Shelby Alsup, LMFT, PhD candidate
School of Graduate Psychology,
Pacific University, Hillsboro, OR,
USA

Ziya Altug, PT, DPT, MS, OCS, CSCS
Private Practice, Los Angeles, CA,
USA

Jaesung An, PhD candidate
Department of Recreation, Sport &
Tourism, College of Applied Health
Sciences, University of Illinois at Urbana-
Champaign, IL, USA

A. George Awad, MBBCh, PhD
Department of Psychiatry and the
Institute of Medical Science, University of
Toronto, Humber River Hospital, Toronto,
Canada

Awujoola Adeola M.D. MPH(c)
Department of Biostatistics and
Epidemiology College of Public Health East
Tennessee State University Johnson City,
TN, USA

Atef Bakhoum, MD, MSc, PhD
National Hepatology and Tropical
Medicine Research Institute, Cairo, Egypt

Freedom Drugs and HIV Program, Cairo,
Egypt

Ryan Bart, DO, Capt USAF
United States Air Force Medical Corps

Department of Psychiatry and Behavioral
Neurosciences, Cedars-Sinai Medical
Center, Los Angeles, California, USA

Luma Bashmi, MA
Department of Scientific Research
and Development, King Hamad
University Hospital, Muharraq, Kingdom
of Bahrain

Vladimir Bokarius, MD, PhD, MSOM
Psychiatry and Chronic Pain, San Mateo,
California, USA

Michael Bolton, MD
Private practice in Santa Barbara, CA, USA

Department of Psychiatry, Cedars
Sinai Medical Center, Los Angeles,
CA, USA

Eva-Lotta Brakemeier, PhD, Dr Dipl Psych, Dipl Music
Institute for Psychology, Universität
Greifswald, Greifswald, Germany

Eric Brymer, PhD
Australian College of Applied Psychology,
Sydney, Australia

Institute of Sport, Physical Activity and
Leisure, Leeds Beckett University,
Leeds, UK

University of Cumbria, UK

Amy Bucciarelli, MS, ATR-BC, LMHC
Center for Arts in Medicine, University of
Florida, Gainesville, FL, USA

Kayse Budd, MD
Private Practice in San Diego and Los
Angeles, CA, and online, USA

Enrico G. Castillo, MD, MSHPM
Los Angeles County Department of
Mental Health, Los Angeles, CA, USA

Jane and Terry Semel Institute for
Neuroscience and Human Behavior at
UCLA, Los Angeles, CA, USA

Department of Psychiatry and
Biobehavioral Sciences, David Geffen
School of Medicine at UCLA, Los Angeles,
CA, USA

Center for Social Medicine and
Humanities, UCLA, Los Angeles, CA, USA

Tiffany Chang, BS
Department of Psychiatry and
Behavioral Neurosciences,
Cedars-Sinai Medical Center,
Los Angeles, CA, USA

Monika Chaudhry, MD, FAPA
Department of Psychiatry and Behavioral
Neurosciences, Cedars-Sinai Medical
Center, Los Angeles, CA, USA

Robert A. Chernoff, JD, PhD
Department of Psychiatry and
Behavioral Neurosciences,
Cedars-Sinai Medical Center,
Los Angeles, CA, USA

Jennifer M. Christopher, MA
Department of Behavioral Medicine,
Midwestern University, College of Health
Sciences, Downers Grove, IL, USA

Neurobehavioral Medicine Consultants,
Ltd., Elmhurst, IL, USA

Anna M. Ciampanelli, MA
Department of Behavioral Medicine,
Midwestern University, College of Health
Sciences, Downers Grove, IL, USA

Neurobehavioral Medicine Consultants,
Ltd., Elmhurst, IL, USA

Steven Clevenger, DO
Department of Psychiatry and Behavioral
Neurosciences, Cedars-Sinai Medical
Center, Los Angeles, CA, USA

Department of Psychiatry, Western
Michigan University Homer Stryker M.D.
School of Medicine, Kalamazoo,
MI, USA

Samantha Cohen, MA
Department of Psychiatry and Behavioral
Neurosciences, Cedars-Sinai Medical
Center, Los Angeles, CA, USA

Itai Danovitch, MD, MBA
Department of Psychiatry and Behavioral
Neurosciences, Cedars-Sinai Medical
Center, Los Angeles, CA, USA

Julieta Dascal, MSW
Department of Psychiatry and
Behavioral Neurosciences, Cedars-Sinai
Medical Center, Los Angeles,
California, USA

Katherine Dashper, PhD
School of Events, Tourism and Hospitality
Management, Leeds Beckett University,
Leeds, UK

Katrina DeBonis, MD
Jane and Terry Semel Institute for
Neuroscience and Human Behavior at
UCLA, Los Angeles, CA, USA

Department of Psychiatry and
Biobehavioral Sciences, David Geffen
School of Medicine at UCLA, Los Angeles,
CA, USA

Veterans Administration Greater Los Angeles Healthcare System, Los Angeles, CA, USA

Paul Dieppe, MD
University of Exeter Medical School, Exeter, UK

Kevin Ding, BS
Department of Neurosurgery, David Geffen School of Medicine at UCLA, Los Angeles, CA, USA

Karyn S. Eilber, MD
Department of Surgery, Division of Urology, Cedars-Sinai Medical Center, Los Angeles, CA, USA

Gail K. Ellison, PhD
Center for Arts in Medicine, University of Florida, Gainesville, FL, USA

Sabrina A. Esbitt, PhD
Department of Family and Social Medicine, Montefiore Medical Center, Bronx, New York, NY, USA

Lidia Eskander, MD
Department of Psychiatry and Behavioral Neurosciences, Cedars-Sinai Medical Center, Los Angeles, CA, USA

Mona Ezzat-Velinov, MD, ABFM, ABIHM, IFMCP
New Roots, San Diego, CA, USA

Physician, Human Longevity Inc., San Diego, CA, USA

Edward J. Feldman, MD
Division of Digestive Diseases, Cedars-Sinai Medical Center, Los Angeles, CA, USA

Katerina Furman, BA
Department of Psychiatry and Biobehavioral Sciences, David Geffen School of Medicine at UCLA, Los Angeles, CA, USA

University of California, Berkeley, Berkeley, CA, USA

Shaina Ganjian, MD
Department of Pediatrics, Kaiser Permanente Los Angeles Medical Center, Los Angeles, California, USA

Bruce L. Gewertz, MD, FACS
Department of Surgery, Cedars-Sinai Medical Center, Los Angeles, CA, USA

Interventional Services, Cedars-Sinai Medical Center, Los Angeles, CA, USA

Academic Affairs, Cedars-Sinai Medical Center, Los Angeles, CA, USA

Suzanne Gilberg-Lenz, MD, CAS
Private Practice, Beverly Hills, California, USA

Department of Obstetrics and Gynaecology, Cedars-Sinai Medical Center, Los Angeles, CA, USA

Yasmine Gohar, MA
Department of Psychiatry and Behavioral Neurosciences, Cedars-Sinai Medical Center, Los Angeles, CA, USA

Matthew Goldenberg, DO
Department of Psychiatry and Behavioral Neurosciences, Cedars-Sinai Medical Center, Los Angeles, CA, USA

Sarah Goldingay, PhD
Department of Drama, University of Exeter, Exeter, UK

Karl Goodkin, MD, PhD
Department of Psychiatry, University of Nebraska Medical Center in Omaha, Omaha, NE, USA

Alex Gordon, BS Candidate
Department of Psychiatry and Behavioral
Neurosciences, Cedars-Sinai Medical
Center, Los Angeles, CA, USA

Jared M. Greenberg, MD
Jane and Terry Semel Institute for
Neuroscience and Human Behavior at
UCLA, Los Angeles, CA, USA

Department of Psychiatry and Biobehavioral
Sciences, David Geffen School of Medicine
at UCLA, Los Angeles, CA, USA

VA Health Services Research
and Development Center for the
Study of Healthcare Innovation,
Implementation, and Policy, VA Greater
Los Angeles Healthcare System, Los
Angeles, CA, USA

Nicole Van Groningen, MD
Department of Medicine, Cedars-Sinai
Medical Center, Los Angeles, CA, USA

Mimi Guarneri, MD, FACC, ABOIM
Academy of Integrative Health and
Medicine, La Jolla, CA, USA

Pacific Pearl, La Jolla, CA, USA

Physician, Human Longevity Inc., San
Diego, CA, USA

Blaire Heath, DO, PharmD, RD
Department of Psychiatry, Loma Linda
University Health, Loma Linda, CA, USA

Rebecca Hedrick, MD
Department of Psychiatry and Behavioral
Neurosciences, Cedars-Sinai Medical
Center, Los Angeles, CA, USA

Nathalie Herrera, MD
Department of Psychiatry and Behavioral
Neurosciences, Cedars-Sinai Medical
Center, Los Angeles, CA, USA

Nora Hutchinson, MD
Department of Medicine, McGill
University, Montreal, Quebec, Canada

Tom A. Hutchinson, MB, FRCP(C)
McGill Programs in Whole Person Care,
Montreal, Quebec, Canada

Sindhu A. Idicula, MD
Menninger Department of Psychiatry,
Baylor College of Medicine, Houston,
TX, USA

Waguih William IsHak, MD, FAPA
Department of Psychiatry and
Biobehavioral Sciences, David Geffen
School of Medicine at UCLA, Los Angeles,
CA, USA

Department of Psychiatry and
Behavioral Neurosciences, Cedars-Sinai
Medical Center, Los Angeles,
California, USA

Kristina Jones MD, MA
Consultation-Liaison Psychiatry,
Cedars-Sinai Medical Center,
Los Angeles, CA, USA

Anna Klimowicz, DO
Department of Psychiatry, Icahn
School of Medicine at Mount Sinai
Morningside & West, New York,
NY, USA

Samuel Korouri, BA
Department of Psychiatry and Behavioral
Neurosciences, Cedars-Sinai Medical
Center, Los Angeles, CA, USA

University of California Los Angeles, Los
Angeles, CA, USA

Una J. Lee, MD
Female Pelvic Medicine and Reconstructive
Surgery, Section of Urology and
Renal Transplantation, Virginia

Mason Medical Center, Seattle, WA, USA

Soo Liang Ooi, BHSc (Comp Med), MMath
School of Biomedical Sciences, Charles Sturt University, Bathurst, Australia

Tiffany Lin, MD
Department of Psychiatry, Kaiser Permanente San Jose Medical Center, San Jose, CA, USA

Angela Liu, BS candidate
Department of Psychiatry and Behavioral Neurosciences, Cedars-Sinai Medical Center, Los Angeles, California, USA

Ingrid Lobben, MSW, MEd
Social work, Lakewood Regional Medical Center, Lakewood, CA, USA

James Lomax, MD
Menninger Department of Psychiatry, Baylor College of Medicine, Houston, TX, USA

Natalie Lorea, BS candidate
Department of Psychiatry and Behavioral Neurosciences, Cedars-Sinai Medical Center, Los Angeles, CA, USA

Charles Louy, MD, PhD, MBA
Department of Anesthesiology, Cedars-Sinai Medical Center, Los Angeles, CA, USA

Zara Louy, MA, NBC-HWC
Private Practice, Los Angeles, CA, USA

James Lundy, DPT
Head 2 Toe Physical Therapy, Manhattan Beach, CA, USA

Dermot P. Maher, MD, MS, MHS
Department of Anesthesiology and Critical Care Medicine, Johns Hopkins School of Medicine, Baltimore, MD, USA

Amy Mann, LCSW
Inflammatory Bowel Disease Program, Division of Digestive Diseases, Cedars-Sinai Medical Center, Los Angeles, California, USA

Vicki Manoukian, MA
Department of Psychiatry and Behavioral Neurosciences, Cedars-Sinai Medical Center, Los Angeles, California, USA

Allison M. Mays MD, MAS
Section of Geriatric Medicine, Division of Internal Medicine, Department of Medicine, Cedars-Sinai Medical Center, Los Angeles, CA, USA

Timothy P. Melchert, PhD
Department of Counselor Education and Counseling Psychology, Marquette University, Milwaukee, WI, USA

Asbasia A. Mikhail, MD, FACEP
Department of Emergency Medicine, Huntington Memorial Hospital, Pasadena, CA, USA

Exer Urgent Care, Pasadena and La Canada, CA, USA

Jeff Moe, PhD, LPC, NCC, CCMHC
Department of Counseling & Human Services, Old Dominion University, Norfolk, VA, USA

Lancer Naghdechi, DO
Department of Psychiatry and Behavioral Neurosciences, Cedars-Sinai Medical Center, Los Angeles, CA, USA

Piyush Peter Nayyar, MD
Department of Medicine, David Geffen School of Medicine at UCLA, Los Angeles, CA, USA

Ashley Ngor, BS candidate
Department of Psychiatry and Behavioral
Neurosciences, Cedars-Sinai Medical
Center, Los Angeles, CA, USA

UCLA, Los Angeles, CA, USA

John B. O'Hara, PsyD
Institute of Living/Hartford Hospital,
Hartford, CT, USA

Department of Medicine, University of
Wisconsin School of Medicine and Public
Health, Madison, WI, USA

Neurobehavioral Medicine Consultants,
Ltd., Elmhurst, IL, USA

Dotun Ogunyemi, MD, FACOG, MFM
Obstetrics & Gynecology, California
University of Science & Medicine, San
Bernardino, CA, USA

Michael K Ong, MD, PhD
Department of Medicine, David
GeffenSchool of Medicine at UCLA,
Los Angeles, CA, USA

Veterans Administration Greater
LosAngeles Healthcare System, Los
Angeles, CA, USA

Sylvester Olubolu Orimaye, PhD, MPH
Department of Health Services
Management and Administration College
of Public HealthEast Tennessee State
UniversityJohnson City, TN, USA

Sok Cheon Pak, PhD
School of Biomedical Sciences,
Charles Sturt University, Bathurst,
Australia

Sarin Pakhdikian, DO candidate
Western University of Health Sciences,
College of Osteopathic Medicine, Pomona,
CA, USA

Department of Psychiatry and
Behavioral Neurosciences, Cedars-Sinai
Medical Center, Los Angeles,
California, USA

Thomas Parisi, DO, MA
Department of Psychiatry, Loma
Linda University Health, Loma Linda,
CA, USA

Laura L. Payne, PhD
Department of Recreation, Sport &
Tourism, College of Applied Health
Sciences, University of Illinois at Urbana-
Champaign, IL, USA

Dilani M. Perera, PhD, LPC-S, LCDC, NCC, MAC
Department of Counselor Education,
Fairfield University, Fairfield, CT, USA

Patricia A. Pimental, PsyD, ABN, AAPM, FACPN
Department of Behavioral Medicine,
Midwestern University, Downers Grove,
IL, USA

Neurobehavioral Medicine Consultants,
Ltd., Elmhurst, IL, USA

Demetria R. Pizano, MA
Department of Psychiatry and Behavioral
Neurosciences, Cedars-Sinai Medical
Center, Los Angeles, California, USA

Gabriel Pollock, MD
Department of Anesthesiology, Cedars-
Sinai Medical Center, Los Angeles, CA, USA

Lucy Postolov, DACM, LAc, DiplAc
Postolova Acupuncture Group and
Cannapy Health LLC, Los Angeles,
CA, USA

Cedars-Sinai Medical Center, Los Angeles,
CA, USA

Physicians Advisory Board for the Cancer
Support Community, Los Angeles,
CA, USA

Tom Pruzinsky, PhD
Department of Psychology, Quinnipac
University, Hamden, CT, USA

Ossama Riaz, MD
Department of Psychiatry and Behavioral
Sciences, James H. Quillen College of
Medicine, East Tennessee State University,
Johnson City, TN, USA

Lori A. Robbins, MD
Division of Digestive Diseases, Cedars-Sinai
Medical Center, Los Angeles, CA, USA

Sonja Rosen, MD
Section of Geriatric Medicine, Division of
Internal Medicine, Department of
Medicine, Cedars-Sinai Medical Center,
Los Angeles, CA, USA

Harry C. Sax, MD
Department of Surgery, Cedars-Sinai
Medical Center, Los Angeles, CA, USA

Lorne Schussel, PhD
Department of Counseling and
Clinical Psychology, Teachers
College Columbia University, New York,
NY, USA

Vinathe Sharma-Brymer, PhD
Independent researcher, Brisbane, Australia

Daniel J. Siegel, M.D.
Mindsight Institute, Santa Monica, CA
David Geffen School of Medicine at UCLA
Mindful Awareness Research Center at
UCLA Los Angeles, CA, USA

Wendelin Slusser, MD
Semel Healthy Campus Initiative Center,
UCLA, Los Angeles, CA, USA

Patrick Sodeke M.D. MPH(c)
Department of Biostatistics and
Epidemiology College of Public Health East
Tennessee State University Johnson City,
TN, USA

Lubna Somjee, PhD
Private Practice Poughkeepsie,
New York, USA

Eleanor K. Sommer, MSc
Center for Arts in Medicine, University of
Florida, Gainesville, FL, USA

Brennan Spiegel, MD
Center for Outcomes Research and
Education, Cedars-Sinai Medical Center,
Los Angeles, CA, USA

David Geffen School of Medicine at UCLA,
Los Angeles, CA, USA

Heather Spooner, MA, ATR-BC
Center for Arts in Medicine, University of
Florida, Gainesville, FL, USA

Alexander J. Steiner, PsyD
Department of Psychiatry and
Biobehavioral Sciences, David Geffen
School of Medicine at UCLA, Los Angeles,
California, USA

Theodore A. Stern, MD
Avery D. Weisman Psychiatric
Consultation Service, Massachusetts
General Hospital, Boston, MA, USA

Thomas P. Hackett Center for Scholarship
in Psychosomatic Medicine, Massachusetts
General Hospital, Boston, MA, USA

Office for Clinical Careers,
Massachusetts General Hospital, Boston,
MA, USA

Department of Psychiatry, Harvard
Medical School, Boston, MA, USA

Margaret L. Stuber, MD
Department of Psychiatry, David Geffen
School of Medicine at UCLA, Los Angeles,
CA, USA

Veterans Administration Greater Los
Angeles Healthcare System, Los Angeles,
CA, USA

Carrian Sun, MD, PhD
Department of Psychiatry and
Behavioral Neurosciences,
Cedars-Sinai Medical Center,
Los Angeles, CA, USA

David Geffen School of Medicine at UCLA
Los Angeles, California, USA

Andrea Svicher, PhD candidate
Department of Health Sciences, University
of Florence, Florence, Italy

Chona Sweet, DrNP, MSN, RN, FNP-C
Department of Anesthesiology,
Cedars-Sinai Medical Center, Los Angeles,
CA, USA

Emile Tadros, BS, MD Candidate
Wayne State University School of
Medicine, Detroit, Michigan, USA

Natasha Thrower, MD
Menninger Department of Psychiatry,
Baylor College of Medicine, Houston,
TX, USA

Gabriel Tobia, MD
Department of Psychiatry, Brigham
and Women's Hospital, Harvard
Medical School, Boston, MA, USA

Jennice Vilhauer, PhD
Live Forward Psychological, Inc.,
Los Angeles, CA, USA

Talya Vogel, MS, PsyD candidate
PGSP – Stanford PsyD Consortium, Palo
Alto, CA, USA

Dax Volle, MD
Jane and Terry Semel Institute for
Neuroscience and Human Behavior at
UCLA, Los Angeles, CA, USA

Department of Psychiatry and
Biobehavioral Sciences, David Geffen

School of Medicine at UCLA, Los Angeles,
CA, USA

Sara L. Warber, MD
Department of Family Medicine,
University of Michigan School of Medicine,
Ann Arbor, MI, USA

Elli Weisbaum, MES, PhD candidate
Institute of Medical Science, Faculty of
Medicine, University of Toronto, Toronto,
Canada

Neuroscience and Mental Health
Department, The Hospital for Sick
Children, Toronto, Canada

Jeanne M. Weiss, MD
Private Practice, Santa Monica, CA, USA

Kenneth Wells, MD, MPH
Jane and Terry Semel Institute for
Neuroscience and Human Behavior at
UCLA, Los Angeles, CA, USA

Department of Psychiatry and Biobehavioral
Sciences, David Geffen School of Medicine
at UCLA, Los Angeles, CA, USA

VA Health Services Research and
Development Center for the Study of
Healthcare Innovation, Implementation,
and Policy, VA Greater Los Angeles
Healthcare System, Los Angeles, CA, USA

Center for Health Services and
Society, UCLA, Los Angeles, CA, USA

UCLA, Jonathan Fielding School
of Public Health, Los Angeles, CA, USA

Raymond Wen, PharmD candidate
Department of Psychiatry and Behavioral
Neurosciences, Cedars-Sinai Medical
Center, Los Angeles, CA, USA

Elizabeth Whiteman, MD
Section of Geriatric Medicine,
Division of Internal Medicine,
Department of Medicine, Cedars-Sinai
Medical Center, Los Angeles, CA, USA

Isaac Yang, MD
Department of Neurosurgery, David Geffen
School of Medicine at UCLA, Los Angeles,
CA, USA

Catherine de Zagon
Catherine de Zágon Balance + Wellbeing
Naturopath Health Counseling, Rome, Italy

Cassidy Zanko, MD
Department of Psychiatry, David Geffen
School of Medicine at UCLA, Los Angeles,
CA, USA

Veterans Administration Greater Los
Angeles Healthcare System, Los Angeles,
CA, USA

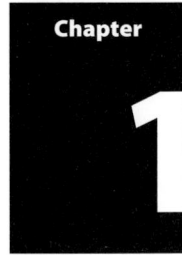

Defining Wellness

Waguih William IsHak, Amy Mann, Vicki Manoukian, Sarin Pakhdikian, Monika Chaudhry, Angela Liu, and Ryan Bart[*]

Introduction

Imagine a society comprising individuals who realize their maximal potential in every facet of their lives. In this society, people work together to better their communities and the lives of others. Individually, the citizens are free of disease, physically fit, well-educated masters of their craft, and they engage in a life of recreation and interconnectedness with family, neighbors, and friends while living with purpose and passion. Is this utopia too good to be true? The voice of reason may say life is not perfect; there are too many ever-changing variables. We are familiar with the physical law of entropy stating that randomness, or disorder, increases with time. However, why not aim toward a society as described above? We can strive to be the best version of ourselves, both on the micro, individual level and on the macro, societal level.

Wellness is the integration of this notion into all dimensions of our lives. It is not necessarily something to achieve, but rather something to be constantly moving toward. There will always be space for growth and improvement. Understanding the multiple facets of wellness helps guide us toward an optimal life as individuals and as a society [1]. In order to pursue wellness, we must first understand what it is. Notions of wellness emerged after the end of World War II. This is because health needed to be transformed. Medical and technological advances were made allowing for the successful treatment of infectious diseases, which were previously the leading cause of death [2]. Since then, the focus of medicine and health has turned to chronic illnesses such as heart disease, diabetes, and cancer [3]. Heart disease is now the number one cause of death in the USA for both men and women [4]. These illnesses are directly associated with lifestyle factors such as chronic stress, physical activity, and nutrition, to name a few. This realization helped us begin to recognize the multifactorial nature of our overall health.

Psychiatrist George L. Engel coined the term *biopsychosocial health* in the 1970s. Biopsychosocial health recognizes the important interplay of biological, psychological, and social factors in the prevention and treatment of our most prevalent illnesses. In fact, according the American College of Lifestyle Medicine (ACLM), 85 percent of chronic diseases are caused by unhealthy lifestyle choices. Additionally, 80 percent or more of the total healthcare-related expenses in the USA are associated with treating ailments that stem from poor lifestyle choices [5]. This increased prevalence of chronic, preventable disease has led to increased focus on wellness. The concept of wellness has long existed under the

---

[*] Disclaimer: The views expressed in this material are those of the author, and do not reflect the official policy or position of the US Government, the Department of Defense, or the Department of the Air Force.

umbrella of "health." However, the term wellness has more recently come to the forefront. In order to offer the recommendations in this textbook that promote wellness, we must first understand what wellness is.

Wellness Definitions

The World Health Organization (WHO) has defined health as "a state of complete physical, mental and social well-being and not merely the absence of disease or infirmity" [6]. This definition laid out the foundation of not only health but also what it means to be well [7]. The three dimensions of wellness are physical, mental, and social. These dimensions not only emphasize the presence of each individual dimension for wellness but also depend on achieving a balance of the dimensions into an integrated whole [8] in order to reach an optimal state of well-being [9]. However, it is important to distinguish that wellness is different from health [10].

The definition of health has made a lateral transition that differentiates health and wellness since the original definition postulated by the WHO. Wellness is more comprehensive and is interrelational, with an emphasis on optimal human functioning [11], whereas health is limited to an individual's overall state of illness or lack thereof [12].

There have been numerous iterations of the working definition of wellness. In 1964, the WHO moved forward from their original definition of health and developed a definition for wellness that included the same three key dimensions from the 1949 definition: physical, mental, and social. It also asserted that multiple subdimensions can be established, which further expanded the definition. The WHO again updated their definition in 2004 and published a working definition of wellness: "the optimal state of health of individuals and groups. There are two focal concerns: the realization of the fullest potential of an individual physically, psychologically, socially, spiritually, and economically, and the fulfillment of one's role expectations in the family, community, place of worship, workplace, and other settings"[13] (Figure 1.1).

In 1981, Ng et al. distinguished that wellness and illness were two independent variables, not two opposite ends of a spectrum. They proposed that wellness is measured as a direct correlation of the degree that one feels positive and enthusiastic [14]. Their definition included wellness facets such as the development of autonomy, realistic self-assessment, emotional intelligence, and stress management. Another definition proposed wellness as a way of life that establishes harmony of mind, body, and spirit, and is harnessed through a healthy lifestyle [15]. Wellness has also been defined as the ability to creatively adapt in order to reach optimal function [16].

There are numerous other proposed definitions similar to the aforementioned. The numerous efforts to define wellness reflect its complex and multifactorial nature. Now, with multiple wellness definitions at hand, let's examine what wellness is not. This will help us understand how wellness is distinct from other related terminology. As discussed previously, wellness is distinct from health [10]. Wellness should also be distinguished from well-being. Well-being is described as a balance between one's challenges and one's resources [10]. While well-being points toward wellness, it is not as comprehensive as wellness itself [8]. Well-being is more transient than wellness. Thus, one can be in a state of well-being but prevented from harnessing wellness due to limitations in psychological, social, or physical resources [10].

On a similar note, wellness is distinct from quality of life (QOL). Quality of life is a measure of an individual's functionality in the setting of the disease status, whereas,

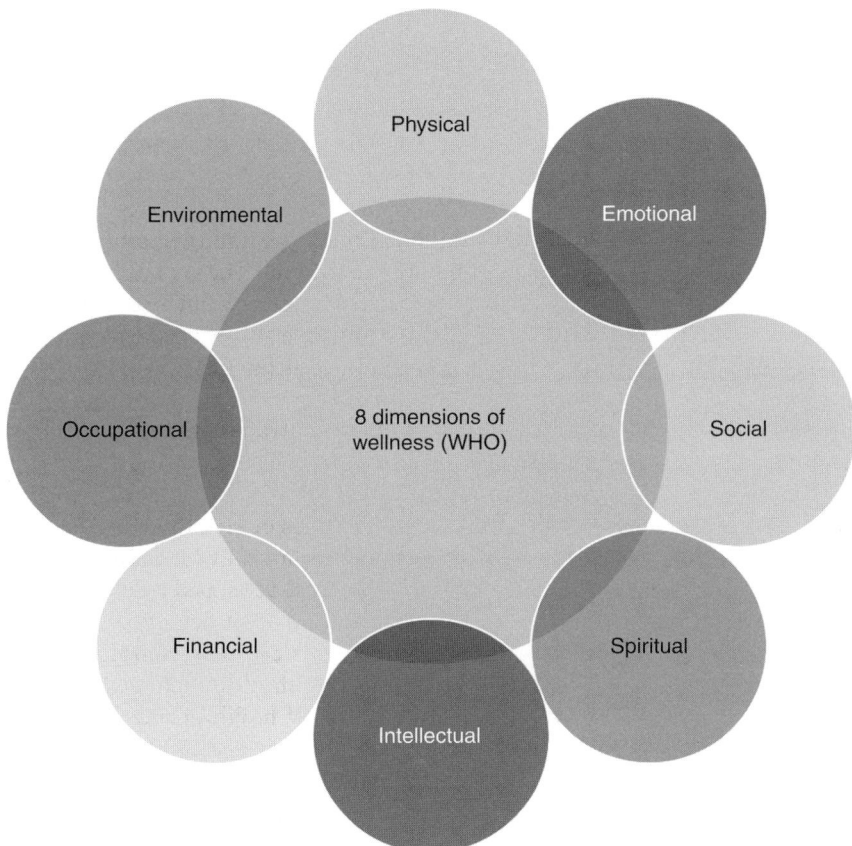

Figure 1.1 WHO dimensions of wellness.

according to the WHO's definition, wellness requires the absence of disease [8]. To further distinguish, QOL is a measure of disease burden and an evaluation of the efficacy of medical treatment [7]. However, wellness exists without the presence of disease. To summarize, wellness is distinct from health, well-being, and QOL because wellness focuses on the lifestyle choices that promote the actualization of optimal function and fulfillment [10].

Now that we have reviewed the distinctness of wellness, let's examine how its definitions can be incorporated into various dimensions and models of wellness.

Wellness Models and Dimensions

While the WHO has been at the forefront of, first, recognizing the importance of wellness and, second, establishing a working definition, it is important to examine additional applications of the concept. A well-known model for wellness is the Wheel of Wellness (WoW; Figure 1.2), which defined wellness as a "way of life oriented towards optimal health and well-being in which mind, body, and spirit are integrated by the individual to live life more fully within the human and natural community" [17, 18].

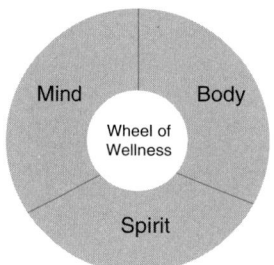

Figure 1.2 The Wheel of Wellness.

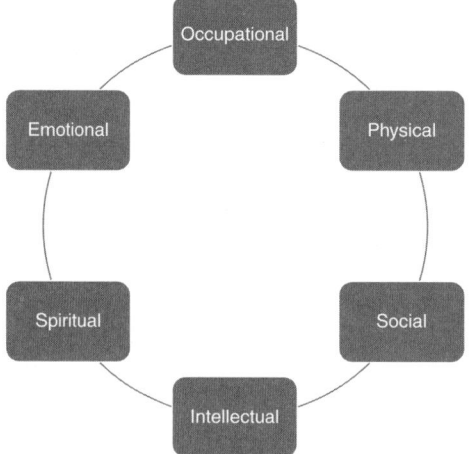

Figure 1.3 Six dimensions of wellness.

Furthermore, the WoW model integrates five second-order and 17 third-order dimensions of wellness. The second-order dimensions include: creative self, coping self, social self, essential self, physical self.

Another wellness model is that of the National Wellness Institute (NWI). They define wellness as the "active process through which people become aware of, and make choices toward, a more successful existence" [19]. This involves manifesting a holistic, positive, and affirming outlook on life. Note that they use the terminology "make choices toward," again supporting the aforementioned concept that wellness is not necessarily an achievement, but rather an ideal to move toward. The NWI dissects wellness into six dimensions: emotional, physical, social, intellectual, occupational, and spiritual [19] (Figure 1.3). These dimensions encompass the facets of our daily lives. The NWI asserts that each dimension is interdependent with the others. The application of the NWI model helps people understand the various components that comprise wellness and how they relate to one another.

As described in the definition section, wellness is distinct from health, well-being, and QOL. It has been asserted that wellness is holistic and multidimensional; research has also addressed that the various wellness dimensions are interrelated. According to Roscoe [20], the core dimensions of wellness are social, emotional, physical, intellectual, and spiritual. These five dimensions are what most college health textbooks use to describe wellness [21].

Wellness, however, is a determinant of the integrated whole, not a sum of its individual dimensions. Stephen Covey, in his book *The 7 Habits of Highly Effective People*, asserted that "The whole is greater than the sum of its parts." This holds true in the context of the dimensions of wellness. It is also important to highlight that Rachele and colleagues emphasize that wellness is determined by lifestyle behaviors that direct one toward optimization across multiple domains. While the dimensions above promote wellness, wellness – in turn – also results in positive outcomes within the various dimensions. Thus, wellness and its various dimensions are a cyclical continuum that feed into one another and build resilience and momentum. This concept highlights the multidimensionality of wellness and helps to emphasize that this multifaceted nature must be accounted for when measuring wellness [10].

For example, the mere presence of an individual influences his/her environment and can help build better communities and social networks. Our belief systems, values, and worldviews allow us to make meaningful interactions with others and enrich life through work, community, and recreation. The benefits of physical activity are endless; they promote strength, endurance, and vitality. A strong sense of self-worth and self-control also determine the sense of direction we obtain in our lives. To find oneself in an enriching and creative environment stimulates mental activity and the ability to share one's skills with others. All of these facets are interconnected and comprise wellness according to both the WoW and NWI models. There is no concrete distinction as to how much of each dimension should encompass a person's life. Rather, it is the ability to holistically balance these virtues that enables us to move toward wellness.

In constructing an operational definition of wellness, there is ongoing complexity and difficulty when it comes to language and definition overlap, specifically when trying to promote, measure, and develop new evidence-based wellness programs based on the individual's functioning across physical, psychological, social, spiritual, economic, familial, community, religious, and workplace dimensions. Traditional literature review and current social beliefs tend to use wellness, well-being, quality of life, and health interchangeably at various times and settings, causing much confusion. The goal of an operational definition of wellness is to develop clear parameters, so that it may be analyzed and discussed in a standardized way. "While it is inevitable that cross-over exists between similar constructs, wellness does have distinctly identifiable features" [10].

The traditional definition of health has been primarily focused on the disease state and is illness based. Thus, someone who has a controlled chronic illness would be deemed not well under conventional beliefs, and unable to achieve an optimal state of life satisfaction. Because health has been historically grouped into, and a prerequisite to, wellness, workplace wellness programs have focused almost all their attention on employee physical health programs, giving little attention to the other dimensions of wellness, including spiritual, intellectual, and emotional constructs. Instead, aerobic fitness, activity, sleep monitoring and weight management programs are being utilized. Although longitudinal program studies show positive BMI, blood pressure, and cholesterol health outcomes, they fail at nurturing the deeper human pathways toward a meaningful life beyond absence of illness [10].

Rachele et al. formulated an operational understanding of wellness that is of significant importance [10]. Their work emphasizes that wellness is truly a multifaceted model, and it should be promoted and practiced as such. It differs from the notion of health, quality of life, and well-being in that wellness focuses on individual lifestyle behaviors that promote achievement of optimal function and fulfillment. It goes beyond constraining oneself to the "rearview mirror" in which the individual is moving away from chronic disease or conditions.

Rather, it puts the individual in the driver's seat, looking forward and engaging in the present with all aspects of their life. Rachele et al. explore the framework of operational understanding of wellness by showing the efficacy of wellness programs in the organizational or workforce setting, while addressing the need to broaden the scope of wellness outside of just physical health. Wellness programs require collaboration for better outcomes for all participants. They should be designed and carried out specifically by all members who can come to a consensus of a common goal. This can complicate things, given the multidimensional concept of wellness, which includes spirit, emotion, social, physical, intellectual, and psychological domains. Currently, in the workplace dynamic, employers have created opportunities for their employees to implement physical fitness. However, they can improve in enhancing mentorship, coaching, and career planning to manage stress and enrich the future plans of their employees. Much like Rachele and colleagues, both Depken [21] and Renger et al. [9] named the same five dimensions for wellness: physical, emotional, social, intellectual, and spiritual. Renger also added a sixth dimension: environmental. This is to recognize the influence that one's surroundings can have on our reality both in the present and in the future, as one's environment can directly play a role in the decisions that one makes. Renger et al. also addressed the value of knowledge, attitude, perception, behavior, and skill as important factors for the implementation of each wellness dimension. They also commented on the importance of balance and how the dimension are interrelated. This again highlights the importance of understanding that wellness is multifactorial.

Adams proposed four key wellness principles [22]: (1) wellness is multidimensional; (2) research and practice related to wellness should be geared toward optimization instead of causes of illness; (3) balance is crucial to wellness; and (4) wellness is relative, subjective, and perceptual. In regard to principle four, there are currently a number of validated tools to assess an individual's comprehensive wellness. Of course, there will always be a layer of subjectivity as the wellness measurement tools rely on an individual's own self-evaluation. Again, this highlights the importance of the concept of balance in wellness. It is hard to be well when life is not in a state of equilibrium. Much like the human body, the optimal is homeostasis; or for the spirit, equanimity. Another important point to re-emphasize from Adam's wellness principles is that wellness is distinct from illness.

Synthesis

Well-being is a theory and term commonly used interchangeably when discussing wellness. Well-being is an outcome measure of how people perceive their lives to be going, most commonly evaluated in self-reported QOL surveys. There is no single consensus when it comes to defining well-being, but there is general agreement that it involves a balance between the demands of our lives and the amount of resources we have to sustain, accomplish, and cultivate conditions for us to thrive [4]. A mother may have a career, multiple children with multiple academic and social obligations, attend night classes, need a new car, be managing an elderly parent, and trying to lose weight. Well-being necessitates positive emotions such as joy, pleasure, and happiness, and implies the absence of continuous negative emotions such as sadness and depression. There are two central principles of well-being, hedonic and eudaimonic, which are not mutually exclusive and describe pleasure stemming from different motives and joy eliciting experiences [10]. The positive emotions one gets from these two diverse avenues of pleasure, researchers found, interestingly enough, affect the body differently on a cellular level. Hedonic perspective "stems from the pleasure you get from a satisfying yet superficial experience such as a massage or eating delicious food." Eudaimonic well-being is pleasure originating from an action that contributes to greater society, for example volunteering or giving a friend advice [23]. Well-being is best fostered as a result of both hedonic and eudaimonic aspects, multidimensional phenomena, and resource accessibility.

In Jerome Rachele's operational definition of wellness, he explains and clarifies how the concept's uniqueness sets it apart from the other constructs discussed above. Wellness includes "being both holistic and multidimensional, being focused on lifestyle behaviors, being about actions or processes, recognizing the interrelatedness between person and environment, and being unique by way of goal and context" [10]. This idea of wellness expresses the opposite of an all-or-nothing perspective, but that if someone is lacking in one dimension, physical health for example, their other dimensions, like spirituality or social or emotional dimensions, become stronger, larger, and solidified. For example, an individual gets diagnosed with a treatable form of cancer. The experience will take them on a journey of appointments, scans, and medications. But in this process, they may join a support group, start journaling, join a yoga class at the church, decide to attend services, befriend participants, and foster new friendships. A chain reaction has been set in motion, and their illness no longer defines their sense of life satisfaction and fulfillment. Wellness is process- and behavior-driven. It's about the journey to get to optimal functioning, not about the outcome. One may argue that an individual may not fully arrive at optimal wellness as it is a quest that continues indefinitely. This operational definition of wellness recognizes the multitude of negative and complex lifestyle constraints we experience, and emphasizes creative, unique, and personalized lifestyle choices and practices to engage the mind and nurture the spirit.

The application of wellness prompts the dialog of confrontation with reality and the assessment of the degree to which wellness is achieved in one's life. People must understand how to achieve their full potential and whether or not their current path will lead them there. The feeling of discomfort within one's own comfort zone is a trying time to discover how the emotional, intellectual, occupational, physical, social, environmental, and spiritual states interplay in reaching said potential. There is no concrete distinction as to how much of each dimension should encompass a person's life. Rather, it is the ability to holistically balance these virtues that enables us to achieve and apply wellness in a way that is authentic to the individual.

Self-actualization is a key factor in wellness. Abraham Maslow was an American psychologist best known for establishing Maslow's hierarchy of needs. His theory asserts that in order to reach maximum human potential, one must first fulfill more basic human needs. These needs begin with the most basic principles of physiological needs. These are our basic biological requirements for survival. Do we have a roof over our heads? Are we fed? Warm? Sleeping well? It is important to understand how crucial these basic necessities are. If these basic needs are not satisfied, wellness will be far beyond reach. It would then become more of a conversation using language such as QOL with a goal toward health.

According to Maslow's hierarchy, after physiological needs come safety needs. One must feel protected and safe. Social and physical environments intersect to create this sense of order and security. The next tier is love and belonging. This acknowledges how our social and emotional relationships play into our overall functionality and, ultimately, into our wellness. Meaningful connections with others in the workplace, family, and day-to-day interactions enhance one's self-worth and experience of life. According to Maslow, after belongingness needs come esteem needs. For wellness to be present, one must have positive self-esteem. Grounded confidence emanates to others and has a significant impact on our

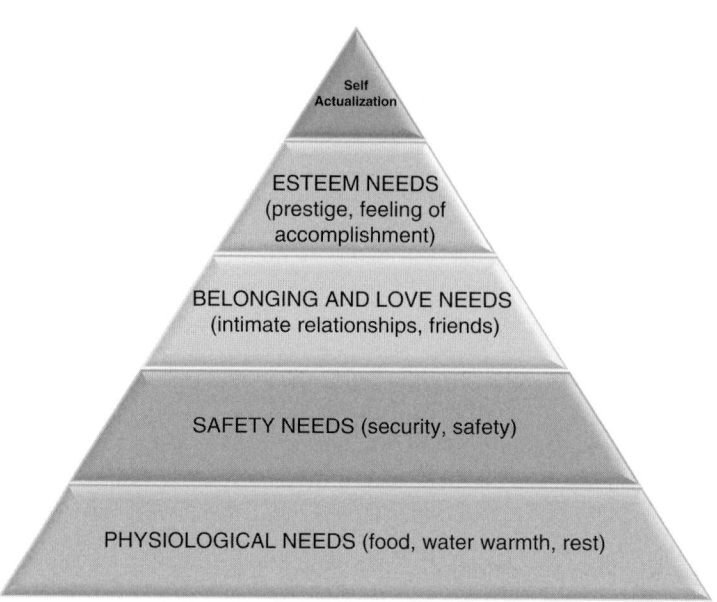

Figure 1.4 Maslow's hierarchy of needs.

social interactions. This again highlights the interconnected nature of wellness. Interpersonal relationships influence behavior, resulting in friendship, intimacy, trust, acceptance, affection, and love. These social interactions are opportunities to engage and connect, and can enhance one's wellness.

Maslow's hierarchy (Figure 1.4) culminates in self-actualization. Self-actualization is a critical component to wellness. It is all-encompassing and does not necessarily fit into a single dimension of wellness, but is ideally present in all dimensions of one's wellness. For example, in the physical dimension, actualization can mean hitting one's target time in the marathon one has been training for. In professional life, it can mean studying or working diligently for years to obtain expertise in a skill set or knowledge base. Both of these examples share a common theme: commitment and dedication. In order to self-actualize, one must have a goal. From there he/she must be focused and disciplined enough to see that goal through. This requires grit. Grit is essential to self-actualization and to wellness. Sometimes, short-term sacrifices are required for long-term growth. This may lead to transient deficits in one's well-being (e.g., sleep deprivation required to reach an academic goal) but will ultimately contribute to one's occupational/professional wellness through self-actualization. When wellness is present in one's occupational life, this success will feed into the other wellness dimensions of that person's life. This example can be translated to any of the other dimensions.

To understand wellness holistically, it is worthwhile to examine underlying emotions. Our experience of life is subjective. Two people can share the same objective experience; however, they may have completely different perspectives on what happened. This is because every experience is impacted by our outlook, or lens, through which we encounter each situation. The key component that impacts our experiential lens is our emotions. Our emotions are responses to natural, instinctive feelings. Knowledge and reason are what allow us to apply experiences, feelings, and thoughts to our emotions. The way we respond emotionally affects the psyche and the body. The mind is a powerful and complex unit. It allows us to strategize and then respond to events in our lives. In the 1970s, psychologist Paul Eckman identified six basic emotions said to be experienced universally. These are happiness, sadness, disgust, fear, surprise, and anger.

Happiness is an emotion we all strive to attain and maintain. It is defined as a pleasant emotional state that exemplifies content, joy, and satisfaction. There are different depths of happiness. More superficially, it can be considered as the "honeymoon" state of happiness. This might come as a result of a new purchase or reward. Going deeper, happiness is best when it comes from within. This type of happiness is what leads one toward wellness. It is more permanent and innate versus the subjective moment-to-moment shifts in emotion associated with a more transient state of happiness. Hope is a key component of this more in-depth concept of happiness, according to philosopher Annie Dillard. Hope that no matter what difficulty comes our way, everything will be okay. This eternal trust in the universe is what leads to an innate sense of happiness, which ultimately guides one toward wellness. Happiness, joy, and hope can be expressed through facial expression, body language, and tone of voice. It radiates to others and is contagious.

As alluded to with the discussion of hope, there are many aspects of our lives that contribute to or complicate happiness. Along with a variety of contributing factors, our emotional state may be influenced by culture, interpersonal relationships, and one's self-worth. Countless research studies have supported the idea that happiness plays a definitive role in mental and physical health.

In contrast, sadness, another basic emotion, is linked to poorer health and wellness outcomes. Sadness can be defined as hopelessness, disinterest, grief, or disappointment. It is normal and almost expected to feel sadness at some point in time. However, much like the discussion with happiness, there is a difference between the transient, short-term emotion of sadness and the prolonged state. Prolonged states of sadness can turn into depression. In fact, Barsky et al. demonstrated that negative affect (anxiety, hostility, guilt, and depression) is directly correlated to somatic symptoms, both in number and severity [24]. The authors describe this phenomenon as somatosensory amplification, which has shown that somatic symptoms are subjective to one's perception of the symptom itself and that this perception is directly related to one's emotional state. Additionally, they noted that more medical visits are associated with emotional dysphoria. Persistent sadness can be detrimental to wellness because it can impact the way people cope and engage with reality and those they interact with. Isolation, avoidant behaviors, self-medicating, and negative thoughts can have adverse outcomes in regard to one's overall wellness.

A powerful emotion that plays a vital role in survival is fear. Perceiving danger and experiencing fear generally triggers the fight-or-flight sympathetic nervous system response. During this response, the muscles in the body become tense, heart and respiration rates increase, and the mind is hyper-alert, priming the body to run from danger or to fight. This innate physiologic response is a prime example of biopsychosocial health in action. In this response, our physiology is greatly altered by our rapid emotional response to a perceived danger or fear.

The emotion of fear is one that traces back to our primal instincts and has developed throughout evolution. As centuries have passed and technology advanced, our responses to danger and fear have changed based on circumstances. Naturally, this emotional response is triggered when one feels threatened or experiences stress. This response was geared toward the hunter-gatherer lifestyle. The challenge with modern society is that most of us are in a chronic state of stress. Stress triggers the sympathetic nervous system and activates the hypothalamic–pituitary–adrenal axis (HPA axis). Chronically engaging the HPA axis eventually wears it out and has negative consequences. Our fight-or-flight response is not optimally primed to engage when acutely needed because it is operating on overdrive at baseline. This makes the body and mind more prone to illness and disease. Thus, they become less resilient and responsive when acute insults occur.

Unpleasant tastes, sights, or smells can provoke disgust. The evolution of our species transformed as appropriate reactions were made to things that might be harmful or fatal. This notion can be applied to food, hygiene, infections, and death, which can affect one's sustainability with their surroundings. Disgust is experienced in the context of morals and values as well. When we observe and engage with others, we may agree or disagree with their behaviors, thus feeling a sense of distaste or loathing. Anger is another powerful emotion. Hostility, agitation, and frustration culminate in the feelings associated with anger. This emotion can be constructive in the short term. It can motivate people to take action and make the appropriate changes toward their ideal path to wellness. Conversely, it can be detrimental when anger is expressed wildly, uncontrolled, or for a prolonged period. It poses a threat to oneself and others. The mental and physical consequences that result from anger can deter a person from making rational decisions. Anger is linked to coronary heart disease and diabetes, as well as aggressive driving, drinking, and smoking. A brief yet startling emotional response known as surprise was the final basic human emotion described by Eckman. The effects of surprise can be positive, negative, or neutral, and impact human behavior. Unusual or surprising events stand out in long-term memory.

The above emotions play a central role in modulating one's interaction with the world. They have a direct impact on one's wellness. It is crucial to recognize how emotions play a role in wellness. Emotions, both positive and negative, can promote and/or deter one from wellness. It all depends on how we choose to respond to such emotions.

Conclusion

Wellness is a thoughtful, profound, unique, and evolving process, balancing physical, mental, and social dimensions. As the area of practicing wellness medicine grows, it allows us as practitioners to have a much larger toolkit to call upon to empower and improve a patient's QOL. In this chapter, we have learned that the impact of medical illness could well be mitigated in the pursuit of wellness, thus liberating us from the confines of one-dimensional thinking. Wellness is about adopting healthy habits, practicing self-care, connecting to one's community, having meaningful relationships, being mentally stimulated, having resources to live within one's means, seeking a purpose in life connected to the greater universe, and having a safe, comfortable, and happy home environment. Wellness terms have become buzzwords "because they capture something particularly salient about a culture at a moment in time and come to stand in for wide agreement about how something should be characterized. Wellness captures the sense that the era of combating diseases has given way to a more complex problem of success in modernity: living well" [25]. Wellness means different things to different people, and it is important as healthcare providers to pull the term from its buzzword status of being large and vague and to give it practical, applicable use within our crucial medical evaluations, conversations, and treatment plans.

After thorough review of the various models and definitions of wellness, it is clear that wellness is multifactorial and too complex to succinctly define. This is because wellness is all-encompassing, thus making it in essence larger than life. Our goal with this textbook is to provide a comprehensive resource for healthcare professionals and individuals to learn about the nuances and the large array of dimensions and subdimensions that comprise wellness. In order to do this, it is beneficial to reach a consensus on the working definition of wellness. We will use the definition proposed by Bart et al. [8]. The authors synthesized a definition from the WHO's 2004 definition with the addition of a clause from the WHO 1964 definition (also present in the original 1949 definition of health) clarifying that wellness is "not merely the absence of disease or infirmity." Bart and colleagues' definition of wellness as synthesized from the various WHO definitions is:

> The optimal state of health of individuals and groups, and not merely the absence of disease or infirmity. There are two focal concerns: the realization of the fullest potential of an individual physically, psychologically, socially, spiritually and economically, and the fulfillment of one's role expectations in the family, community, place of worship, workplace and other settings.

To this definition, we will also add, just as the WHO did in 1964, that multiple subdimensions can be addressed under the umbrella of each of the above dimensions. This is not dissimilar to the WoW model composed of second- and third-order dimensions. This working definition now helps build the platform needed to conceptualize wellness and subsequently make recommendations for how to promote wellness.

The purpose of this book is to serve as a comprehensive reference for healthcare professionals and/or individuals for how to optimize their lives and move toward wellness. These concepts can be applied on the micro, individual level, as well as the macro, societal level. We hope you find the information useful and practical and are able to implement it in a way that helps to transform the lives of others.

References

1. G Miller, LT Foster. Critical synthesis of wellness literature. 2010. http://dspace .library.uvic.ca:8443/bitstream/1828/2894/5 /Critical_Synthesis%20of%20Wellness%20 Update.pdf (accessed May 15, 2019).

2. LT Foster, CP Keller. *Atlas of Wellness*. Georgetown, ON, University of British Columbia Press; 2007.

3. BL Seaward. *Managing Stress: Principles and Strategies for Health and Wellbeing* (9th ed.). Boston, MA: Jones and Bartlett Learning; 2017.

4. Centers for Disease Control (CDC). Heart disease facts & statistics. 2019. www.cdc.gov/h eartdisease/facts.htm (accessed May 15, 2019).

5. American College of Lifestyle Medicine (ACLM). Lifestyle medicine. www .lifestylemedicine.org/What-is-Lifestyle-Medicine (accessed May 15, 2019).

6. World Health Organization (WHO). Constitution. 1949. www.loc.gov/law/help/ us-treaties/bevans/m-ust000004-0119.pdf (accessed May 15, 2019).

7. WW IsHak, JM Greenberg, K Balayan, et al. Quality of life: the ultimate outcome measure of interventions in major depressive disorder. *Harv Rev Psychiatry* 2011; **19**: 229–239.

8. R Bart, WW IsHak, S Ganjian, et al. The assessment and measurement of wellness in the clinical medical setting: a systematic review. *Innov Clin Neurosci* 2018; **15**: 14–23.

9. R Renger, M Soto, T Erin, et al. Optimal living profile: an inventory to assess health and wellness. *Am J Health Behav* 2000; **24**: 403–412.

10. J Rachele, W Cockshaw, E Brymer. Towards an operational understanding of wellness. *JSLaM* 2013; **7**: 3–12.

11. CE Westgate. Spiritual wellness and depression. *J Counsel Dev* 1996; **75**: 26–35.

12. L Breslow. A quantitative approach to the World Health Organization definition of health: physical, mental and social well-being. *Int J Epidemiol* 1972; **1**: 347–355.

13. B Smith, K Tang, D Nutbeam. WHO health promotion glossary: new terms. *Health Promot Int* 2006; **21**: 340–345.

14. LK Ng, DL Davis, RW Manderscheid. Toward a conceptual formulation of health and wellbeing. In: LK Ng, DL Davis, RW Manderscheid, eds., *Strategies for Public Health: Promoting Health and Preventing Disease.* New York, Van Nostrand Reinhold Co.; 1981; 44–58.

15. ID Coulter. A wellness system: the challenge for health professionals. *J Can Chiropr Assoc* 1993; **37**: 97–103.

16. MI Gatterman, J Brimhall. CCE adopts health promotion and wellness competencies. *Dynam Chiroprac* 2006; **24**: 1–5.

17. JE Myers, TJ Sweeney, JM Witmer. *The Wellness Evaluation of Lifestyle.* Palo Alto, CA, Mindgarden Press; 1998.

18. JE Myers, TJ Sweeney, JM Witmer. The wheel of wellness counseling for wellness: a holistic model for treatment planning. *J Counsel Dev* 2000; **78**: 251–266.

19. National Wellness Institute (NWI). The six dimensions of wellness. www .nationalwellness.org/page/AboutWellness (accessed May 15, 2019).

20. LJ Roscoe. Wellness: a review of theory and measurement for counselors. *J Counsel Dev* 2009; **87**: 216–226.

21. D Depken. Wellness through the lens of gender: a paradigm shift. *Wellness Perspec* 1994; **70**: 54–69.

22. T Adams. The power of perceptions: measuring wellness in a globally acceptable, philosophically consistent way. 2003. www .hedir.org (accessed May 15, 2019).

23. JW Yeung, Z Zhang, TY Kim. Volunteering and health benefits in general adults: cumulative effects and forms. *BMC Public Health* 2018; **18**: 1–8.

24. AJ Barsky, JD Goodson, RS Lane, PD Cleary. The amplification of somatic symptoms. *Psychosom Med* 1988; **50**: 510–519.

25. A Kirkland. What is wellness now? *J Health Politics Policy Law* 2014; **39**: 957–970.

Chapter

2

Screening and Assessment Methods for Wellness

Jared M. Greenberg, Enrico G. Castillo, Waguih William IsHak, and Kenneth Wells

Introduction: Why Wellness?

There are multiple movements within medicine, public health, and health policy that have expanded the measurement of well-being and wellness and made such practices imperative. Medicine continues to grow more highly specialized and focused on biomedical treatments. Physicians' roles have become more siloed, and our knowledge of the effects of illness and medical treatments on patients' lives is limited. Simultaneously, public health research has elucidated the importance of contexts, connectedness, and functioning to health. Biomedical treatments and the absence of illness do not define health. Well-being, social connectedness, and one's ability to function in essential domains of life are essential components of health. In response, health policy has begun to prioritize patient-reported outcomes, including well-being and health-related quality of life (QOL).

There is a large body of research on patient-reported outcome measures (PROMs), namely surveys that capture information about patients' QOL and functional status. Implementation of PROMs in routine clinical practice has the potential for numerous benefits. Patient-reported outcome measures can: enrich our understanding of how health-care affects outcomes that may be most meaningful to patients; guide treatment planning, such as by helping to track a patient's functional status over time; serve as benchmarks, giving us a way to compare treatments, providers, and healthcare systems; be helpful to communities and policy-makers, tracking the effects of healthcare systems and large initiatives; and serve as helpful information for patients about health status, helping with goal-setting and with decision-making about treatments and providers [1, 2].

When used as a screening tool, PROMs can serve a function similar to traditional screening practices, such as those for diabetes, hypertension, or certain cancers. Screening for well-being helps providers to focus on a dimension of health that we can no longer afford to overlook, given ample evidence for the links between emotional well-being and overall health and longevity [3]. To this end we will describe evidence-supported PROMs that can be used as wellness screening tools in clinical settings, as well as considerations for their implementation.

How to Screen

Before we present options for screening tools, it is important to discuss several considerations regarding the screening or assessment process. The specific goals of assessment (not only for wellness screening but for other PROMs as well) can include one or more of the following: screening for problems (e.g., poor QOL), monitoring progress over time, facilitating patient-centered care, aiding decision-making, facilitating communication within

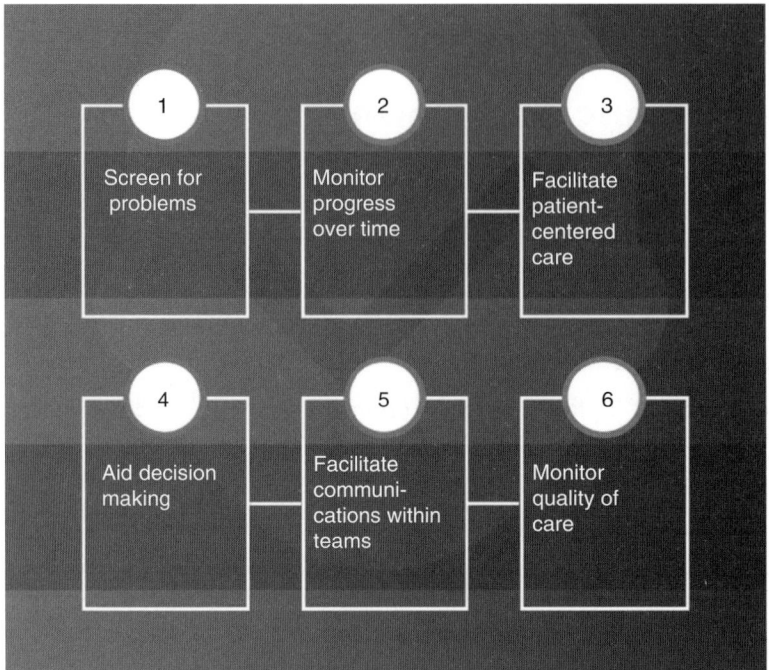

Figure 2.1 Goals of patient-reported outcome assessment [3].

1 Screen for problems

2 Monitor progress over time

3 Facilitate patient-centered care

4 Aid decision making

5 Facilitate communi-cations within teams

6 Monitor quality of care

teams, and monitoring the quality of care [4] (Figure 2.1). Resource requirements increase with increasing scope of the intervention. The purpose of screening will influence decisions about what to measure (i.e., which instrument or instruments to use) and how to go about gathering the information.

The method of administration of assessments can take many forms, depending on the care setting, staffing, workflow, time demands, and available equipment. In terms of setting, assessments can be completed at home (or elsewhere) prior to clinic visits, in the waiting room at visits, or while meeting with a clinician [5]. Assessments can be filled out on paper by patients, administered verbally in person by a provider or member of the clinic staff who records the responses, completed on a computer or smart phone, or administered over the phone by a staff member or using interactive voice response (IVR) technology. Computerized assessment facilitates incorporation into electronic health records (although paper assessments can be keyed in) and also offers the possibility of recent advancements in computerized adaptive testing [2], in which item responses determine subsequent questions or prompts, so that the total number of items differs based on an individual's responses.

Another consideration is whom to screen. As an example, it may be desirable to assess the wellness of all patients in an outpatient clinic, who are more likely to be independent and have time for completing assessments [6], but in addition to the potential adminis-trative and clinical burden of this "catch all" approach, such patients may not be in the greatest need of monitoring. More targeted strategies, such as screening patients with certain mental or physical health conditions, psychosocial risk factors, or other charac-teristics (e.g., adolescents in a pediatric practice, elderly patients in general practice), can focus efforts on those with greater needs for monitoring [2]. Assessment of inpatients entails such considerations as whether patients require assistance in completing surveys, the fact that the hospital environment can itself affect responses [7], and the question of whether short stays and lack of post-discharge assessment will render the information useful. It should also be recognized that, regardless of setting, the specific reason for a clinical encounter can affect ratings of well-being in a way that is more acute or situational (consider the difference between a routine physical and the initiation of cancer therapy) and therefore may be open to misinterpretation [2]. Some questionnaires (e.g., WHO-5, presented below) account for this by asking about an average over a recent period of time, but many do not.

Assessment Instruments

Well-being is most commonly formally assessed using questionnaires that ask about a person's self-reported sense of wellness. As discussed in greater detail in Chapter 4, a number of related concepts and terms are currently in use for describing well-being as experienced and reported from an individual's own perspective. Commonly used terms include *subjective well-being, emotional well-being, psychological well-being, quality of life, life satisfaction, flourishing,* and *thriving.* While definitions and boundaries differ among these concepts, a high degree of conceptual and psychometric overlap has been demonstrated among them, and research has yet to establish any of these constructs as being superior to the others. Countless instruments with differing characteristics have been developed for measuring subjective well-being and related constructs, a complete accounting of which is beyond the scope of this handbook and could fill several volumes. Here we present a few noteworthy instruments for measuring self-reported well-being, with consideration given to those that are readily available and particularly suitable for screening activities. Table 2.1 presents a summary of instruments mentioned in this chapter.

WHO-5 Well-Being Index

The five-item WHO Well-Being Index, or WHO-5, is among the most widely used questionnaires for assessing respondents' subjective sense of well-being. Originally published in 1998, the WHO-5 has been translated into more than 30 languages and has been used in research and clinical settings worldwide [8]. The scale presents five statements assessing positive affect, energy, and meaningful activity, and asks respondents to indicate their degree of concurrence with each statement during the preceding two-week period, from "At no time" (0 points) to "All of the time" (5 points). The raw score is simply the sum of all ratings, with a score of 25 corresponding to the best possible sense of well-being. A percentage score is calculable by multiplying the raw score by 4. A raw score below 13 indicates poor well-being and is considered an indication for additional screening for depression. The percentage score is useful for monitoring changes in well-being, with a 10 percent difference indicating a significant change [9]. A systematic literature review concluded that the WHO-5 is highly valid for clinical use, useful as an outcome measure balancing the wanted and unwanted effects of treatments, both sensitive and specific as a screening tool for depression, and applicable across a wide range of fields [8]. The WHO-5 is available as a downloadable PDF at www.psykiatri-regionh.dk/who-5/Documents/WHO5_English.pdf.

Table 2.1 Noteworthy assessment instruments

Instrument	Number of items	What it measures	Where to access	Notes
WHO-5	5	Positive affect, energy/vigor, meaning	www.psykiatri-regionh.dk/who-5/Documents/WHO5_English.pdf	Easy to score as a raw sum or percentage score; 10 percent change is considered meaningful.
SF-36	36	Clinical status, physical functioning and well-being, mental functioning and well-being, social/role functioning and well-being, general health perceptions	www.optum.com/solutions/life-sciences/answer-research/patient-insights/sf-health-surveys.html	Requires special software to score.
SWLS	5	Life satisfaction	http://labs.psychology.illinois.edu/~ediener/SWLS.html	Straightforward scoring by summation.
PERMA-Profiler	23	Positive emotions, engagement, relationships meaning, accomplishment, negative emotions, health, overall well-being	www.authentichappiness.sas.upenn.edu/questionnaires/perma	Can be taken online. Also available in an adolescent version, the EPOCH Measure.
PROMIS	Varies	More than 300 measures spanning global, physical, mental, and social health	www.healthmeasures.net/explore-measurement-systems/promis	Available in adult and pediatric versions, and fixed length or computer adaptive testing versions.
WMI/HowsYourHealth.org	9	Pain, emotional issues, polypharmacy, adverse medication effects, low confidence in managing health problems	https://howsyourhealth.org/static/professional.html	Can be taken online. Providers can create an account and receive reports based on patient responses.

EPOCH = Engagement, Perseverance, Optimism, Connectedness, and Happiness; PERMA = Positive emotion, Engagement, Relationships, Meaning, Accomplishment; PROMIS = Patient Reported Outcomes Measurement System; SF = Short Form; SWLS = Satisfaction with Life Survey; WHO = World Health Organization; WMI = What Matters Index.

SF-36

For more robust measurement of well-being, albeit more cumbersome to implement and interpret, the 36-item Short-Form Health Survey, or SF-36, is the most utilized measure of generic (as opposed to disease-specific) health-related QOL [10]. Developed for the RAND Corporation's Medical Outcomes Study of the 1980s and early 1990s, the SF-36 comprises the underlying dimensions of physical and mental health, with five categories of indicators across the two dimensions: clinical status, physical functioning and well-being, mental functioning and well-being, social/role functioning and well-being, and general health perceptions. The developers of the SF-36 considered its ability to compare patients with different medical and psychiatric conditions to be an important feature. The well-being items are intended to capture "subjective internal states not observable by others." Items on the SF-36 span eight domains: vitality, physical functioning, bodily pain, general health perceptions, physical role functioning, emotional role functioning, social role functioning, and mental health [11]. Shorter scales derived from the SF-36 include the widely used SF-12, which assesses the same eight domains. Scoring of both the SF-36 and SF-12 entails weighting and transformation of the eight scaled scores and requires special software [12].

Frendl and Ware conducted a systematic review of randomized clinical trials to determine how often efficacious treatments were associated with meaningful change in functioning and well-being as measured by the SF-36. Clinical and SF-36 outcomes were concordant in more than 80 percent of trials, though SF-36 changes were often modest, with 58 percent meeting the threshold for minimal important difference (MID). The impact of treatments on QOL varied among medical conditions. For example, treatments for rheumatoid arthritis, psoriatic arthritis, and psoriasis showed the largest SF-36 improvements, whereas no efficacious therapies for peripheral arterial disease or chronic obstructive pulmonary disease achieved MID [10]. A license to use the SF-36 (in updated form, SF-36v2) or one of its derived measures can be obtained at www.optum.com/solutions/life-sciences/answer-research/patient-insights/sf-health-surveys.html.

Satisfaction with Life Scale

Many well-being experts have conceived of subjective well-being as consisting of an emotional (or affective) component and a cognitive (or judgmental) component, with the latter described as one's overall satisfaction with life. This aspect of well-being may be more stable over time than one's emotional state. One of the most commonly used measures of life satisfaction is the Satisfaction with Life Scale (SWLS) developed by Diener and colleagues [13]. The SWLS presents five statements related to life satisfaction (e.g., "The conditions of my life are excellent"; "I am satisfied with my life") and asks respondents to indicate their degree of agreement with each statement on a scale from "Strongly disagree" (1 point) to "Strongly agree" (7 points). The scale is scored by simply summing the responses, and total scores are divided into five-point ranges, from "Extremely dissatisfied" (5–9 points) to "Extremely satisfied" (31–35 points). The SWLS has been shown to be a valid and reliable measure of life satisfaction, suitable for use with a wide range of age groups and applications, and less time- and resource-intensive than many other measures of life satisfaction [14]. The scale is available to use without charge or need for permission at http://labs.psychology.illinois.edu/~ediener/SWLS.html.

PERMA and the PERMA-Profiler

In his 2011 book *Flourish: A Visionary New Understanding of Happiness and Well-being*, psychologist Martin Seligman, a leader in the field of positive psychology, defined well-being (also termed *flourishing*) in terms of five pillars: *positive emotion, engagement, relationships, meaning,* and *accomplishment,* forming the acronym PERMA [15]. One of the more recently developed instruments for measuring well-being is the PERMA-Profiler, a 23-item survey that assesses the five PERMA domains as well as overall well-being, negative emotion, loneliness, and physical health. Items are worded as questions, including: "In general, how often do you feel joyful?" (positive emotion); "In general, to what extent do you feel excited and interested in things?" (engagement); "How satisfied are you with your personal relationships?" (relationships); "In general, to what extent do you feel that what you do in your life is valuable and worthwhile?" (meaning); and "How often do you achieve the important goals you have set for yourself?" (accomplishment). A series of eight studies including approximately 32,000 participants established the acceptability of the scale's psychometric properties, including model fit, internal and across-time consistency, and content, convergent, and divergent validity. Results of the PERMA-Profiler can be visually represented as a colorful bar graph (Figure 2.2), with bars corresponding to the different domains, reflecting the multidimensional nature of flourishing [16]. The University of Pennsylvania's Authentic Happiness website (www.authentichappiness.sas.upenn.edu) provides free access to a number of well-being measures, including an online version of the PERMA-Profiler (www.authentichappiness.sas.upenn.edu/questionnaires/perma). The measure was also adapted for use with adolescents, with the five domains of *engagement, perseverance, optimism, connectedness,* and *happiness* combining to form the EPOCH Measure of Adolescent Well-being [17]. A printable version of the EPOCH measure, along with explanation and scoring instructions, is available for download at www.peggykern.org/uploads/5/6/6/7/56678211/epoch_measure_of_adolescent_well-being_102014.pdf.

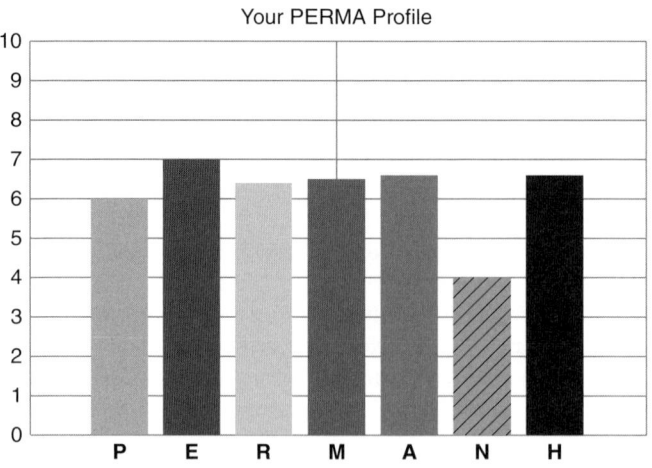

Figure 2.2 Example of PERMA-Profiler results.

PROMIS

The Patient-Reported Outcomes Measurement Information System (PROMIS) developed by the National Institutes of Health (NIH) is the most comprehensive approach to standardizing assessment of health-related QOL in acute and chronic health conditions, and is rapidly becoming the industry standard for assessment of patient-reported outcomes [18]. It consists of a comprehensive set of more than 300 individual measures grouped under the broad categories of *global health*, *physical health*, *mental health*, and *social health*, and is available in adult and pediatric versions, as well as translations into numerous languages. The *mental health* measures include scales for *positive affect* (15- or 34-item versions), *general life satisfaction* (5 or 10 items), and *meaning and purpose* (4, 6, 8, or 34 items), as well as measures of cognitive function, emotional distress, self-efficacy, and substance-use. The *physical health* measures focus on functional and QOL issues such as fatigue, pain intensity, pain interference, physical function, and sleep disturbance, whereas the *social health* measures focus on ability to participate in social roles and activities, satisfaction with relationships, social isolation, and social support. PROMIS measures are available online as fixed-length, short-form measures, computer adaptive tests (also called item banks), batteries (a combined set of measures, also called profiles), and performance tests. The PROMIS measures are available free of charge for download or administration via computer or iPad app at www.healthmeasures.net/explore-measurement-systems/promis.

Screening for Lifestyle Factors Related to Well-Being

One of the many drivers of an individual's wellness is the set of choices and behaviors which may either promote or diminish health and well-being. With this in mind, one approach to wellness screening entails assessment of healthy (or unhealthy) lifestyle factors such as diet, exercise, and use of substances, including tobacco. Such information can be used to identify individuals whose choices and habits place them at greater risk of ill-health and lower QOL and can in turn prompt interventions ranging from education to motivational interviewing to more elaborate individual and group interventions focused on promoting a healthy lifestyle.

Much of the existing work in this area relates to screening for levels of physical activity and diet. Physical activity may be of particular interest, not only because of its well-known benefits for physical and mental health and QOL, but also because it has been shown that people who engage in regular exercise are more likely to choose to change an unhealthy habit and demonstrate greater discipline in adhering to the chosen change. This results in greater success in reducing health risks [19].

A number of screening instruments for physical exercise have been developed. An Australian study of screening for physical activity in family practice [20] evaluated the feasibility, reliability, and validity of two brief assessment tools, one consisting of two questions and one consisting of three questions. Validity was assessed via concurrence with the Active Australia Questionnaire as well as seven-day accelerometer counts. Both tools were found to be reliable, feasible to administer by physicians in family practice clinics, and suitable for identifying the least active patients, using only one to two minutes of a physician's time. Physicians tended to prefer the two-question assessment:

1. How many times a week do you usually do 20 minutes or more of vigorous-intensity physical activity that makes you sweat or puff and pant? (e.g., heavy lifting, digging, jogging, aerobics, or fast bicycling).
   - 3 or more times
   - 1–2 times
   - None

2. How many times a week do you usually do 30 minutes or more of moderate-intensity physical activity or walking that increases your heart rate or makes you breathe harder than normal? (e.g., carrying light loads, bicycling at a regular pace, or doubles tennis)
   - 5 or more times
   - 3–4 times
   - 1–2 times
   - None

More recently, technological approaches to lifestyle and health behavior screening have included the use of patient-facing kiosks and computer or smart phone apps. Advantages of such approaches include convenience, less use of providers' time, increased disclosure, and appeal to patients (particularly younger patients), resulting in increased use. As one of several examples, Check Up GP, a health and lifestyle screening app designed for adolescents and young adults, has been tested in general practice clinics in Australia. Domains covered by the app include diet, exercise, sleep, safety, stress, bullying, sexuality, substance-use, mood, home life, and school/work. Use of the app, which patients could access either prior to a doctor visit or on a tablet in the waiting room, resulted in greater disclosure of sensitive health issues, and higher ratings by patients of their general practitioners on communication, partnership, personal relationship, and health promotion [21]. It was also found to be valued by staff. It was noted, however, that successful implementation requires adequate time and intensive facilitation, which may entail resources beyond existing staff [22].

Yet another method of screening is the use of an IVR system. Rose et al. [23] noted that although many international governing bodies recommend screening of primary care patients for unhealthy behaviors and mental health, such screening is not routine practice in the USA. They conducted a study in which primary care patients at academic medical centers were contacted 1–3 days prior to their doctor visit and were invited to complete a questionnaire using an IVR system. The questionnaire asked patients about physical activity, smoking, alcohol use, concern about weight, mood, and pain. Of two-thirds of patients who accepted the questionnaire, 96 percent completed it, 87 percent screened positive on at least one item, and 59 percent reported multiple problems. While consistent with studies of screening using other methods, these results stood in stark contrast to low rates of screening and intervention for these issues in typical primary care practice. Additionally, the screening facilitated participation in a brief treatment for unhealthy drinking, which serves as a model for the linkage between screening and intervention during routine care [23].

The What Matters Index and HowsYourHealth.org

The What Matters Index (WMI) was developed by John Wasson to capture information that guides care toward outcomes that matter most to patients. The index is based on five patient-reported measures – pain, emotional issues, polypharmacy, adverse medication effects, and low confidence in managing health problems – and was found to be a good indicator of QOL [24]. The WMI can be used to predict risk for subsequent costly care, and in fact has been shown to be as effective for this purpose as complex, computer-generated risk models constructed from insurance claims and medical records data. It also presents the advantage of providing information that is immediately actionable for addressing the needs of a particular patient [25]. The WMI is accessible at https://howsyourhealth.org by selecting the "Quick Health Checkup" option, which due to its brevity is especially well suited to completion via smart phone (privacy is maintained, and information is not shared or stored). Responses are used to provide respondents with pertinent information such as tips for communicating with providers, information about emotional care, pain and pain management, or an online problem-solving tool. Depending on their WMI results, users may be directed to complete a "full check-up" survey by clicking a link. This "full" survey emphasizes wellness topics such as daily functioning, emotional state, social activities and social support, diet and exercise, substance use, violence/abuse, and finances, in addition to questions about physical health symptoms and experiences with medical care. Once the survey is completed, users receive a summary tailored to their responses; a "personal action plan" with assets, needs, risk considerations, and links to suggested reading and education; and finally a detailed "Personal Health Plan" which can be edited, saved, shared with providers, and even accessed directly by registered providers. A controlled trial of 1651 older adults found that patients who used HowsYourHealth reported benefits for daily activities, emotional well-being, and social support as well as overall quality of care [26]. Professionals can register with HowsYourHealth .org, create a customized registry for patients to use, receive reports based on patient responses, and access other features at https://howsyourhealth.org/static/professional.html.

Conclusion

If the ultimate goal of healthcare is to improve people's lives in a meaningful and holistic way, assessment must go beyond clinical and symptomatic improvement, and screening must entail more than the detection of specific disease states and their risk factors. Screening for well-being can help to identify those at greatest risk of poor outcomes and, if monitored over time, can help ensure that treatments and services are oriented toward improving patients' QOL. This chapter has presented the rationale, practical considerations, and options for conducting assessment of well-being. While an important first step, such assessment is but the beginning of the wellness journey. Subsequent chapters will continue along the path to well-being by presenting strategies and interventions for its enhancement across a range of populations, settings, and scenarios. You may wish to return to this chapter for guidance in gauging the impact of any wellness intervention or strategy you employ.

References

1. EC Nelson, E Eftimovska, C Lind, et al. Patient reported outcome measures in practice. *BMJ* 2015; **350**: g7818.

2. CF Snyder, NK Aaronson, AK Choucair, et al. Implementing patient-reported outcomes assessment in clinical practice: a review of the options and considerations. *Qual Life Res* 2012; **21**(8): 1305–1314.

3. E Diener, MY Chan. Happy people live longer: subjective well-being contributes to health and longevity. *Appl Psychol Health Well Being* 2011; **3**(1): 1–43.

4. J Greenhalgh. The applications of PROs in clinical practice: what are they, do they work, and why? *Qual Life Res* 2009; **18**(1): 115–123.

5. KN Lohr, BJ Zebrack. Using patient-reported outcomes in clinical practice: challenges and opportunities. *Qual Life Res* 2009; **18**(1): 99–107.

6. SJ Ackerley, HJ Gordon, AF Elston, LM Crawford, KM McPherson. Assessment of quality of life and participation within an outpatient rehabilitation setting. *Disabil Rehabil* 2009; **31**(11): 906–913.

7. M Veenstra, T Moum, AM Garratt. Patient experiences with information in a hospital setting: associations with coping and self-rated health in chronic illness. *Qual Life Res* 2006; **15**(6): 967–978.

8. CW Topp, SD Ostergaard, S Sondergaard, P Bech. The WHO-5 Well-Being Index: a systematic review of the literature. *Psychother Psychosom* 2015; **84**(3): 167–176.

9. Psychiatric Research Unit. *WHO (Five) Well-Being Index (1998 version)*. Hillerød, Denmark: WHO Collaborating Center for Mental Health; 1998.

10. DM Frendl, JE Ware, Jr. Patient-reported functional health and well-being outcomes with drug therapy: a systematic review of randomized trials using the SF-36 health survey. *Med Care* 2014; **52**(5): 439–445.

11. AL Stewart, JE Ware, Jr. *Measuring Functioning and Well-Being: The Medical Outcomes Study Approach*. Durham, NC: Duke University Press; 1992.

12. JE Ware, Jr., M Kosinski, SD Keller. *SF-12: How to Score the SF-12 Physical and Mental Health Summary Scales*. Boston, MA: The Health Institute, New England Medical Center; 1995.

13. E Diener, RA Emmons, RJ Larsen, S Griffin. The Satisfaction with Life Scale. *J Pers Assess* 1985; **49**(1): 71–75.

14. W Pavot, E Diener, CR Colvin, E Sandvik. Further validation of the Satisfaction with Life Scale: evidence for the cross-method convergence of well-being measures. *J Pers Assess* 1991; **57**(1): 149–161.

15. MEP Seligman *Flourish: A Visionary New Understanding of Happiness and Well-Being*. New York: Free Press; 2011.

16. J Butler, ML Kern. The PERMA-Profiler: a brief multidimensional measure of flourishing. *Int J Wellbeing* 2016; **6**(3): 1–48.

17. ML Kern, L Benson, EA Steinberg, L Steinberg. The EPOCH Measure of Adolescent Well-Being. *Psychol Assess* 2016; **28**(5): 586–597.

18. D Cella, W Riley, A Stone, et al. The Patient-Reported Outcomes Measurement Information System (PROMIS) developed and tested its first wave of adult self-reported health outcome item banks: 2005–2008. *J Clin Epidemiol* 2010; **63**(11): 1179–1194.

19. JH Wasson. Regular exercise is strongly associated with anticipated success for reducing health risks. *J Ambul Care Manage* 2014; **37**(3): 273–276.

20. BJ Smith, AL Marshall, N Huang. Screening for physical activity in family practice: evaluation of two brief assessment tools. *Am J Prev Med* 2005; **29**(4): 256–264.

21. MJ Webb, G Wadley, LA Sanci. Improving patient-centered care for young people in general practice with a codesigned screening app: mixed methods study. *JMIR Mhealth Uhealth* 2017; **5**(8): e118.

22. MJ Webb, G Wadley, LA Sanci. Experiences of general practitioners and practice support staff using a health and lifestyle screening app in primary health care: implementation case study. *JMIR Mhealth Uhealth* 2018; **6**(4): e105.

23. GL Rose, TA Ferraro, JM Skelly, et al. Feasibility of automated pre-screening for lifestyle and behavioral health risk factors in primary care. *BMC Fam Pract* 2015; **16**: 150.

24. JH Wasson, L Soloway, LG Moore, P Labrec, L Ho. Development of a care guidance index based on what matters to patients. *Qual Life Res* 2018; **27**(1): 51–58.

25. JH Wasson, L Ho, L Soloway, LG Moore. Validation of the What Matters Index: a brief, patient-reported index that guides care for chronic conditions and can substitute for computer-generated risk models. *PLoS One* 2018; **13**(2): e0192475.

26. JH Wasson, TA Stukel, JE Weiss, et al. A randomized trial of the use of patient self-assessment data to improve community practices. *Eff Clin Pract* 1999; **2**(1): 1–10.

The Biopsychosocial Assessment

Lubna Somjee and Sabrina A. Esbitt

Introduction

In the past few decades we have seen incredible advances in healthcare with respect to technology, research, and interventions. As we continue to research health and healthcare, we have uncovered that the traditional focus on the biomedical model (BM) exclusively has been reductionistic and not robust in assessing and treating patients. Accordingly, it is critical that our work with patients, including the assessment process, needs to reflect these advances in healthcare. This includes a biopsychosocial (BPS) approach to working with patients [1].

Traditionally, the dominant approach to health focused on the body and the ways medicine can assess and intervene. This is the BM model. This model posits that illness is determined by biologically based defects. This approach was incredibly helpful for illnesses like tuberculosis, and other infectious diseases. However, in the twentieth century, people were more likely to die of chronic diseases including – but not limited to – heart disease, cancer, and so forth [2]. While the BM component continues to be important, alone it is reductionistic. The exclusive focus on physiology has been found to be limiting in distinct ways, especially as it relates to chronic illnesses:

- Science has uncovered that the etiology of chronic disease is multifactorial.
- There are disparities in healthcare (socioeconomic, education, income).
- There is a focus on pathology, with little focus on wellness.

In 1977, doctors George Engle and John Romano proposed the BPS model to address some gaps in healthcare. This approach includes the biological, psychological, and social factors in the etiology of health and treatment – and better addressed chronic disease and wellness overall [3, 4]. Given the shift in our understanding of illness and disease, we need to ensure our approach with patients, including our assessment process, captures a more complete picture of our patients.

This chapter will cover the components of a BPS assessment, benefits to the clinician and patient, resources to support the assessment process, as well as the importance of self-reflection in practice.

Assessment of Clinical Issues

Medical Assessment

Traditional approaches to assessment may or may not involve taking an in-depth social history. They do include taking a medical history, and often do so by eliciting the chief complaint and its history, past medical history, including medication, allergies, surgical history, family medical history, and a review of systems [5]. Within an ambulatory care setting, this assessment may be tailored depending on the clinical scenario: new patient arriving with no health issues for the annual physical; new patient out of care for many years with multiple complaints; new patient in your office for a sick appointment; well-known patient with a sick appointment. Of course, all of these scenarios are simplified or complicated by known and unknown social, family, cultural, and structural factors, as well as psychological comorbidities, that shape their everyday lived experience of wellness or illness.

Eliminating or limiting the psychosocial from the assessment of a patient's medical history does not eliminate or limit its impact on the patient's medical history. The BPS approach has been gaining increasing importance in patient care, even as healthcare leaders acknowledge the limitations of time and how essential it is to use it wisely [6, 7].

Front-loading the social history is one way of embedding the assessment of the presenting illness within the larger social context and lived experience of the patient [8]. Using a narrative format and reframing the assessment as a collaborative history-building from the patient – not a history-taking done by the provider – through the use of patient-centered communication skills and enriched social history interviewing is another approach that expands the assessment from BM to fully BPS [9].

Psychological Assessment

Mental health is health. Seventy percent of healthcare resources are used by only 10 percent of the population, the majority of whom have complex comorbid psychiatric and medical conditions [10, 11]. Most people that have mental health issues, up to 70 percent, in fact, receive their mental healthcare – including screening, assessment, and psychopharmacology – from their primary care providers [12]. Medical settings are the first point of contact in the healthcare system for people with psychiatric issues. No medical history is complete without a psychiatric history, which includes a screening for depressive symptoms and querying current mood, mental health history, as well as past and family psychiatric history, including diagnoses, treatment, and individual and social factors that helped or hindered recovery.

Screening of Current Psychiatric Symptoms

A comprehensive overview of psychiatric screening in medical settings is beyond the scope of this chapter. However, a few key points deserve to be mentioned. Universal screening for depression in the general adult population, including pregnant and postpartum women, is recommended by the United States Preventive Services Task Force [13]. As screening for a problem implies intent to treat that problem, health service providers should have plans in place for referrals to additional resources for diagnosis, treatment, recovery support, and relapse prevention. Importantly, screeners cannot diagnose depression without contextual assessment, degree of distress/disability, mental health history, and the integration of the medical history to first rule-out medical causes.

Evidence-based screening tools for depression include the Patient Health Questionnaire (PHQ-2, a two-item brief screen, and the PHQ-9, a full nine-item screener), based on the DSM-5 criteria for a major depressive episode [14]. The Geriatric Depression Scale (GDS), which includes fewer somatic items and more cognitive, affective, and behavioral symptoms of depression, is often recommended for use with older adults, whose more common medical comorbidities may lead to false-positives on the PHQ-9 [15].

When taking a comprehensive history, as with a new outpatient or admission, providers also often conduct brief screening for current anxiety, trauma, and alcohol- or substance-use disorder. The Generalized Anxiety Disorder 7-item screener (GAD-7) is a brief self-report screening measure that also maps onto DSM-5 criteria [16]. The Primary Care PTSD Screen for DSM-5 (PC-PTSD-5) is a five-item screen that was designed for use in primary care settings [17, 18]. The Patient Checklist-5 (PCL-5) is a 20-item pen-and-paper self-report measure of DSM-5 symptoms of posttraumatic stress disorder (PTSD) that is recommended for follow-up assessment for patients who screen positive on the PC-PTSD-5 [19, 20]. Multiple screening tools exist for alcohol and drug use. The CAGE-AID is a very brief validated three-item screener that allows providers to screen for both alcohol- and substance-use disorders [21].

Should patients endorse symptoms of current psychological or substance-use disorders, providers should assess severity, duration, impact, and distress associated with their symptoms. Contextual factors that indicate severity and offer clues as to areas of urgent intervention include details of impairment – if any domains are more or less impacted, impact on family context, including what supports are offered and accessed or not. Family history of mental illness, including severity, chronicity, impact on the patient and family, and treatment outcomes all guide diagnosis and treatment planning. Barriers to treatment engagement and shared decision-making include the patient's mental health literacy and beliefs about mental illness, and internalized individual and social/cultural stigma, and often emerge through the building of the psychiatric history.

Assessment of Psychosocial Factors

A BPS assessment is reflective of a BPS approach to patient care. It allows for the various factors contributing to someone's health, including the biological, but also attending to the psychological and social/environmental issues contributing to one's medical and mental health. It takes into account the ecological and contextual environment of the patient, which is the domain in which almost all wellness and disease prevention activity occurs. The BPS assessment also locates the patient within the developmental and lifespan context, understanding that at different ages and stages, individuals and their families negotiate different opportunities, challenges, and changes, all of which impact health and wellness. Clinicians with more information about a patient will be able to home in on a proper diagnosis, and treatment that is more targeted. Additionally, patient-centered communication, which is helpful in doing a BPS assessment, can in and of itself help with patient outcomes, patient satisfaction, and improved outcomes in patients with chronic medical issues [22].

Case Illustration

The patient is a 65-year-old black male, cisgender, heterosexual, married with two children, and recently retired engineer. He was enjoying retirement and was busy with travel, hobbies, and social activities. He has an implantable cardioverter defibrillator (ICD), and approximately a year into retirement it discharged due to a faulty lead. Since then he has experienced significant anxiety – he is worrying excessively and fears being away from home in the event that the device discharges again. He is no longer traveling, only going to places within a few miles from home, and rarely ventures out unless someone accompanies him. Over time, he has also developed some symptoms of PTSD and increased hypertension. He sees his primary care physician and is given anxiolytics; however, unsurprisingly the anxiety continues. This patient has reluctantly sought a health psychologist after pressure from his wife.

After a BPS assessment, the health psychologist noted that: (1) his anxiety was longstanding although symptoms became more severe post cardiac event; (2) his anxiety was further exacerbated by the fact that his cardiologist was not taking the time to explain things to him, or was using highly technical language he did not understand; (3) he felt some of his medical professionals were not treating him appropriately based on race (not answering his questions, taking significantly less time with him than with other patients, asking him to look things up on the Internet versus answering questions about his condition, minimizing his health concerns); and (4) the patient's retirement, overall a happy event, also involves some unforeseen challenges. Unwilling to travel due to fears about his ICD device, he finds himself home alone, without the structure, social support, and sense of purpose that work provided. Additionally, (5) one of his children was experiencing stress while at college, which was adding to the patient's stress levels.

This assessment allowed the clinician to understand the roots feeding his anxiety and hypertension versus simply recognizing some of his symptoms. The psychologist was able to address all the sources of his anxiety and provide tools to help decrease his hypertension. The psychologist was also able to work with his medical providers to get him on more appropriate medications, and the patient was able to better address the concerns above using a multitude of approaches, including but not limited to finding a new cardiologist. This led to decreased anxiety, decreased hypertension, and the ability to enjoy his family and his retirement activities again.

Psychosocial History

When we examine psychosocial factors that impact medical illness – certain types of depression [23], stress, support systems [24], socioeconomic status, race [25], and unhealthy workplaces [26] just to name a few – we increase our ability to better address our patients' needs and provide more complete and targeted treatment. The BPS model allows for the complexity of each individual, thereby allowing us to provide comprehensive rather than reductionistic treatment.

This model is not only a philosophy of care, but also a practical clinical guide. There is no universally agreed upon single BPS assessment as domains and questions vary depending on the setting, the population being assessed, and the healthcare professional's background. However, there are some domains useful to assess regardless of one's specialty. These domains provide patient context which influences health-related actions and how health information is conveyed and understood. Context can also influence how we proceed with assessments and treatment. The information gleaned can also be used by an organization to track trends and disparities in healthcare. Expanding the medical genogram to include the family and social history (Figure 3.1) is one way to capture contextual and ecological information in an accessible and structured format [7].

Before discussing these domains, it is useful to note the importance of self-reflection – to recognize how our upbringing, life experiences, individual characteristics, and our own individual privileges shape our views, assumptions, and biases of others and events. This is critical to keep in mind as it shapes how we observe, understand, and behave with others, including our patients.

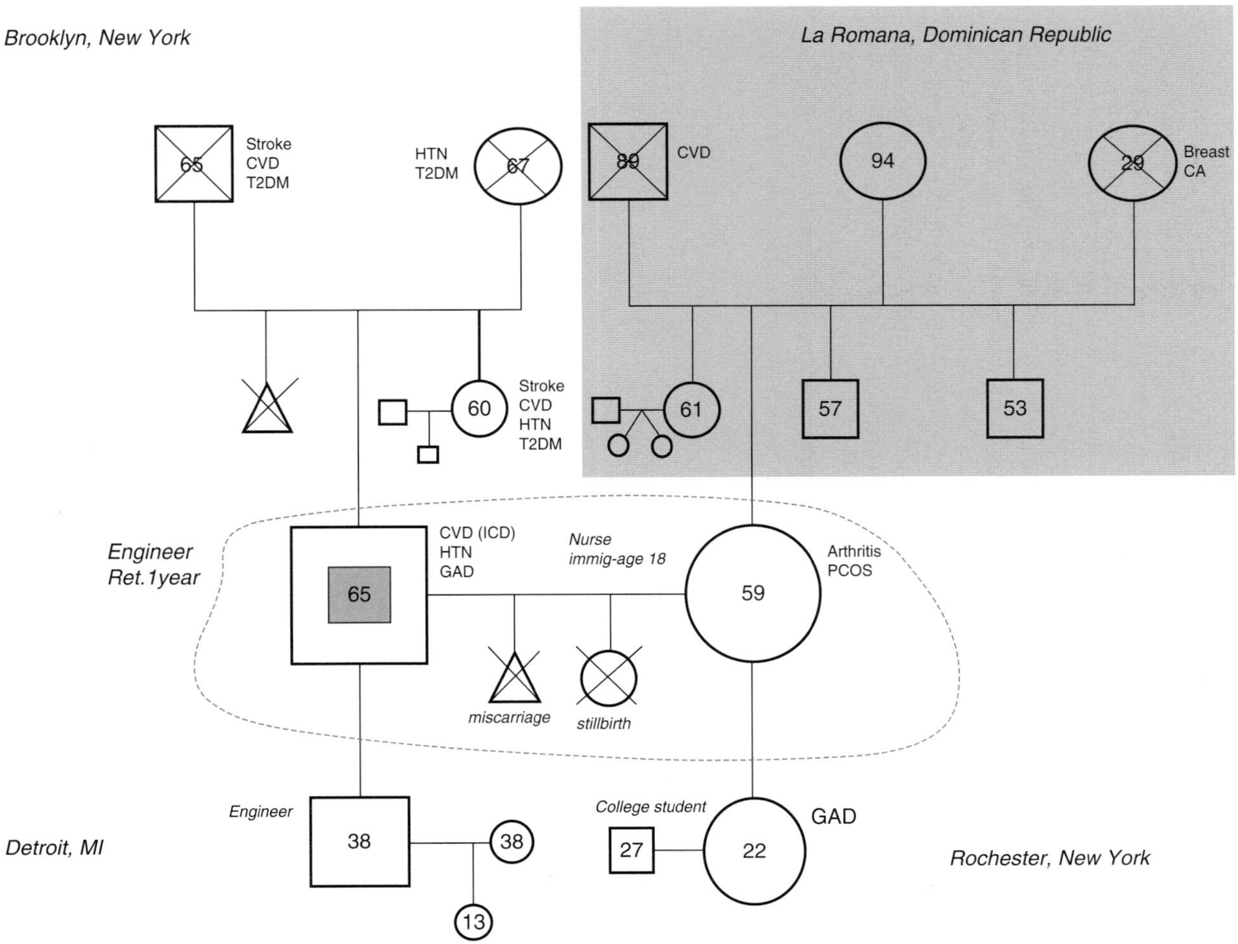

Figure 3.1 Expanding the medical genogram to capture contextual and ecological information.

Components of a Psychosocial Assessment

- Structural determinants of health
- Religion/spiritual beliefs
- Life experiences/lifespan-developmental perspective
- Language
- Race/ethnicity
- Gender identity and sexual orientation

Structural Determinants of Health

A patient's state of wellness is molded by the environment in which they and their family live. The elements that make up this environment are called the social, or structural, determinants of health. As defined by the World Health Organization, "structural mechanisms are those that generate stratification and social class divisions in the society and that define individual socioeconomic position within hierarchies of power, prestige and access to resources" [27].

Income, education, employment (including not only employment status but also employment conditions), social class, as well as gender, race, and ethnicity are core elements of the structural determinants of health. Housing and neighborhood resources, food security, immigration history and documentation status, family resources, organization, and social support, as well as access to and engagement with the health system itself, are additional social-contextual factors that are structurally driven and often intersect, i.e., structural racism impacts social and economic status, neighborhood, access to food, education, and health resources, etc. Routine assessment of these structural determinants of health is increasingly common, as providers and healthcare systems shift perspectives from an individually determined model of health to one that understands the power of structural forces to shape health and wellness, and the role of the healthcare system in addressing health inequities on a patient and population level.

Social Determinants of Health: Employment History

A 41-year-old white, cisgender, bisexual female, employed mother of three, with a primary medical history of type-2 diabetes, has an HbA1C < 10, which been steadily rising over the past several years. Before we move on to making recommendations about diet or exercise, or changing medications, we need to understand how structural factors, like employment, shape her self-management of her diabetes [28]. Without this knowledge, we may well end up making a general treatment plan that is a poor fit for this specific patient. Our patient, like us, spends the lion's share of her life at work, and work is a social structure that informs her health and wellness. An employment history in the context of the BPS assessment captures if and where our patient is employed, as well as her experience of her employment. If a patient is not employed, that also has implications for their health and well-being, as well as that of their family. Schedules (flexible, allowing for doctors' appointments and family caregiving; inflexible with little time off; known or unpredictable, variable shifts, night shifts), hours and days worked, benefits (salary, insurance), workplace safety, sedentary versus active tasks, commuting, and workplace culture (support, mentorship, opportunity for growth, toxicity, harassment, or discrimination) all impact our patient's diet, sleep, activity, access to healthcare resources, including medications, and emotional and social well-being, and play a vital role in her diabetes self-management.

When we ask patients about their life circumstances as part of our BPS assessment, we are aware of how this data will ultimately inform our history of the present illness (HPI) and our approach to intervention. We develop our conceptualization and diagnosis based on our biopsychosocial assessment of the patient's own preferences, beliefs, and values as they operate within the structures in which they live, allowing us to tailor our interventions to the patient's own lived experience, resources, and health goals.

Life Experiences

Certain key life experiences are critical to assess in helping to better understand a patient. Childhood experiences can include family experiences growing up, education, job history, military history, abuse or trauma history, mental health issues in the family, and legal history. We also know trauma is widespread and can impact one's overall well-being even outside of a DSM diagnosis. It is important to keep in mind that adverse childhood experiences (ACEs) can contribute to negative medical [29] and mental health outcomes in adults [30].

Adverse childhood experiences can include physical, sexual, or psychological abuse or neglect, including physical, emotional, healthcare, or educational neglect, inadequate supervision, or exposure to violent environments [31]. The impact of ACEs can be far-reaching medically and mentally, and can include cardiovascular disease, gastrointestinal, respiratory, neurological, and musculoskeletal disorders [32]. The impact of ACEs can also include moderate to heavy drinking, drug use, depressed affect, and suicide attempts [33].

Race/Ethnicity

Race (socially constructed categories) or ethnic background (groups that share a common identity-based ancestry or culture) alone do not tell a professional much about a patient. When assessed dynamically along with the interplay of socioeconomic status, culture, nationality, acculturation levels, and so forth, they can provide the clinician a jumping-off point to assess cultural reference, including healthcare behaviors, how a patient may utilize healthcare, complementary approaches, and understanding and communicating healthcare issues. Additionally, people facing discrimination are at greater risk for health issues, and this is important to keep in mind when working with people of color [34].

Increased contextual information can also help with increasing patient–provider communication, given that both healthcare provider demographics and patient demographics play a role in communication. Culturally competent knowledge can help with avoiding bias and misdiagnosis. Additionally, there are healthcare disparities among people of color resulting in higher rates of morbidity and mortality than among their white counterparts. Some of this may have to do with discrimination within the healthcare system [35]. Tracking this information can also help clinics to track and trend any disparities and to address them.

Race and ethnicity can be assessed by taking a thorough history of family of origin, country of origin, migration history, degree of acculturation to the country of residence, and cultural or religious practices. This information may often be gained over time through questionnaires and interviews. Asking about a patient's race can be uncomfortable for healthcare professionals who don't often think or talk about race. As long as they are clear about why it is useful, and can communicate this, it can help professionals feel more grounded and confident in asking appropriate questions.

Patients may be wary if asked certain questions regarding race – or other individual characteristics – given mistrust and incredible discrimination within the healthcare system [36], or the political climate overall. It is important to take the patient's cue as to how much they are comfortable sharing information. Obtaining information can be done in more informal, conversational ways, including open-ended questions. For example, instead of asking where someone was born, a clinician can ask if a patient grew up in the area, which can lead to increased understanding of not only where someone is from, but also levels of acculturation and so forth. It is best to ask for this information rather than attempting to obtain it through observation, as third parties are not good judges of race or ethnicity – especially when someone is bi- or multiracial – and a patient's nuanced response provides richer information [37].

Religion/Spiritual Beliefs

Asking about religion or spiritual beliefs can also help in understanding how a patient makes healthcare decisions, how they cope, the impact on their mental and medical health, and health behaviors [38]. It also needs to be taken into account as it relates to ethical choices and end-of-life decisions.

Language

Language is important to assess, including whether patients speak, write, or read in more than one language, and which one they feel most comfortable using. While a patient may speak the same language as the healthcare professional, taking into account fluency is important especially when it comes to more sophisticated use of language (humor, assertiveness, basic healthcare terms, and so forth). Literacy and numeracy should not be assumed. Multilingual patients may not have equivalent written and verbal literacy across languages.

Gender Identity and Sexual Orientation

Populations facing discrimination are at greater risk for healthcare issues. This includes the LGBTQ community, who face discrimination on a daily basis. Based on a poll by the Harvard Chan School, NPR, and the Robert Wood Johnson Foundation, it was found that 57 percent of LGBTQ adults deal with slurs, 53 percent deal with offensive comments about their identity, and 51 percent say they, a friend, or family member has experienced violence [39].

In order to provide quality care and address health disparities, clinicians need to be aware of a patient's gender identity and sexual orientation [40]. There is bias against the LGBTQ community in healthcare, ranging from the questions asked on intake forms, to implicit preferences toward heterosexual people by heterosexual healthcare professionals [41]. Additionally, increased contextual information on a patient's sex, gender identity, etc. can only help with patient–provider communication, help avoid misdiagnoses, and track, trend, and address disparities.

Healthcare professionals need to be familiar with ways patients may self-identify when it comes to sexual orientation and gender identity. While patients may not always share this information for fear of bias from a healthcare professional, it is useful to become used to gently gathering it as part and parcel of any intake, intake forms, and screening tools. This includes becoming familiar with certain terms, including, but not limited to:

Lesbian: A female who experiences sexual, romantic, or emotional attraction to other females.

Gay: This term is often used to describe men who experience sexual, romantic, or emotional attraction to other men, but lesbians may also be referred to as gay.

Bisexual: Sexual, romantic, or emotional attraction toward both males and females.

Pansexual: Sexual, romantic, or emotional attraction toward a person regardless of the person's sex or gender identity.

Asexual: A lack of sexual attraction and limited or no engagement in sexual activity.

Transgender: People whose gender identity differs from the sex they were assigned at birth.

Cisgender: People whose gender identity corresponds to the sex they were assigned at birth.

There is more information online at: https://ok2bme.ca/resources/kids-teens/what-does-lgbtq-mean [42].

Some people may have sexual, romantic, or emotional attractions toward someone of the same sex, as one example, and may have sexual encounters but may not identify as lesbian or gay due to cultural reasons, fear of negative reactions from others, or other personal reasons. Others may have no sexual attraction to anyone; as reduced sexual desire can be a sign or symptom of mental or medical illness, it is important to distinguish between asexuality, which is normative, and a change in sexual desire, which may warrant further investigation.

While there are obviously no specific LGBTQ diseases, LGBTQ people may be more likely to experience certain health issues, and care must be taken to screen for those issues. According to the Office of Disease Prevention and Health Promotion [43], these can include: increased risk for suicide; lesbians are less likely to obtain preventive services for cancer, such as pap smears and mammograms; lesbian and bisexual females are more likely to be overweight or obese and to have eating disorders; transgender and gay men have a higher level of HIV/STDs; and transgender individuals are more likely to be victimized.

To enrich your history, shift your format: Chronologically oriented questions can allow providers to capture multiple and intersecting aspects of a patient's past and present life experiences, and gain important insights into the development and maintenance of their health environment, health behaviors, and health beliefs (Figure 3.2) [44]. Many providers find that starting with "where were you born?" can easily segue into family makeup, immigration history, childhood socioeconomic status, ACEs, education history, relationship history, and early experiences with health/illness and the healthcare system. However, for providers used to capturing history through a clinician-centered review of systems, shifting format can mean shifting paradigms. As an analysis of 112 recorded patient–provider transcripts found that providers on average gave patients 11 seconds to speak about their presenting issues before interrupting [45], taking a chronological approach to the BPS history requires a commitment to a patient-centered approach in which a BPS history is collaboratively built, and power is shifted to and shared with our patients [8, 9].

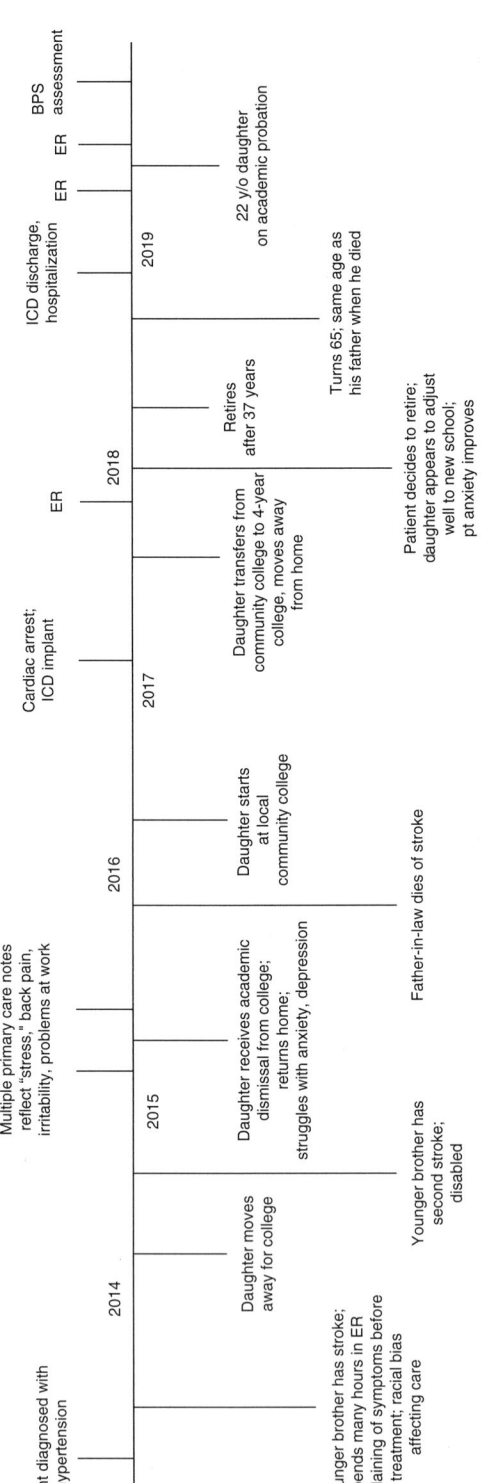

Figure 3.2 The chronological approach to the BPS history.

Patient diagnosed with hypertension

Multiple primary care notes reflect "stress," back pain, irritability, problems at work

ICD discharge, hospitalization

ER

ER

BPS assessment

2014

2015

2016

2017

2018

2019

Cardiac arrest; ICD implant

ER

22 y/o daughter on academic probation

Daughter moves away for college

Daughter receives academic dismissal from college; returns home; struggles with anxiety, depression

Daughter starts at local community college

Daughter transfers from community college to 4-year college, moves away from home

Retires after 37 years

Younger brother has stroke; spends many hours in ER complaining of symptoms before treatment; racial bias affecting care

Younger brother has second stroke; disabled

Father-in-law dies of stroke

Turns 65; same age as his father when he died

Patient decides to retire; daughter appears to adjust well to new school; pt anxiety improves

Challenging Topics in the BPS History

Even the most seasoned and psychosocially skilled health service providers find aspects of the social history challenging. Common areas of the social history that providers struggle with include sexual history, alcohol- and substance-use disorder, poverty, education, race and racism, employment, gender and sexual identity, immigration history and documentation status, and trauma history. Considering how rarely frank and open conversations about these issues occur in our training or in our personal lives, and the taboos surrounding them, it is only to be expected that even highly skilled providers are inexperienced in talking about sensitive subjects with our patients. However, there are several steps providers can take to increase not only their comfort, but the patient's comfort with the psychosocial assessment.

- Take a minute to self-reflect and calibrate. Self-reflection is a lifelong learning task. Over time and with practice, providers can become aware of their own emotions, and the physical and behavioral "tells" that indicate they may have strong personal beliefs or feelings about an issue. Awareness of these beliefs and biases allows providers to thoughtfully calibrate themselves to approach even the most sensitive questions with intention and openness.
- Many providers find it helpful to have a script prepared that introduces to their patient the rationale behind the social history. They might suggest that, "in order to take the best care of you, I need to know more about you: your family, your lifestyle, your culture, and the important life experiences that have made you who you are."
- Asking permission before broaching sensitive topics lets the patient know that you are aware of the sensitive nature of these topics, and that they are in control of the amount and kind of information they share with you. "I know that some of these questions may feel personal or private; you don't have to answer anything you don't wish to talk about."
- Universalizing statements are also helpful in normalizing the social history assessment and its place within the medical visit: "I ask these questions of all my patients."
- When patients share deeply sensitive or stigmatizing material, such as trauma history, the best thing providers can do is listen closely and empathetically. Validating the patient's strength for overcoming hardships and thanking them for their honesty and trust demonstrates that you are someone they can trust and turn to, should future difficulties arise.

Resources in the Assessment Process

When you consider the assessment process, it is useful to think about all patient touchpoints from the time they make an appointment to the appointment itself. Those touchpoints can be helpful in contributing to a robust BPS assessment.

For example, having a patient fill out forms prior to their appointment might allow them more time and to be more forthcoming in their responses. Your forms can convey much about your practice based on what you ask, what you do not ask, and how you ask it. Inclusive wording informs the patient that the practice is open to diversity and focused on individualized care. When the patient first arrives at the appointment, it is important that the waiting room experience is positive. Patient emotions might be running high, and the waiting room can set the tone and allow healthcare professionals to connect well with that patient. This can include clarity and ease of check-in and comfortable seating. Many patients will connect with their healthcare professionals but leave practices due to staff rudeness or inefficiencies. Ensuring front-desk staff greet everyone warmly and are empathetic, and the check-in process is smooth, is important.

Having flyers or brochures about non-clinical services your practice offers, or behavioral health services and health-related community services available, sends a message that complete care is important to the practice. Pictures of people on magazines, flyers, and brochures should represent diverse groups.

Various healthcare professionals can also obtain patient information to help complete the assessment. Medical technicians and nurses can obtain more detailed information based on the forms patients have filled out. They can assess not only why the patient is coming in and do some physical assessments, based on the scope of their license, but can also query about potential stressors or changes in their lives, discuss their history, assess and discuss a patient's network to see how they may be supported at home or beyond, get a sense of how their cognitive or psychosocial history may impact a patient's response to medical or mental health issues, and assess the potential impact of cultural or spiritual issues on their health. This allows the practice to get to know the patient beyond a basic medical assessment, and can allow physicians to drill down and obtain additional detailed information that can help with diagnosis and treatment.

Beyond leveraging the patient experience, various clinicians, and questionnaires, using various interview approaches can be helpful. When interviewing patients, many medical professionals use clinician-centered interviewing, which involves the clinician leading the discussion and often asking closed-ended questions. While this is often helpful in later parts of an assessment, when used throughout clinicians can often miss crucial details – especially psychosocial details that can help with providing targeted treatment. Instead, using patient-centered interviewing at the start is ideal in most cases.

Patient-centered interviewing includes the patient leading the interview and directing the conversation, with the clinician asking open-ended questions, engaging in active listening, and nonverbal responses that encouraging talking, reflection, and other cues that encourage the patient to continue to share so the clinician can understand their perspective [46].

As the interview continues, the clinician would then ask more follow-up questions and more clinician-centered questions in order to drill down for more specific information. Patient-centered communication in assessment is crucial and research shows it is correlated with positive perceptions about patient visits, which is associated with better health status and fewer diagnostic tests and referrals, and better recovery from discomfort and concern [47]. Bickley's *Bates' Guide to Physical Examination and History Taking* is a useful resource on more detailed interviewing skills [48].

Conclusion

A BPS assessment can be done efficiently, involves numerous touchpoints, and lays a solid foundation for all the work that follows. A complete picture of your patient not only conveys your interest in individualized care, but also provides you with more detailed information that can go a long way toward diagnosis, treatment, and patient adherence to the medical regimen.

References

1. GL Engel. The biopsychosocial model and the education of health professionals. *Ann N Y Acad Sci* 1978; **310**: 169–181.

2. J Fuller. The new medical model: a renewed challenge for biomedicine. *CMAJ* 2017; **189**: E640–E641.

3. GL Engel. The need for a new medical model: a challenge for biomedicine. *Science* 1977; **196**: 129–136.

4. RC Smith. The biopsychosocial revolution: interviewing and provider–patient relationships becoming key issues for primary care. *J Gen Int Med* 2002; **17**: 309–310.

5. A Phillips, A Frank, C Loftin, et al. A detailed review of systems: an educational feature. *J Nurse Pract* 2017; **13**: 681–686.

6. HL Behforouz, PK Drain, JJ Rhatigan, et al. Rethinking the social history. *N Engl J Med* 2014; **371**: 1277–1279.

7. S McDaniel, TI Campbell, DB Seaburn. *Family-Oriented Primary Care: A Manual for Medical Providers*. New York, Springer-Verlag; 1989.

8. B Wu. History taking in reverse: beginning with the social history. *Consultant* 2013; **53**: 34–36.

9. P Haidet, DA Paterniti. "Building" a history rather than "taking" one. *Arch Intern Med* 2003; **163**(10): 1134.

10. ML Berk, AC Monheit. The concentration of healthcare expenditures, revisited. *Health Affairs* 2001; **20**(2): 9–18.

11. JA Schoenman. NIHCM Foundation data brief: the concentration of healthcare spending. 2012. www.nihcm.org/pdf/Data Brief3%20Final.pdf.

12. RC Kessler, O Demler, RG Frank, et al. Prevalence and treatment of mental disorders, 1990 to 2003. *N Engl J Med* **352**: 2515–2523.

13. U.S. Preventive Services Task Force. Final recommendation statement: depression in adults: screening. 2016. www.uspreventive servicestaskforce.org/Page/Document/Rec ommendationStatementFinal/depression-i n-adults-screening1.

14. K Kroenke, RL Spitzer, JBW Williams. The PHQ-9. *J Gen Intern Med* 2001;**16**(9): 606–613.

15. PA Parmelee, IR Katz. Geriatric Depression Scale. *J Am Geriatr Soc* 1990; **38** (12): 1379.

16. RL Spitzer, K Kroenke, JBW Williams, B Löwe. A brief measure for assessing generalized anxiety disorder. *Arch Intern Med* 2006; **166**(10): 1092.

17. A Prins, MJ Bovin, R Kimerling, et al. The Primary Care PTSD Screen for DSM-5 (PC-PTSD-5). 2015 [Measurement instrument].

18. A Prins, MJ Bovin, DJ Smolenski, et al. The Primary Care PTSD Screen for DSM-5 (PC-PTSD-5): development and evaluation within a veteran primary care sample. *J Gen Intern Med* 2016; **31**(10): 1206–1211.

19. FW Weathers, BT Litz, TM Keane, et al. PTSD. 2018. www.ptsd.va.gov/professional/a ssessment/adult-sr/ptsd-checklist.asp.

20. CA Blevins, FW Weathers, MT Davis, TK Witte, JL Domino. The Posttraumatic Stress Disorder Checklist for DSM-5 (PCL-5): development and initial psychometric evaluation. *J Trauma Stress* 2015; **28**: 489–498.

21. RL Brown, LA Rounds. Conjoint screening questionnaires for alcohol and other drug abuse: criterion validity in a primary care practice. *Wis Med J* 1995; **94**(3): 135–140.

22. W Levinson. Patient-centred communication: a sophisticated procedure. *BMJ Qual Saf* 2011; **20**(10): 823–825.

23. MM Burg, D Abrams. Depression in chronic medical illness: the case of coronary heart disease. *J Clin Psychol* 2001; **57**(11): 1323–1337.

24. BN Uchino, K Bowen, R Kent de Grey, J Mikel, EB Fisher. Social support and physical health: models, mechanisms, and opportunities. In: E Fisher, L Cameron, A Christensen, et al., eds., *Principles and Concepts of Behavioral Medicine*. New York, Springer; 2018; 341–372.

25. DR Williams, N Priest, NB Anderson. Understanding associations among race, socioeconomic status, and health: patterns and prospects. *Health Psychol* 2016; **35**(4): 407–411.

26. J Goh, J Pfeffer, SA Zenios. The relationship between workplace stressors and mortality and health costs in the United States. *Manage Sci* 2016; **62**(2): 608–628.

27. DD Moortel, H Vandenheede, C Muntaner, C Vanroelen. Structural and

intermediary determinants of social inequalities in the mental well-being of European workers: a relational approach. *BMC Public Health* 2014; **14**(1).

28. Lifestyle Management: Standards of Medical Care in Diabetes – 2019. *Diabetes Care* 2018; **42**(Supplement 1).

29. HL Wegman, C Stetler. A meta-analytic review of the effects of childhood abuse on medical outcomes in adulthood. *Psychosom Med* 2009; **71**(8): 805–812.

30. American Academy of Pediatrics. Adverse childhood experiences and the lifelong consequences of trauma. www.aap.org/en-us/Documents/ttb_aces_consequences.pdf.

31. RT Leeb, LJ Paulozzi, C Melanson, TR Simon, I Arias. Child maltreatment surveillance: uniform definitions for public health and recommended data elements 2008. www.cdc.gov/violenceprevention/pdf/cm_surveillance-a.pdf.

32. HL Wegman, C Stetler. A meta-analytic review of the effects of childhood abuse on medical outcomes in adulthood. *Psychosom Med* 2009; **71**(8): 805–812.

33. MT Merrick, KA Ports, DC Ford, et al. Unpacking the impact of adverse childhood experiences on adult mental health. *Child Abuse Negl* 2017; **69**: 10–19.

34. Robert Wood Johnson Foundation. Race, racism and health. www.rwjf.org/en/library/collections/racism-and-health.html.

35. BD Smedley, AY Stith, AR Nelson. Unequal treatment: confronting racial and ethnic disparities in health care. 2003. www.nap.edu/read/12875/chapter/1.

36. NE Adler, DH Rehkopf. U.S. disparities in health: descriptions, causes, and mechanisms. *Annu Rev Public Health* 2008; **29**(1): 235–252.

37. R Hasnain-Wynia, DW Baker. Obtaining data on patient race, ethnicity, and primary language in health care organizations: current challenges and proposed solutions. *Health Serv Research* 2006; **41**(4 Pt 1): 1501–1518.

38. HG Koenig. Religion, spirituality, and health: the research and clinical implications. *ISRN Psychiatry* 2012; **2012**: 1–33.

39. A Powell, ed. *Proceedings from Harvard Chan School of Public Health: Health in the LGBTQ Community: Improving Care and Confronting Discrimination.* 2018. https://news.harvard.edu/gazette/story/2018/03/health-care-providers-need-better-understanding-of-lgbtq-patients-harvard-forum-says.

40. Institute of Medicine (US) Board on the Health of Select Populations. *Collecting Sexual Orientation and Gender Identity Data in Electronic Health Records: Workshop Summary.* Washington, DC, National Academies Press; 2013.

41. JA Sabin, RG Riskind, BA Nosek. Health care providers' implicit and explicit attitudes toward lesbian women and gay men. *Am J Public Health* 2015; **105**(9): 1831–1841.

42. KW Counseling services. What does LGBTQ+ mean? https://ok2bme.ca/resources/kids-teens/what-does-lgbtq-mean.

43. Office of Disease Prevention and Health Promotion. Lesbian, gay, bisexual, and transgender health. www.healthypeople.gov/2020/topics-objectives/topic/lesbian-gay-bisexual-and-transgender-health.

44. LM Mazer, T Storage, S Bereknyei, J Chi, K Skeff. A pilot study of the chronology of present illness: restructuring the HPI to improve physician cognition and communication. *J Gen Intern Med* 2016; **32**(2): 182–188.

45. N Singh Ospina, KA Phillips, R Rodriguez-Gutierrez, et al. Eliciting the patient's agenda: secondary analysis of recorded clinical encounters. *J Gen Intern Med* 2019; **4**(1): 36–40.

46. J Hashim. Patient-centered communication: basic skills. *J Am Fam Phys* 2017; **95**(1): 29–34.

47. M Stewart, JB Brown, A Donner, et al. The impact of patient-centered care on outcomes. *Fam Pract* 2000; **49**(9),796–804.

48. LS Bickley. *Bates' Guide to Physical Examination and History Taking* (12th ed.). Philadelphia, PA, Lippincott, Williams & Wilkins; 2017.

Chapter 4

Wellness Measurement

Timothy P. Melchert

Introduction

Incorporating wellness into considerations of health, healthcare, and social policy has reached an exciting point. Aristotle, Buddha, and other philosophers, sages, and religious leaders throughout history developed great insights into the topic, but only in recent decades has the construct of wellness been examined and clarified through systematic empirical research. There are still major debates regarding several aspects of the topic, but it is now widely considered a measurable construct that should play a role in healthcare and social policy. This volume represents another step forward in bringing wellness into the mainstream of health and healthcare.

Wellness often means different things to different people, and the causes of wellness and the components that comprise well-being continue to be vigorously debated. Philosophical and theological arguments dominated the debate for centuries, with little resolution on important aspects of the subject, and up until recently it was widely believed that too little was known to include considerations of wellness in healthcare practice or policy. Much, of course, still needs to be learned, but empirical research has now clarified several issues, including how wellness can be usefully measured and incorporated into clinical practice, research, and social policy. It is exciting to begin realizing ancient dreams and aspirations of humankind regarding what is most important in life by systematically incorporating these considerations into healthcare. Doing so has the potential to improve well-being for patients and society in general.

What to Measure

The most difficult question to answer when considering the measurement of wellness for clinical, research, or policy purposes concerns what to measure. There have been debates about the nature of wellness, well-being, happiness, health, meaning and purpose in life, flourishing, and related concepts probably ever since *Homo sapiens* developed language. However, as a result of more systematic empirical investigation into these concepts in recent years, some clarity is emerging. Though there is no doubt that human wellness is multi-faceted and complex, some consensus has emerged regarding several aspects of the topic. (In this chapter, I use the terms "wellness" and "well-being" synonymously.)

The primary question debated across history concerns the nature and meaning of wellness, happiness, and "the good life." Answers to this question varied markedly across time and place. In Western culture, the ancient debate often focused on the importance of pleasure as the goal of life (hedonia, primarily associated with Epicurus in ancient Greece) versus the pursuit of a virtuous and excellent life in which one is able to achieve one's full potential (eudaimonia, typically associated with Aristotle). After the rise of Christianity, Christian religious teachings often provided the answers to these types of questions. Following the Scientific Revolution and the Enlightenment, infectious disease gradually became to be understood in scientific terms, and positive, humanistic attitudes began taking hold that emphasized the use of science and reason to solve problems and improve the human condition, in terms of both physical and mental health. The emergence of the disciplines of psychiatry and psychology in the nineteenth century was also a reflection of this trend. During the Great Depression, however, concerns about getting basic needs met focused attention on income and employment as foundational for well-being. Following the devastation and horror of World War II, the founders of the World Health Organization [1] advocated for a remarkably positive and modern conceptualization of well-being that they incorporated into the WHO mission statement in 1948, namely, "a state of complete physical, mental, and social well-being and not merely the absence of disease and infirmity."

Starting in the 1990s, the positive psychology movement gained traction as dissatisfaction grew with the focus on pathology and "what is wrong" rather than "what is right." Seligman and Csikszentmihalyi in 2000 [2] defined positive psychology as "the scientific study of positive human functioning and flourishing on multiple levels that include the biological, personal, relational, institutional, cultural, and global dimensions of life." Just recently, concern has grown that large numbers of people are sensing that conventional approaches to achieving security and well-being are being threatened by technological and societal changes, and populist political movements in several wealthy countries have been growing as a result.

The evolving conceptualizations of wellness over the centuries reflect the difficulty people have had in identifying the nature of well-being, for individuals or communities. There has been growing consensus, however, on these issues. At the most basic level, there is consensus that the most useful perspective for conceptualizing and measuring wellness involves a biopsychosocial approach. There are, of course, times when one's biological functioning is the top priority, but at other times one's psychological, family, or vocational functioning, or even the economic or political functioning of the community, become top considerations. For people in general, however, the measurement of wellness is best accomplished through a comprehensive biopsychosocial perspective. Though Engel [3] argued that the conceptualization of health and healthcare needed to incorporate psychological and social as well as biological perspectives, clearly a person also exists in a fourth dimension of time as well. From conception to death, the biopsychosocial processes that play out across time are critical to understanding virtually any health or developmental outcome. In fact, the three biopsychosocial dimensions plus time are so basic to understanding human development that they are analogous to the three spatial dimensions plus time that are fundamental to understanding the physical universe [4]. The time dimension is particularly important for understanding wellness, such as when a young person sacrifices pleasant leisure activities (hedonia) so that she/he might develop academic skills to increase chances of later career security and life meaning (eudaimonia), or a person eats healthily and exercises regularly, which may be less pleasant in the moment but helps to ensure stronger physical health over the long term.

A second critical consideration in the measurement of wellness concerns the importance of including both objective and subjective perspectives. For example, it might seem that objective measures showing strong physical health and high income would generally be associated with high levels of life satisfaction and well-being, but of course that frequently is not the case (e.g., elite athletes, individuals with quadriplegia or terminal illness, or those living with little or great wealth fall at many different points with regard to emotional well-being, life satisfaction, meaning, and fulfillment). Correlations between many objective and subjective aspects of well-being are actually surprisingly low. Consequently, both perspectives need to be considered.

For some purposes, objective measures of health and wellness are clearly superior, while subjective perspectives provide little useful information (e.g., measuring blood pressure). But the opposite is true as well. Some very important aspects of life can be assessed only by asking people how they feel. How one feels in terms of mood, the quality of one's social support, or the sense of meaning and purpose in life are frequently considered critical to evaluating wellness, and one's subjective judgment regarding those experiences is typically the important measure. One can objectively observe and rate a person's behaviors or take various physiological measures across situations and time and then make inferences based on that data, but the results will often be inferior and far costlier than those obtained by simply asking a person how they feel about these things.

Research on the association between loneliness and mortality highlights the importance of considering both objective and subjective perspectives on well-being. Meta-analyses have found that loneliness substantially increases the risk of mortality by roughly the same amount as being obese, smoking 15 cigarettes a day, or drinking more than six alcoholic drinks per day [5]. The increase in mortality associated with loneliness was also found to be essentially the same if social isolation was measured objectively (in terms of having infrequent social contact and living alone) or subjectively (in terms of *feeling* lonely, even if one has frequent social contact). Further, and contrary to popular stereotypes, the increased risk for mortality due to loneliness was actually greater for populations younger than 65 years than it was for older individuals. Surveys also suggest widespread problems involving loneliness: one large national 2018 survey by Cigna [6], a health services company, found that 47 percent of Americans felt alone and 13 percent reported there were zero people who knew them well. Nonetheless, issues such as obesity, cigarette smoking, and alcoholism are widely considered to be major public health concerns, while loneliness is not.

It is also important to note that the relationship between objective and subjective measurements of wellness is often complicated. For example, an objective measure of income is typically considered important to understanding well-being, given the importance of getting basic needs met. In fact, low and moderate levels of income do have reliable and fairly strong positive correlations with emotional well-being and happiness, but that relationship weakens considerably as income rises above the point at which people's basic needs are met [7]. In fact, the correlation between income and emotional well-being is essentially zero at levels above approximately $75,000 (in the USA; the amount varies depending on the cost of living across countries). The importance of measuring subjective aspects of well-being in addition to objective ones is evident when caring for a variety of medical populations, such as patients with brittle diabetes whose quality of life may be low but whose HbA1C counts are reasonably well controlled; patients with medically unexplained pain that causes disability; adolescents and young adults with good physical health but very low life satisfaction; or elderly individuals with terminal disease who nonetheless develop a strong sense of meaning in life and life satisfaction. The health and well-being of these individuals cannot be captured by focusing on either subjective or objective measurement approaches alone.

There is widespread agreement regarding the importance of a biopsychosocial perspective that incorporates both objective and subjective measures of wellness, but there is less agreement about which particular components to include. Nonetheless, there are examples representing high levels of consensus regarding how the construct can be conceptualized. A very prominent example was developed by the Organization for Economic Cooperation and Development (OECD). The 35 member countries of the OECD reached a consensus on a definition of subjective well-being that encompasses assessments of life evaluation, emotional states, and meaning and purpose. The OECD then developed a set of questionnaire items to measure these variables and evaluated their psychometric reliability and validity, usefulness for informing policy, and their international comparability [8]. They recommend that all member countries use five core questions to assess these elements in national surveys. These items ask individuals to respond on a scale from 0 to 10 in terms of "Overall, how satisfied are you with life as a whole these days?"; "Overall, to what extent do you feel the things you do in your life are worthwhile?"; and, with regard to how they felt yesterday, "How about happy?" "How about worried?" and "How about depressed?" (p. 253). The OECD also recommends additional questions when a more detailed assessment is desired to further assess life satisfaction, affect, meaning and purpose, and how individuals felt during the time they were engaged in particular daily activities, along with satisfaction with specific life domains such as one's standard of living, health, personal relationships, and personal safety. Outcomes regarding each of these areas across the OECD member states are published annually.

Another influential perspective on measuring wellness focuses on *quality of life* (QOL). This construct is also considered to be multidimensional. The most widely used generic measure of QOL in medical research is the 36-item Short Form Health Survey (often referred to as the SF-36) [9]. This instrument includes eight subscales measuring physical functioning, social functioning, emotional functioning, sexual functioning, cognitive functioning, pain/discomfort, vitality, and overall well-being. This instrument is also available in various shortened forms. Another prominent international effort to assess QOL was undertaken by the World Health Organization [10]. Their WHOQOL instrument included 100 items that covered 10 areas across the biopsychosocial domains and has since been shortened by different research groups.

Meaning in life (eudaimonia) has also been considered an important component of wellness, but was long thought to be too elusive and idiosyncratic to be measured in a reliable or valid manner. Recently, however, there has been major research progress regarding this construct as well. Heintzelman and King [11] asked why meaning in life is widely believed to be both a necessity, something required to make one's life livable and worthwhile, but also extremely difficult to attain and chronically lacking. They argued that "Nothing that human beings require to survive can be next to impossible to obtain" (p. 561). Their comprehensive review of the research included three conclusions: (1) lonely, socially isolated individuals consistently report lower meaning in life and that "Social relationships are a foundational source of meaning in life" (p. 562); (2) experiencing positive emotion is consistently related to meaning in life; and (3) viewing life as making sense, as having coherence and regularity, is associated with life feeling more meaningful. They also noted that most surveys find that large majorities of individuals report that their lives are meaningful (e.g., the 2007 Gallop Global Poll of 137,678 individuals across 132 nations found 91 percent responded affirmatively). That meaning in life may be a common experience might be objectionable to French existentialists and others attracted to the mystique of the construct, but Heintzelman and King [11] noted that this finding also calls into question the notion of whether meaning in life is a *constructed* experience that individuals must search for and create. Instead, perhaps people do need meaning in life to survive, and that is why it is commonplace [11, 12]. Further, even though people may commonly feel that they have meaning and purpose in their lives, they may at the same time also seek to find more meaning and purpose in their lives – the latter pursuit does not negate the former experience.

The two most commonly used measures for assessing meaning in life for research purposes are the Purpose in Life Test and the Meaning in Life Questionnaire. In addition to the OECD measure mentioned above, a very widely used approach to measuring subjective well-being is the five-item Satisfaction with Life Scale, developed by Diener and colleagues [13]. This scale has been widely used in research and commercial surveys (including worldwide through Gallup) and provides a global self-assessment of one's satisfaction with life based on one's personally chosen criteria. Reviews of many more instruments for measuring a variety of aspects of wellness are also available [14, 15].

Measurement Accuracy

A critical issue when using any test or measure in clinical practice or research concerns its accuracy. Almost all measures used in clinical practice are imperfect, whether they assess subjective or objective characteristics, and so the main concern becomes whether measures are sufficiently accurate to be useful for particular clinical or other purposes. The accuracy of many medical tests is very good, even though the sensitivity and specificity of other commonly used tests are less than desirable. The accuracy of psychometric measures is typically assessed by examining their reliability (i.e., their precision of measurement or reproducibility and repeatability) and their validity (i.e., whether they actually measure what they purport to measure or whether they are measuring the right thing). Many measurements in medicine and psychology have reasonably high levels of reliability but weaker evidence regarding their validity (e.g., blood pressure, cholesterol, and cardiac rhythms can be measured reliably, but their relation to disease is less clear; several psychiatric disorders can be diagnosed with reasonably high levels of reliability but the exact nature of particular disorders and their relation to neurophysiological dysfunction can be unclear).

Many measures of subjective well-being, affect, and eudaimonic well-being have reasonably strong evidence regarding their reliability. Reliability coefficients for many instruments indicate that they are clearly suitable for research purposes and can reliably be used to inform clinical assessments as well [8]. Establishing validity is generally more challenging than establishing reliability, particularly for measures of subjective psychological constructs. But even when there are no objective measures of QOL, meaning in life, or emotion to which to compare individuals' subjective judgments, these concepts are still critical to assessing health and wellness. Of course, this is true of many other variables in medicine and behavioral health, such as pain, energy, vitality, and many psychiatric symptoms, so this is not a new problem for healthcare providers and researchers. Ongoing research will clarify these issues but there is already ample evidence supporting the validity of these measures for informing our understanding of health and wellness [8, 11, 16].

Administration Issues

It is important when measuring complex variables such as health and well-being to adopt a consistent and standardized measurement approach in order to reduce bias and increase the comparability of results across individuals and groups. Particularly when assessing subjective variables, there are a variety of response biases and styles that can introduce error into individuals' responses, including a tendency to agree positively to questions, or to disagree, or to give the socially desirable answer that puts respondents in a favorable light. These response biases can be conscious or unconscious, and can occur whether people are responding to in-person interviews or to printed or computer-administered questionnaires. To minimize the effects of response bias, consistently employing a standardized approach across individuals is recommended. To reduce error further, it is generally important to use multiple-item surveys rather than single-item ones because measurement errors across items tend to cancel each other out.

When asking people about their life satisfaction or feelings, the reference period is another important consideration. Asking a person to rate their life satisfaction at the present time or over their whole life course can cause measurement problems, so life satisfaction questions typically ask respondents about their lives in the recent past (e.g., "overall these days" is commonly used). When inquiring about one's emotions, responses may vary significantly if one answers with regard to "right now" versus "yesterday" versus "the past month." As a result, many emotion questions ask about feelings experienced yesterday or over the last 24 hours. Surveys that inquire about meaning and purpose in life typically include no reference period. Because asking about sensitive topics such as stressful life events may influence subsequent responses, it is generally recommended that questions about life satisfaction, emotion, and meaning and purpose in life are asked first. For some purposes, computerized administration can also be an ideal choice for these questionnaires [8]. The particular purpose of a measure will dictate how items are constructed and how the measure is administered, but in general it is important to remain consistent in one's approach in order to maximize reliability and interpretability of responses.

An issue of growing importance in behavioral health treatment concerns measurement-based care [17]. This approach obviously has long been critical in the care of chronic medical conditions such as diabetes and hypertension, but consistently monitoring treatment progress to inform treatment planning has not been widely used in behavioral healthcare. The benefits and importance of measurement-based care for behavioral health are rapidly becoming evident, however. The quality, consistency, and accountability of behavioral healthcare can all suffer without consistently gathered patient-outcome data. Negative patient outcomes and deterioration in clinicians' skills can be missed, as can the ability to demonstrate effectiveness and value to patients, insurers, and taxpayers. Measurement-based care can improve the therapeutic relationship and foster collaboration among care team members. But most importantly, it has the potential to improve treatment effectiveness, reduce symptoms, and improve QOL and well-being for patients. The assessment of symptoms has commonly been included in past measurement-based care approaches, but an important question at this point is the extent to which general functioning, quality of life, and wellness should also be regularly assessed to inform the effectiveness of treatment. This issue should receive more research attention.

Culture also needs to be taken into account when measuring well-being. Well-being can be understood very differently across cultures, and the role of family, religion, spirituality, community, and other factors can vary greatly. Clinicians and researchers need to be culturally sensitive and informed when assessing this construct, just as they must when working with all culturally and socioeconomically diverse populations. When working with older populations, wellness assessment often focuses on quality of life and reducing suffering on a day-to-day basis. At the other end of life, some believe that children as young as 11 can be reliably assessed for subjective well-being, though it is much more common to assess wellness in adolescents age 15 and over [8].

Discussion

The conceptualization and measurement of wellness are relatively new areas of empirical investigation, and so clinicians and researchers need to keep current with the evolving literature in this area. For example, resilience, or the ability to "bounce back" to a baseline level of functioning while facing stress, adversity, or trauma, is a critical quality, but its relation to wellness is still unclear. For victims of trauma to go further beyond their baseline capacities to find benefit and reach even higher levels of functioning has been referred to as "posttraumatic growth" [18]. The relation of these concepts to wellness needs further investigation, but clearly they can be vitally important to recovery and health maintenance for many physical and mental health conditions.

Clinicians, researchers, and individuals in general are also advised to avoid assuming causation when correlations are found between physical health and subjective well-being. For example, it might be assumed that the correlation commonly found between positive emotion and strong physical health reflects the effect of positive emotions on promoting physical health. But current research has not yet advanced enough to rule-out the possibility that stronger physical health leads to more positive emotion and well-being. More comprehensive biopsychosocial data and more longitudinal and neuroscience research are needed before causal conclusions can be drawn regarding these questions. It is perhaps likely that causation actually goes in either direction, and is perhaps also reciprocal, depending on individual biopsychosocial characteristics and circumstances. It may be some time before clear conclusions are reached regarding these questions.

Given that empirical research in this area is still in its early stages, it is also important to continue questioning the ways that wellness has been conceptualized. Ever since ancient Greeks debated the nature of wellness and the good life, Western discussions on the topic often revolved around the importance of pursuing pleasure (hedonism) versus a virtuous and excellent life focused on fulfilling one's potential (eudaimonia). But evolutionary theory suggests that both of these perspectives are likely incomplete because the ultimate goal of living organisms is survival and reproduction, not maximizing happiness, virtue, or fulfillment. If organisms with particular characteristics have greater reproductive success, they will leave greater numbers of descendants and their characteristics will eventually come to dominate in a population. At present, research suggests that the achievement of happiness or virtuousness, or fulfilling one's potential, does not necessarily result in adaptive advantages and greater reproductive success [18, 19]. Hedonism and eudaimonia have long been central to discussions of the good life, but evolutionary research finds that humans are highly social animals very focused on a variety of social and other survival goals. As with everything else in the organic world, evolutionary theory has advanced our understanding of all the biopsychosocial dimensions of human life and has overturned conventional thinking regarding several aspects of human nature. This could happen with regard to wellness in human life as well.

References

1. World Health Organization. *Constitution of the World Health Organization.* Geneva, World Health Organization; 1948.

2. MEP Seligman, M Csikszentmihalyi. Positive psychology: an introduction. *Am Psychologist* 2000; **55**(1): 5–14.

3. G Engel. The need for a new medical mode: a challenge for biomedicine. *Science* 1977; **196**: 129–136.

4. TP Melchert. *Biopsychosocial Practice: A Science-Based Framework for Behavioral Health Care.* Washington, DC, American Psychological Association; 2015.

5. J Holt-Lundstad, TB Smith, M Baker, T Harris, D Stephenson. Loneliness and social isolation as risk factors for mortality: a meta-analytic review. *Perspect Psychol Sci* 2015; **10**: 227–237.

6. Cigna. New Cigna study reveals loneliness at epidemic levels in America. 2018. www.cigna.com/newsroom/news-releases/2018/new-cigna-study-reveals-loneliness-at-epidemic-levels-in-america (accessed April 21, 2020).

7. D Kahneman, A Deaton. High income improves evaluation of life but not emotional well-being. *PNAS* 2010; **107**: 16489–16493.

8. OECD. *OECD Guidelines on Measuring Subjective Well-Being.* Paris, OECD Publishing; 2013.

9. JE Ware, CD Sherbourne. The MOS 36-item Short-Form Health Survey (SF-36): I. Conceptual framework and item selection. *Med Care* 1992 **30**(6): 473–483.

10. WHOQOL Group. The World Health Organization Quality of Life Assessment (WHOQOL): development and general psychometric properties. *Soc Sci Med* 1998; **46**(12): 1569–1585.

11. SJ Heintzelman, LA King. Life is pretty meaningful. *Am Psychologist* 2014; **69**: 561–574.

12. RF Baumeister, MJ Landau. Finding the meaning of meaning: emerging insights on four grand questions. *Rev Gen Psychol* 2018; **22**: 1–10.

13. ED Diener, RA Emmons, RJ Larsen, S Griffin. The Satisfaction with Life Scale. *J Personality Assess* 1985; **49**(1): 71–75.

14. PJ Cooke, TP Melchert, K Connor. Measuring well-being: a review of instruments. *Counsel Psychologist* 2016; **44**(5): 730–757.

15. M Linton, P Dieppe, A Medina-Lara. Review of 99 self-report measures for assessing well-being in adults: exploring dimensions of well-being and developments over time. *BMJ Open* 2016; **6**: 1–16.

16. SA Hooker, KS Masters, CL Park. A meaningful life is a healthy life: a conceptual model linking meaning and meaning salience to health. *Rev Gen Psychol* 2018; **22**: 11–24.

17. JC Fortney, J Unützer, G Wrenn, et al. A tipping point for measurement-based care. *Psychiatric Serv* 2017; **68**(2): 179–188.

18. W von Hippel. *The Social Leap: The New Evolutionary Science of Who We Are, Where We Come From, and What Makes Us Happy.* New York, Harper Wave; 2018.

19. R Wrangham. *The Good Paradox: The Strange Relationship Between Virtue and Violence in Human Evolution.* New York, Pantheon; 2019.

The Wellness Treatment Plan

Dilani M. Perera and Jeffry Moe

Introduction

Considering the principle of holism, a wellness treatment plan requires addressing at least the physical, mental, and social well-being of a client/patient irrespective of medical illness. According to the World Health Organization, "Health is a state of complete physical, mental and social well-being and not merely the absence of disease or infirmity" [1]. A wellness treatment plan may be organized and developed based on the conceptualization of the client/patient's strengths and challenges (i.e., the premise) and supporting material based on a theoretical model [2]. For the target audience, including physical and mental healthcare providers, we suggest treatment plan considerations from two models of wellness: Six Dimensions of Wellness by Dr. Bill Hettler, and Indivisible Self: An Evidence Based Model of Wellness (IS-WEL) by Drs. Jane Myers and Thomas Sweeney [3, 4]. Irrespective of the model, wellness is multidimensional and holistic, moving an individual toward optimal functioning [3, 4]. Seeking wellness requires conscious, self-directed, and mindful decision-making [3]. Wellness requires a desire for a positive state of being [4]. Therefore, wellness is an active positive process in which a person makes a conscious decision to develop optimal functioning across multiple domains of health and well-being, including the mind, body, and social relationships.

Two Wellness Models

It has not been unusual for treatment providers specialized in their various fields to function and provide treatment in isolated components. For example, a physician may not consider the influence of mental, spiritual, or social aspects of a person in treating the presenting physical issue. Similarly, a spiritual leader may not consider the mental or physical aspects of the person beyond the presenting spiritual concern. However, from a holistic wellness point of view, a person is more than the sum of their parts and, therefore, the problems of one facet will influence the functioning of other aspects of the self. Wellness models are predicated on this holism, and in fact consider treatment based on reductionism to be at best incomplete. The experience of dual or multi-diagnostic complexity, where individuals are considered resistant to traditional forms of treatment because of multiple presenting issues, is one example of how a holistic wellness perspective can complement or even supersede reductionist forms of evidence-based practice.

The first model we present, Hettler's Six Dimensions of Wellness (see Figure 5.1), includes emotional, intellectual, occupational, physical, social, and spiritual components [3].

The emotional dimension includes awareness and acceptance of one's own feelings. The development of self-esteem, self-control, and determination as a sense of direction is

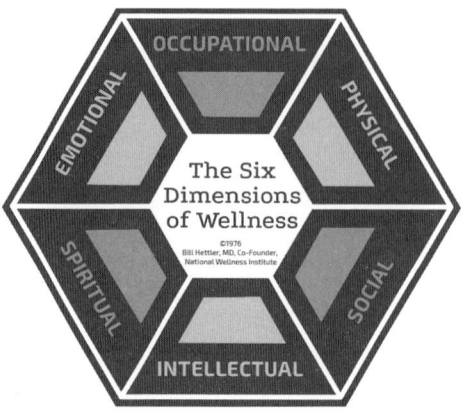

Figure 5.1 Six Dimensions of Wellness. Dimensions of Wellness Model ©1976 Bill Hettler, MD. Reprinted with permission from the National Wellness Institute, Inc., NationalWellness.org.

considered in this emotional dimension. The intellectual dimension involves creative and stimulating mental activity, as well as sharing one's abilities with others. The occupational dimension is based on the premise that people's lives are enriched through satisfaction at work, and that work is interconnected to living and playing. The physical dimension recognizes the benefits of regular physical activity and healthy eating, as well as personal responsibility in self-care decisions, such as when to seek medical attention. The social dimension focuses on involvement and contribution to one's environment and community. Finally, the spiritual dimension is search for meaning and purpose in existence through the development of belief systems, values, and creating a worldview [3].

The Myers and Sweeney IS-WEL model includes an overall wellness factor; five second-order factors, and 17 third-order factors (see Figure 5.2). These 17 third-order factors interrelate with specific second-order factors.

The Creative Self includes thinking, emotions, control, work, and positive humor. The Coping Self encompasses leisure, stress management, self-worth, and realistic beliefs. The Social Self comprises friendship and love. The Essential Self incorporates spirituality, gender identity, and self-care. Lastly, the Physical Self integrates exercise and nutrition [4]. More explanation of each of these factors is provided in Table 5.1.

Research on Wellness Treatment Planning

Next, we focus on the research that supports the use of a wellness treatment plan focused on an integrated healthcare perspective. Issues related to construct definition, measurement, and stability of findings over time continue to obscure the evidence base on wellness interventions [5]. Evidence-based paradigms related to wellness, such as the trauma-focused model and the integrated behavioral health framework, are predicated on the mind–body connection and the concept of treating individuals as unified wholes who are more than the sum of their parts. The tenets of wellness theory have broad empirical support, found in research linking physical and mental health generally [6], and research on the relationship between overall well-being and constructs such as hope, posttraumatic growth [7], self-efficacy, and mindfulness [8].

Findings from several meta-analytic studies support the link between physical activity and psychological well-being [6], including the preventive effects of exercise in relation to

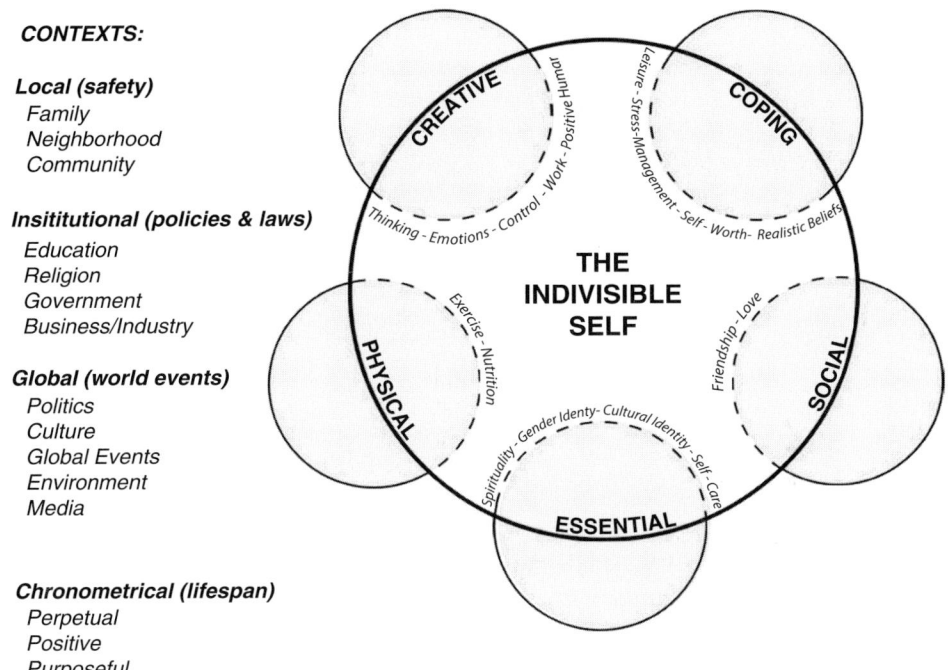

THE INDIVISIBLE SELF:
An Evidence-Based Model Of Wellness

CONTEXTS:

Local (safety)
Family
Neighborhood
Community

Insititutional (policies & laws)
Education
Religion
Government
Business/Industry

Global (world events)
Politics
Culture
Global Events
Environment
Media

Chronometrical (lifespan)
Perpetual
Positive
Purposeful

Figure 5.2 The Indivisible Self: An Evidence-Based Model of Wellness. Reprinted with permission.

depression [9], anxiety, and posttraumatic stress disorder (PTSD) [10]. Behavioral interventions can promote adherence to treatment for chronic physical illness, and for conditions such as cardiovascular disease and HIV sero-conversion [6]. The link between physical health and psychological well-being appears to be robust in both adults and children [11], with higher rates of physical activity (or less sedentary living) protective against negative physical and mental health.

The link between physical and mental health, while supported empirically, is better understood in relation to specific traits and outcomes as opposed to a general, mutually influential relationship [12]. Links between family functioning and physical health [13], or self-esteem and both physical and mental health [5], extend the mind–body connection into the social environment and provide further evidence for approaching treatment through a wellness lens. Research on career development and satisfaction also supports wellness theory, as links between hope, job satisfaction, workplace commitment, the phenomena associated with burnout, and both physical and mental health outcomes all have empirical support [14].

Some researchers have specifically focused on spirituality, a key component of wellness theory, though a difficult construct to operationalize. Spirituality has been found to relate positively to active coping, hopefulness, and optimism, and to be protective against clinical

Table 5.1 Abbreviated definitions of components of the Indivisible Self Model

Wellness factor	Definition
Total Wellness	The sum of all items on the 5F-Wel; a measure of one's general well-being or total wellness
Creative Self	The combination of attributes that each of us forms to make a unique place among others in our social interactions and to positively interpret our world.
Thinking	Being mentally active, open-minded; having the ability to be creative and experimental, having a sense of curiosity; a need to know and to learn; the ability to solve problems.
Emotions	Being aware of or in touch with one's feelings; being able to experience and express one's feelings appropriately, both positive and negative.
Control	Belief that one can usually achieve the goals one sets for oneself; having a sense of planfulness in life; being able to be assertive in expressing one's needs.
Work	Being satisfied with one's work; having adequate financial security; feeling that one's skills are used appropriately; the ability to cope with workplace stress.
Positive humor	Being able to laugh at one's own mistakes and the unexpected things that happen; the ability to use humor to accomplish even serious tasks.
Coping Self	The combination of elements that regulate one's responses to life events and provide a means to transcend the negative effects of these events.
Leisure	Activities done in one's free time; satisfaction with one's leisure activities; having at least one activity in which "I lose myself and time stands still."
Stress management	General perception of one's own self-management or self-regulation; seeing change as an opportunity for growth; ongoing self-monitoring and assessment of one's coping resources.
Self-worth	Accepting who and what one is, positive qualities along with imperfections; valuing oneself as a unique individual.
Realistic beliefs	Understanding that perfection and being loved by everyone are impossible goals, and having the courage to be imperfect.
Social Self	Social support through connections with others in friendships and intimate relationships, including family ties.
Friendship	Social relationships that involve a connection with others individually or in community, but that do not have a marital, sexual, or familial commitment; having friends in whom one can trust and who can provide emotional, material, or informational support when needed.
Love	The ability to be intimate, trusting, and self-disclosing with another person; having a family or family-like support system characterized by shared spiritual values, the ability to solve conflict in a mutually respectful way, healthy communication styles, and mutual appreciation.

Table 5.1 (cont.)

Wellness factor	Definition
Essential Self	Essential meaning-making processes in relation to life, self, and others.
Spirituality	Personal beliefs and behaviors that are practiced as part of the recognition that a person is more than material aspects of mind and body.
Gender identity	Satisfaction with one's gender; feeling supported in one's gender; transcendence of gender identity (i.e., ability to be androgynous).
Cultural identity	Satisfaction with one's cultural identity; feeling supported in one's cultural identity; transcendence of one's cultural identity.
Self-care	Taking responsibility for one's wellness through self-care and safety habits that are preventive in nature; minimizing the harmful effects of pollution in one's environment.
Physical Self	The biological and physiological processes that compose the physical aspects of a person's development and functioning.
Exercise	Engaging in sufficient physical activity to keep in good physical condition; maintaining flexibility through stretching.
Nutrition	Eating a nutritionally balanced diet, maintaining a normal weight (i.e., within 15 percent of the ideal), and avoiding overeating.
Contexts	
Local context	Systems in which one lives most often – families, neighborhoods, and communities – and one's perceptions of safety in these systems.
Institutional context	Social and political systems that affect one's daily functioning and serve to empower or limit development in obvious and subtle ways, including education, religion, government, and the media.
Global context	Factors such as politics, culture, global events, and the environment that connect one to others around the world.
Chronometrical context	Growth, movement, and change in the time dimension that are perpetual, of necessity positive, and purposeful.

5F-Wel = Five Factor Wellness Inventory.
From JE Myers, TJ Sweeney. The Indivisible Self: An Evidence-Based Model of Wellness. *J Individ Psychol* 2004; 60(3): 234–245. Reprinted with permission.

anxiety [15]. Religious and spiritual beliefs produce positive, negative, and at times a mixed effect on adherence to pharmacological treatment in people with HIV/AIDS, psychiatric disorders, or cystic fibrosis [16]. While religious and spiritual beliefs have mixed relationships to physical health outcomes [16] largely depending on the content of belief, spiritual beliefs can provide the narrative framework and subsequent behavioral reinforcements for promoting treatment adherence, coping with chronic pain, and engaging in positive self-care behavior [17]. An issue not addressed in this compilation of existing research on religious and spiritual influence on physical and mental health treatment is the meaning or definition of spirituality. While religion is more easily defined based on the beliefs of the person served, understanding a person's spirituality can be more challenging. However, based on these findings, the authors suggest that treatment providers receive training to be sensitive to religious and spiritual issues of their clients/patients.

Wellness and well-being manifest in all domains of life, whether in relationships, physical health, mental health, career or vocational satisfaction, and spirituality; the realization of achievement in one area can augment resilience and support coping with dissatisfaction in another area. Generalizing from evidence affirming the connections between mind, body, spirituality, work, and social environment, treatment providers seeking to work from a wellness or strength-based framework can develop effective treatment plans based on specific, evidence-informed relationships.

Establishing a Treatment Plan

Prior to delving into specifics of the wellness treatment plan we first focus on general considerations for the development of any treatment plan. A treatment plan should consider and include extra-therapeutic factors, which facilitate 40 percent of desired change [18], and contribute to successful outcomes. First, incorporating client/patient strengths and resources enables the client/patient to own the treatment plan. Next, developing treatment goals that the client/patient accepts as relevant and credible improves the client/patient's likelihood of executing the treatment plan. Third, building hope and expectancy for success and trust in the professional relationship with the practitioner facilitates successful attainment of goals [18].

We propose developing a treatment plan using the three key features method [2]. First, develop a treatment plan overview – a brief paragraph – with the intent written in client/patient-friendly language that permits the client/patient to understand, own, and be responsible for executing the treatment plan [2]. This feature of the treatment plan is also useful if and when a referral is made and the treatment plan is shared with another practitioner. Next, develop long-term goals; these are the ideal goals a client/patient may achieve if conditions are optimal [2]. Finally, establish short-term goals that are attainable in a brief time frame to instill hope for change and chart treatment progress [2]. Goals must be derived in a collaborative effort with the client/patient for a positive treatment outcome [5]. It is helpful to establish short-term goals that are both observable and measurable so that both the client/patient and practitioner can identify when the goal is met. An alternative is to formulate broad goals with observable and measurable objectives that lead to achieving the stated goal. Hope derived from early positive change is a necessary component for the trajectory toward a positive outcome [18]. Therefore, intentionally crafted, achievable goals and objectives are key to a successful outcome.

While both long-term and short-term treatment goals are developed to alleviate client/patient challenges, it is necessary to also connect the client/patient's strengths to the treatment plan to facilitate client/patient ownership of the change process [2]. Goals may be worked through simultaneously or at times sequentially as required by the client/patient's circumstances. Goals are informed by the practitioner's wellness orientation. Long-term goals are normally generated based on the premise, and short-term goals can be derived from supportive material in the case conceptualization [2]. The format for writing goals can vary based on the practitioner and the clinical setting. Three of the most common forms are writing goals based on what the client/patient needs to improve (i.e., achieve, develop, learn); what the client/patient needs to reduce (i.e., maladaptive behavior); and SOAP (subjective, objective, assessment, and plan) format [2]. The SOAP format develops short-term goals for each session. Developing goals that are written specifically in language the client/patient can understand, congruent with client/patient wishes and desires, and viewed as attainable by the client/patient may yield the best outcome [5].

Even within a specific wellness model, there are many styles through which a treatment plan may be conceptualized and executed. These styles include: (1) assumption-based; (2) symptom-based; (3) interpersonally based; (4) historically based; (5) thematically based; and (6) diagnosis-based [2]. Of these, the assumption-based and thematically based styles are the best for developing a wellness treatment plan because the former allows choice of a specific wellness model through which to develop the treatment plan while the latter facilitates a plan based on the themes of wellness relative to the client/patient.

Multicultural Variables and Treatment Planning

Considering the multicultural pluralistic society in which we exist, the multidimensional and holistic nature of wellness or optimal living cannot be achieved without consideration of client/patient multicultural variables. These variables influence the definition of optimal living. Further, goals, expectations, and the process of achieving goals vary based on client/patient variables. These individual factors that influence the development of a wellness treatment plan include demographics such as age, gender, race and ethnicity, sexual orientation, religion and/or spirituality, education, and socioeconomic status. Other features that may influence the wellness treatment plan are client/patient personality variables and life experiences. A discussion of the finer details of individual human complexities is not appropriate for this chapter. However, with mindful attention to individual variables and their influence, an intentionally designed wellness treatment plan needs to be established.

Steps to Wellness Treatment Planning

In the preceding chapters, the authors have shared screening and assessment methods, as well as wellness measurement. Here we introduce the concepts of collaborative treatment planning for wellness with clients/patients through (1) introduction of the wellness model; (2) assessment of wellness; (3) design and implementation of interventions; and (4) evaluation and follow-up [19]. This model has shown evidence for improvement in wellness with children, adolescents, and adults. We assert that this four-phase model can be integrated for wellness treatment planning with a new or existing client/patient.

Phase One: Orientation to Wellness

Begin the discussion about wellness by inquiring from the client/patient instances in which they experienced the connection between mind and body. Their own stories will facilitate information to introduce the concepts of holism and optimal functioning. Once the provider verifies client/patient understanding of wellness tenets, the chosen wellness model can be introduced. For instance, if choosing Hettler's Six Dimensions model, explain the six dimensions and verify that the client/patient either has experienced or understands the connection between the presenting problem and the other dimensions. If using the IS-WEL model, consider the impact of the local, institutional, global, and chronometrical contexts and client/patient understanding of wellness across the lifespan. The provider may have to educate the client/patient on wellness, holism, and optimal functioning, relating it to the client/patient's experiences that demonstrate interconnection between mind and body, to build hope in the treatment plan, and to optimize the follow-through of wellness-based treatment goals.

Phase Two: Assessing Wellness

Once the client/patient understands the wellness treatment planning concepts, assessment of client/patient wellness in the different dimensions should occur. Assessment could be informal and/or formal. For instance, informal assessment can take the form of an interview protocol based on the six dimensions when utilizing Hettler's model, or based on the five main factors and their related 19 subfactors for those utilizing the IS-WEL model. For more formal assessments, the National Wellness Institute provides the Dimensions of Life, Wellness Focus Survey Tool, Wholeness-Wellness Exercise, Wheel of Wellness Assessment, and a variety of other measures. For those committed to the IS-WEL model, the revised 5 Factor Wellness Evaluation of Lifestyle (WEL), a psychometric instrument developed to assess strengths and areas for growth within each domain and subdomain of the Indivisible Self framework, is available. Scaling the client/patient's subjective awareness of their own wellness level across each domain of functioning can be a useful technique both to further orient clients/patients to wellness thinking, and to prioritize treatment foci. Clients/patients can be asked to assess their perception of their own wellness using a 1–10 scale, with 10 being optimized wellness and 1 representing a lack of functioning in the particular domain. It is important to rebalance the needs of each domain, too, even though scaling may reveal more severe issues in one area. For example, using the IS-WEL model, a client/patient may identify lower functioning in the area of stress management, and comparable functioning in the area of exercise and leisure activities. Following the principle of holism, and the research on the relationship of physical activity to overall well-being, it would be appropriate to encourage development of exercise and leisure routines even if stress management has the lowest subjective rating.

Phase Three: Wellness-Based Lifestyle Planning

Once the assessment is completed and the results are shared, facilitate the client/patient to set goals to achieve a more wellness-based lifestyle. Further, focus the client/patient on a few areas where strengths are not optimized and set short-term goals in client/patient-friendly language that are both observable and measurable to begin the journey toward wellness. Wellness treatment planning is based on the concepts of holism. In essence, the improvement of underdeveloped strengths and assets in one area of the client/patient's capacity improves the overall functioning. Interventions for achieving goals will vary depending on the model and areas chosen for improvement. However, it is vital that the provider mobilize extra-therapeutic factors, or focus the discussion on client/patient behaviors between provider visits that will contribute to a successful wellness outcome.

Phase Four: Evaluation and Follow-Up

Once the long-term and short-term goals are in place, it is necessary to evaluate client/ patient progress toward those goals. Adjustment to short-term goals may be necessary once the client/patient begins to better understand the holistic and optimal functioning of self. Continual discussion during provider visits on how the wellness treatment goals are progressing, how they are affecting the different facets of the client/patient, and contributing to growth toward optimal functioning will indicate if fine-tuning of the treatment plan is required. To understand how client/patient variables influence wellness treatment planning, two different case studies are presented here.

Case Vignettes

Vignette 1

Your new client/patient goes by both the names Pedro and Lucia. When dressed as a male, he goes by Pedro; when dressed as a female, she goes by Lucia. According to the client/ patient, the pronouns change based on the outward expression of gender. Pedro/Lucia is a 50-year-old of Hispanic descent. The client/patient is heterosexual and has been married for 35 years to a cisgender female. Pedro/Lucia's gender identity is known to his family and to those around him. The client/patient states a belief in Christ but not a religious affiliation. Pedro/Lucia has a master's degree and is employed as an engineer, placing the family in the middle class. The client/patient appears shy yet friendly. The presenting concern is high blood pressure.

Short-Term Goals Using the Six Dimensions of Wellness Model

Once the client/patient is oriented to the Six Dimensions of Wellness model, a formal or informal assessment should follow. Depending on the assessment, one or more of the six areas may need wellness treatment planning. Scaling is a useful option to understand the client/patient's subjective wellness awareness and experience. Assuming the client/patient rates different intensity levels on the six dimensions of wellness and applying the concepts of holism and optimal functioning, some possible short-term goals for Pedro/Lucia using the six dimensions are provided below. Notice these short-term goals are observable and measurable.

1. Emotional dimension: Identify three prominent feelings from which the client/patient regularly operates.
2. Intellectual dimension: Generate a list of creative and mentally stimulating activities the client/patient enjoys outside of work.
3. Occupational dimension: Identify two stressors and two rewards related to work.
4. Physical dimension: Develop a plan that includes regular physical activity (i.e., at least three times per week) and healthy eating.
5. Social dimension: Identify three relationships that contribute to the client/patient interconnectedness to the environment and community.
6. Spiritual dimension: Identify at least one personal value and belief that is currently at odds with client/patient lifestyle.

Vignette 2

Niranjan is a 33-year-old cisgender Asian male who is an immigrant employed at a gas station. He is an active Buddhist. He completed high school but did not go further in education. He presents himself as an extroverted individual. His presenting concern is depression, with related concerns of self-worth and hopes for the future. He was close to his mother and father, both of whom have died within the past 18 months. He states he has many close relationships with family and friends in his home country, but has struggled to create friendships in the USA despite his outgoing nature.

Short-Term Goals Using the IS-WEL Model

After orienting Niranjan to the IS-WEL model, including exploring areas of cross-culture resonance and potential incongruence, the domains and subdomains are explored to identify potential focus areas. The client/patient identifies high ratings in the areas of the Essential Self related to cultural identity, gender identity, and spirituality, and similar high ratings in the domain of the Physical Self related to exercise and nutrition. Ratings in the areas of the Coping Self and the Creative Self were revealed to be more moderate, with lower ratings in the subdomains of self-worth (Coping Self) and sense of control (Creative Self). Finally, the domain of the Social Self was associated with the lowest ratings, primarily based on the client/patient's sense of loss of connection to otherwise healthy friendships, family relationships, and potential romantic relationships with individuals in his home country. Again, organizing treatment goals around the concepts of holism and of optimal functioning, short-terms goals for each domain were developed:

1. Creative Self: Identify 10–20 interests, competencies, strengths, and talents that the client/patient values about himself and can rely on to develop wellness in other areas.
2. Coping Self: This area will have two main goals:

    a. Identify five coping strategies and stress management activities that have worked in the past, and five potentially new strategies that the client/patient would like to try.
    b. Identify two unrealistic beliefs related to coping, well-being, or happiness, and identify at least one refuting belief that is more realistic or adaptive.

3. Social Self: Identify traits in friends and potential romantic partners; link a list of interests and talents from the Creative Self with potential areas to explore meeting people.
4. Essential Self: Identify areas of strength that the client/patient can generalize to promote coping in other areas, including ways to connect with others around shared spiritual, cultural, or gender socialization habits.
5. Physical Self: Identify three ways each that exercise and nutrition are already supporting wellness for the client/patient. Since this is another strength area, attempt to link optimal functioning here with coping strategies to promote higher wellness in other areas. For example, exercise routines can be modified to incorporate more social activities.

Conclusion

As research continues to support the mind–body connection, and as society continues to embrace wellness as a core tenet of human development, organizing treatment around evidence-based wellness concepts will become more expected. With heightened scrutiny on ways to reduce healthcare costs through prevention, promote lifelong health and well-being, and empower individuals in supporting their own wellness across the lifespan, incorporating the philosophy of wellness can help practitioners depathologize their case conceptualization and also tap into the power of synergy across domains of human functioning.

Rather than being a source of cross-cultural misunderstanding or tension, a wellness-oriented case conceptualization has the potential to increase cultural competency, especially when links between physical, mental, and spiritual and/or family functioning are honored and explored.

References

1. World Health Organization. The constitution of the World Health Organization: principles. 2019. www.who.int/about/mission/en/ (accessed January 13, 2019).

2. PS Berman. *Case Conceptualization and Treatment Planning* (3rd ed.). Los Angeles, CA, Sage; 2014.

3. National Wellness Institute. The Six Dimensions of Wellness. www.nationalwellness.org/page/Six_Dimensions (accessed January 13, 2019).

4. JE Myers, TJ Sweeney. Wellness counseling: the evidence-base for practice. *J Counsel Dev* 2008; **86**: 482–493.

5. JL Moe. Wellness and distress in LGBTQ populations: a meta-analysis. *J LGBT Issues Counsel* 2016; **10**: 112–129.

6. CD Patnode, CV Evans, CA Senger, et al. Behavioral counseling to promote a healthful diet and physical activity for cardiovascular disease prevention in adults without known cardiovascular disease risk factors: updated evidence report and systematic review for the U.S. preventive services task force. *JAMA* 2017; **318**: 175–193.

7. GA Casellas, C Ochoa, C Ruini. Psychological and clinical correlates of posttraumatic growth in cancer: a systematic and critical review. *Psycho-Oncology* 2017; **26**: 2007–2018.

8. L Smith-MacDonald, JM Norris, S Raffin-Bouchal, et al. Spirituality and mental well-being in combat veterans: a systematic review. *Military Med* 2017; **182**: e1920–e1940.

9. AL Rebar, R Stanton, D Geard, et al. A meta-meta-analysis of the effect of physical activity on depression and anxiety in non-clinical adult populations. *Health Psychol Rev* 2015; **9**: 366–378.

10. JW Whitworth, JT Ciccolo. Exercise and post-traumatic stress disorder in military veterans: a systematic review. *Military Med* 2016; **181**: 953–960.

11. DJ Korczak, S Madigan, M Colasanto. Children's physical activity and depression: a meta-analysis. *Pediatrics* 2017; **139**: 1–14.

12. J Ohrnberger, E Fichera, M Sutton. The relationship between physical and mental health: a mediation analysis. *Soc Sci Med* 2016; **195**: 42–49.

13. M Cousino, K Rea, K Schumacher, et al. A systematic review of parent and family functioning in pediatric solid organ transplant populations. *Pediatr Transplant* 2017; **21**: e12900.

14. RJ Reichard, JB Avey, S Lopez, et al. Having the will and finding the way: a review and meta-analysis of hope at work. *J Posit Psychol* 2013; **8**: 292–304.

15. JPB Gonçalves, G Lucchetti, PR Menezes, et al. Religious and spiritual interventions in mental health care: a systematic review and meta-analysis of randomized controlled clinical trials. *Psychol Med* 2015; **45**: 2937–2949.

16. B Badanta-Romero, R de Diego-Cordero, E Rivilla-García. Influence of religious and spiritual elements on adherence to pharmacological treatment. *J Relig Health* 2018; **57**: 1905–1917.

17. A Kelly-Hanku, P Aggleton, P Shih. I shouldn't talk of medicine only: biomedical and religious frameworks for understanding antiretroviral therapies, their invention and their effects. *Glob Public Health* 2018; **13**: 1454–1467.

18. MA Hubble, BL Duncan, SD Miller. *The Heart and Soul of Change*. Washington, DC, American Psychological Association Press; 1999.

19. JE Myers, TJ Sweeney, M Witmer. The wheel of wellness, counseling for wellness: a holistic model for treatment planning. *J Counsel Dev* 2000; **78**: 251–266.

6

The Concept of Wellness in Psychiatric and Substance-Use Disorders

A. George Awad

Introduction

Though the concept of wellness had its origins several decades back, in recent years it has gained considerable interest and wide popularity. The massive rise in the number of publications in the popular and scientific press by advocates and critics has moved the concept into becoming a major public issue, further enhanced by its attractiveness as a commercial target [1–5].

The economic prosperity that followed World War II, and the expectations of improved standards of living in Western countries, led to the emergence of new societal concepts such as quality of life and related constructs, including satisfaction, preferences, and well-being [6]. The 1948 redefinition, by the World Health Organization (WHO), of the state of health to include psychosocial issues such as satisfaction, feelings of well-being, and fulfillment added a significant impetus toward recognition of mental health as part of health [7].

As a follow-up, the WHO's Expert Committee on Mental Health in its meeting in September 1950 defined mental health as "a condition, subject to fluctuations due to biological and social factors, which enables the individual to achieve a satisfactory synthesis of his own, potentially conflicting, instinctive drives to form and maintain harmonious relations with others, and to participate in constructive changes in his social and physical environment" [8]. In other words, mental health resonates more with the state of wellness, as it provides an approach and a process for healthy living. Frequently, the terms *mental health* and *psychiatric disorders* have been used synonymously. The WHO definition of mental health in 1950 clarified some of the conceptual confusion. Psychiatry, being a major part of mental health, is a medical specialty that deals with the study, diagnosis, treatment, and prevention of psychiatric disorders, while mental health, besides psychiatry as its major component, deals with other societal, ideological, and political attributes. The difference, then, between health and mental health is more than semantics and tends to indicate from where issues like wellness have come about. For clarity, I am adopting the WHO definition of mental health, in the use of the term "mental health" whenever it is mentioned in this chapter.

Overall, then, the WHO redefinition of health, as well as the subsequent definition of mental health, seems to open the door in healthcare, to go beyond improvements in symptoms or absence of disease into expectations of more encompassing concepts such as wellness, which represents a broad and continuous approach of improvements toward healthy living. Applying the broad concept of wellness for use in psychiatric and substance-use disorder populations poses several challenges and requires special considerations to make it appropriate for the lives of these patients. Psychiatric disorders, by virtue of their psychopathology, are frequently long term and disabling, particularly in the case of psychotic disorders such as schizophrenia, or severe bipolar or depressive disorders [9]. Similarly, substance-use disorders are chronic relapsing conditions, characterized by an inability to reduce or control drug use [10]. The prevalence of comorbid drug abuse in psychotic disorders such as schizophrenia is 2–4 times higher than in the general population [10]. Stigmatizing attitudes toward psychiatric and substance-use disorder patients add to the disability and increase its morbidity.

In essence, persons with psychiatric and/or addictive disorders frequently confront major challenges – emotional, physical, social, economic, and attitudinal – the same issues that figure highly in the concept of wellness. For all these reasons, the concept of wellness is not just desirable, but also important and necessary for achieving improved quality of life and quality of living. On the other hand, the concept of wellness as a scientific field requires rigorous scientific inquiry, not only for its application in psychiatric and addictive populations, but also to develop conceptual models that can inform the determinants that underpin the concept and lead the way to developing more appropriate concept-based measurement tools.

Validation of the Concept of Wellness as Applied to Psychiatric Disorders

In validation of a scientific concept, such as wellness, a number of issues related to the concept need to be explored: the multiplicity of definitions; the lack of informative conceptual models that can inform the process of development of reliable measurement tools; and the demonstration of the reliability and consistency of persons with psychiatric and substance-use disorders when providing self-reports, since a good deal of the concept of wellness is subjective in nature [11].

Multiplicity of Definitions of Wellness

The popularity of wellness as a term stems from its simplicity and the ease of its understanding. Yet, when it comes to its definition, wellness proves to be a challenge, compounded by the many theoretical, political, ideological, philosophical, and commercial points of view. Inevitably, such a broad array of diverse orientations has led to a proliferation of definitions. The increasing number of definitions has, in turn, influenced the conceptual thinking of wellness as an independent entity. Wellness has been referred to at times as a holistic medicine, integrative medicine, complementary medicine, or alternative medicine, among others. As frequently happens, a definition of any concept dictates what follows in terms of its content. Not surprising, then, that the multiplicity of definitions can easily impede the process of development of clear conceptual thinking that can better enhance the understanding of the concept.

Among the many proposed definitions, several have defined wellness in psychological terms, such as feeling positive about life [12]. Many definitions include cognitive attributes, such as development of autonomy and self-assessment, as well as the ability to cope effectively with stress [13]. Other definitions propose that wellness is a balance between various dimensions representing physical, mental, social, vocational, and environmental factors [3]. Others have equated wellness with happiness or have described it as healthy functioning [14]. In reviewing the plethora of definitions, the majority on balance include aspects that reflect upon physical, mental, affective/cognitive, and social/vocational states. It is also becoming clear that such broad concepts of wellness encompass several other life and society-related factors beyond the impact of psychiatric and substance-use disorders' deficits. That leads to the question of whether it is more useful for the concept of wellness, in order to be applied to psychiatric and substance-use disorder populations, to be narrow in scope and limited to health-related issues? As experienced previously in similar areas such as quality of life, limiting it to health-related quality of life provides more focus and research depth in the development of the concept [6]. I believe there needs to be a serious expert discussion about such a proposal in terms of its application to psychiatric and substance-use disorder practices. There needs to be a balance between what is ideal and what is achievable under optimum conditions. Failing to do so may lead to unfulfilled expectations that may undermine the concept of satisfaction and wellness.

At the end, it may be that there will not be forthcoming agreement on one definition in the near future. In such a situation, it is then incumbent on researchers and opinion leaders to define in their publications or presentations what they mean by the term "wellness."

Development of Conceptual Models of Wellness Applicable to Psychiatric Populations

The importance of the development of conceptual models appropriate for psychiatric populations is that it not only defines the concept or its boundaries, but also allows for the exploration of the factors underpinning the concept and how much they contribute to the variance. As discussed before, the multiplicity of definitions is a clear reflection of the broad and diverse conceptual thinking. The attractiveness of the concept of wellness for commercial interests has also added a different dimension and tends at times to blur the lines between its use in science and its popular public use. In spite of the huge increase in published reports, there is a clear lack of tested and validated conceptual models that can inform better understanding, specific to psychiatric and substance-use disorders. In a study of the conceptualization and measurement of perceived wellness, results suggested that perceptions of wellness in various dimensions are intertwined by their affective nature [15]. Another proposed model attempted to link clinical variables with health-related quality of life [16]. Another study suggested that illness and wellness are two independent continuums rather than two ends of the same continuum [17]. Another model proposed wellness as a balance of five factors: physical, psychological/emotional, social, intellectual, and spiritual [3]. Others expanded such models by adding two more factors: occupational and environmental [18]. Several concepts emphasize the subjective and perceptual nature of wellness. Recently, wellness has been viewed as a process that can be non-dependent on health or illness, being a purposeful process of individual growth leading to the achievement of the state of wellness [19].

Overall, the majority of proposed conceptual models perceived wellness as a multidimensional construct, with its dimensions well-integrated with each other and interacting in a dynamic process. Wellness is construed as a continuum that has no end and thus becomes more of a movement or a process toward ever higher levels of wellness, dependent on self-motivation. Such a conceptualization seems to entrust the person with some responsibility in their own recovery and the achievement of wellness.

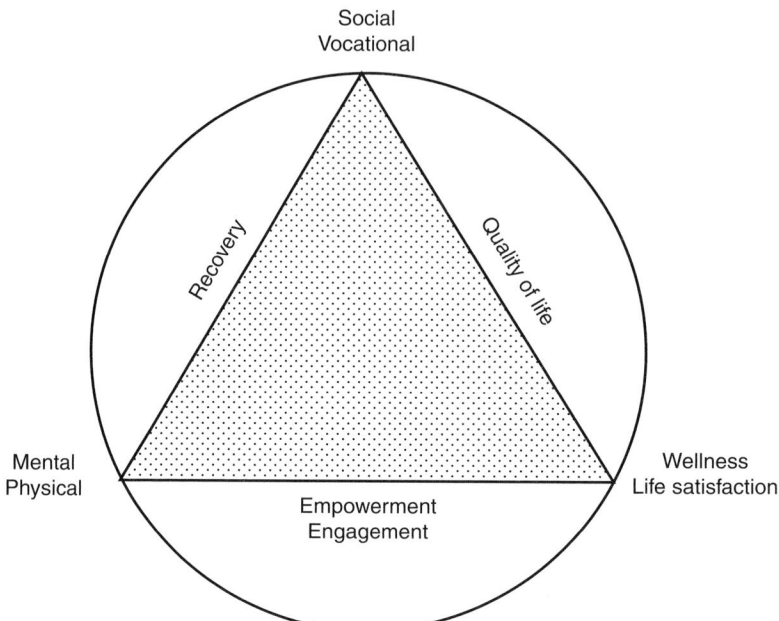

Figure 6.1 The circle of wellness in psychiatric disorders.

In a recent effort to stimulate scientific discourse in the field of psychiatric wellness, we proposed our conceptual working model based on the principles that we advocate: narrowing the concept, making it more applicable to the psychiatric population, and ensuring its components can be evaluated by currently available valid measuring tools. As depicted in Figure 6.1, the three major dimensions proposed include mental/physical, social/vocational, and general feelings of satisfaction/wellness.

The three major dimensions are depicted in a circular fashion, to emphasize their interconnectedness and how each factor can impact on other factors. We postulated that the mental/physical factors can influence the social/vocational factor through the process of recovery, while the social/vocational factors impact on wellness and life satisfaction, largely through improved quality of life and quality of living. Empowerment and engagement are considered to be the tools that link the mental/physical factors to achievement of wellness and life satisfaction.

For the assessment of the mental/physical dimensions, the modified Sickness Impact Profile (SIP-83) has been selected [20]. The original Sickness Impact Profile (SIP) is a well-validated and extensively used health status index [21]. It includes 12 subcategories representing three dimensions: three physical categories, four psychosocial categories, and five independent categories. The scale is designed to measure impact of the illness on performance rather than capacity. In 1983 we were granted permission by the author of the SIP to adapt it for specific use in psychiatry. The modified SIP-83 is much briefer, self-administered, and takes about 10 minutes to complete. It covers aspects of physical and emotional health, including side effects of medication. Since then, the SIP-83 has been extensively used in our studies of quality of life and other clinical trials [20].

The Personal and Social Performance Scale (SPS) is chosen to evaluate social functioning [22]. It is a well-validated and extensively used scale to measure social activities, personal and social relationships, and self-care. For wellness, the perceived wellness survey is used [15]. It is well-validated, but not yet extensively used in a clinical population. It includes 36 items and covers six categories: physical, spiritual, intellectual, psychological, social, and emotional dimensions. Additionally, there is a global measure of life satisfaction based on the original Gurin Global Likert Scale that asks one question: "How would you describe your present feeling of life satisfaction?" The response is recorded in a five-point Likert format rating from very good to very poor [23].

At the conclusion of this study, items to emerge as significant and contributory are folded together for further testing as an omnibus single scale.

Appropriate Measurement Tools

As generally required in constructing measuring tools, they have to prove the tests for reliability and validity in capturing the core features of the disorder or the concept under investigation. They have to be practical and user-friendly in terms of their complexity and the time needed for completion. Scales need to be sensitive enough to detect small changes at a time, as expected in long-term psychiatric or substance-use disorders. Applying such requirements to the presently available measures for wellness, the majority of them seem to be inappropriate for use in a psychiatric population. The majority of them are too long and could tax the limited cognitive abilities of many psychiatric patients. Most of the measures are based on validation in non-clinical populations. According to a recent review [24], very few – only five – measures have been used in medical settings, and even fewer, or unknown if ever used, in a psychiatric population. The five scales include: Wellness Evaluation of Lifestyle (WEL), [25], Five Factor Wellness (FF-WEL) [3], the Perceived Wellness Survey (PWS) [15], the Optimal Living Profile (OLP), and the Body–Mind Spirit Wellness Behaviour and Characteristics Inventory (BMS-WBCI) [26]. Though the five scales are not completely informative, the PWS seems to be the more appropriate for use in psychiatric disorders. As we did in testing our working model of wellness, we recommended its use and supplanted it with another global scale such as the Gurin Likert Scale, described above.

For the concept of wellness to be applicable and useful in the management of psychiatric and substance-use disorders, there is a need for development of purpose-specific, reliable and valid, but brief, scales for regular clinical use. The availability of such practical measurement instruments can make it much easier and possible to integrate the concept of wellness in clinical care and care plans. For research purposes, longer and more detailed instruments are likely to be required.

Reliability of Psychiatric Patients' Self-Reports

Since a good part of the concept of wellness is subjective in nature and depends on patients' ability to provide reliable and consistent self-reports, it is then imperative to demonstrate that the majority of psychiatric patients can do so. Over the past few years, we and others have demonstrated that psychiatric patients' self-reports can be reliable, consistent, and quantified [20]. In an early study, we demonstrated the consistency and reliability of self-reports over four weeks by patients with schizophrenia, about their level of satisfaction and inner feelings [27]. Repeated measures of analysis of variance (ANOVA) failed to detect any group bi-weekly interaction effects for severity of illness, side effects, neurocognitive deficits, or doses of antipsychotic medication. Based on such extensive data, we believe that the majority of stable psychiatric patients are capable of informing about their feelings of well-being and wellness. Obviously, that cannot be applied to extreme clinical presentation, such as during the acute disorganized phase, nor in the very chronic and significantly deteriorated psychotic phase.

Enhancing Wellness in Psychiatric and Substance-Use Disorders

Enhancing Wellness

Wellness, being multidimensional, requires also multimodal integrative approaches related to mental, physical, psychological, and social factors. Persons with psychiatric and substance-use disorders frequently require lifelong treatment approaches, reflecting the chronic nature and mostly unknown etiology of their illness. Over recent decades, medications have become the cornerstone of clinical management. Medications have to be prescribed rationally and wisely to maintain benefits and reduce the likelihood of side effects. Adherence to prescribed medications has been recognized as a major issue behind frequent relapses and the need for hospitalizations, which interrupt patients' tenure in the community and impede the process of recovery. Using long-acting injectable forms of medications can prove helpful for some of the patients who frequently default in taking their medications regularly. The frequent comorbidity of addictive behavior with psychiatric disorders, particularly in psychotic disorders, requires special attention to treat both psychiatric disorder and addictive behavior at the same time [28].

In addition to medications, the majority of people with psychiatric or addictive disorders require a good deal of psychosocial support by engaging in individual and group therapies. They need to enroll in rehabilitative programs that train and prepare them for a productive and fulfilling active role that can enhance feelings of self-worth. Availability of stress management services can enhance patients' abilities to cope with stress. Particular attention has to be paid to economic and housing needs. One of the frequent deficits is in the area of social relationships. A few years ago, in an informal survey of patients attending one of our psychiatric outpatient clinics, patients were asked what was the number one issue that could make a difference in their lives. Having a friend to meet regularly with emerged surprisingly as the number one need. All efforts have to be directed toward improving patients' safe community tenure and averting the need for frequent visits to emergency rooms or hospitalization.

Promoting healthy living in nutrition, physical exercise, and healthy habits, such as not smoking and no substance use, can prove important and helpful. As in chronic conditions, persons with psychiatric and addiction problems require regular booster educational sessions in order for them to maintain healthy habits and life skills. Obviously, the best that can happen to persons with psychiatric and addictive disorders is the discovery of the etiology of the major psychiatric disorders, such as schizophrenia and depression, which can lead to more effective treatments.

Tips to Enhance the Development and Maintenance of Wellness

- Recognize not only deficits, but also areas of strength.
- Accept patients not just as recipients of care, but also as partners in care.

- Empower patients to share responsibility in their own recovery.
- Wellness is not an all-or-nothing phenomenon; it is a long and continuous process.
- Goals have to be realistic, achievable, and revisited periodically.

Synthesis and Concluding Remarks

It is clear that the concept of wellness is not only important as a process of care in psychiatric and substance-use disorders, but also on its own as a valuable and cherished goal. It represents what patients and their families, their doctors, and the society at large aspire to achieve. Yet, to adapt the concept of wellness for use in a psychiatric and substance-use disorder population requires a good deal of tidying.

The several designations given to the concept over the decades of its development, from holistic to alternative medicine and much more in between, tend to impede the scientific development of the concept of wellness. Wellness is not an alternative to medicine, but an extension of traditional medicine. In psychiatric as well as substance-use disorders, not only the illness disorder needs to be attended to, but also the person behind the illness needs to be recognized and attended to. Historically and traditionally, persons with psychiatric and substance-use disorders have been provided with psychosocial and economic support. The emergence of concepts such as wellness makes the process of care more focused, continuous, and well-integrated, and taps into the individual's strength and potential. The concept of wellness has to rise above ideology and commercialism, and attain the scientific status it deserves. For this to happen, particularly in its application to psychiatric and substance-use disorders, is to narrow its scope and goals to make it achievable by the majority of patients. There needs to be more conceptual thinking specific to this population. Learning more about the major determinants of wellness in such disorders can enhance the pursuit of wellness, as well as improve the development of more appropriate and purpose-specific measurement tools. Having appropriate evaluative tools not only can provide a reliable gauge of the value of various interventions, but can also facilitate the search for neurobiological markers that can enrich our understanding.

Development of informative conceptual thinking and more reliable measuring tools by themselves is not enough, as the field has to go beyond measurements into how to integrate wellness in regular clinical care and care plans. In essence, the concept of wellness has to be entrenched in the cultural ethos of clinical management.

Key Points

- Wellness is an important concept in the management of psychiatric and substance-use disorders.
- Psychiatric and substance-use disorders impose significant and long-term limitations and disabilities.
- The concept of wellness needs to adapt to the limitations in the lives of psychiatric and substance-use disorder populations.
- In its application to psychiatric and substance-use disorder populations, there is need for development of specific conceptual thinking and more purpose-specific measurement tools.

- For the concept of wellness to be continuous, it has to be integrated with clinical care and care plans.
- Wellness is a lifelong approach that requires regular reevaluation and a periodic booster of professional care and educational support.

References

1. A Kirkland. What is wellness now? *J Health Polit Policy Law* 2014; **39**: 957–970.

2. J Myers. The indivisible self: an evidence based model of wellness. *J Individ Psychol* 2004; **60**: 234–245.

3. J Mayers, R Luecht, T Sweeny. The factor structure of wellness: reexamining theoretical and empirical models underlying the Wellness Evaluation of Life Style (WEL) and the Five Factor Wel. *Meas Eval Couns Dev* 2004; **36**: 194–208.

4. L Roscoe. Wellness: a review of theory and measurement for counselors. *J Couns Rev* 2003; **87**: 216–226.

5. T Adams, J Bezner, M Drabbs et al. Conceptualization and measurement of the spiritual and psychological dimensions of wellness in a college population. *J Am Coll Health*, 2000; **48**: 165–173.

6. AG Awad, LNP Voruganti, RJ Heselgrave. Measuring quality of life in patients with schizophrenia. *Pharmacoeconomics* 1997; **11**: 32–47.

7. World Health Organization. The constitution of the World Health Organization. *WHO Chronicle* 1947;**1**: 9.

8. World Health Organization. *Mental Health: Report on the Second Session of the Expert Committee*. Geneva, World Health Organization; 1951.

9. M Seeman. Schizophrenia and its sequelae. In: AG Awad, LNP Voruganti, eds., *Beyond Assessment of Quality of Life in Schizophrenia*. Gland, Springer; 2016; 3–13.

10. T George, HI Crystal. Comorbidity of psychotic and substance abuse disorders. *Curr Opin Psychiat* 2000; **13**: 327–331.

11. AG Awad, LNP Voruganti. The impact of newer atypical antipsychotics on patient reported outcomes in schizophrenia. *CNS Drugs* 2013; **27**: 625–636.

12. C Ruff, C Keyes. The structure of psychological well-being revisited. *J Pers Soc Psychol* 1995; **69**: 719–727.

13. M Schier, C Carver. Optimism, coping and health: assessment and implications of generalized outcome experiences. *Health Psychol* 1985; **4**: 219–247.

14. RM Ryan, V Huta. Wellness as healthy functioning or wellness as happiness: the importance of eudaimonic thinking (response to the Kashdan et al., and Waterman discussion). *J Posit Psychol* 2009; **4**: 302–304.

15. T Adams, J Bezner, M Steinhardt. The conceptualization and measurement of perceived wellness integrating balance across and within domains. *Am J Health Promot* 1997; **11**: 208–218.

16. I Wilson, P Cleary. Linking clinical variables with health-related quality of life. *JAMA* 1995; **273**: 59–65.

17. R Manderscheid, C Ruff, E Freeman, et al. Evolving definitions of mental illness and wellness. *Prev Chronic Dis* 2010; **7**: 1–8.

18. R Reneger, M Soto, T Erin, et al. Optimal living profile: an inventory to assess health and wellness. *Am J Health Behav* 2000; **24**: 403–412.

19. S McMahon, J Fleury. Wellness in older adults: a concept analysis. *Nurs Forum* 2012; **47**: 39–51.

20. AG Awad, LNP Voruganti, RJ Heselgrave. Preliminary validation of a conceptual model to assess quality of life in schizophrenia. *Qual Life Res* 1997; **11**: 32–47.

21. M Bergner, RA Bobbit, WB Carter, et al. The sickness impact profile development and final version of a health status measure. *Med Care* 1981; **19**: 787–803.

22. PI Morrosini, L Magliano, L Brambilla, et al. Development, reliability and

acceptability of new version of the DSM IV social and occupational functioning assessment scale (SOFAS) to assess routine social functioning. *Acta Psychia Scand* 2000; **101**: 323–329.

23. J Ankar, K Saket, C Satish, et al. Likert scale explored and explained. *Brit J Appl Sci Technol* 2015; **7**: 396–403.

24. R Bart, W Ishak, S Ganjian, et al. The assessment measurement of wellness in the clinical medical setting: systematic review. *Innov Clin Neurosci* 2018; **15**: 14–23.

25. B Naydeck, J Pearson, R Ozminkowski, et al. The impact of the Highmark employee wellness program on four year

health costs. *J Occup Environ Med* 2008; **50**: 146–156.

26. D Hermon, R Hazler. Adherence to a wellness model and perceptions of wellness. *J Couns Rev* 1999; **77**: 339–343.

27. AG Awad. Antipsychotic medication in schizophrenia: how satisfied are our patients? In: JSE Hellwell, ed., *Clear Perspectives in Management Issues in Schizophrenia*. London, Shire Hall International; 1999; 1–6.

28. AG Awad. The neurobiology of comorbid drug abuse in schizophrenia and psychotic disorder. In: V Preedy, ed., *Neuropathology of Drug Addictions and Substance Misuse*, vol. I. Amsterdam, Elsevier; 2016; 82–88.

Neurological and Neurosurgical Disorders and Wellness

Kevin Ding and Isaac Yang

Introduction

Neurological and neurosurgical disorders represent a particularly salient area for interventions using practices of wellness medicine. Due to the complex physiology and functions of the nervous system, disease processes can have a wide range of clinical presentations, each with unique hardships. Because the nervous system itself provides individuals with cognition, sense of self, and identity, the loss of normal neurological function in day-to-day activities can elicit substantial emotional distress. Neurological disorders are also somewhat unique in that a large number of conditions lack curative treatments and require lifelong symptom management and supportive care [1]. Medical and surgical interventions for such diseases often come with their own set of complications, side effects, and impacts on quality of life [2]. It is therefore important for care providers to understand the ways in which patients can improve their health by seeking personalized cognitive, behavioral, physical, and spiritual interventions alongside their standard course of treatment. Exercise, for example, has been shown to directly improve cognitive outcomes by stimulating muscle memory, and its ability to decrease stress levels and provide opportunities for social interaction can provide an overall sense of self-efficacy and empowerment [3]. As providers work with patients to bring wellness medicine into the plan of care, patients can achieve a more complete picture of health and well-being.

This chapter provides an overview of wellness medicine interventions for neurological and neurosurgical disorders, organized by categories of practice. Such categories include mind–body therapies, psychosocial therapies, biologically based supplements, exercise, and manual body therapies. Although the different types of wellness medicine interventions often have indications for specific neurological diseases, they share a common purpose of providing patients with a greater sense of autonomy with regards to their course of treatment, and emphasize the importance of developing a holistic perspective of health and wellness.

Current Usage for Neurological Conditions

According to the 2007 National Health Interview Survey, it is estimated that the proportion of US adults with neurological conditions who use complementary and alternative medical (CAM) practices is 44.1 percent, a higher rate than in patients without neurological conditions (32.6 percent) [1, 3]. Notably, over 50 percent of these patients who use CAM practices do so without consulting or discussing it with their healthcare provider [3]. Because these treatments have the potential to work synergistically with traditional biopharmaceutical interventions, it is important to educate healthcare providers on these practices. In the same survey, it was shown that among patients with neurological conditions, the highest rate of CAM usage was seen in adults 25–44 years old. Of the various CAM categories, mind–body interventions had the highest frequency of use. Common neurological conditions for which patients often use CAM interventions include back pain with sciatica, memory loss, migraines, regular headaches, seizures, stroke, and dementia [3].

Mind–Body Therapies for Neurological Disorders

Because stress can often be an exacerbating factor for neurological conditions, mind–body interventions can have notable therapeutic effects for patients. Self-directed implementation of such practices allows for a greater quality of life by re-empowering patients with a sense of control amid the uncertainties of chronic neurological diseases.

Mind–body therapies were reportedly used by 24.5 percent of adults with neurological conditions [4]. According to the NCCAM, mind–body medicine is defined as practices that "enhance the mind's capacity to affect bodily function and symptoms" [4]. Such practices have a growing body of evidence supporting their effectiveness in improving neurological symptoms and include deep breathing exercises, progressive relaxation, meditation, neurofeedback, and yoga [5].

Progressive Relaxation and Focused Breathing

Progressive relaxation involves techniques geared toward reducing the body's physiological response to stress and increasing parasympathetic tone. For example, Jacobson's progressive muscular relaxation involves a systematic relaxation of major muscle groups throughout the body, often accompanied by a redirection of attention toward the rhythm, rate, and depth of breathing [5]. According to a National Institute of Health panel, there is strong evidence that relaxation techniques can effectively reduce chronic pain [6]. Based on clinical trials with a highest-level evidence rating, the US Headache Consortium recommended relaxation training, among other mind–body therapies, for clinically effective migraine relief [5]. Progressive relaxation has also repeatedly been shown to reduce seizure frequency in patients with epilepsy. In a randomized controlled trial, progressive relaxation effectively reduced seizure frequency by 29 percent compared to 3 percent in patients who simply did quiet sitting [7].

Meditation and Mindfulness

Similar to progressive relaxation techniques, meditation helps reduce physiological stress through increased awareness of one's physical and mental state. Effective meditation involves the development of a mental space that encourages awareness and acceptance of one's thoughts and feelings [8]. The positive effects of meditation on neurological disease are thought to occur through increased levels of GABAergic cortical inhibition in the brain, along with decreased systemic levels of norepinephrine. These physiological effects are known to be associated with decreased levels of stress and anxiety [9]. In the clinical context, meditation has been shown to improve symptoms for patients with neurological diseases. For example, the 10-week Mindfulness-Based Stress Reduction Program effectively improved pain ratings in participants and has become a standard in meditation-based clinical intervention [10]. In the context of multiple sclerosis, several randomized controlled trials have shown that mindfulness training can improve quality of life, depression, and fatigue [11]. In addition, meditation was shown to correlate with decreased incidence of nonfatal stroke and acute coronary events that put patients at increased risk of future stroke [12].

Neurofeedback

Neurofeedback is an operant-conditioning-based intervention that involves more direct awareness of brain functionality through measuring brain activity and providing patients with visual or auditory feedback [13] (Figure 7.1). The goal is to provide patients with a medium through which they can perceive and self-regulate region- and frequency-specific brain activity, similar to how meditation allows for awareness and self-regulation of thoughts and feelings [14]. Such activity is measured through various parameters of electroencephalogram (EEG) recording, electromagnetic signal, cerebral blood flow, electromagnetic tomography, and functional magnetic resonance imaging (fMRI) [14]. There is robust evidence on the benefits of these techniques to train neurological activity in the management of a wide variety of neurological diseases. Neurofeedback training of the sensorimotor cortex, for example, has been shown to improve functional outcomes for patients with stroke, paralysis, or disorders of sensory/motor integration [14]. In particular, multiple studies have shown that neurofeedback interventions that enhance sensorimotor

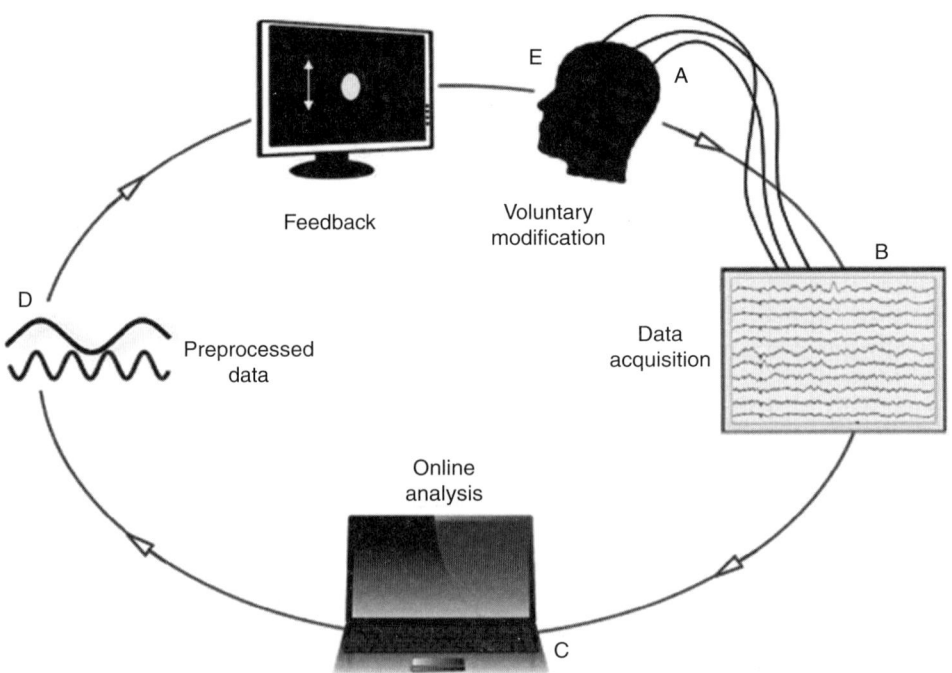

Figure 7.1 Overview of a neurofeedback setup, in which patient EEG data is acquired, processed, presented to the patient, and voluntarily modified by the patient. Reprinted from J Bagdasaryan, Mle V Quyen. Experiencing your brain: neurofeedback as a new bridge between neuroscience and phenomenology. *Front Hum Neurosci* 2013; **7**: 680, with permission from Frontiers Media SA.

rhythm (12–15 Hz) effectively reduce seizure frequency in adult and pediatric patients [14–16]. Additionally, various permutations of neurofeedback interventions can alleviate pain sensations in chronic pain syndromes and improve motor function in patients with Parkinson's disease [14, 17, 18].

Yoga

Yoga is a healing practice of ancient Indian origin that incorporates physical poses with meditation and spiritual connection to achieve a holistic sense of health and well-being. Similar to other mind–body interventions, many of its benefits as a non-pharmaceutical intervention for neurological conditions stem from its ability to reduce physiological stress [19]. As a mode of therapy, yoga has been shown to reduce mean blood pressure and decrease respiratory rate through a reduction of autonomic "fight-or-flight" activity [19]. Secondary to such a reduction of physiological stress is an improvement in symptoms and quality of life for patients with neurological conditions. Many studies have shown that yoga effectively decreases seizure frequency – one randomized controlled trial showed that 19/20 subjects demonstrated a significant reduction in seizure frequency after three months of yoga meditation protocol [20, 21]. For patients with peripheral neuropathies, such as diabetic neuropathy and carpal tunnel syndrome, yoga has been shown through randomized controlled trials to increased nerve conduction velocities, improve grip strength, and reduce pain compared to control subjects who did not perform yoga [22, 23]. For patients with pain syndromes such as fibromyalgia, yoga has been shown to provide clinically significant improvements in pain, stiffness, and strength [19, 24].

Psychosocial Therapies

Wellness medicine focuses not only on improving the disease-specific symptoms of neurological conditions, but also on achieving a more holistic picture of health for the patient. Adoption of the "sick role," especially from an early age in pediatric patients, can produce a decreased sense of resiliency, and can contribute to the development of depressive symptoms later in life [25]. Especially in the case of neurological diseases, patients can experience significant decline in psychological well-being, whether directly due to neurological disease processes and the side effects of pharmaceutical treatment, or simply due to the hardships of living with a chronic, functionally impairing disease. Thus, psychological interventions can help patients with neurological conditions achieve a greater sense of health and well-being beyond symptom control. The implementation of psychological interventions includes positive reinforcement of behaviors and thought processes that promote optimism and self-empowerment. Some examples that have been shown to effectively improve patient well-being in the context of neurological diseases include cognitive-behavioral therapy, art and expression-based therapy, positive savoring, and life summary [2].

Cognitive-Behavioral Therapy

Cognitive-behavioral therapy (CBT) is a collaborative practice in which therapists help guide clients through their thoughts, attitudes, and behavioral responses to certain difficulties or events in their lives [26]. Cognitive appraisal of these responses and the administration of techniques to encourage more positive behaviors allow individuals to achieve improved mood and quality of life. These behavioral modifications can indirectly improve disease outcomes by encouraging positive health behaviors and adherence to medically prescribed treatments, in addition to decreasing physiological stress [26]. In the context of neurological diseases, response modifications are often geared toward specific challenges brought on by neurological symptoms or medication side effects, such as coping with public perceptions of motor or speech impairments. Therapy is therefore targeted at helping patients develop an individualized toolkit of skills and behaviors to limit maladaptive thinking [26]. Such therapies ultimately serve to reduce anxious and depressive thoughts and behaviors that stem from disease-related disability. Specifically, CBT for patients with multiple sclerosis and Parkinson's disease has been shown to improve symptoms of fatigue, behavioral outbursts from cognitive impairments, depression, and anxiety [26–28].

Art and Expression

Art and expression-based therapies involve a variety of creative and performing arts to provide sensory and emotional stimulation while also promoting joy, creativity, and social interaction [29]. In patients with Parkinson's disease, music therapy has been shown to improve deficits in motor control through rhythmic auditory cues [30]. Through the synchronization of rhythmic stimuli with motor movements, patients can improve coordination, gait pattern, and movement timing. Such improvements have been attributed to compensation by the cerebello-thalamocortical network for dopaminergic degeneration in the basal ganglia [30]. For pediatric brain tumor patients undergoing chemotherapy, creative arts therapies including dance, music, and visual arts have resulted in improved scores for parent-reported hurt, parent-reported nausea, mood, happiness, and nervousness [31]. In patients with Alzheimer's disease, movement, rhythm, and singing helped stimulate emotional recall and a strengthened sense of identity [29]. One unique form of creative expression that has recently gained popularity is TimeSlips, an activity in which patients with dementia are asked to build stories and narratives around a staged photograph [32]. The activity allows for social interaction, collaboration, and mutual validation in a group setting and was shown to improve pleasure and social communication ratings [32]. These various modes of creative expression ultimately provide patients with an improved sense of well-being and contribute to a more holistic experience of health.

Positive Savoring

Positive savoring is a relatively simple psychological exercise in which participants are asked to document and reflect on favorable events, benevolence, and general experiences of gratitude on a consistent basis as a means for improving mood and well-being [33]. In a study of a cohort of adults diagnosed with neuromuscular diseases, gratitude and positive savoring led to increased measures of subjective well-being and improved sleep duration and restfulness compared to the non-treatment control group [33]. In a randomized study on traumatic brain injury patients, writing down three positive events each day for 12 weeks led to significantly higher happiness ratings on the Seligman's Authentic Happiness Inventory (SAHI) [34]. The evidence suggests that despite its relative simplicity, positive savoring as a psychological intervention can help patients achieve significantly higher levels of happiness in life.

Life Summary

Life summary refers to a psychological intervention in which patients experiencing dementia-related cognitive decline reminisce on major events and accomplishments in their lives [2]. As dementia patients experience cognitive decline, difficulty recalling important life events and experiences can lead to frustration, stress, and further cognitive and behavioral exacerbations. Such exacerbations can make family visits and social interactions rather difficult, for both loved ones and patients [35]. The goal of life summary interventions is to provide a platform where family members or facilitators can help patients recall important experiences and events in their past through photos, familiar items, music, and other salient tokens from their lives [2]. One such intervention involved 60-minute sessions led by two facilitators with different themes, such as music, family, youth, and achievements. After eight weeks of intervention, one session per week, patients experienced significant improvement in cognitive function and a decrease in depressive symptoms [36]. In another application of life summary, patients' families were invited to play a game involving a recollection of the patient's major life events, which proved to be a positive experience for family members while reducing signs of depression in patients [35].

Biologically Based Therapies

In the context of wellness medicine, biologically based therapies refer to the use of nutritional supplements, plant-based therapies, and dietary modifications that can either directly or indirectly improve disease symptoms. Many of these biological supplements have antioxidant properties that target inflammation and can consequently improve disease states that are autoimmune in nature. The use of biological therapies for neurological diseases has a growing body of evidence, especially in pathologies related to nutrient deficiencies. Because these supplements often come at a low cost and usually do not have significant side effects, they offer patients alternative modes of treatment to supplement their pharmaceutical interventions. However, due to the risk of possible interactions with prescribed drugs, it is important that care providers are informed of patients' use of dietary supplements and modifications.

Dietary Supplements

Vitamin D is a molecule that has been the subject of increased investigation for its actions beyond calcium and bone homeostasis, including its effects on glucose homeostasis, autoimmunity, inflammation, and cardiovascular health [37]. Unbalanced vitamin D homeostasis has been linked to neurodegenerative and autoimmune diseases such as multiple sclerosis (MS), amyotrophic lateral sclerosis (ALS), Alzheimer's disease, and Parkinson's disease [37] (Figure 7.2). Particularly in patients with MS, epidemiological data suggests that increased sun exposure and vitamin D levels are associated with lower incidence of MS. On the other hand, vitamin D deficiency has been linked with a twofold increase in risk of developing MS [37]. In a phase II double-blind randomized controlled trial, the use of vitamin D hormone supplement, cholecalciferol, as an add-on treatment with subcutaneous interferon β-1a for relapsing-remitting MS led to fewer new combined unique active lesions [38]. It is important, however, that care providers appropriately titrate vitamin D dosages according to the patient's present vitamin D status. Although vitamin D deficiencies have frequently been seen in patients with Alzheimer's disease, Parkinson's disease, and ALS, it is unclear whether they

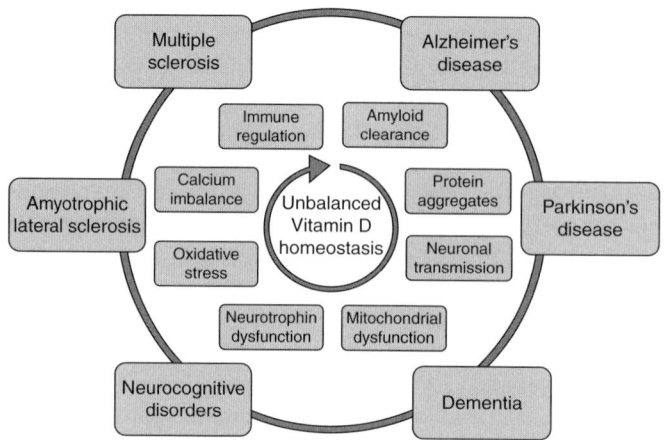

Figure 7.2 Diagram of the underlying mechanisms of unbalanced vitamin D. Reprinted from C Di Somma, E Scarano, L Barrea, et al. Vitamin D and neurological diseases: an endocrine view. *Int J Mol Sci* 2017; 18(11), with permission from MDPI.

are mechanistically linked to the disease or a consequence of decreased mobility leading to a lack of sun exposure [37]. Notwithstanding, appropriate vitamin D supplementation may still be beneficial in reducing risk of osteoporosis in this population [39].

A variety of other dietary supplements have been shown to improve symptoms of neurological diseases. In the pediatric population, prophylactic supplementation of oral magnesium oxide reduces migraine headache frequency and intensity, according to a double-blind, placebo-controlled study [40]. The same effect was seen with riboflavin (vitamin B2) in a retrospective study of pediatric and adolescent migraine patients [41].

Herbal and Plant-Based Therapies

In recent years, studies have begun to elucidate the effectiveness of cannabinoid treatment for neurological disorders [42]. The most robust evidence exists for cannabidiol, a plant-derived cannabinoid, for treatment of seizures in children with Lennox–Gastaut syndrome and Dravet syndrome. Smaller studies have also provided evidence showing that cannabidiol effectively reduces seizure frequency in childhood epilepsy syndromes of other etiologies. Although there is still a lack of evidence demonstrating cannabinoid treatment efficacy in other neurodegenerative disorders, it has been approved in many countries for the treatment of MS-related spasticity and pain. These treatments usually exist in the form of nabiximol, which is a mixture of Δ9-tetrahydrocannabinol (THC) and cannabidiol in the form of an oral mucosal spray. Nabilone, a synthetic THC, has been used for the treatment of pain and chemotherapy-associated nausea [42].

Polyphenols are dietary molecules found in a variety of fruits, vegetables, teas, and spices that have antioxidant and radical scavenging activity in the body. Due to their ability to reduce oxidative stress from reactive oxygen species, these molecules can provide neuroprotection from inflammation-mediated neuronal death [43]. Dietary polyphenols include quercetin, resveratrol, curcumin, and catechins. Resveratrol can be found in chocolate, red wine, and peanuts, while quercetin can be found in berries, red wine, Ginkgo biloba, and onions. Curcumin is a yellow-pigmented molecule extracted from turmeric [44]. Consumption of green tea, which contains epigallocatechin-3-gallate (EGCG), a subtype of the polyphenol catechin, has been epidemiologically associated with lower incidence of

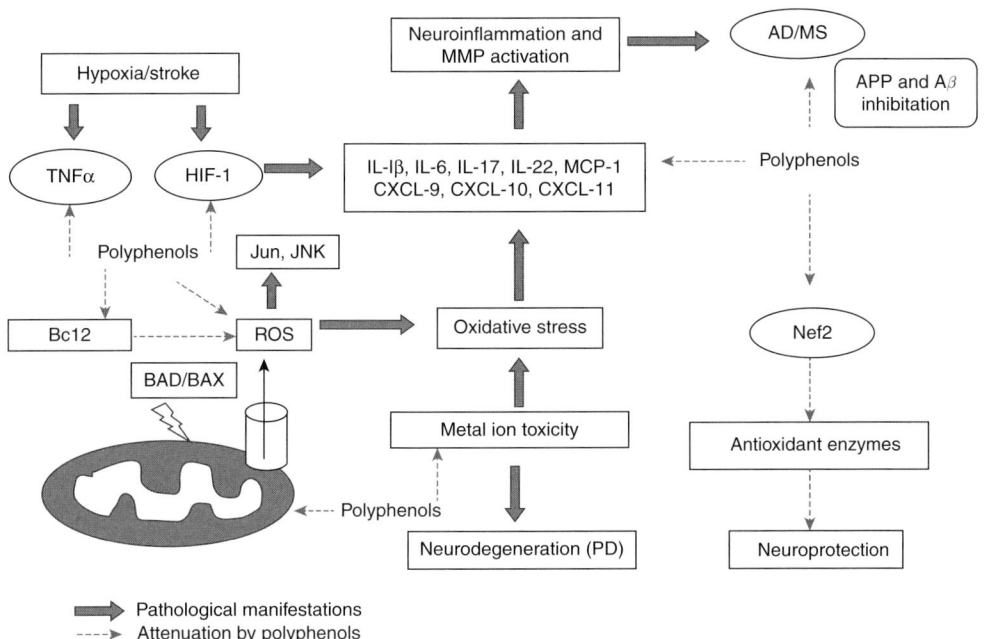

Figure 7.3 Diagrammatic representation of the mechanisms by which polyphenols attenuate neuropathologies and function as a neuroprotectant. Reprinted from KS Bhullar, HP Rupasinghe. Polyphenols: multipotent therapeutic agents in neurodegenerative diseases. *Oxid Med Cell Longev* 2013; 2013: 89174, with permission from Hindawi.

Parkinson's disease [43]. In animal models of Parkinson's disease, green tea extract and EGCG have been shown to provide neuroprotective effects by acting as an iron chelator [43]. Other neuroprotective mechanisms of polyphenols include anti-acetylcholinesterase activity, prion inhibition, and modulation of immune response pathways [43] (Figure 7.3). Due to the multitude of potential neuroprotective mechanisms and limited side effects, consumption of polyphenol-rich foods can be an excellent supplement to medical management of neurological diseases.

Specialized Diets

In recent years, the ketogenic diet has been gaining popularity as an effective form of short-term weight loss. It is defined as a high-fat and -protein diet with minimal carbohydrate intake. However, its application in the context of neurological diseases has been around for decades, in particular for the treatment of seizure disorders [45]. Robust evidence from multiple randomized clinical trials has shown that ketogenic diets effectively reduce seizure frequency at a rate comparable to currently available anti-epileptic drugs. In one such study, patients experienced a 50 percent or greater reduction of seizure frequency after three months of adopting a ketogenic diet [46]. Recent studies have also suggested that ketogenic diets may be effective therapies for other neurological disorders, including Alzheimer's, ALS, traumatic brain injury, and pain [45].

Variants of the ketogenic diet have also shown to be effective in treating epilepsy disorders, such as the medium-chain triglyceride (MCT) diet, modified Atkins diet

(MAD), and low glycemic index treatment (LGIT). These diets tend to have better patient adherence in older children and adults, though the evidence for their effectiveness in reducing seizure frequency is not as robust as the classic ketogenic diet [45].

Exercise Therapies

Physical exercise is considered a mainstay of adjunctive therapy for patients with neurological conditions if the patient has adequate motor function to safely execute physical exercise regimens. Apart from the systemic benefits of exercise for improving cardiovascular health, lowering cholesterol, and decreasing the risk of metabolic syndrome, exercise can have very direct effects on improving brain function. In the context of neurological diseases, robust evidence suggests that aerobic exercise improves disease-specific neurological function in patients with dementia, Parkinson's disease, and multiple sclerosis [47].

It is suggested that patients with Parkinson's disease undergo aerobic training therapy on a treadmill with proper safety measures and support. Patients should start at a comfortable intensity and duration, and progressively increase intensity and duration to 10 minutes [47]. It is also recommended that patients combine aerobic exercise with strength and balance training to improve overall motor function. Studies have shown that this combination of training improves walking speed, balance, and quality of life [47]. Supplementation of exercise therapy with previously mentioned musical rhythm therapy can also help patients improve gait patterns and speed [30]. In animal models, exercise has been shown to slow down the rate of dopaminergic cell death and restore the functionality of the basal ganglia [47, 48].

In patients with dementia, exercise therapy has been shown to improve cognitive function, gait function, and ability to perform activities of daily living [49]. Physical exercise in the form of brisk walking three times a week for 40 minutes has been shown to significantly increase hippocampal volume after a year [47]. Mechanistically, these benefits are thought to occur as a result of elevated brain-derived neurotropic factor (BDNF), which is a hippocampal growth factor involved in adult neurogenesis [47]. Types of exercise therapy for patients with dementia can vary based on mobility and level of independence, and must be tailored according to the patient's mental and physical status.

Multiple sclerosis is a condition characterized by a progressive decline of motor function due to autoimmune demyelinating attacks on the nervous system. Deficits often occur in the form of flare-up episodes, or relapses, that result in paresis, ataxia, weakness, loss of autonomic function, and fatigue, among other symptoms [47]. Physical exercise has been shown to effectively improve MS-related motor deficits, as well as strength, mobility, exercise tolerance, and overall quality of life measures [50]. Effective exercises for MS patients include a combination of aerobic exercises, such as cycling, treadmill walking or running, and swimming, with isometric and isokinetic muscle resistance exercises [47].

Manual Body Therapies

Therapies involving manual interventions on the body, such as massage, spinal manipulation, and acupuncture, are often relevant to the treatment of neurological conditions in the context of pain management. In particular, there has been growing favor for integrated medical approaches to pain management among care providers in light of the risks of overprescribing opioid painkillers.

Massage

Standard massage therapies for patients with neurological diseases should be carried out by licensed massage therapists in a quiet room on a comfortable massage table. Such routines usually consist of effleurage, petrissage, friction, and static compression strokes [51]. In a pilot study, it was found that standardized massage therapy effectively improved levels of fatigue, pain, and perceived health and quality of life in patients with MS. However, it was not effective in reducing MS-related spasticity [51]. In a randomized controlled trial, massage therapy was shown to significantly decrease the frequency of migraine attacks in patients who underwent six weeks of therapy but did not influence the intensity of migraine episodes [52].

Acupuncture

Acupuncture is a therapy that originated in China and has been practiced for thousands of years. It involves the precise insertion of needles into the skin on different acupuncture points across the body in line with the Chinese medical concept of qi flow and regulation [53]. Currently, acupuncture is used as an effective mode of analgesia, and in 1998 was stated to be effective for the treatment of stroke rehabilitation by the NIH Consensus Development Panel [54]. Other studies have provided evidence that acupuncture effectively improves chronic low back pain and headache syndromes [54]. A number of randomized controlled trials have also touted its efficacy in managing polyneuropathies, including diabetic neuropathy, Bell's palsy, and carpal tunnel syndrome [54].

Spinal Manipulation

Spinal manipulation is a therapy performed by chiropractors and osteopathic doctors in which the vertebral joints are stretched beyond their usual resistance limits to release synovial gases with an audible popping sound. Such manipulations are thought to temporarily increase the vertebral range of motion [55]. Both osteopathic and chiropractic spinal manipulation have been shown through randomized controlled trials to be effective in alleviating acute and subacute lower back pain [55, 56]. In the context of lower back pain related to radiculopathy or sciatica, spinal manipulation has been shown to have moderate benefits for improving pain, functional status, and work status [57].

Conclusion

Wellness medicine offers a diverse repertoire of interventions that can positively impact the physical, mental, and emotional health of patients with neurological diseases. Mind–body therapies offer patients the ability to create coherence between thoughts, feelings, and physiology. Meanwhile, psychological interventions take into account the importance of maintaining mental health in patients with chronic diseases, creating a more holistic concept of health for patients. Such practices often positively impact the outcomes for medical treatment of neurological diseases by improving physiological stress and quality of life measures. Additionally, biologically based therapies provide patients with supplemental treatment options that can improve neurological function with minimal cost and side effects. Exercise therapies, in addition to improving mood and quality of life, can lead to direct neurological improvements. Finally, manual body therapies such as massage, acupuncture, and spinal manipulation can provide significant alleviation of pain associated with neurological conditions.

Because therapies for neurological conditions that are included under the umbrella of wellness medicine have a lesser-known basis in scientific evidence, it is important for physicians and care providers to be well informed of their relative efficacies. By integrating wellness interventions discussed in this chapter, providers can effectively re-empower patients diagnosed with neurological conditions to have more control over their journey through treatment and recovery.

References

1. RE Wells, V Baute, HST Wahbeh. Complementary and integrative medicine for neurologic conditions. *Med Clin North Am* 2017; **101**(5): 881–893.

2. Lai, KS Lim, WY Low, V Tang. Positive psychological interventions for neurological disorders: a systematic review. *Clin Neuropsychol* 2019; **33**(3): 490–518.

3. RE Wells, RS Phillips, SC Schachter, EP McCarthy. Complementary and alternative medicine use among US adults with common neurological conditions. *J Neurol* 2010; **257**(11): 1822–1831.

4. R Erwin Wells, RS Phillips, EP McCarthy. Patterns of mind–body therapies in adults with common neurological conditions. *Neuroepidemiology* 2011; **36**(1): 46–51.

5. H Wahbeh, SM Elsas, BS Oken. Mind–body interventions: applications in neurology. *Neurology* 2008; **70**(24): 2321–2328.

6. Integration of behavioral and relaxation approaches into the treatment of chronic pain and insomnia. NIH Technology Assessment Panel on Integration of Behavioral and Relaxation Approaches into the Treatment of Chronic Pain and Insomnia. *JAMA* 1996; **276**(4): 313–318. (No authors listed.)

7. CA Puskarich, S Whitman, J Dell, et al. Controlled examination of effects of progressive relaxation training on seizure reduction. *Epilepsia* 1992; **33**(4): 675–680.

8. EA Hoge, E Bui, L Marques, et al. Randomized controlled trial of mindfulness meditation for generalized anxiety disorder: effects on anxiety and stress reactivity. *J Clin Psychiatry* 2013; **74**(8): 786–792.

9. D Krishnakumar, MR Hamblin, SJ Lakshmanan. Meditation and yoga can modulate brain mechanisms that affect behavior and anxiety: a modern scientific perspective. *Anc Sci* 2015; **2**(1): 13–19.

10. J Kabat-Zinn. An outpatient program in behavioral medicine for chronic pain patients based on the practice of mindfulness meditation: theoretical considerations and preliminary results. *Gen Hosp Psychiatry* 1982; **4**(1): 33–47.

11. AB Levin, EJ Hadgkiss, TJ Weiland, GA Jelinek. Meditation as an adjunct to the management of multiple sclerosis. *Neurol Res Int* 2014; **2014**: 704691.

12. GN Levine, RA Lange, CN Bairey-Merz, et al. Meditation and cardiovascular risk reduction: a scientific statement from the American Heart Association. *J Am Heart Assoc* 2017; **6**(10).

13. J Bagdasaryan, V Quyen Mle. Experiencing your brain: neurofeedback as a new bridge between neuroscience and phenomenology. *Front Hum Neurosci* 2013; **7**: 680.

14. H Marzbani, HR Marateb, MJE Mansourian. Neurofeedback: a comprehensive review on system design, methodology and clinical applications. *Basic Clin Neurosci* 2016; **7**(2): 143–158.

15. JE Walker, GP Kozlowski. Neurofeedback treatment of epilepsy. *Child Adolesc Psychiatr Clin N Am* 2005; **14**(1): 163–176, viii.

16. WW Finley, HA Smith, MD Etherton. Reduction of seizures and normalization of the EEG in a severe epileptic following sensorimotor biofeedback training: preliminary study. *Biol Psychol* 1975; **2**(3): 189–203.

17. M Rossi-Izquierdo, A Ernst, A Soto-Varela, et al. Vibrotactile neurofeedback balance training in patients with Parkinson's disease: reducing the number of falls. *Gait Posture* 2013; **37**(2): 195–200.

18. VLDLG Ibric Neurofeedback in pain management. In: TH Budzyknski,

JR Evans, A Abarbanel, eds., *Introduction to Quantitative EEG and Neurofeedback: Advanced Theory and Applications* (2nd ed.). Amsterdam, Elsevier; 2009; 417–451.

19. SK Mishra, P Singh, SJ Bunch, R Zhang. The therapeutic value of yoga in neurological disorders. *Ann Indian Acad Neurol* 2012; **15**(4): 247–254.

20. B Rajesh, D Jayachandran, G Mohandas, K Radhakrishnan. A pilot study of a yoga meditation protocol for patients with medically refractory epilepsy. *J Altern Complement Med* 2006; **12**(4): 367–371.

21. T Lundgren, J Dahl, N Yardi, L Melin. Acceptance and commitment therapy and yoga for drug-refractory epilepsy: a randomized controlled trial. *Epilepsy Behav* 2008; **13**(1): 102–108.

22. V Malhotra, S Singh, OP Tandon, et al. Effect of yoga asanas on nerve conduction in type 2 diabetes. *Indian J Physiol Pharmacol* 2002; **46**(3): 298–306.

23. MS Garfinkel, A Singhal, WA Katz, et al. Yoga-based intervention for carpal tunnel syndrome: a randomized trial. *JAMA* 1998; **280**(18): 1601–1603.

24. JW Carson, KM Carson, KD Jones, et al. A pilot randomized controlled trial of the Yoga of Awareness program in the management of fibromyalgia. *Pain* 2010; **151**(2): 530–539.

25. L Treat, J Liesinger, JY Ziegenfuss, et al. Patterns of complementary and alternative medicine use in children with common neurological conditions. *Glob Adv Health Med* 2014; **3**(1): 18–24.

26. L Dennison, R Moss-Morris. Cognitive-behavioral therapy: what benefits can it offer people with multiple sclerosis? *Expert Rev Neurother* 2010; **10**(9): 1383–1390.

27. I Berardelli, M Pasquini, V Roselli, et al. Cognitive behavioral therapy in movement disorders: a review. *Mov Disord Clin Pract* 2015; **2**(2): 107–115.

28. C Swalwell, NA Pachana, NN Dissanayaka. Remote delivery of psychological interventions for Parkinson's disease. *Int Psychogeriatr* 2018; **30**(12): 1783–1795.

29. MJ Marshall, SA Hutchinson. A critique of research on the use of activities with persons with Alzheimer's disease: a systematic literature review. *J Adv Nurs* 2001; **35**(4): 488–496.

30. A Raglio. Music therapy interventions in Parkinson's disease: the state-of-the-art. *Front Neurol* 2015; **6**: 185.

31. JR Madden, P Mowry, D Gao, PM Cullen, NK Foreman. Creative arts therapy improves quality of life for pediatric brain tumor patients receiving outpatient chemotherapy. *J Pediatr Oncol Nurs* 2010; **27**(3): 133–145.

32. LJ Phillips, SA Reid-Arndt, Y Pak. Effects of a creative expression intervention on emotions, communication, and quality of life in persons with dementia. *Nurs Res* 2010; **59**(6): 417–425.

33. RA Emmons, ME McCullough. Counting blessings versus burdens: an experimental investigation of gratitude and subjective well-being in daily life. *J Pers Soc Psychol* 2003; **84**(2): 377–389.

34. HE Andrewes, V Walker, B O'Neill. Exploring the use of positive psychology interventions in brain injury survivors with challenging behaviour. *Brain Inj* 2014; **28**(7): 965–971.

35. GD Cohen, KM Firth, S Biddle, MJ Lloyd Lewis, S Simmens. The first therapeutic game specifically designed and evaluated for Alzheimer's disease. *Am J Alzheimers Dis Other Demen* 2008; **23**(6): 540–551.

36. JJ Wang. Group reminiscence therapy for cognitive and affective function of demented elderly in Taiwan. *Int J Geriatr Psychiatry* 2007; **22**(12): 1235–1240.

37. C Di Somma, E Scarano, L Barrea, et al. Vitamin D and neurological diseases: an endocrine view. *Int J Mol Sci* 2017; **18**(11): 2482.

38. R Hupperts, J Smolders, R Vieth, et al. High dose cholecalciferol (vitamin D3) oil as add-on therapy in subjects with relapsing-remitting multiple sclerosis (RRMS) receiving subcutaneous interferon β-1a (scIFNβ-1a) (S44.005). *Neurology* 2017; **88**(16 Supplement): S44.005.

39. MJ Bagur, MA Murcia, AM Jimenez-Monreal, et al. Influence of diet in multiple sclerosis: a systematic review. *Adv Nutr* 2017; **8**(3): 463–472.

40. M Condo, A Posar, A Arbizzani, A Parmeggiani. Riboflavin prophylaxis in pediatric and adolescent migraine. *J Headache Pain* 2009; **10**(5): 361–365.

41. F Wang, SK Van Den Eeden, LM Ackerson, et al. Oral magnesium oxide prophylaxis of frequent migrainous headache in children: a randomized, double-blind, placebo-controlled trial. *Headache* 2003; **43**(6): 601–610.

42. D Friedman, JA French, M Maccarrone. Safety, efficacy, and mechanisms of action of cannabinoids in neurological disorders. *Lancet Neurol* 2019; **18**(5): 504–512.

43. KS Bhullar, HP Rupasinghe. Polyphenols: multipotent therapeutic agents in neurodegenerative diseases. *Oxid Med Cell Longev* 2013; **2013**: 891748.

44. P Riccio, R Rossano, GM Liuzzi. May diet and dietary supplements improve the wellness of multiple sclerosis patients? A molecular approach. *Autoimmune Dis* 2011; **2010**: 249842.

45. CE Stafstrom. Dietary therapies for epilepsy and other neurological disorders: highlights of the 3rd international symposium. *Epilepsy Curr* 2013; **13**(2): 103–106.

46. K Martin, CF Jackson, RG Levy, PN Cooper. Ketogenic diet and other dietary treatments for epilepsy. *Cochrane Database Syst Rev* 2016; **2**.

47. BK Pedersen, B Saltin. Exercise as medicine: evidence for prescribing exercise as therapy in 26 different chronic diseases. *Scand J Med Sci Sports* 2015; **25**(Suppl 3): 1–72.

48. LM Shulman, LI Katzel, FM Ivey, et al. Randomized clinical trial of 3 types of physical exercise for patients with Parkinson disease. *JAMA Neurol* 2013; **70**(2): 183–190.

49. D Forbes, SC Forbes, CM Blake, EJ Thiessen, S Forbes. Exercise programs for people with dementia. *Cochrane Database Syst Rev* 2015; **4**: CD006489.

50. AE Latimer-Cheung, LA Pilutti, AL Hicks, et al. Effects of exercise training on fitness, mobility, fatigue, and health-related quality of life among adults with multiple sclerosis: a systematic review to inform guideline development. *Arch Phys Med Rehabil* 2013; **94**(9): 1800–1828.

51. D Backus, C Manella, A Bender, M Sweatman. Impact of massage therapy on fatigue, pain, and spasticity in people with multiple sclerosis: a pilot study. *Int J Ther Massage Bodywork* 2016; **9**(4): 4–13.

52. SP Lawler, LD Cameron. A randomized, controlled trial of massage therapy as a treatment for migraine. *Ann Behav Med* 2006; **32**(1): 50–59.

53. K Kawakita, K Okada. Acupuncture therapy: mechanism of action, efficacy, and safety: a potential intervention for psychogenic disorders? *Biopsychosoc Med* 2014; **8**(1): 4.

54. A Dimitrova, C Murchison, B Oken. Acupuncture for the treatment of peripheral neuropathy: a systematic review and meta-analysis. *J Altern Complement Med* 2017; **23**(3): 164–179.

55. TJ Kaptchuk, DM Eisenberg. Chiropractic: origins, controversies, and contributions. *Arch Intern Med* 1998; **158**(20): 2215–2224.

56. JC Licciardone, ST Stoll, KG Fulda, et al. Osteopathic manipulative treatment for chronic low back pain: a randomized controlled trial. *Spine (Phila Pa 1976)* 2003; **28**(13): 1355–1362.

57. R Chou, LH Huffman, American Pain Society, American College of Physicians. Nonpharmacologic therapies for acute and chronic low back pain: a review of the evidence for an American Pain Society/American College of Physicians clinical practice guideline. *Ann Intern Med* 2007; **147**(7): 492–504.

Cardiovascular and Pulmonary Wellness

Waguih William IsHak and Nathalie Herrera

Introduction

Cardiovascular diseases include coronary artery disease, stroke, hypertensive heart disease, valvular heart disease, cardiac arrhythmias, heart failure, aortic aneurysm and dissection, peripheral arterial disease, and deep venous thrombosis [1]. Pulmonary diseases include asthma, bronchitis, chronic obstructive pulmonary disease (COPD), cystic fibrosis, idiopathic pulmonary fibrosis, lung cancer, pneumonia, pulmonary embolism, pulmonary hypertension, sarcoidosis, and tuberculosis [2]. Both cardiovascular and pulmonary disorders share symptoms of chest pain, shortness of breath, palpitations, fatigue, and leg swelling. The literature is rich in interventions that aim to prevent or treat cardiovascular and pulmonary disorders. This chapter not only reviews the evidence for wellness interventions that can be implemented beyond traditional methods that are utilized to address cardiovascular and pulmonary symptom severity, but also explores the evidence for interventions that primarily improve wellness in patients with cardiovascular and pulmonary pathology. Prior research substantiates the belief that there are 10 such interventions that are supported by evidence: nutrition, exercise, meditation, yoga, massage, humor, music, meaningful relations, positive thinking, and supplements.

Nutrition

Nutrition has been shown to boost wellness in patients with heart and lung diseases [1,2]. Of particular interest is the Mediterranean diet, which includes vegetables and fruits, fish (rich in omega-3 polyunsaturated fats), whole grains (high in fiber), olive oil (rich in unsaturated fats), nuts, and legumes [3]. Evidence shows that the Mediterranean diet is associated with high self-rated wellness [4]. Moreover, research studies have shown that the following food items are associated with improved wellness: mushrooms, seaweed, legumes, plant-based proteins, coffee, tea, modest alcohol intake, and fermented foods such as kimchi, sauerkraut, tempeh, milk-based kefir, yogurt, and kombucha [5]. Likewise, previous studies have suggested the beneficial effects of following healthy dietary patterns, with a diet rich in fiber from whole plant foods. These benefits include decreasing cardiovascular disease, coronary heart disease, and mortality risks, as well as improving psychological well-being [6, 7]. Although more research is needed, available studies support the sustained intake of whole fruits, and fruit fiber is associated with a reduced rate of vascular aging, a lower risk of mortality from cardiovascular disease, and a reduced risk of hypertension [6]. In spite of the fact that evidence supports a favorable relation between healthy nutrition and a positive effect in patients with heart and lung disease [7–11], research studies are still needed to examine and compare the impacts of different dietary interventions on wellness as the primary outcome in this population.

Exercise

Exercise, especially brisk walking for 30 minutes per day, has been proven to improve wellness ratings in patients with cardiovascular and pulmonary disorders [12]. Increasing physical activity levels, especially in association with cardiorespiratory physiotherapy interventions, are linked to improved wellness in chronic pulmonary disorders [13]. In a 2017 randomized controlled trial of previously sedentary postmenopausal women, Vélez-Toral et al. found that with an exercise plus health-promotion intervention, participants experienced enhancements in several health-related quality of life (HRQoL) dimensions, particularly mental well-being [14].

Similarly, a 2006 study by Heppner et al. showed that participation in regular exercise such as walking after the completion of pulmonary rehabilitation is associated with slower declines in overall HRQoL [15].

Meditation

Meditation has gained much traction in recent years as an intervention for symptom relief in chronic disease, including cardiovascular and pulmonary disorders [16]. In a 2019 study of patients with heart failure, Viveiros et al. concluded that meditation is a useful intervention to improve quality of life, psychosocial wellness, and biophysical factors, and to reduce overall symptom burden [17]. Despite variations in practice that depend on the particular type of meditation, mindful meditation seems of be of benefit in cardiovascular and pulmonary wellness [17, 18]. More studies are needed to examine the effects in patients with cardiovascular and pulmonary disorders specifically, beyond the effects shown in stress management and improvement in quality of life [19].

Yoga

Yoga and other movement-based meditative practices have shown promise in improving wellness ratings in patients with cardiovascular and pulmonary disorders [20]. There is a significant number of reported physiologic effects of yoga [21], as highlighted in Figure 8.1.

Yoga appears to be a relatively safe intervention that can be incorporated into primary and secondary prevention strategies for cardiovascular disease [21]. The effects of yoga in cardiac diseases are detailed in Table 8.1.

Because of its mind–body approach to decreasing stress, positively impacting cardiovascular risk factors, and improving an overall sense of well-being, yoga is a potentially important tool in the armamentarium of cardiac rehabilitation programs. Guddeti et al. in 2019 created a "comprehensive approach" model to cardiac rehabilitation [21], which includes interventions such as yoga, meditation, and exercise, as shown in Figure 8.2.

Massage

Few studies have examined the effect of massage therapy in heart and lung disease. Massage has been used as a safe and cost-effective intervention in prehypertensive women, although the effects did not persist long-term [22]. More studies are needed to examine the potential for massage to improve wellness in cardiac and pulmonary disorders.

Table 8.1 The effects of yoga in cardiac diseases. Adapted from Guddeti et al. 2019 [21]

Cardiac disease	Effect
Autonomic dysfunction	Increased heart rate variability, increased vagal output, decreased sympathetic arousal
Arrhythmias	Reduced atrial fibrillation episodes, decreased atrial fibrillation-related symptoms and anxiety, reduced number of nonfatal device-treated ventricular events, no proven mortality benefit
Coronary artery disease	Reduced angina episodes, increased exercise time, no decrease in recurrent coronary events such as myocardial infarction, no mortality benefit
Heart failure	Longer exercise time, greater maximal oxygen consumption, improved physical function like strength and balance, no mortality benefit

From RR Guddeti, G Dang, MA Williams, VM Alla. Role of yoga in cardiac disease rehabilitation. *J Cardiopul Rehabil Prev* 2019; 39: 146–152; doi: 10.1097/HCR.0000000000000372 [21]. Reprinted with permission of Wolters Kluwer Health.

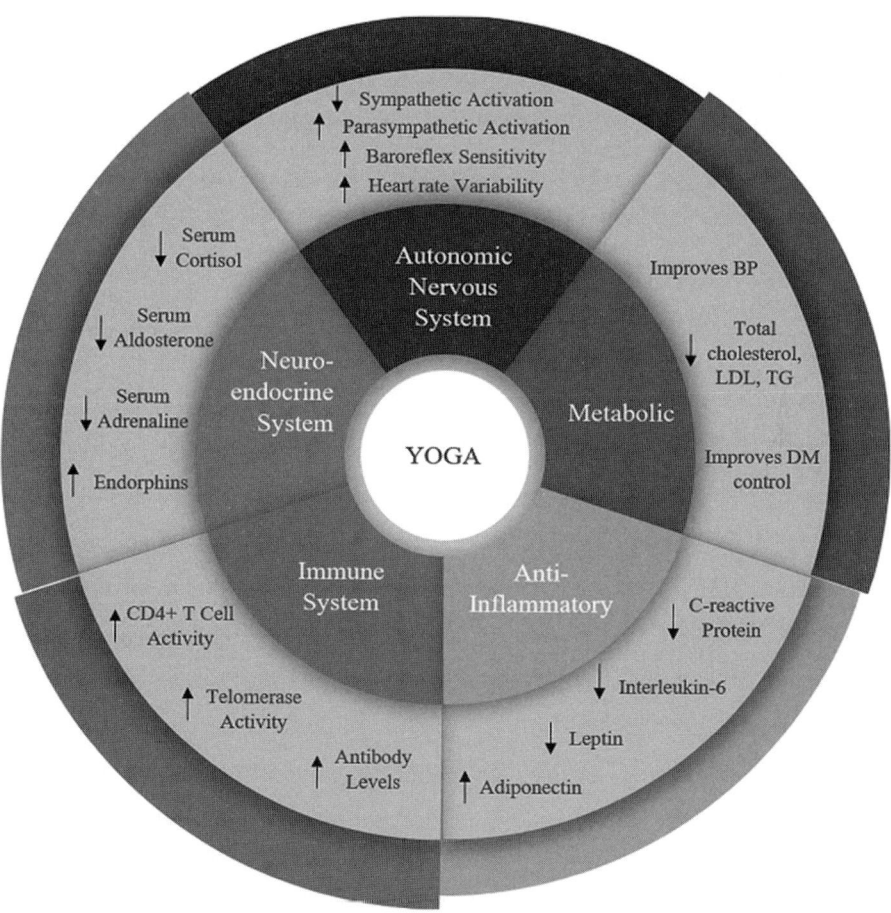

Figure 8.1 Reported physiologic effects of yoga. Reprinted from Guddeti et al. 2019 [21]. From RR Guddeti, G Dang, MA Williams, VM Alla. Role of yoga in cardiac disease rehabilitation. *J Cardiopul Rehabil Prev* 2019; 39: 146–152; doi: 10.1097/HCR.0000000000000372 [21]. Reprinted with permission of Wolters Kluwer Health.

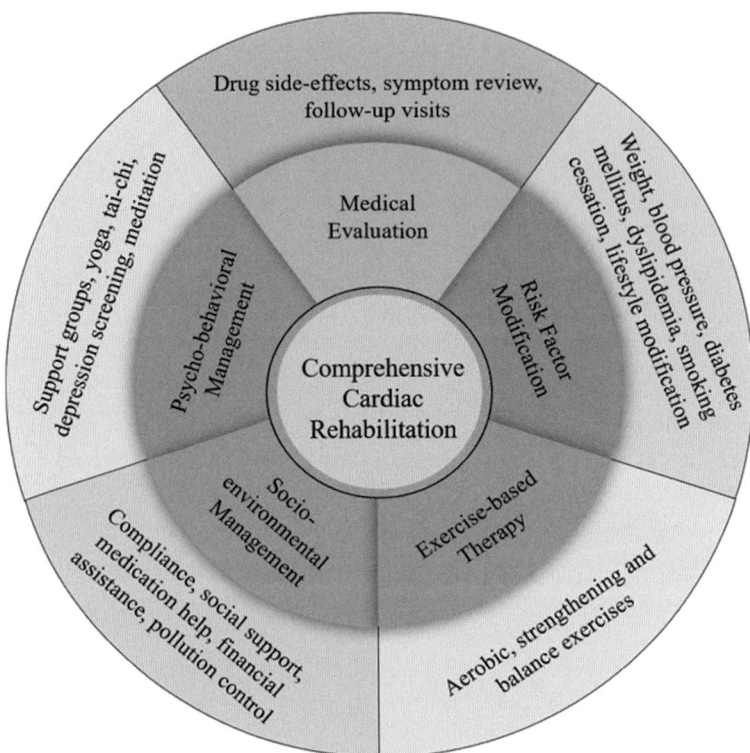

Figure 8.2 "Comprehensive approach" model to cardiac rehabilitation. Includes interventions such as yoga, meditation, and exercise. Reprinted from Guddeti et al. 2019 [21]. From RR Guddeti, G Dang, MA Williams, VM Alla. Role of yoga in cardiac disease rehabilitation. *J Cardiopul Rehabil Prev* 2019; 39: 146–152; doi: 10.1097/HCR.0000000000000372 [21]. Reprinted with permission of Wolters Kluwer Health.

Humor

Positive health benefits have been observed with humor, and research shows that even depressed patients are open to its use as a therapeutic tool [23]. Lockwood and Yoshimura in 2014 showed that self-ratings of social and psychological well-being significantly improved in patients recovering from cardiovascular disease from two national support groups [24]. More studies are needed to examine the wellness effects of humor in patients with pulmonary disorders.

Music

Music has been shown to improve wellness ratings in patients with cardiovascular disorders [25]. Although music and dance seem to have positive effects in chronic lung disease, more rigorous studies need to be conducted to establish their effects on wellness [26].

Meaningful Relations

Meaningful relations and social connections have a positive impact on wellness in patients with cardiovascular and pulmonary disorders. Kok et al. showed that positive perceptions of social connections are associated with increases in vagal tone and improvements in wellness ratings [27].

Positive Thinking

An important wellness intervention is increasing positive thinking and positive emotions. According to Kok et al., the effects of positivity and positive social connections are mediated through increases in vagal tone resulting in a "self-sustaining upward-spiral dynamic" [27].

Supplements

Omega-3 fatty acids and vitamin B12 in moderate amounts have an established role in improving wellness in patients with cardiovascular and pulmonary disorders [5]. Although the list of supplements to improve wellness in this population has expanded in recent years, evidence of health and wellness benefits need to be produced using rigorous research methodology.

Conclusion

Research studies showing the evidence of the above wellness interventions in specific cardiovascular diseases are highlighted in Table 8.2.

Research studies showing the evidence of the above wellness interventions in specific pulmonary diseases are highlighted in Table 8.3.

As can be seen, there are a number of notable interventions that have been shown to improve wellness in patients with cardiovascular and pulmonary disorders. Despite their potential benefits, incorporating these interventions still needs more research and higher-quality evidence. Larger controlled studies are needed that are designed specifically to examine wellness as the primary outcome in this population, focusing on each disease state within the cardiovascular and pulmonary domain, especially during and after recovery from severe illness.

References

1. DP Zipes, P Libby, RO Bonow, O Robert, DL Mann, GF Tomaselli. *Braunwald's Heart Disease: A Textbook of Cardiovascular Medicine* (11th ed.). Philadelphia, PA, Elsevier, 2018.
2. SE Weinberger, BA Cockrill, J Mandel. *Principles of Pulmonary Medicine* (7th ed.). Philadelphia, PA, Elsevier, 2018.
3. RJ Widmer, AJ Flammer, LO Lerman, A Lerman. The Mediterranean diet, its components, and cardiovascular disease. *Am J Med* 2015; **128**: 229–238.
4. T Govindaraju, BW Sahle, TA McCaffrey, JJ McNeil, AJ Owen. Dietary patterns and quality of life in older adults: a systematic review. *Nutrients* 2018; **10**: E971.
5. AM Freeman, PB Morris, K Aspry, et al. A clinician's guide for trending cardiovascular nutrition controversies: part II. *J Am Coll Cardiol* 2018; **72**: 553–568.
6. ML Dreher. Whole fruits and fruit fiber emerging health effects. *Nutrients* 2018; **10**: E1833.
7. RS Najjar, CE Moore, BD Montgomery. A defined, plant-based diet utilized in an outpatient cardiovascular clinic effectively treats hypercholesterolemia and hypertension and reduces medications. *Clin Cardiol* 2018; **41**: 307–313.
8. RT Ahnen, SS Jonnalagadda, JL Slavin. Role of plant protein in nutrition, wellness and health. *Nutr Rev* 2019; **77**: 735–747.

Table 8.2 Research studies showing the evidence of wellness interventions in specific cardiovascular diseases

Pathology	Nutrition	Exercise	Meditation	Yoga	Massage	Humor	Music	Meaningful relations	Positive thinking	Supplements
Coronary artery disease	X [5,9]	X [12]	X [19]	X [21]						X [5,9]
Stroke	X [5]									X [5]
Hypertensive heart disease						X [24]				
Valvular heart disease										
Cardiac arrhythmias				X [21]						
Heart failure			X [17]	X [20,21]						
Aortic aneurysm and dissection										
Peripheral artery disease	X [3,6]	X [12]	X [19]					X [27]	X [27]	X [3,6]
Deep venous thrombosis										

Table 8.3 Research studies showing the evidence of wellness interventions in specific pulmonary diseases

Pathology	Nutrition	Exercise	Meditation	Yoga	Massage	Humor	Music	Meaningful relations	Positive thinking	Supplements
Asthma	X [6,10,11]									X [6,10,11]
Bronchitis										
Chronic obstructive pulmonary disease	X [6,10,11]	X [15]					X [26]			X [6,10,11]
Cystic fibrosis										
Idiopathic pulmonary fibrosis										
Lung cancer	X [6,10]									X [6,10]
Pneumonia										
Pulmonary embolism										
Pulmonary hypertension										
Sarcoidosis										
Tuberculosis	X [10]									X [10]

9. F Marangoni, G Corsello, C Cricelli, et al. Role of poultry meat in a balanced diet aimed at maintaining health and wellbeing: an Italian consensus document. *Food Nutr Res* 2015; **59**: 27606.

10. I Romieu. Nutrition and lung health. *Int J Tuberc Lung Dis* 2005; **9**: 362–374.

11. I Romieu, C Trenga. Diet and obstructive lung diseases. *Epidemiol Rev* 2001; **23**: 268–287.

12. SS Bassuk, JE Manson. Physical activity and the prevention of cardiovascular disease. *Curr Atheroscler Rep* 2003; **5**: 299–307.

13. L Denehy, CL Granger, D El-Ansary, SM Parry. Advances in cardiorespiratory physiotherapy and their clinical impact. *Expert Rev Respir Med* 2018; **12**: 203–215.

14. M Vélez-Toral, D Godoy-Izquierdo, NML de Guevara, et al. Improvements in health-related quality of life, cardio-metabolic health, and fitness in postmenopausal women after an exercise plus health promotion intervention: a randomized controlled trial. *J Phys Act Health* 2017; **14**: 336–343.

15. PS Heppner, C Morgan, RM Kaplan, AL Ries. Regular walking and long-term maintenance of outcomes after pulmonary rehabilitation. *J Cardiopul Rehabil* 2006; **26**: 44–53.

16. RR Chan, JL Larson. Meditation interventions for chronic disease populations: a systematic review. *J Holist Nurs* 2015; **33**: 351–365.

17. J Viveiros, B Chamberlain, A O'Hare, KA Sethares. Meditation interventions among heart failure patients: an integrative review. *Eur J Cardiovasc Nurs* 2019; **18**: 1–9.

18. RA Heckenberg, P Eddy, S Kent, BJ Wright. Do workplace-based mindfulness meditation programs improve physiological indices of stress? A systematic review and meta-analysis. *J Psychosom Res* 2018; **114**: 62–71.

19. JO Younge, RA Gotink, CP Baena, JW Roos-Hesselink, MG Hunink. Mind–body practices for patients with cardiac disease: a systematic review and meta-analysis. *Eur J Prev Cardiol* 2015; **22**: 1385–1398.

20. GA Kelley, KS Kelley. Meditative movement therapies and health-related quality-of-life in adults: a systematic review of meta-analyses. *PLoS One* 2015; **10**: e0129181.

21. RR Guddeti, G Dang, MA Williams, VM Alla. Role of yoga in cardiac disease rehabilitation. *J Cardiopul Rehabil Prev* 2019; **39**: 146–152.

22. M Givi, M Sadeghi, M Garakyaraghi, et al. Long-term effect of massage therapy on blood pressure in prehypertensive women. *J Educ Health Promot* 2018; **7**: 54.

23. A Bokarius, K Ha, R Poland, et al. Attitude toward humor in patients experiencing depressive symptoms. *Innov Clin Neurosci* 2011: **8**(9): 20–23.

24. NL Lockwood, SM Yoshimura. The heart of the matter: the effects of humor on well-being during recovery from cardiovascular disease. *Health Commun* 2014; **29**: 410–420.

25. ER Gasenzer, R Leischik. [Music, pulse, heart and sport]. *Herz* 2018; **43**: 43–52.

26. K Philip, A Lewis, NS Hopkinson. Music and dance in chronic lung disease. *Breathe (Sheff)* 2019; **15**: 116–120.

27. BE Kok, KA Coffey, MA Cohn, et al. How positive emotions build physical health: perceived positive social connections account for the upward spiral between positive emotions and vagal tone. *Psychol Sci* 2013; **24**: 1123–1132.

Gastrointestinal System and Wellness

Lori A. Robbins and Edward J. Feldman

Introduction

Gastrointestinal (GI) symptoms such as pain, heartburn, abdominal bloating, diarrhea, and constipation occur in most individuals at some time or another. Numerous diagnostic studies and medical interventions are available, but often the problems continue. Eager for relief, nearly half of all patients with chronic GI symptoms turn to the many "complementary" or "alternative" approaches available to the public [1]. This chapter reviews the options that have undergone testing, and summarizes those that are most likely to be of clinical benefit based on the quality of the studies. Many of the alternative approaches have undergone one form or another of clinical trial, but most often the data was either of poor quality or the studies were poorly controlled. Table 9.1 lists those approaches that are low risk and may be beneficial or have some supportive evidence. Table 9.2 lists those approaches that are clinically interesting but have insufficient supportive data to make a recommendation. Recommendations are based on searches performed using Pubmed, MEDLINE, and the Cochrane Database of Systematic Reviews. Multiple abstracts were identified and then reduced after reviewing the study design. There have been numerous attempts in the literature to better understand the usefulness of any one approach, but few were able to reasonably overcome the difficulties presented in their study design. The authors have attempted to "digest" the literature and summarize the field as of now. This chapter is organized into four primary areas of common GI symptoms and concerns.

Gastroesophageal Reflux Disorder (GERD)

Gastroesophageal reflux is experienced on a frequent, ongoing basis by 20 percent of the US public, and is the most common complaint in outpatient visits [2]. GERD has been defined as a disorder "associated with troublesome symptoms and/or complications on account of reflux of stomach contents in the esophagus" [3]. Left untreated, chronic acid reflux can result in complications including Barrett's esophagus and esophageal adenocarcinoma. For patients with nonerosive reflux disease (NERD), however, nontraditional therapies such as acupuncture and lifestyle modifications may be useful for symptom management.

Lifestyle

Lifestyle modifications are frequently recommended as therapy for GERD. Dietary recommendations such as eliminating fatty foods, spicy foods, citrus, alcohol, and chocolate have been commonly suggested based on their effects on the lower esophageal sphincter.

Table 9.1 Wellness therapies with some supportive evidence for various GI disorders

Gastroesophageal reflux disease

Lifestyle changes: weight loss, head-of-the-bed elevation, avoidance of late-night meals

Acupuncture

Functional dyspepsia

Peppermint/caraway oil combination

STW5

Acupuncture

Inflammatory bowel disease

Curcumin*

Acupuncture and moxibustion

Psychological therapies: CBT, mindfulness training

Exercise and yoga

Exclusive enteral nutrition**

VSL #3 Probiotic*

Irritable bowel syndrome

Low FODMAP diet

Soluble fiber

Peppermint oil

Probiotics

Psychological therapies: CBT, relaxation therapy, multicomponent psychological therapy, hypnotherapy, dynamic psychotherapy

Exercise

* Ulcerative colitis only
** Crohn's disease only

Table 9.2 Wellness therapies with insufficient supportive evidence for various GI disorders

Gastroesophageal reflux disease

Melatonin

High-quality patient–provider interactions

Breathing training

Functional dyspepsia

Red pepper powder

Artichoke leaf extract

Rikkunshito

Table 9.2 (cont.)

Inflammatory bowel disease
Wormwood*
Andrographis paniculata
Cannabis
Indigo naturalis
Wheatgrass
Hypnotherapy
Specific carbohydrate diet
Partial enteral nutrition
Irritable bowel syndrome
Gluten-free diet
STW5
Padma lax
Chinese herbal medicine

* Crohn's disease only

However, a systematic review failed to show that avoidance of these foods led to improved symptoms of GERD or pH testing [4]. Only weight loss and head-of-the-bed elevation proved to be effective treatments. Based on this evidence, most experts now recommend that patients avoid only the foods they have identified as triggers for their symptoms. A more recent review by Ness-Jensen et al. suggested avoidance of late-evening meals, smoking cessation, and dietary fiber may also be efficacious in improving GERD, based on small clinical trials and a large prospective cohort study [5].

Acupuncture

There is some evidence that acupuncture may be beneficial as an adjunctive therapy for GERD. In a study of patients with GERD who did not respond to single-dose proton pump inhibitor (PPI), 30 patients were randomized to receive either double-dose PPI or single-dose PPI plus acupuncture. The PPI-plus-acupuncture group showed significant improvement in daytime heartburn, nighttime heartburn, and acid regurgitation scores at the end of treatment. In contrast, the twice daily PPI group did not significantly change [6]. In addition, a meta-analysis of 12 studies found that patients treated with acupuncture along with traditional medicine had global symptom improvement compared to those receiving traditional medicine alone [7]. All of these studies should be interpreted with caution, however, as they are limited by lack of blinding for the acupuncture. Despite this shortcoming, given the low risk of serious adverse effects with acupuncture, this may be a reasonable option as adjunctive therapy to improve symptomatic response in patients with NERD.

Functional Dyspepsia

Functional dyspepsia is defined as one or more of the following symptoms: postprandial fullness, early satiation, epigastric pain and/or burning, which are unexplained after routine clinical evaluation [8]. Dyspepsia is common, accounting for 5 percent of all primary care visits, although most patients self-manage and do not seek medical care. The pathophysiology is poorly understood and likely multifactorial. Proposed mechanisms include delayed or accelerated gastric emptying, visceral hypersensitivity, impaired gastric accommodation, and psychological distress [9]. Given the heterogeneous nature of this disorder, it is difficult to treat and traditional Western medicine often does not offer satisfactory results, so many patients turn to alternative approaches. Treatments with the most evidence to support their use include combination therapy with peppermint and caraway oils, STW5, and acupuncture.

Peppermint/Caraway Oil

There have been a few randomized controlled trials (RCTs) that have shown benefits of a peppermint and caraway oil combination in functional dyspepsia. Peppermint and caraway oil are anti-spasmodics that block calcium channels, thereby leading to smooth muscle relaxation. In a double-blind RCT by Rich et al., 144 patients with functional dyspepsia received a peppermint and caraway oil preparation or a placebo for four weeks. In the treatment group, the average pain symptom score decreased by 62 percent, versus 26 percent in the control group ($p < 0.0001$). Significantly more patients in the treatment group (86 percent) had an improvement of at least 10 percent versus patients in the placebo group (57 percent). Similarly, the mean symptom score was reduced by 57 percent in the treatment group versus 20 percent in the placebo group [10]. In another study, by May et al., 96 patients with nonulcer dyspepsia were randomized to placebo versus a combination caraway oil and peppermint oil capsule for 29 days. The average pain intensity decreased significantly by 40 percent in the treatment group versus 22 percent in the placebo group. In particular, the sensations of pressure, heaviness, and fullness were improved in the treatment group versus placebo [11].

STW5

STW5 (Iberogast[R]) is a combination of nine herbal extracts. Although the exact mechanism of action in functional dyspepsia is unclear, potential mechanisms include effects on GI motility and microbiome, inhibition of inflammation, improvement of visceral hypersensitivity, and decreased gastric acid secretion. The largest study included 315 patients who received STW5 or placebo for eight weeks. Patients who received STW5 had significant improvement in GI symptom scores compared to placebo [12]. In addition, a meta-analysis including three RCTs pooled data to show that STW5 was significantly more effective than placebo at improving the severity of the most bothersome GI symptoms in patients with functional dyspepsia [13].

Acupuncture

There is some evidence that acupuncture may be beneficial in functional dyspepsia patients. The exact pathophysiology is unclear, but proposed mechanisms of action include acceleration of gastric emptying, improvement in gastric accommodation, decrease of visceral hypersensitivity, and modulation of the brain–gut axis. In a Cochrane review of acupuncture versus sham acupuncture for functional dyspepsia, acupuncture was shown to significantly decrease symptom scores and improve quality of life, although notably all included studies were low quality [14]. Ma et al. completed a larger RCT with 712 patients to assess the efficacy of acupuncture at specific and nonspecific sites versus sham acupuncture or a prokinetic medication for four weeks. All groups had improvement in dyspepsia symptoms and quality of life after 4 and 12 weeks. Overall response rate was significantly higher in the acupuncture groups and prokinetic group versus the sham acupuncture group. The highest response was in the group receiving acupuncture on specific points of the stomach meridian (71 percent) [15].

Inflammatory Bowel Diseases (IBD)

Ulcerative colitis (UC) and Crohn's disease (CD) are chronic inflammatory disorders of the gut characterized by immune system dysregulation. Since symptoms often do not correlate with mucosal inflammation, endoscopic remission is suggested as the goal of therapy. Ongoing active inflammation in IBD patients can lead to severe complications such as stricturing, bowel obstruction, perforation, or the development of colon cancer. Therefore, as of now, alternative approaches are typically considered to be adjunctive rather than primary management tools.

Curcumin

Curcumin is present in turmeric and has anti-inflammatory properties. In a study of 89 patients with quiescent UC, patients received mesalamine or sulfasalazine plus curcumin 1 g twice daily versus mesalamine or sulfasalazine plus placebo for six months. There was a significantly lower relapse rate in patients receiving curcumin (4.6 percent) versus placebo (20.5 percent) [16]. Additionally, there was a significant improvement in the clinical activity index and endoscopic index from baseline in the curcumin group. In contrast, the clinical activity index worsened and the endoscopic index was not significantly changed from baseline in the placebo group. Six months after the trial had ended, there was no significant difference in relapse rates between the two groups.

Another RCT included 50 patients with mild to moderately active UC despite mesalamine therapy [17]. Patients were treated with 3 g per day of curcumin plus mesalamine versus placebo plus mesalamine therapy for four weeks. In the curcumin group, 53 percent achieved remission at week 4 based on the Simple Clinical Colitis Activity Index, versus 0 percent in the placebo group. Significantly more patients in the curcumin group had a clinical response, achieved endoscopic remission, or achieved endoscopic improvement versus the placebo group.

Acupuncture and Moxibustion

There is some evidence that acupuncture may exert anti-inflammatory effects by inhibiting inflammatory cytokines and may therefore have some utility in the treatment of IBD. Ninety-two patients with mild to moderately active CD were randomized to herb-partitioned moxibustion plus acupuncture versus a control group of wheat bran-partitioned moxibustion with superficial acupuncture for 12 weeks [18]. Patients in the treatment group had significantly improved Crohn's Disease Activity Index scores, quality of life ratings, histopathological scores, increased hemoglobin, and decreased C-reactive protein (CRP) versus the control group. True assessment of endoscopic response is difficult to interpret as only selected patients received a colonoscopy and the protocol for taking biopsies was not clearly stated. It is also unclear if the endoscopist was blinded with respect to treatment group.

Another trial included 51 patients with mild to moderately active CD who received acupuncture or control treatment at non-acupuncture points for four weeks [19]. Patients in the traditional acupuncture group had a significant improvement in disease activity compared to the control group, but remission rates and changes in quality of life were not different between the groups. Endoscopic assessment was not performed.

A meta-analysis of 10 trials with UC patients suggested that acupuncture alone, moxibustion alone, or combined therapy was superior to oral sulfasalazine therapy for UC [20]. However, it is notable that the included studies had poor methodological quality.

Psychological Therapy

Cognitive-behavioral therapy and mindfulness interventions may improve quality of life in IBD patients, and may therefore be useful in combination with traditional therapy. A meta-analysis including 14 trials was performed to assess the effect of psychological therapy in IBD patients. The analysis concluded that psychological therapies, particularly cognitive-behavioral therapy, may improve quality of life and depression scores. However, there is not sufficient evidence to suggest a benefit for achieving remission, preventing relapse, or improving anxiety or stress in IBD patients [21]. Studies on mindfulness have shown similar results. A review that included eight studies evaluating mindfulness-based interventions in IBD concluded that mindfulness seemed to improve quality of life, anxiety, and depression [22]. There was no effect on disease activity, cytokine levels, or fecal calprotectin. Two of the studies showed an improvement in CRP in the mindfulness groups. An additional study suggested that psychological therapy may decrease healthcare utilization and sick days [23].

Exercise

It is difficult to determine the true impact of exercise in IBD as such studies cannot feasibly be blinded. One trial involved 30 patients with mild to moderate CD who were randomized to moderate-intensity running for 10 weeks versus no prescribed exercise [24]. Patients in the exercise group had significantly improved health-related quality of life compared to the control group. Another trial of 77 patients with UC randomized patients to weekly yoga versus written self-care advice for 12 weeks [25]. Disease-specific quality of life and clinical activity index were improved in the yoga group compared to the control group.

Diet

Diet may affect the microbiome and the immune system, and there is accumulating evidence suggesting that certain foods may modulate inflammation. Almost half of IBD patients have attempted some type of dietary therapy [26]. Exclusive enteral nutrition (EEN) has been shown to be effective in induction of remission in children with CD. Although EEN is equivalent to steroids for inducing remission in children with CD, a meta-analysis showed that corticosteroids were superior to EEN in adults [27]. For this reason, EEN is only recommended as induction therapy for adult patients with CD in whom steroids are contraindicated. There is not sufficient evidence to suggest that EEN is effective in the treatment of UC.

Probiotics

The pathogenesis of IBD is not completely understood, but there is some supporting evidence that the disease process may involve gut dysbiosis. Probiotics have therefore been proposed as a potential treatment for IBD. A meta-analysis that included 23 RCTs with 1763 patients suggested that probiotics may help induce and maintain remission in patients with UC and may prevent clinical relapse in patients with pouchitis [28]. Subgroup analysis suggested that VSL#3^R was the only probiotic that was efficacious. However, it is notable that none of the trials in UC patients assessed endoscopic relapse. Since symptoms do not always correlate with endoscopic findings, the role of probiotics in improving endoscopic findings or preventing the development of active inflammation remains unclear. There is insufficient evidence to suggest that probiotics are efficacious for the treatment of CD.

Irritable Bowel Syndrome (IBS)

Irritable bowel syndrome is a chronic disorder in which patients report abdominal pain and a change in defecation pattern. Most patients with IBS associate their symptoms with particular food item intake and they often limit their dietary options without a clear plan or evidence that such changes are useful.

Low FODMAP Diet

One of the most popular and well-studied diets for IBS is the low fermentable oligosaccharides, disaccharides, monosaccharides, and polyols (FODMAP) diet. FODMAPs are poorly absorbed carbohydrates that induce osmotic effects and undergo fermentation to produce gas, therefore leading to luminal distention and symptoms. Multiple meta-analyses evaluating the low FODMAP diet in IBS patients suggest it may be efficacious, particularly for abdominal pain and bloating. However, once again, the quality of evidence is low. One recent meta-analysis included 9 RCTs using various control groups such as Western diet, habitual diet, and high FODMAP diet. The authors found that low FODMAP diet improved GI symptoms, abdominal pain, and health-related quality of life [29]. Another meta-analysis included 7 RCTs with similar control groups and found that low FODMAP diet reduced global IBS symptoms [30]. It is difficult to perform blinding with dietary interventions, which limits the rigorousness of these trials.

Fiber

Increasing fiber is often used as first-line therapy in IBS patients. Fiber is typically classified into two groups: soluble and insoluble. Soluble fiber dissolves in water to form a gel, and can be found in foods such as oat bran, barley, nuts, and psyllium. Insoluble fibers, such as wheat bran, corn bran, and various vegetables, add bulk to the stool and do not dissolve in water. There is evidence that soluble fiber may be beneficial in IBS patients. One controlled trial to assess the effect of fiber intake on IBS patients included 275 patients with IBS who were randomized to 10 g of psyllium, bran, or placebo for 12 weeks [31]. Patients in the psyllium group had significantly decreased IBS symptom severity score versus the placebo group. The group that received bran did not have any benefit versus placebo. Similarly, a meta-analysis including 14 RCTs and 906 patients with IBS also concluded that soluble fiber was an effective treatment for IBS. Insoluble fiber was not found to be effective [32].

Peppermint Oil

Several RCTs and meta-analyses have reported a benefit of peppermint oil for IBS. Peppermint oil contains menthol, which works as an analgesic and reduces smooth muscle contractility of the gut. A recent meta-analysis including 12 RCTs with 835 patients suggested that peppermint oil improves both abdominal pain and global symptoms in IBS patients [33].

Probiotics

Multiple studies have assessed the efficacy of different probiotics in IBS. A large meta-analysis by Ford et al. included 53 RCTs of probiotics with 5545 patients. The authors concluded that combinations of probiotics seemed to be beneficial for overall IBS symptoms and abdominal pain. Despite this evidence for an overall benefit, there is not yet enough data to make a conclusion regarding which specific combinations or species should be recommended [34].

Psychological Therapies

Irritable bowel syndrome seems to be a heterogeneous disease and the exact pathophysiology remains unclear, although there is some suggestion that dysregulation of the brain–gut axis may be involved. Anxiety and depression are more common in IBS patients than controls, and various studies have shown that psychological therapies may provide some benefit in IBS patients. A meta-analysis from 2019 included 36 RCTs comparing various psychological therapies in IBS [35]. The authors found that cognitive-behavioral therapy, relaxation therapy, multicomponent psychological therapy, hypnotherapy, and dynamic psychotherapy were all beneficial when data was pooled. Out of all the therapies, cognitive-behavioral therapy and relaxation training were the most studied, with the highest number of trials evaluating these therapies.

Exercise

Physical activity is an effective therapy for multiple diseases, including fibromyalgia (FM) and depression, and there is some evidence that exercise is beneficial for IBS patients as well. Given that physical activity promotes colonic motility, exercise may be particularly beneficial in patients with constipation-predominant IBS. In an RCT of 102 patients with IBS, patients increased physical activity as instructed by a physiotherapist or maintained their normal lifestyle for 12 weeks. The group with increased physical activity had significant improvement of the overall IBS score and there were significantly fewer patients who had increased severity of IBS symptoms in the physical activity group [36]. Multiple studies have addressed the effect of yoga specifically on IBS symptoms, and while results have been somewhat mixed, the two largest controlled studies suggested a benefit of yoga for IBS symptoms and quality of life [37, 38].

Conclusion

Many herbal and "mind–body" therapies have been evaluated for various GI disorders. Numerous trials using these approaches have been published, but tend to be of low quality. Either a small number of subjects used and/or difficulty in blinding the subjects in therapies such as exercise and acupuncture are significant problems. A true assessment of efficacy is difficult to obtain. However, some therapies are low risk and could be recommended since they may provide the patient with some benefit.

If "wellness" is the goal, then low-risk options become potentially useful resources in improving symptoms and related concerns. Furthermore, patient participation in both choosing the options and then actively consuming an agent and/or participating in an activity can reduce anxiety and subsequently encourage the patient's participation in the healing process. Though no one therapeutic approach is likely to help all patients, informed dialog with the provider on these topics will encourage self-awareness and hopefully motivate the patient to be active in their healthcare.

References

1. A Hung, N Kang, A Bollom, JL Wolf, JE Lembo. A complementary and alternative medicine use is prevalent among patients with gastrointestinal diseases. *Dig Dis Sci* 2015; **60**: 1883–1888.

2. JE Richter, JH Rubenstein. Presentation and epidemiology of gastroesophageal reflux disease. *Gastroenterology* 2018; **154**: 267–276.

3. N Vakil, SV van Zanten, P Kahrilas, et al. The Montreal definition and classification of gastroesophageal reflux disease: a global, evidence-based consensus paper. *Z Gastroenterol* 2007; **45**: 1125–1140.

4. T Kaltenbach, S Crockett, LB Gerson. Are lifestyle measures effective in patients with gastroesophageal reflux disease? An evidence-based approach. *Arch Intern Med* 2006; **166**: 965–971.

5. E Ness-Jensen, K Hveem, H El-Serag, J Lagergren. Lifestyle intervention in gastroesophageal reflux disease. *Clin Gastroenterol Hepatol* 2016; **14**: 175–182. e1-3.

6. R Dickman, E Schiff, A Holland, et al. Clinical trial: acupuncture vs. doubling the proton pump inhibitor dose in refractory heartburn. *Aliment Pharmacol Ther* 2007; **26**: 1333–1344.

7. J Zhu, Y Guo, S Liu, et al. Acupuncture for the treatment of gastro-oesophageal reflux disease: a systematic review and meta-analysis. *Acupunct Med* 2017; **35**: 316–323.

8. V Stanghellini, FK Chan, WL Hasler, et al. Gastroduodenal disorders. *Gastroenterology* 2016; **150**: 1380–1392.

9. M Camilleri, V Stanghellini. Current management strategies and emerging treatments for functional dyspepsia. *Nat Rev Gastroenterol Hepatol* 2013; **10**: 187–194.

10. G Rich, A Shah, N Koloski, et al. A randomized placebo-controlled trial on the effects of Menthacarin, a proprietary peppermint- and caraway-oil-preparation, on symptoms and quality of life in patients with functional dyspepsia. *Neurogastroenterol Motil* 2017; **29**.

11. B May, S Köhler, B Schneider. Efficacy and tolerability of a fixed combination of peppermint oil and caraway oil in patients suffering from functional dyspepsia. *Aliment Pharmacol Ther* 2000; **14**: 1671–1677.

12. U von Arnim, U Peitz, B Vinson, KJ Gundermann, P Malfertheiner. STW 5, a phytopharmacon for patients with functional dyspepsia: results of a multicenter, placebo-controlled double-blind study. *Am J Gastroenterol* 2007; **102**: 1268–1275.

13. J Melzer, W Rösch, J Reichling, R Brignoli, R Saller. Meta-analysis: phytotherapy of functional dyspepsia with the herbal drug preparation STW 5 (Iberogast). *Aliment Pharmacol Ther* 2004; **20**: 1279–1287.

14. L Lan, F Zeng, GJ Liu, et al. Acupuncture for functional dyspepsia. *Cochrane Database Syst Rev* 2014; **10**: CD008487.

15. TT Ma, SY Yu, Y Li, et al. Randomised clinical trial: an assessment of acupuncture on specific meridian or specific acupoint vs. sham acupuncture for treating functional dyspepsia. *Aliment Pharmacol Ther* 2012; **35**: 552–561.

16. H Hanai, T Iida, K Takeuchi, et al. Curcumin maintenance therapy for ulcerative colitis: randomized, multicenter, double-blind, placebo-controlled trial. *Clin Gastroenterol Hepatol* 2006; **4**: 1502–1506.

17. A Lang, N Salomon, JC Wu, et al. Curcumin in combination with mesalamine induces remission in patients with mild-to-moderate ulcerative colitis in a randomized controlled trial. *Clin Gastroenterol Hepatol* 2015; **13**: 1444–1449.e1.

18. CH Bao, JM Zhao, HR Liu, et al. Randomized controlled trial: moxibustion and acupuncture for the treatment of Crohn's disease. *World J Gastroenterol* 2014; **20**: 11000–11011.

19. S Joos, B Brinkhaus, C Maluche, et al. Acupuncture and moxibustion in the treatment of active Crohn's disease: a randomized controlled study. *Digestion* 2004; **69**: 131–139.

20. J Ji, Y Lu, H Liu, et al. Acupuncture and moxibustion for inflammatory bowel diseases: a systematic review and meta-analysis of randomized controlled trials. *Evid Based Complement Alternat Med* 2013; **2013**: 158352.

21. DJ Gracie, AJ Irvine, R Sood, et al. Effect of psychological therapy on disease activity, psychological comorbidity, and quality of life in inflammatory bowel disease: a systematic review and meta-analysis. *Lancet Gastroenterol Hepatol* 2017; **2**: 189–199.

22. MM Hood, S Jedel. Mindfulness-based interventions in inflammatory bowel disease. *Gastroenterol Clin North Am* 2017; **46**: 859–874.

23. HC Deter, W Keller, J von Wietersheim, et al. Psychological treatment may reduce the need for healthcare in patients with Crohn's disease. *Inflamm Bowel Dis* 2007; **13**: 745–752.

24. P Klare, J Nigg, J Nold, et al. The impact of a ten-week physical exercise program on health-related quality of life in patients with inflammatory bowel disease: a prospective randomized controlled trial. *Digestion* 2015; **91**: 239–247.

25. H Cramer, M Schafer, M Schols, et al. Randomised clinical trial: yoga vs written self-care advice for ulcerative colitis. *Alimentary Pharmacol Therapeut* 2017; **45**: 1379–1389.

26. S Kakodkar, EA Mutlu. Diet as a therapeutic option for adult inflammatory bowel disease. *Gastroenterol Clin North Am* 2017; **46**: 745–767.

27. M Zachos, M Tondeur, AM Griffiths. Enteral nutritional therapy for induction of remission in Crohn's disease. *Cochrane Database Syst Rev* 2007; **4**: CD000542.

28. J Shen, ZX Zuo, AP Mao. Effect of probiotics on inducing remission and maintaining therapy in ulcerative colitis, Crohn's disease, and pouchitis: meta-analysis of randomized controlled trials. *Inflamm Bowel Dis* 2014; **20**: 21–35.

29. D Schumann, P Klose, R Lauche, et al. Low fermentable, oligo-, di-, mono-saccharides and polyol diet in the treatment of irritable bowel syndrome: a systematic review and meta-analysis. *Nutrition* 2018; **45**: 24–31.

30. J Dionne, AC Ford, Y Yuan, et al. A systematic review and meta-analysis evaluating the efficacy of a gluten-free diet and a low FODMAPs diet in treating symptoms of irritable bowel syndrome. *Am J Gastroenterol* 2018; **113**: 1290–1300.

31. CJ Bijkerk, NJ de Wit, JW Muris, et al. Soluble or insoluble fibre in irritable bowel syndrome in primary care? Randomised placebo controlled trial. *BMJ* 2009; **339**: b3154.

32. P Moayyedi, EM Quigley, BE Lacy, et al. The effect of fiber supplementation on irritable bowel syndrome: a systematic review and meta-analysis. *Am J Gastroenterol* 2014; **109**: 1367–1374.

33. N Alammar, L Wang, B Saberi, et al. The impact of peppermint oil on the irritable bowel syndrome: a meta-analysis of the pooled clinical data. *BMC Complement Altern Med* 2019; **19**: 21.

34. AC Ford, LA Harris, BE Lacy, EMM Quigley, P Moayyedi. Systematic review with meta-analysis: the efficacy of prebiotics, probiotics, synbiotics and

antibiotics in irritable bowel syndrome. *Aliment Pharmacol Ther* 2018; **48**: 1044–1060.

35. AC Ford, BE Lacy, LA Harris, EMM Quigley, P Moayyedi. Effect of antidepressants and psychological therapies in irritable bowel syndrome: an updated systematic review and meta-analysis. *Am J Gastroenterol* 2019; **114**: 21–39.

36. E Johannesson, M Simrén, H Strid, A Bajor, R Sadik. Physical activity improves symptoms in irritable bowel syndrome: a randomized controlled trial. *Am J Gastroenterol* 2011; **106**: 915–922.

37. V Kavuri, P Selvan, A Malamud, N Raghuram, S Selvan. Remedial yoga module remarkably improves symptoms in irritable bowel syndrome patients: a 12-week randomized controlled trial. *Eur J Integrative Med* 2015; **7**: 595–608.

38. S Evans, KC Lung, LC Seidman, et al. Iyengar yoga for adolescents and young adults with irritable bowel syndrome. *J Pediatr Gastroenterol Nutr* 2014; **59**: 244–253.

Wellness and the Genito-Urinary System

Karyn S. Eilber and Una J. Lee

Introduction

The focus of this chapter about the genito-urinary (GU) system is evidence-based information on how to support health and wellness of the urinary system in general, as well as during recovery from a urologic condition. It is widely accepted that diet, exercise, lifestyle, and behavior affect overall health by impacting organ systems. The impact of wellness medicine on the GU tract is less recognized and less robustly studied, but the principles remain important and impactful. This chapter will discuss: bladder health, including overactive bladder, urinary incontinence, and urinary tract infections; sexual health; prostate health, including benign prostatic hyperplasia and prostate cancer; and kidney health, including kidney stones.

Bladder Health

Bladder health is a key component of one's overall health. Bladder health has recently been defined by a National Institutes of Health (NIH) transdisciplinary research team as "A complete state of physical, mental, and social well-being related to bladder function, and not merely the absence of lower urinary tract symptoms"[1]. Healthy bladder function permits daily activities, adapts to stressors, and allows travel, exercise, social, and occupational activities. The strength of this definition is the incorporation of the physical, environmental, social, economic, and psychological aspects of bladder health, which have previously not been recognized as critical determinants of bladder health.

General Bladder Health

Voiding Habits

Voiding frequency is related to many contributing factors, including responsiveness to normal or abnormal physiologic sensations, fluid intake, habits, opportunity to void, fear of leakage, and others [2]. The bladder is designed to fill, store, and empty urine on a regular basis and when socially acceptable.

Some people may have adopted dysfunctional voiding behavior such as bearing down to void and/or failing to relax the pelvic floor. Many women also report hovering over public toilets to avoid contact for hygiene purposes [3]. Men and women also report situational awareness, including challenges when traveling and voiding in public places [4]. Healthy voiding includes a relaxed position for voiding, relaxation of the pelvic floor, and allowing time to allow the bladder to empty adequately [2].

Physical Activity

High levels of exercise have been associated with less nighttime voiding, as well as lower blood levels of an inflammation marker [5]. Physical activity has also been inversely related to urinary incontinence in women, and is beneficial for men with lower urinary tract symptoms related to benign prostatic hyperplasia (BPH). There is some evidence that high-impact competitive sports such as gymnastics are associated with pelvic floor muscle changes, including urinary incontinence in women.

Nutrition

High-quality nutrition has been shown to be associated with less bothersome urinary symptoms, including nocturia [6]. Dietary intake has a potentially powerful effect on preventing disease, supporting urinary anatomy and function, and improving bothersome urinary symptoms. While there is a great deal of information on diet and nutrition in general, there is limited evidence specifically promoting bladder and/or urinary health in the absence of disease. Some nutritional recommendations are targeted to prevent urinary infections, prevent cancer, or alleviate urinary pain or symptoms. Principles of nutrition that target pain pathways, decrease inflammation, and support bowel health will in turn support urinary health.

Bladder Cancer

Cigarette smoking is a strong risk factor for bladder cancer. Smokers have a three times greater risk of bladder cancer, and this risk increases with age and with duration of smoking. Smoking cessation decreases the risk of bladder cancer, and it is important to counsel smokers on these risks to promote lifelong bladder health.

Occupational carcinogenic exposures associated with bladder cancer were highest among workers exposed to aromatic amines (tobacco, dye, and rubber workers; hairdressers before the 1980s; printers; and leather workers) and polycyclic aromatic hydrocarbons (PAHs) (chimney sweeps, nurses, waiters, aluminum workers, seamen, and oil/petroleum workers) [7]. While occupational contact is long-term exposure, it stands to reason that one should limit exposure to potentially carcinogenic substances to avoid the development of an unhealthy bladder.

Overactive Bladder

Overactive bladder (OAB) is a prevalent and costly urinary condition that impairs the quality of life of women and men of all ages. Overactive bladder is a diagnosis based on symptoms in the absence of obvious pathology. The hallmark of OAB is urinary urgency with or without associated urinary incontinence. "Urgency" is the strong, overwhelming sensation to urinate that cannot be delayed and may interfere with one's daily activities and is different from "urge," which is the non-pathologic sensory messaging signaling the need to urinate. Urgency is often accompanied by bothersome urinary frequency and urgency incontinence.

Behavioral Modification for OAB

Fluid Management

If one has overactive bladder symptoms, the first step is to examine one's fluid intake. Increased fluid intake is associated with urinary frequency. Correspondingly, when one decreases fluid intake by 25 percent, frequency decreases by 23 percent, urgency by 34 percent, and nocturia by 7 percent [8]. A voiding diary can help identify patterns and quantify intake. The type of fluid also correlates with urinary symptoms.

Caffeine

Beverages containing caffeine can aggravate OAB. Caffeine causes urgency and frequency through diuresis, and increased flow rate and voided volumes. Caffeine also decreases the threshold at which a sensation is felt when filling the bladder, promoting the sensation of urgency [9]. Caffeine has also been shown to increase the excitability of the urinary bladder by inducing transient contractions of smooth muscle [10]. One study found that high caffeine intake (> 400 mg/dl) was associated with uncontrolled contractions of the bladder, compared to moderate intake (100–400 mg/day), so moderation or elimination is key when bothersome OAB symptoms are present.

Alcohol

Alcohol promotes urinary urgency and frequency by acting as a diuretic, causing dehydration, and interfering with the signaling involved with micturition. High alcohol consumption has been positively associated with moderate to severe bothersome urinary symptoms in men.

Weight Loss

Obesity (BMI > 30 kg/m^2) has been independently associated with OAB and urinary incontinence in various patient populations. Studies have demonstrated the positive impact of even modest weight loss (5 percent of total body weight) on bothersome OAB symptoms [11]. Sharing the information that modest weight loss can improve urinary symptoms can be motivating for patients who desire to both lose weight and improve their bladder health.

Bladder Training

Bladder training has been shown to be an effective intervention for OAB symptoms. Bladder training requires motivation and commitment by the patient and can break the cycle of frequent voiding through increasing the time between voids. Women are encouraged to inhibit the urge to urinate by either distraction, positive affirmation, or pelvic floor contraction (see "urge suppression" in the next section).

Pelvic Floor Muscle Therapy

"Kegel exercises" refers to identifying, contracting, and strengthening pelvic floor muscles. Contraction of the pelvic floor muscles is a key component of "urge suppression" and management of urinary incontinence. The functional application of these contractions to suppress urgency and/or incontinence is critical to successful bladder training. The efficacy of pelvic floor muscle therapy is well-established and is most effective when integrated in combination with behavioral modifications. Additionally, the instruction of a trained pelvic floor physical therapist has been shown to enhance the effectiveness of the intervention through individualized structured therapy.

Mindfulness

A positive correlation exists between psychological stress levels and OAB. There is demonstrated benefit of mindfulness as a treatment modality for bladder symptoms. Mindfulness-based stress reduction has been shown to reduce urge incontinence episodes after an eight-week program. A similar study demonstrated a decrease in urge incontinence episodes with mindfulness-based stress reduction after up to one year of follow-up [12, 13]. Another study showed the benefit of the mind over the bladder. Older women living independently in a retirement community were subjectively improved with an educational intervention to self-manage urinary incontinence through mindfulness, bladder diaries, and bladder health education [14].

Psychological Health

There is an important connection between the bladder/pelvic floor and psychological health. A history of GU trauma or abuse is prevalent in patients with pelvic floor dysfunction. There may be a level of shame, stress, pain, and/or dysfunction associated with this intimate GU area of the body, so it may help to counsel patients with sensitivity and acknowledge this mind–pelvic area connection.

Urinary Tract Infections

Urinary tract infections (UTIs) are a prevalent and costly healthcare problem, estimated to cost more than $2.47 billion per year [15] and to be responsible for 8.1 million visits to healthcare providers annually. They are the second most common type of infection, with 40 percent of women and 12 percent of men experiencing at least one UTI in their lifetime [16].

The current definition of UTI relies on laboratory and clinical findings, but we now have a deeper knowledge of the urinary microbiome [17]. Contrary to popular belief, current evidence demonstrates that urine is not sterile [18]; the urinary tract hosts a complex, generally beneficial microbiome. Gene-sequencing techniques have identified a ubiquitous, diverse community of bacterial species in the urinary tract that cannot be cultured using standard techniques [19]. Currently, a positive urine culture in the presence of acute dysuria is treated with a course of antibiotics and is considered the standard of care. But there is data that challenges this dogma.

It is possible for acute urinary symptoms to resolve without a course of antibiotics [20], and it is uncommon for a lower urinary tract infection to cause serious illness [21]. Bacteriuria and urinary symptoms are common entities that often occur together and have the potential to resolve spontaneously. Neither is strongly linked to serious urinary tract disease, and there are appreciable risks, benefits, and alternatives for antibiotic treatment, given the specific situation and patient group.

One of the key areas in the evaluation and treatment of urinary symptoms is discriminating between asymptomatic bacteriuria and symptomatic UTI [22]. Urinary symptoms are certainly real to patients, and a source of concern and distress. Urinary symptoms can occur in the presence of significant bacteriuria or without. Dysuria is considered central to the diagnosis of a UTI. Urine odor, debris, cloudiness, or discoloration are not reliable signs of a UTI. Urine is a bodily waste product and varies in appearance and odor according to many contributing factors. The opportunity within healthcare encounters to have thorough, informed-consent discussions on the risks, benefits, and alternatives to antibiotic treatment for symptomatic and/ or asymptomatic bacteriuria would likely decrease overuse and overtreatment of antibiotics. In the setting of mild urinary symptoms, consideration should be given to treatment with analgesics, hydration, and rest, and the symptomatic episode may resolve on its own.

When women see healthcare providers, they often want to know *why* they are getting UTIs or recurrent UTIs. Some women have a vulnerability to UTIs due to many factors, including sexual activity, biologic factors, as well as external factors. Their UTIs may or may not be related to a behavior or to hygiene. It is important not to speak to women with UTIs in a way that can be interpreted as condescending or critical, as this can lead to self-blame and even measures of extreme hygiene that can strip the GU tract of its natural defenses. Counseling patients in a patient-centered manner on the pathophysiology of UTIs is important for a patient's greater understanding of the condition.

Alternative Treatments for Prevention of UTI

Various non-antimicrobial treatments for prevention of UTIs have theoretical benefit and minimal risk (Table 10.1) and are highly utilized by women with UTI and UTI-like symptoms; however, herbal supplements are not regulated by the Food and Drug Administration (FDA), and therefore there is no guarantee of strength, safety, or purity. Clinical evidence for non-antimicrobial prevention of urinary tract infections is limited and sometimes conflicting. Safety, efficacy, cost, and biologic plausibility should be taken into account, and an individual can choose what they feel best supports their urinary health.

Water

Increased water intake is generally a safe, inexpensive, and effective method of reducing UTIs and maintaining bladder health. One recent randomized controlled trial assigned healthy premenopausal female participants with a history of three or more UTIs in the past year and self-reported drinking of less than 1.5 liters daily to drink an additional 1.5 liters of water daily versus no additional water over a one-year time period. The water-drinking group had

Table 10.1 Non-microbial treatment options for recurrent urinary tract infection: theoretical benefit, minimal harm, and limited clinical data

Treatment	Dosage*
Vaginal estrogen	Applied vaginally twice weekly at night
Cranberry	36 mg proanthocyanidin (PAC) orally daily (1–3 capsules/tablets depending on formulation)
Probiotics/ Lactobacillus	Intravaginal lactin-V probiotic five days, then once per week; 10^9 CFU L. rhamunosus or L. reuteri orally twice daily
Vitamin C	Doses range from 100 mg to 2000 mg orally daily
Methenamine	Methenamine mandelate or methenamine hippurate 1 g orally bid
D-mannose	2 g of D-mannose powder daily
Acupuncture	Treatment consisted of insertion of needles and obtaining of *deqi* (a sensation described as numbness, heaviness, and distention). Acupuncture points were chosen according to the patient's traditional Chinese medicine diagnosis. Points were located on the lower abdomen or back or on the lower extremities. Treatments were twice weekly for four weeks.
Vaccine therapy	Not currently commercially available

*Dosages listed are based on available clinical trial data, but many alternative doses exist.

a 50 percent reduction in cystitis episodes, 50 percent fewer antibiotics, and longer time between cystitis episodes [23]. It should be noted that this research was supported by Danone Research, France, which sells Evian bottled water. The benefit of increased water intake is thought to be through dilution and flushing of bacteriuria, thereby reducing attachment to urothelial cells, reducing nutrients for growth, and improving clearance. The Institute of Medicine recommends a daily water intake from fluids of 2.2 liters [24].

Estrogen

Vaginal estrogen has been associated with colonization of the vagina with *Lactobacillus*, which is protective against UTIs. Menopause, with the associated change in vaginal pH and flora, increases the risk of UTIs. A 1999 study compared an estradiol-releasing silicone vaginal ring to no treatment; women treated with vaginal estrogen were found to have a decreased number of recurrent urinary tract infections and a longer time between infections [25]. A 2008 Cochrane systematic review demonstrated vaginal estrogen to be safe and effective in the prevention of recurrent UTIs in postmenopausal women, whereas oral estrogen is not effective for UTI prevention [26].

Probiotics

Studies have examined the use of *Lactobacilli*, either orally or vaginally, to prevent UTIs. The use of *Lactobacillus crispatus* intravaginal suppository works to prevent recurrence of UTIs by replenishing naturally occurring bacteria, as shown by phase II randomized clinical trial data. A 2015 Cochrane review [27] showed no benefit for probiotics compared with placebo or no treatment in UTI prevention, but a benefit cannot be ruled out as the data were limited and based on small studies with poor methodological reporting. At this time, there is no FDA-approved vaginal probiotic available in the USA. The role of oral probiotics in prevention of UTIs has no significant supporting evidence, but people do take them for the theoretical benefit.

Cranberry

Cranberry has been used for centuries in the treatment of urinary conditions. The proanthocyanidin (PAC) of cranberry inhibits adherence of *Escherichia coli* uropathogens to urothelial cells [28]. Proanthocyanidin does not eradicate bacteria, but rather inhibits the first step in the infection process. Prophylactic efficacy of various cranberry products (juices, cranberry powders enriched with PACs, extracts, and capsules) has been largely uncharacterized in terms of chemical composition, making it difficult to assess their bioefficacy [29]. In a 2012 Cochrane review, four of five studies (with a combined total of 594 participants) provided data that could be combined in a meta-analysis specific to the population of women with recurrent UTIs [30–33]. This meta-analysis showed a small, non-statistically significant reduction in risk of repeat symptomatic UTI with cranberry treatment compared to placebo or no treatment.

One of the limitations of the current body of clinical studies of non-juice cranberry products is the lack of reporting of the amount of active ingredients in the tablets or capsules. The effective dose of cranberry products and the variability in patient populations studied likely contribute to the inconsistency of the clinical data [34]. The level of PAC varies in cranberry products on the market, and the amount of the active ingredient is not regulated. In general, risks of using cranberry supplements are minimal; some can be associated with gastrointestinal distress and cranberry juice often has high levels of sugar. The 2012 Cochrane review analysis showed no benefit in most population groups, with a small benefit is some subgroups, whereas a 2012 meta-analysis found a reduction in urinary infections [35, 36]. It is important to be educated on the nuances of the data on cranberry so individuals can utilize this natural option if they desire at its full potency.

Alternative Botanical Supplements

Alternative botanical therapies most commonly used in UTI prevention include *Vaccinium macrocarpon* (cranberry), cranberry–lingonberry, berberine sulfate (a plant alkaloid), and the herb uva ursi (bearberry leaf). There is an array of other home remedies and supplements that patients may use, but many lack clear scientific evidence.

Vitamin C

Ascorbic acid (vitamin C) acidifies the urine, which theoretically has a bacteriostatic effect. However, strong clinical data supporting this intervention is not available.

Methenamine

Methenamine is an "antiseptic" medication that hydrolyzes ammonia and formaldehyde in acidic urine, thus acting as a potent bactericidal agent. This medication, which is not an antibiotic, has been prescribed for over 100 years and is well tolerated, with a low rate of adverse events (less than 4 percent report nausea or diarrhea). Methenamine has been shown to be effective in suppressing recurrent UTIs in two placebo-controlled trials in women with recurrent cystitis [37]. This FDA-approved prescription medication is a viable non-antibiotic option in the prevention of UTIs.

D-mannose

The mechanism of action of D-mannose is inhibition of uropathogenic *E. coli* (UPEC) adherence to urothelial cells. Uropathogenic *E. coli* is the primary cause of UTIs. D-mannose appears to be more effective *in vitro* or when introduced directly into the bladder. Higher dosages required to achieve an *in vivo* effect may be associated with pre-diabetic conditions. There are limited clinical studies, and further investigation is needed.

Acupuncture

Clinical studies are limited but show some potential. In one 2002 study, half as many UTI episodes per person-month occurred in the acupuncture group compared to the control group. Stimulation of the posterior tibial nerve, which is a known treatment for OAB, may explain the improvement in symptoms.

Vaccine Therapy

The development of a safe and effective systemic or vaginal vaccine to prevent recurrent UTIs would be an important breakthrough. Uropathogenic *E. coli* strains utilize structural and secreted virulence factors that contribute to their capacity to cause disease, although the adherence of the *E. coli* bacteria to the host epithelial cells is the most important factor. These vaccines target these biological mechanisms. Investigational studies have been conducted, but currently no licensed vaccine is available.

Chinese Herbal Medicines

Chinese herbal medicines (CHMs) have been used to treat UTI symptoms for over 2000 years. The biological plausibility of CHMs is supported by *in vitro* research suggesting that some Chinese herbs may have diuretic, antibiotic, immune-enhancing, antipyretic, anti-inflammatory, and pain-relieving effects. A 2015 Cochrane review [38] found limited evidence from seven randomized controlled trials on the possible role of CHMs as a treatment for recurrent UTIs, either as the sole intervention or as an adjunct to antibiotic treatment for postmenopausal women.

Urinary Symptoms in the Absence of a UTI

Individuals can experience symptoms that seem exactly *like* a bladder infection but are *not* caused by bacteria. Symptoms like urgency, frequency, burning, urinary pain, or discomfort can be due to other causes, such as inflammation or irritation of the urinary tract and/or vaginal atrophy. Increased sensitivity of the nerves that inhabit the urethra and bladder can occur when bladder irritants such as caffeine or alcohol, sexual activity, dehydration, and stress occur, or it can simply happen spontaneously.

When these UTI-like episodes occur, the strategy is to support the body and immune system so that it can heal from this inflammatory process: increasing hydration, getting adequate amounts of restorative high-quality sleep, eating nourishing foods, managing one's stress, and avoiding activities that are irritating to this sensitive area of the body. Avoiding unnecessary antibiotics will help decrease the unwanted side effects and impact on one's microbiome. Understanding the delicate balance and function of microorganisms is important for maintaining our body's natural defenses.

Sexual Health

The World Health Organization partially defines sexual health as "a state of physical, emotional, mental and social well-being in relation to sexuality; it is not merely the absence of disease, dysfunction or infirmity" [39]. On the contrary, sexual dysfunction is when an individual or couple's normal sexual activity is negatively impacted over 75 percent of the time for a minimum of six months' duration and it causes significant distress [40]. Sexual dysfunction is more prevalent for women (43 percent) than men (31 percent) and is more likely to occur in the presence of poor physical and emotional health [40, 41]. Furthermore, sexual health contributes to wellness and quality of life, with 62.2 percent of male and 42.8 percent of female US adults attributing a high importance of sexual health for quality of life [42].

The evaluation and management of sexual dysfunction must be patient-centered, unbiased, and non-judgmental. Clinicians must respect the patient's concerns, sexual preferences, and expectations in order to provide the best treatment and maximize positive outcomes as impaired sexual health can have significant negative effects on quality of life and overall health and wellness.

Female Sexual Dysfunction

Female Sexual Interest/Arousal Disorder

Female sexual interest/arousal disorder is a condition in which there is a deficiency or absence of sexual interest, thoughts, or fantasies resulting in a failure to initiate or respond to sexual activity [40]. This condition was previously referred to as hypoactive sexual desire disorder (HSDD). It is the most common female sexual disorder and affects 8.9 percent of women aged 18–44 years, 12.3 percent aged 45–64, and 7.4 percent over age 65 [43]. The disorder is further categorized into general (present with any partner or situation) versus situational (present only with a specific partner or situation). Treatment is aimed at any identifiable underlying disorder and includes education, modification of influencing factors, sex therapy (behavioral and cognitive therapy), hormonal therapy, and/or the addition or discontinuation of medications that affect the central nervous system [44].

Loss of sexual interest commonly occurs after menopause, and hormone replacement therapy should be considered for women in a postmenopausal state. In general, systemic estrogen replacement improves symptoms of vulvovaginal atrophy such as vaginal dryness, and it has been shown to improve vaginal lubrication as well as sexual desire [45]. Although it is used "off-label," current data supports the use of transdermal testosterone replacement with or without concomitant estrogen replacement for the treatment of HSDD as important for libido, arousal, genital sensation, and orgasm [45, 46]. Phosphodiesterase inhibitors (sildenafil) have not been shown to have a significant effect on improving female sexual dysfunction [47].

Flibanserin is the only medication approved by the FDA indicated for HSDD in premenopausal women. It is a serotonin agonist/antagonist that increases dopamine and norepinephrine while decreasing serotonin [48, 49]. The combination of increased dopamine and norepinephrine levels with decreased serotonin promotes sexual desire. In clinical trials, flibanserin has been shown to increase the number of satisfying sexual events; however, it has significant side effects, including insomnia, somnolence, and dizziness, and when combined with alcohol has significant risk of hypotension and syncope [50, 51].

Female Orgasmic Disorder

Female orgasmic disorder is the difficulty or inability for a woman to achieve orgasm during sexual stimulation when this causes distress and/or interpersonal difficulty [40]. It is the second most common female sexual disorder, with prevalence estimates of 4–7 percent in the general population and 5–42 percent in the primary care setting [52]. This condition can be lifelong (woman has never had an orgasm) or acquired (woman has difficulty reaching orgasm although orgasm has been attained before), is not secondary to an obvious medical condition or substance, and can be generalized versus situational.

Female orgasmic disorder can be treated with cognitive-behavioral therapy, sensate focus, and directed masturbation [53, 54]. Success rates for sex therapy range from 65 to 85 percent, with younger, emotionally healthy women in a loving relationship portending a better prognosis [55].

Genito-Pelvic Pain/Penetration Disorder

Genito-pelvic pain/penetration disorder (GPPPD) is a new diagnosis in the DSM-5 that encompasses the previously individual diagnoses of vaginismus and dyspareunia. The diagnosis of GPPPD includes at least one of the following criteria: (1) difficulty with vaginal penetration during intercourse; (2) genito-pelvic pain during vaginal intercourse or penetration attempts; (3) fear or anxiety associated with genito-pelvic pain or vaginal penetration, or tightness of the pelvic floor muscles during attempted vaginal penetration [40]. The prevalence of GPPPD is not known as the diagnosis was recently established; however, prevalence rates of dyspareunia and vaginismus are 3–25 percent and 0.4–6.6 percent, respectively [56, 57].

The etiology of GPPPD is usually a complex combination of psychological, social, cultural, and relationship factors, and can correlate with male partners' sexual dysfunction [58, 59]. As the etiology of GPPPD is multifactorial, the treatment is multidisciplinary, including pain management, pelvic floor physical therapy, cognitive therapy, desensitization, and sensate focus [60, 61].

Male Sexual Dysfunction

Erectile Disorder

When assessing a man for erectile dysfunction (ED), it is important to assess whether the disorder is psychogenic (situational and morning erections present) or organic (generally gradual and in the presence of chronic illness such as diabetes or vascular disease).

Treatment for psychogenic ED includes sensate focus, cognitive-behavioral therapy, and psychological reassurance, but it is often amenable to treatments for organic ED as well. Pharmacologic treatment of ED is based on increasing blood flow to the penis. Although testosterone can improve libido and response to phosphodiesterase-5 (PDE-5) inhibitors, testosterone replacement alone usually is not sufficient to treat ED. Non-pharmacologic treatments include constriction rings, vacuum erection devices, and penile prostheses.

Male Hypoactive Sexual Desire Disorder

Male hypoactive sexual desire disorder is characterized by decreased or absent sexual thoughts or fantasies and/or desire for sexual activity. Not surprisingly, this disorder can be associated with erectile and/or ejaculatory dysfunction. The National Health and Social Life Survey found that 15 percent of men between the ages of 18 and 59 years lacked sexual interest for several months within the last year [41]. Treatment includes addressing any underlying medical or psychiatric disorders, psychotherapy, and pharmacotherapy. Exercise and management of stress can also support libido.

Premature (Early) Ejaculation

Premature ejaculation (PE) is the most common sexual disorder in men, affecting up to 30 percent of the male population, and yet it is poorly understood [62]. The lack of understanding of PE is in part due to the absence of a standard definition of PE until relatively recently. In 2014, the International Society of Sexual Medicine defined PE as "(i) ejaculation that always or nearly always occurs prior to or within about 1 minute of vaginal penetration from the first sexual experience (lifelong PE) or a clinically significant and bothersome reduction in latency time, often to about 3 minutes or less (acquired PE); (ii) the inability to delay ejaculation on all or nearly all vaginal penetrations; and (iii) negative personal consequences, such as distress, bother, frustration, and/or the avoidance of sexual intimacy" [63]. Treatment includes psychotherapy, behavioral therapy such as the "stop–start" or "squeeze" techniques, and topical anesthetics. There are no FDA-approved medications for PE, although some antidepressants that are known to delay orgasm are used off-label to treat PE.

Delayed Ejaculation

Delayed ejaculation (DE) is defined in the DSM-5 as a persistent difficulty or inability to achieve orgasm despite the presence of adequate desire, arousal, and stimulation [40]. While there is no universal definition of normal time for reaching orgasm, generally latencies beyond 25–30 minutes are considered DE [64]. Delayed ejaculation has an estimated prevalence of 1–4 percent, making it the least common of the male sexual disorders [41, 65].

In addition to psychogenic or biologic (age, neurologic conditions, chronic medical conditions) causes of DE, medications associated with DE include antidepressants, benign prostatic hyperplasia (BPH) medications, selective serotonin reuptake inhibitors (SSRIs), tricyclic antidepressants, and monoamine oxidase inhibitors [66, 67].

As with the other sexual disorders, treatment includes psychosexual therapy as well as pharmacotherapy. There are no FDA-approved medications for DE; however, cabergoline, yohimbine, and buproprion are often used off-label.

Sexual dysfunction in both men and women often results from a combination of medical and psychological conditions, thus requiring multimodal therapy for effective treatment. Clinicians should be aware of the different types of sexual disorders in order to guide therapy. It is imperative that treatment be thoughtful, unbiased, and non-judgmental, with the goal of allowing patients to have fulfilling sexual experiences, as sexual health contributes to overall health and wellness.

Prostate Health

The prostate is a gland, normally about the size of a walnut, that sits at the base of the bladder and surrounds the prostatic urethra. Its main function is to secrete an alkaline fluid that provides nutrition for sperm. The majority of the ejaculate volume is prostatic secretions rather than sperm. The prostate gland is under the hormonal influence of testosterone, specifically dihydrotestosterone. The most common disorders affecting the prostate are BPH, prostatitis (inflammation), and prostate cancer.

Benign Prostatic Hyperplasia

Benign prostatic hyperplasia refers to the non-cancerous growth of the prostate and affects approximately one-third of men over the age of 50 years, and estimates indicate that up to 14 million men in the USA have symptoms of BPH [68]. Common symptoms of BPH include intermittent or decreased force of urinary stream, frequency, urgency, nocturia (waking at night to void), and inability to urinate.

Men who are not bothered by symptoms of BPH do not require treatment; however, men with bothersome symptoms can be treated with medical therapy or surgery. Medications for BPH include alpha-blockers that relax the smooth muscle of the prostate to facilitate the flow of urine, and 5-alpha reductase inhibitors that decrease prostatic volume.

Saw palmetto is a phytotherapeutic supplement for BPH that is widely prescribed in Europe and available over the counter for men to use in the USA, with minimal to no side effects. The most popular agent is *Serenoa repens* (saw palmetto berry extract). The possible mechanisms of action are proposed to be antiandrogenic, inhibition of 5-alpha-reductase, inhibition of growth factors, an anti-estrogenic effect, an anti-edema effect, and an anti-inflammatory effect [69]. Definitive clinical data supporting its efficacy is limited [70]. Saw palmetto is first-line therapy in Europe for mild to moderate BPH with lower urinary tract symptoms, and in Italy 50 percent of the medications used for BPH are phytotherapies [71]. In the USA, herbal medicines and dietary supplements are not regulated and undergo no efficacy or safety testing per the 1994 Dietary Supplement Health and Education Act. Therefore, it may be useful to utilize medical grade formulations of saw palmetto to optimize the potency and potential benefits.

There are a variety of minimally invasive procedures for BPH, some of which can be performed in the office setting. Most of the minimally invasive procedures utilize an energy source (microwave, radiofrequency, high-intensity ultrasound) to heat and destroy prostate tissue. Transurethral resection of the prostate is still considered the gold standard for treatment of BPH.

Prostatitis

Prostatitis refers to inflammation of the prostate gland that can be due to infection or other causes. Symptoms of prostatitis can include frequency, urgency of urination, pain with urination and/or ejaculation, and difficulty urinating. The NIH has classified prostatitis into four categories: Category I, acute bacterial prostatitis; Category II, chronic bacterial prostatitis; Category III, chronic prostatitis/chronic pelvic pain syndrome; and Category IV, asymptomatic inflammatory prostatitis [72].

Acute bacterial prostatitis is associated with a sudden onset of urinary symptoms and/or systemic infection. It is the least common form of prostatitis and responds to antimicrobial therapy. On the other hand, chronic bacterial prostatitis is usually associated with recurrent urinary tract infections. Chronic prostatitis/chronic pelvic pain syndrome is not associated with infection, but can have variable urinary symptoms and a variety of pelvic pain, including perineal, penile, and ejaculatory pain. Finally, asymptomatic inflammatory prostatitis, by definition, has no associated symptoms; however, treatment may be considered for select patients, such as those with elevated PSA or infertility.

Prostate Cancer

Prostate cancer is the most common cancer among men after skin cancer, and is the second leading cause of cancer death in American men [73]. The lifetime risk of being diagnosed with prostate cancer is approximately 11 percent; however, most men with prostate cancer do not succumb to the disease [74]. In autopsy studies of men who died of other causes, over 33 percent of men age 70–79 years were incidentally found to have prostate cancer [75]. As a significant proportion of men who have prostate cancer are unaware they even have it, the US Preventive Services Task Force has discouraged routine screening [76].

Treatment for prostate cancer is dependent on patient age, functional status, and prostate cancer grade and clinical stage. Except for watchful waiting, other treatments for prostate cancer, including radiation, surgery, and androgen deprivation, all have the potential to negatively impact quality of life. Radiation and surgery are associated with voiding dysfunction, urinary incontinence, and erectile dysfunction, while common side effects of androgen deprivation include hot flashes, decreased libido, osteoporosis, loss of muscle mass, and anemia.

Alternative Prostate Treatments

Interest in complementary and alternatives therapies (CAMs), including neutraceuticals, is high in men with prostate conditions. In North America, 30 percent of men with prostate disease use some form of complementary and alternative medical therapy, primarily herbal, vitamins, supplements, and dietary modifications. Phytotherapies used in BPH include extract of the berries of *Serenoa repens* (saw palmetto), *Pygeum africanum* (from the bark of the African plum tree), pumpkin seed, rye pollen (also known under the brand name Cernilton), stinging nettle, South African star grass, and quercetin. In prostatitis, quercetin has been studied for its anti-inflammatory and antioxidant properties and may be lacking in the diet of some prostatitis patients because levels of this bioflavonoid are high in many of the foods patients tend to avoid – onions, tea, spices, red wine, cranberry, and citrus fruits – because they trigger symptoms [77]. Clinical and basic research is demonstrating that inflammation may play a critical role in the progression of BPH and prostate cancer; therefore, there is potential for dietary changes and agents that have anti-inflammatory properties.

Lifestyle risk reduction, caloric restriction, omega-3 fatty acids/fish oil, fiber, and bio-flavonoids have been studied in prostate cancer patients, with the goal of reducing cardiac risk and therefore promoting longevity. The leading cause of death in men is cardiovascular disease, and this has been shown to be the case in large-scale prostate cancer prevention trials. Therefore, approaches that support both cardiovascular health and prostate health will have the greatest impact on survival [78, 79].

Kidney Health

The purpose of the renal system is the ultrafiltration of the blood that results in excretion of waste products and excess fluid in the urine, thereby regulating electrolyte levels, maintaining acid–base equilibrium, and regulating fluid homeostasis. The kidneys also synthesize hormones that control blood pressure (renin), stimulate red blood cell production (erythropoietin), and maintain bone health (calcitriol).

Chronic Kidney Disease

The most common kidney disease is chronic kidney disease (CKD) [80], with diabetes and hypertension being the two most common underlying conditions causing CKD. Other conditions that can cause CKD include glomerulonephritis (a group of diseases that cause inflammation of the kidney's filtration system), polycystic kidney disease, congenital anomalies, recurrent pyelonephritis, and autoimmune diseases such as lupus [80]. Chronic use of over-the-counter medications such as aspirin or ibuprofen can also cause kidney damage. Early detection of CKD, controlling any underlying medical condition, avoiding dehydration, maintaining a healthy diet and weight, and avoiding smoking can help prevent progression. There is no evidence to support the use of kidney cleanses or other homeopathic treatments to reverse or delay progression of CKD. In fact, there are documented reports of kidney toxicity related to herbs and supplements, pointing to the potential risks, and some are no longer sold in the USA [81].

Kidney Stones

Over 500,000 emergency room visits annually are due to kidney stones, and estimates indicate that 1 in 11 people will have a kidney stone in their lifetime [82]. Kidney stones are often incidentally diagnosed by radiologic imaging for unrelated reasons, while in other situations symptoms ranging from vague abdominal to excruciating flank pain can be experienced.

Dietary and lifestyle factors play a significant role in the development of stones, with weight gain, obesity, and diabetes being strongly associated with kidney stones [83]. The majority of kidney stones are calcium oxalate, but simply lowering calcium intake usually does not decrease the risk of stone formation. In fact, adequate calcium intake with meals is important to bind with oxalate in the gut. Additionally, dietary salt and animal protein reduction are recommended as avoidance of these can lower urine calcium and oxalate levels, respectively. Low fluid intake is often a risk factor for the formation of kidney stones, and adequate hydration is one of the most effective methods of kidney stone prevention, with the goal of drinking enough fluids to produce 2 liters of urine output per day.

Conclusion

When one's overall physical, psychological, and social health is supported and functioning well, then one's urologic health also functions well. The interconnectedness of the GU system with other body systems is important to recognize and support. Further research is needed on optimal methods for maintaining and promoting the health of the urinary system.

Acknowledgment

We would like to thank Virginia M. Green, PhD, for her assistance in preparing this chapter.

References

1. ES Lukacz, TG Bavendam, A Berry, et al. A novel research definition of bladder health in women and girls: implications for research and public health promotion. *J Womens Health (Larchmt)* 2018; **27**: 974–981.

2. KL Burgio, DK Newman, MT Rosenberg, C Sampselle. Impact of behaviour and lifestyle on bladder health. *Int J Clin Pract* 2013; **67**: 495–504.

3. CG Kowalik, A Daily, S Delpe, et al. Toileting behaviors of women: what is healthy? *J Urol* 2019; **201**: 129–134.

4. MH Palmer, JM Wu, CS Marquez, et al. "A secret club": focus groups about women's toileting behaviors. *BMC Womens Health* 2019; **19**: 44.

5. J Dagenais, SL Chang. The impact of exercise on nocturia: breaking down the inflammatory cycle. *J Urol* 2016; **195**: e970.

6. J Dagenais, SL Chang. Eat right and wake up less? Exploring the link between socioeconomic and dietary factors and nocturia. *J Urol* 2016; **195**: e969–e970.

7. MG Cumberbatch, A Cox, D Teare, JW Catto. Contemporary occupational carcinogen exposure and bladder cancer: a systematic review and meta-analysis. *JAMA Oncol* 2015; **1**: 1282–1290.

8. H Hashim, P Abrams. How should patients with an overactive bladder manipulate their fluid intake? *BJU Int* 2008; **102**: 62–66.

9. S Lohsiriwat, M Hirunsai, B Chaiyaprasithi. Effect of caffeine on bladder function in patients with overactive bladder symptoms. *Urol Ann* 2011; **3**: 14–18.

10. JG Lee, AJ Wein, RM Levin. The effect of caffeine on the contractile response of the rabbit urinary bladder to field stimulation. *Gen Pharmacol* 1993; **24**: 1007–1011.

11. RR Wing, JM Creasman, DS West, et al. Improving urinary incontinence in overweight and obese women through modest weight loss. *Obstet Gynecol* 2010; **116**: 284–292.

12. J Baker, D Costa, JM Guarino, I Nygaard. Comparison of mindfulness-based stress reduction versus yoga on urinary urge incontinence: a randomized pilot study. With 6-month and 1-year follow-up visits. *Female Pelvic Med Reconstr Surg* 2014; **20**: 141–146.

13. J Baker, D Costa, I Nygaard. Mindfulness-based stress reduction for treatment of urinary urge incontinence: a pilot study. *Female Pelvic Med Reconstr Surg* 2012; **18**: 46–49.

14. JE Long, S Khairat, E Chmelo, MH Palmer. Mind over bladder: women, aging, and bladder health. *Geriatr Nurs* 2018; **39**: 230–237.

15. TL Griebling. Urologic diseases in America project: trends in resource use for urinary tract infections in women. *J Urol* 2005; **173**: 1281–1287.

16. Urology Care Foundation. Urinary tract infections: learn how to spot and treat them. 2014. www.urologyhealth.org/patient-magazine/magazine-archives/2014/summer-2014/urinary-tract-infections-learn-how-to-spot-and-treat-them (accessed April 21, 2020).

17. TE Finucane. "Urinary tract infection": requiem for a heavyweight. *J Am Geriatr Soc* 2017; **65**: 1650–1655.

18. EE Hilt, K McKinley, MM Pearce, et al. Urine is not sterile: use of enhanced urine culture techniques to detect resident bacterial flora in the adult female bladder. *J Clin Microbiol* 2014; **52**: 871–876.

19. AJ Wolfe, E Toh, N Shibata, et al. Evidence of uncultivated bacteria in the adult female bladder. *J Clin Microbiol* 2012; **50**: 1376–1383.

20. SA Ferry, SE Holm, H Stenlund, R Lundholm, TJ Monsen. The natural course of uncomplicated lower urinary tract infection in women illustrated by a randomized placebo controlled study. *Scand J Infect Dis* 2004; **36**: 296–301.

21. TM Hooton. Clinical practice: uncomplicated urinary tract infection. *N Engl J Med* 2012; **366**: 1028–1037.

22. MA Averbeck, A Rantell, A Ford, et al. Current controversies in urinary tract infections: ICI-RS 2017. *Neurourol Urodyn* 2018; **37**: S86–S92.

23. TM Hooton, M Vecchio, A Iroz, et al. Effect of increased daily water intake in premenopausal women with recurrent rrinary tract infections: a randomized clinical trial. *JAMA Intern Med* 2018; **178**: 1509–1515.

24. Institute of Medicine. *Dietary Reference Intakes for Water, Potassium, Sodium, Chloride, and Sulfate.* Washington, DC: The National Academies Press; 2005. www.nap.edu/read/10925/chapter/1 (accessed April 21, 2020).

25. B Eriksen. A randomized, open, parallel-group study on the preventive effect of an estradiol-releasing vaginal ring (Estring) on recurrent urinary tract infections in postmenopausal women. *Am J Obstet Gynecol* 1999; **180**: 1072–1079.

26. C Perrotta, M Aznar, R Mejia, X Albert, CW Ng. Oestrogens for preventing recurrent urinary tract infection in postmenopausal women. *Cochrane Database Syst Rev* 2008; **2**: CD005131.

27. EM Schwenger, AM Tejani, PS Loewen. Probiotics for preventing urinary tract infections in adults and children. *Cochrane Database Syst Rev* 2015; **12**: CD008772.

28. D Zafriri, I Ofek, R Adar, M Pocino, N Sharon. Inhibitory activity of cranberry juice on adherence of type 1 and type P fimbriated *Escherichia coli* to eucaryotic cells. *Antimicrob Agents Chemother* 1989; **33**: 92–98.

29. J Vostalova, A Vidlar, V Simanek, et al. Are high proanthocyanidins key to cranberry efficacy in the prevention of recurrent urinary tract infection? *Phytother Res* 2015; **29**: 1559–1567.

30. T Kontiokari, K Sundqvist, M Nuutinen, et al. Randomised trial of cranberry–lingonberry juice and *Lactobacillus* GG drink for the prevention of urinary tract infections in women. *BMJ* 2001; **322**: 1571.

31. C Barbosa-Cesnik, MB Brown, M Buxton, et al. Cranberry juice fails to prevent recurrent urinary tract infection: results from a randomized placebo-controlled trial. *Clin Infect Dis* 2011; **52**: 23–30.

32. L Stothers. A randomized trial to evaluate effectiveness and cost effectiveness of naturopathic cranberry products as prophylaxis against urinary tract infection in women. *Can J Urol* 2002; **9**: 1558–1562.

33. K Sengupta, KV Alluri, T Golakoti, et al. A randomized, double blind, controlled, dose dependent clinical trial to evaluate the efficacy of a proanthocyanidin standardized whole cranberry (*Vaccinium macrocarpon*) powder on infections of the urinary tract. *Current Bioactive Compounds* 2011; **7**: 39–46.

34. S Micali, G Isgro, G Bianchi, et al. Cranberry and recurrent cystitis: more than marketing? *Crit Rev Food Sci Nutr* 2014; **54**: 1063–1075.

35. RG Jepson, G Williams, JC Craig. Cranberries for preventing urinary tract infections. *Cochrane Database Syst Rev* 2012; **10**: CD001321.

36. CH Wang, CC Fang, NC Chen, et al. Cranberry-containing products for prevention of urinary tract infections in susceptible populations: a systematic review and meta-analysis of randomized controlled trials. *Arch Intern Med* 2012; **172**: 988–996.

37. TS Lo, KD Hammer, M Zegarra, WC Cho. Methenamine: a forgotten drug for preventing recurrent urinary tract infection in a multidrug resistance era. *Expert Rev Anti Infect Ther* 2014; **12**: 549–554.

38. A Flower, LQ Wang, G Lewith, JP Liu, Q Li. Chinese herbal medicine for treating recurrent urinary tract infections in women. *Cochrane Database Syst Rev* 2015; **6**: CD010446.

39. World Health Organization. Defining sexual health. 2019. www.who.int/repro ductivehealth/topics/sexual_health/sh_de finitions/en (accessed April 21, 2020).

40. American Psychiatric Association. *Diagnostic and Statistical Manual of Mental Disorders: DSM-5*. Arlington, VA: American Psychiatric Publishing; 2013.

41. EO Laumann, A Paik, RC Rosen. Sexual dysfunction in the United States: prevalence and predictors. *JAMA* 1999; **281**: 537–544.

42. KE Flynn, L Lin, DW Bruner, et al. Sexual satisfaction and the importance of sexual health to quality of life throughout the life course of U.S. adults. *J Sex Med* 2016; **13**: 1642–1650.

43. SJ Parish, SR Hahn. Hypoactive sexual desire disorder: a review of epidemiology, biopsychology, diagnosis, and treatment. *Sex Med Rev* 2016; **4**: 103–120.

44. AH Clayton, I Goldstein, NN Kim, et al. The International Society for the Study of Women's Sexual Health process of care for management of hypoactive sexual desire disorder in women. *Mayo Clin Proc* 2018; **93**: 467–487.

45. SL Davison, SR Davis. Androgens in women. *J Steroid Biochem Mol Biol* 2003; **85**: 363–366.

46. BB Sherwin, MM Gelfand. Differential symptom response to parenteral estrogen and/or androgen administration in the surgical menopause. *Am J Obstet Gynecol* 1985; **151**: 153–160.

47. SA Kaplan, RB Reis, IJ Kohn, et al. Safety and efficacy of sildenafil in postmenopausal women with sexual dysfunction. *Urology* 1999; **53**: 481–486.

48. JN Clements, B Thompson. Flibanserin for hypoactive sexual desire disorder in premenopausal women. *JAAPA* 2018; **31**: 51–53.

49. SM Stahl. Mechanism of action of flibanserin, a multifunctional serotonin agonist and antagonist (MSAA), in hypoactive sexual desire disorder. *CNS Spectr* 2015; **20**: 1–6.

50. Sprout Pharmaceuticals. Flibanserin package insert. Sprout Pharmaceuticals, Inc.

51. DM Stevens, JM Weems, L Brown, KA Barbour, SM Stahl. The pharmacodynamic effects of combined administration of flibanserin and alcohol. *J Clin Pharm Ther* 2017; **42**: 598–606.

52. JS Simons, MP Carey. Prevalence of sexual dysfunctions: results from a decade of research. *Arch Sex Behav* 2001; **30**: 177–219.

53. CM Meston, E Hull, RJ Levin, M Sipski. Disorders of orgasm in women. *J Sex Med* 2004; **1**: 66–68.

54. Psychology Today. Orgasmic disorder. www.psychologytoday.com/us/conditions/o rgasmic-disorder (accessed April 21, 2020).

55. MA Farmer, CM Meston. Predictors of genital pain in young women. *Arch Sex Behav* 2007; **36**: 831–843.

56. RD Hayes, CM Bennett, CK Fairley, L Dennerstein. What can prevalence studies tell us about female sexual difficulty and dysfunction? *J Sex Med* 2006; **3**: 589–595.

57. P Latthe, M Latthe, L Say, M Gulmezoglu, KS Khan. WHO systematic review of prevalence of chronic pelvic pain: a neglected reproductive health morbidity. *BMC Public Health* 2006; **6**: 177.

58. CF Pukall, AT Goldstein, S Bergeron, et al. Vulvodynia: definition, prevalence, impact, and pathophysiological factors. *J Sex Med* 2016; **13**: 291–304.

59. K Oberg, K Sjogren Fugl-Meyer. On Swedish women's distressing sexual dysfunctions: some concomitant conditions and life satisfaction. *J Sex Med* 2005; **2**: 169–180.

60. CR Dunkley, LA Brotto. Psychological treatments for provoked vestibulodynia: integration of mindfulness-based and cognitive behavioral therapies. *J Clin Psychol* 2016; **72**: 637–650.

61. S Bergeron, M Morin, M-J Lord. Integrating pelvic floor rehabilitation and cognitive-behavioural therapy for sexual pain: what have we learned and where do we go from here? *Sex Relat Ther* 2010; **25**: 289–298.

62. RC Rosen. Prevalence and risk factors of sexual dysfunction in men and women. *Curr Psychiatry Rep* 2000; **2**: 189–195.

63. EC Serefoglu, CG McMahon, MD Waldinger, et al. An evidence-based unified definition of lifelong and acquired premature ejaculation: report of the second International Society for Sexual Medicine Ad Hoc Committee for the Definition of Premature Ejaculation. *J Sex Med* 2014; **11**: 1423–1441.

64. CG McMahon. Management of ejaculatory dysfunction. *Intern Med J* 2014; **44**: 124–131.

65. MA Perelman, DN Watter Delayed ejaculation. In: PS Kirana, MF Tripodi, Y Reisman, et al., eds., *The EFS and ESSM Syllabus of Clinical Sexology*. Amsterdam, Medix Publishers; 2014; 660–672.

66. LA Labbate, J Grimes, A Hines, MA Oleshansky, GW Arana. Sexual dysfunction induced by serotonin reuptake antidepressants. *J Sex Marital Ther* 1998; **24**: 3–12.

67. WM Harrison, JG Rabkin, AA Ehrhardt, et al. Effects of antidepressant medication on sexual function: a controlled study. *J Clin Psychopharmacol* 1986; **6**: 144–149.

68. KB Egan. The epidemiology of benign prostatic hyperplasia associated with lower urinary tract symptoms: prevalence and incident rates. *Urol Clin North Am* 2016; **43**: 289–297.

69. E Fagelman, FC Lowe. Saw palmetto berry as a treatment for BPH. *Rev Urol* 2001; **3**: 134–138.

70. J Ricco, S Prasad. The shrinking case for saw palmetto. *J Fam Pract* 2012; **61**: 418–420.

71. K Dreikorn. Complementary and alternative medicine in urology. *BJU Int* 2005; **96**: 1177–1184.

72. JN Krieger, L Nyberg Jr., JC Nickel. NIH consensus definition and classification of prostatitis. *JAMA* 1999; **282**: 236–237.

73. American Cancer Society. Key statistics for prostate cancer. www.cancer.org/cancer/prostate-cancer/about/key-statistics.html (accessed April 21, 2020).

74. National Cancer Institute. Cancer stat facts: prostate cancer. https://seer.cancer.gov/statfacts/html/prost.html (accessed April 21, 2020).

75. JL Jahn, EL Giovannucci, MJ Stampfer. The high prevalence of undiagnosed prostate cancer at autopsy: implications for epidemiology and treatment of prostate cancer in the prostate-specific antigen-era. *Int J Cancer* 2015; **137**: 2795–2802.

76. US Preventive Services Task Force. Final recommendation statement: prostate cancer screening. www.uspreventiveservicestaskforce.org/Page/Document/RecommendationStatementFinal/prostate-cancer-screening (accessed April 21, 2020).

77. J Curtis Nickel, D Shoskes, CG Roehrborn, M Moyad. Nutraceuticals in prostate disease: the urologist's role. *Rev Urol* 2008; **10**: 192–206.

78. MA Moyad, PR Carroll. Lifestyle recommendations to prevent prostate cancer, part I: time to redirect our attention? *Urol Clin North Am* 2004; **31**: 289–300.

79. MA Moyad, PR Carroll. Lifestyle recommendations to prevent prostate cancer, part II: time to redirect our attention? *Urol Clin North Am* 2004; **31**: 301–311.

80. National Kidney Foundation. About chronic kidney disease. www.kidney.org/atoz/content/about-chronic-kidney-disease (accessed April 21, 2020).

81. AC Brown. Kidney toxicity related to herbs and dietary supplements: online table of case reports. Part 3 of 5 series. *Food Chem Toxicol* 2017; **107**: 502–519.

82. KK Stamatelou, ME Francis, CA Jones, LM Nyberg, GC Curhan. Time trends in reported prevalence of kidney stones in the United States: 1976–1994. *Kidney Int* 2003; **63**: 1817–1823.

83. CD Scales Jr., AC Smith, JM Hanley, CS Saigal. Urologic diseases in America: Prevalence of kidney stones in the United States. *Eur Urol* 2012; **62**: 160–165.

Reproductive System
Pregnancy and Postpartum Wellness
Dotun Ogunyemi

Introduction

The focus of this chapter is women's health and the unique domains of reproductive health and pregnancy. For women to be well, measures to prevent disease and to promote and optimize physical, mental, and social health should be widely adopted. Wellness measures should be consistent across the lifespan of women, from adolescence to reproductive age and into menopause. The roles of preventive health, recognition of disparities and improving health equity, and complementary and alternative medicine in optimizing women's wellness are reviewed. Lifestyle includes changeable behaviors that can affect the individual's health in the domains of nutrition, physical activity, stress, self-care, social relationships, and improper health behaviors [1]. Globally the importance of activation of women's empowerment, social networking, and accountability in women's health should be considered. This chapter is arranged to cover the following topics: prevention to improve wellness in women's health; advocacy, disparities, and health equity; mental wellness; non-pharmacologic therapy in pregnancy; non-pharmacologic management of labor and delivery; lifestyle factors and reproductive health, and the impact on wellness; coping mechanisms and interventions; and gynecological health improving wellness by using complementary and alternative therapy safely.

Prevention to Improve Wellness in Women's Health

Well-Women Care

Preventive care visits provide an excellent opportunity for well-woman care for all ages, including screening, evaluation of health risks and needs, counseling, and immunizations. The Well-Woman Chart developed by the Women's Preventive Services Initiative (WPSI) outlines preventive services recommended by the US Preventive Services Task Force (USPSTF) and Bright Futures based on age, health status, and risk factors [2].

General Health of Women

The WPSI General Health section addresses (1) social and community health such as interpersonal violence, alcohol, and tobacco; (2) general physical health including obesity, blood pressure, diabetes, and statins; (3) mental health, i.e., depression and substance-use; (4) reproductive health, including contraceptives and folic acid supplementation; and (5) climacteric/menopausal issues such as urinary incontinence, osteoporosis, and fractures and fall prevention. There are also sections discussing infectious disease and recommendations for cancer screening in addition to the following recommendations.

- All reproductive-aged women should have access to the full range of female-controlled contraceptives to prevent unintended pregnancy and improve birth outcomes.
- It is recommended that all women planning pregnancy take a daily supplement containing 0.4–0.8 mg (400–800 µg) of folic acid. The critical period for supplementation starts at least one month before conception and continues through the first 2–3 months of pregnancy [2].
- Pregnant women and mothers should receive comprehensive lactation support services (including counseling, education, and breastfeeding equipment and supplies) during the antenatal, perinatal, and postpartum periods to ensure the successful initiation and maintenance of breastfeeding.
- Low-dose aspirin taken after 12 weeks of gestation in high-risk pregnancies can reduce risk for preeclampsia.
- Pregnant women should be screened for asymptomatic bacteriuria with urine culture at 12–16 weeks' gestation.
- Women with risk factors for preexisting diabetes should be screened before 24 weeks' gestation, ideally at the first prenatal visit. All postpartum women diagnosed with gestational diabetes mellitus (GDM) should be screened for postpartum diabetes 4–6 weeks after delivery.
- USPSTF recommends women age 65 and older have bone measurement testing to identify osteoporosis. Women between the ages of 50 and 64 years with equivalent or greater 10-year fracture risks based on specific risk factors should also be tested. Women identified with low bone density can reduce their risk of fractures with osteoporosis medications.

Advocacy, Disparities, and Health Equity as Determinants of Women's Health and Wellness

Healthy People 2020 defines health equity as the "attainment of the highest level of health for all people" [3]. Healthy People 2020 defines a health disparity as "a particular type of health difference that is closely linked with social, economic, and/or environmental disadvantage" [4].

Maternal Mortality and Morbidity

To achieve health equity for all women, health disparities must be recognized, and effective processes developed. The USA has the highest maternal mortality rate of any high-resource country and is the only country outside of Afghanistan and Sudan where the rate is rising [5–7]. The five leading causes of maternal mortality are postpartum hemorrhage, preeclampsia, thromboembolism, infection, and cardiac disease. Lessons learned from reviews have shown that the majority of maternal deaths are preventable [8]. The Alliance for Innovation on Maternal Health (AIM) is a national alliance that promotes consistent and safe maternity care to reduce maternal mortality and severe maternal morbidity. It collaborates with states and hospital systems to improve a culture of maternal safety through continuous quality improvement cycles [9]. AIM achieves its goal via maternal safety bundles, which represent best practices for maternity care, developed and endorsed by national multidisciplinary organizations [10]. Each safety bundle has sections on readiness, recognition, response, and reporting. The maternal safety bundles include:

- obstetrical hemorrhage;
- severe hypertension/preeclampsia;
- prevention of venous thromboembolism;
- reduction of low-risk primary cesarean births/support for intended vaginal birth;
- reduction of peripartum racial disparities;
- postpartum care access and standard.

Health Disparities and Inequities in Maternal Care

Contributors to healthcare disparities for women include health system, patient, provider, clinical, and structural factors. Of most concern is the role of poverty and racism. For example, the rate of maternal mortality is 2–3 times higher in African American mothers when corrected for socioeconomic and other factors. To reduce peripartum racial/ethnic disparities, the Disparities Bundle Framework in the Patient Safety bundle has been suggested by the Council of Patient Safety in Women's Healthcare. This framework includes improved communication, cultural competency training, patient education, shared decision-making, system-wide implicit bias training, and a disparity dashboard [11].

Advocacy

Women can benefit from advocacy in areas including contraception, access and autonomy of reproductive care, pregnancy services, and reproductive cancer prevention and early detection. To be competent health advocates, physicians must understand the factors that create health inequities and recognize how they impact the lives of their patients. Additionally, patients and families must be educated to be effective self-advocates.

Mental Wellness, Non-Pharmacologic Therapy, and Pregnancy

Mental Wellness

Stress

Pregnant women experience unique stressors, such as prenatal screenings [12], concerns about infant health and development [12], or having an unwanted pregnancy [13]. Pregnancy represents a state of altered physiology, and in the presence of stress, there is a complex interplay between the internal maternal physiologic environment and the changes induced by the stress response. Prenatal distress has been shown to suppress the lymphocyte activity of the immune system [14], predispose the body to infection [15], and alter cytokine levels [16]. A study of pregnant women during a natural disaster found that those who experienced higher levels of perceived stress were more likely to have children with poorer mental development and language abilities at two years of age [17]. Fetal epigenetic programming may help explain the link between maternal prenatal stress and its negative effects on the child.

Anxiety and Depression

Pregnancy and the period following childbirth are associated with substantial emotional and physical changes for mothers, and increased vulnerability to mental health difficulties. Period prevalence estimates suggest that nearly one-fifth of women experience depression during pregnancy and a similar proportion do so in the first three months after giving birth [18]. Anxiety disorders in the perinatal period have been reported in about 13 percent of pregnant or postpartum women [19]. Perinatal mental health difficulties are associated with serious adverse consequences that include high rates of maternal suicide, poorer pregnancy outcomes [20], and longstanding emotional, social, and cognitive difficulties in children, which appear to be mediated by problematic, early parent–infant interactions.

Many women are fearful about medication harming their developing baby, have guilt about taking medication, and worry about becoming dependent [21]. Mindfulness is "the awareness that emerges through paying attention on purpose, in the present moment, and non-judgmentally to the unfolding of experience moment by moment" [17]. A systematic review that identified 17 studies of mindfulness-based interventions (MBIs) in the perinatal period found no evidence of harm on measured outcomes and some evidence that those who are more vulnerable to depression or anxiety may benefit more from MBIs during the perinatal period [22].

Cognitive-behavioral therapy (CBT) is a psychosocial intervention that challenges and changes unhelpful cognitive distortions and behaviors, improves emotional regulation, and develops personal coping strategies. A systematic review of the efficacy of CBT for treating and preventing perinatal depression that included 40 trials concluded that CBT interventions are effective for treating and preventing depression during the perinatal period [23].

Prenatal Substance-Use

A nurse-administered behavioral intervention for pregnant substance-users that integrates motivational enhancement therapy with CBT (MET-CBT) has been promoted for drug abstinence programs for pregnant women [24].

Insomnia

A recent randomized controlled trial used CBT ($n = 90$) versus imagery exercises ($n = 89$) for treatment of insomnia in pregnant women between 18 and 32 weeks' gestation. Women receiving CBT for insomnia experienced faster remission of the insomnia disorder, a significantly greater reduction in self-reported total wake time, and a small but significantly greater decline in Edinburgh Postnatal Depression Scale scores versus the control group. These results suggest a role for CBT in various psychosocial conditions of pregnancy [25].

Non-Pharmacologic Management of Labor Pain

Safe Reduction of the Primary Cesarean Section Rate

In the USA, the rapid increase in cesarean section (CS) rates without evidence of a concomitant decrease in maternal or neonatal morbidity has raised concern of overuse [26]. Approaches to limit interventions during labor and to support a family-oriented labor experience have been recommended [27]. Admission to labor can be delayed if maternal and fetal statuses are reassuring. The mother can also be offered frequent contact and support, using techniques such as education, oral hydration, comfortable positions, massages, and water immersion [27].

Complementary Practices for Pain Management in Labor

Women's emotional and mental wellness is optimized within a natural, patient-centered, safe, and positive birth experience. Mind–body techniques for relaxation are accessible to women through the teaching of these techniques during antenatal classes. Commonly cited complementary practices associated with providing pain management in labor are mind–body interventions (e.g., yoga, hypnosis, relaxation therapies), alternative medical practices (e.g., homeopathy, traditional Chinese medicine), manual healing methods (e.g., massage, reflexology), pharmacologic and biological treatments, bioelectromagnetic applications (e.g., magnets), and herbal medicines.

Continuous Labor Support

A support person (doula) present during labor is associated with decreased use of analgesia, decreased incidence of operative birth, increased incidence of spontaneous vaginal delivery, and increased maternal satisfaction. Continuous labor support has been shown to be one of the most effective interventions to safely reduce the primary CS rate. If a doula cannot be present or is not desired, women should still be encouraged to invite a family member or friend to be present at the birth and assume this role [28].

Positions of Comfort and Autonomy

Women should be allowed to choose freely regarding the duration of walking during labor. In women without epidural anesthesia, laboring in the upright position in the second stage is associated with a shorter interval to delivery, less pain, and lower incidences of non-reassuring fetal heart rate patterns and of operative vaginal delivery. The upright positions studied include sitting (obstetric chair/stool), semi-recumbent (trunk tilted backward 30° to the vertical), kneeling, squatting (unaided or using squatting bars), and squatting aided with a birth cushion. The benefits of the upright position may be related to gravity, less aortovagal compression, improved fetal alignment, and larger anterior–posterior and transverse pelvic outlets [28].

Dance Labor

The combination of upright position, pelvic movement, back massage, and partner support during the first stage of labor has been termed "dance labor." Specifically, dance labor is beneficial because the upright position enhances the descent of the fetal head; leaning on a labor partner makes it easier for the mother to support her body weight; pelvic tilt exercise appears to be effective in reducing ligament pain intensity and also pain duration; and pelvic movement or rocking, either on a chair or swaying back and forth, allows the woman's pelvis to move and encourages the fetus to descend. Dance labor with music encourages a gentle rhythm and allows the partner to have access to the mother's back for massage or pressure [29].

Water Immersion

Some evidence supports the effectiveness of immersion in water [30]. Research shows that compared with no water immersion, water immersion was associated with decreased use of analgesia, reported maternal pain, labor duration, incidence of perineal trauma, incidence of operative delivery, and better neonatal outcomes [28].

Acupressure and Acupuncture

Acupressure functions in the same way as acupuncture in that it seeks to maintain the balance of energy in the various channels that circulate in the body – called meridians – that are connected to the specific body organs, but without the use of needles. The SP6 point is believed to have the ability to control some aspects of the reproductive organs during childbirth. A randomized clinical trial of 156 laboring mothers confirmed that the use of acupressure on the SP6 point alleviated pain significantly in a noninvasive manner and can improve the quality of care given to pregnant women in labor [31]. In one study, acupuncture significantly reduced labor pain, while it had no effect on labor pain at full dilatation [32].

Lifestyle Factors and Fertility to Enhance Wellness

Approximately 10–15 percent of couples are infertile. To achieve fertility wellness, a couple should assess lifestyle factors that can be potentially modified to optimize fertility [33].

The Reproductive Clock

For women, pregnancy before the age of 30 provides the highest chances of success [34]. A woman is born with a full complement of oocytes. With each menstrual cycle, a cohort of oocytes develops; only one oocyte reaches maturity and ovulates, the others become atretic [35]. As the number of oocytes declines, a woman's menstrual cycle shortens and fertility decreases. Reproductive failure in women older than 35 years is also related to the increased risk of aneuploidy and spontaneous abortion with age [36]. For men, achieving pregnancy before 35 years provides the best chances of success. Semen volume and motility both decrease, and morphology may become increasingly abnormal after the age of 35 years. There is significantly more sperm DNA damage and decline in both sperm motility (40 percent) and viability (below 50 percent) after the age of 40 years [37, 38].

Nutrition

A woman's diet has been shown to particularly affect ovulatory fertility. Women with high "fertility diet" scores of a higher monounsaturated to trans-fat ratio, vegetable protein over animal protein, high-fat over low-fat dairy, a decreased glycemic load, and an increased intake of iron and multivitamins had lower rates of infertility due to ovulation disorders [39].

In men, diet seems to affect sperm quality. A diet rich in carbohydrates, fiber, folate, lycopene [40], fruit, and vegetables [41], but with lower amounts of both proteins and fats, correlates with improved semen quality and is beneficial for fertility. Prior research also shows that men who used oral antioxidants had a significant increase in live birth rate when compared to controls [42].

Weight

The goal set by Healthy People 2010 of reducing obesity in the USA to 15 percent was not met [43]. Instead, adult obesity increased to 35.7 percent in 2010 [44]. In addition to other potential health risks, obesity can have a significant impact on fertility. Obese women have a higher rate of recurrent, early miscarriage, and this may be due to factors such as endometrium receptiveness. But the negative effects of obesity on fertility in women may be reversible. One study found that after losing an average of 10.2 kg, 90 percent of obese previously anovulatory women began ovulating [45]. In men, increased BMI is correlated with decreased sperm concentration [31, 32], decreased sperm motility [46], increased DNA damage [47, 48], and erectile dysfunction [49]. For women, being underweight and having extremely low amounts of body fat are associated with ovarian dysfunction and infertility. Eating disorders such as anorexia nervosa that are associated with extremely low BMI have very high correlations with amenorrhea and oligomenorrhea. Underweight men are at an increased risk of infertility and tend to have lower sperm concentrations than men with a normal BMI [47].

Exercise

Moderate exercise seems beneficial to increased fertility, whereas too vigorous exercise, especially in lean men or women, impairs fertility [50]. Moderately physically active men were shown to have significantly better sperm morphology when compared to men who played in a competitive sport or to elite athletes. Excessive exercise in women can negatively alter energy balance in the body and affect the reproductive system [51]. When energy demand exceeds dietary energy intake, a negative energy balance can result in hypothalamic dysfunction and alterations in gonadotropin-releasing hormone (GnRH) pulsatility, leading to menstrual abnormalities, particularly seen among female athletes [52, 53]. Therefore, it is important for pregnancy-seeking couples to find a balance between exercise and weight in order to maximize successful conception rates.

Psychological Effects

Infertility is stressful due to the societal pressures, testing, diagnosis, treatments, failures, unfulfilled desires, and fiscal costs [54]. Physical stress has been shown to affect female fertility. Women who worked more than 32 hours a week experienced a longer time to conception compared to women who worked 16–32 hours a week [34]. Support and counseling services for women may reduce their anxiety and depression levels, which may increase their chances of becoming pregnant and delivering a live baby [55, 56]. Males who experienced more than two stressful life events before undergoing infertility treatment were more likely to have low sperm concentration, motility, and morphology [57]. Stress and depression are thought to reduce testosterone and luteinizing hormone (LH) pulsing [54, 58], disrupt gonadal function [58], and ultimately reduce spermatogenesis and sperm parameters. Actively coping with stress, such as being assertive or confrontational, may also negatively impact fertility [59, 60] by increasing adrenergic activation, leading to more vasoconstriction in the testes and resulting in lower testosterone levels and decreased spermatogenesis.

Recreational Substances and Environmental Factors

Tobacco Use

Women who smoke have been shown to have significant infertility risks [61] attributable to decreases in ovarian function, a reduced ovarian reserve, and disruption in endocrine function. Chemicals in cigarette smoke may impair oocyte pick up and the transport of fertilized embryos within the oviduct, leading to an increased incidence of ectopic pregnancies, longer times to conception, and infertility among women who smoke [62].

Men who smoke have a decrease in total sperm count, density [63], motility [64, 65], normal morphology [63, 65], semen volume [63], and fertilizing capacity [66], and an increase in DNA damage [64]. Endocrine function may also be affected by smoking, as increases in follicle-stimulating hormone (FSH) and luteinizing hormone (LH) and decreases in testosterone levels have been reported [55].

Marijuana

Marijuana is one of the most commonly used drugs around the world [67], and it acts both centrally and peripherally to cause abnormal reproductive function. Marijuana cannabinoids bind to receptors located on reproductive structures such as the uterus or the ductus deferens. Females who use marijuana are at an increased risk of primary infertility. In women, use of marijuana can negatively impact hormonal regulation and also negatively impact movement through the oviducts, placental and fetal development, and may even cause stillbirth [67–70]. In males, cannabinoids reduce testosterone released from Leydig cells, modulate apoptosis of Sertoli cells, decrease spermatogenesis, decrease sperm motility, decrease sperm capacitation, and decrease acrosome reaction [67].

Cocaine

Cocaine is a stimulant for both the peripheral and central nervous systems, causing vasoconstriction and anesthetic effects. Cocaine decreases sexual stimulation and causes erectile and ejaculation dysfunction [71]. Cocaine has been demonstrated to adversely affect spermatogenesis [72], impair ovarian responsiveness to gonadotropins, and cause placental abruption [73, 74].

Opiates

Opiates are depressants that cause both sedation and decreased pain perception by influencing neurotransmitters [75]. In women, opioid-use disorder is associated with adverse maternal and neonatal outcomes. Neonatal abstinence syndrome and neurobehavioral problems in offspring are a significant consequence. In male heroin users, sexual function becomes abnormal and can remain so even after cessation [76]. Additionally, sperm parameters, most noticeably motility, also decrease with the use of heroin and methadone [77, 78].

Alcohol

Women who had hangovers were more likely to be infertile, suggesting a quantitative effect of alcohol [79]. Amounts of alcohol ranging from one drink a week to five drinks a day have been associated with increasing the time to pregnancy [34], decreasing the probability of conception by over 50 percent [80], decreasing the implantation rate, increasing the risk of spontaneous abortion [81] and fetal death [82], anovulation, luteal phase dysfunction, and abnormal blastocyst development [83]. The mechanism of the adverse fertility effects of alcohol is attributed to hormonal fluctuations including increases in estrogen levels, which reduce FSH and suppress both folliculogenesis and ovulation [83, 84]. In men, alcohol consumption is associated with adverse side effects such as testicular atrophy, decreased libido, decreased sperm count [85, 86], and decreased sperm motility [87].

Coffee

Although considered a harmless habit, caffeine from drinking coffee has powerful effects on many organ systems. Among North American adults, caffeine holds the distinction of being the most widely utilized psychotropic drug. Caffeine is a methylxanthine which is rapidly absorbed by the digestive system. It increases levels of cellular cyclic adenosine monophosphate, which may influence cell development [88, 89]. Caffeine also increases levels of circulating catecholamines that could interfere with uteroplacental circulation through vasoconstriction [88, 90]. It crosses the placenta freely, implying that caffeine concentrations in the fetus are the same as those in the mother's plasma, which is concerning since the fetus has low levels of enzymes to metabolize the molecule [88]. Furthermore, caffeine clearance slows down during pregnancy, and in the second and third trimesters the half-life of caffeine is tripled in comparison with non-pregnant women [88, 90]. Research on caffeine has revealed associations with miscarriage, spontaneous abortion, fetal death, and stillbirth [88, 91]. Based on current evidence, investigators have concluded that abstaining from drinking more than three cups of coffee per day during pregnancy can improve pregnancy outcomes [92].

Heavy Metals, Pesticides, Endocrine Disruptors, Radiation, and Chemicals

Heavy metals include metals such as lead, mercury, boron, aluminum, cadmium, arsenic, antimony, cobalt, and lithium. Lead interrupts the hypothalamic–pituitary axis and has been reported to alter hormone levels [93, 94], alter the onset of puberty, and decrease overall fertility [93]. Lead may alter sperm quality in men, and in women may cause irregular menstruation, induce preterm delivery, and cause miscarriage, stillbirth, and spontaneous abortion [93]. Boron's effects on the hypothalamic–pituitary axis are comparable to those of lead [93]. Ingestion of large quantities of mercury, usually from tainted seafood, can disrupt spermatogenesis and disrupt fetal development [94].

It is important to be careful of exposure to many of the chemicals and pesticides used worldwide, which may mimic natural hormones and dysregulate normal hormone activity, leading to various damaging effects on the reproductive health of both men and women. Men working in agricultural areas that use pesticides have higher concentrations of common pesticides in their urine [95], overall reduced semen parameters [96], oligozoospermia [42], lower sperm counts [97], and sperm concentrations decreased by as much as 60 percent [98].

Radiation in the form of x-rays and gamma rays can be devastating to the sensitive cells of the human body, including germ and Leydig cells. The damage done depends on the age of the patient and the dose of radiation, and ultimately can result in permanent sterility [99].

There have been an increasing number of studies demonstrating negative effects of the radiofrequency electromagnetic waves (RFEMW) utilized by cell phones on fertility. Cell phone usage has been linked with decreases in progressive motility of sperm [100], decreases in sperm viability [100, 101], increases in abnormal sperm morphology, and decreases in sperm counts [100]. Though there is increasing research demonstrating the negative effects of cell phone usage on fertility, there is no clear conclusion as no standard for analyzing cell phone effects is available and many studies have limitations [102, 103]. Many sexually active couples utilize vaginal lubricants to treat vaginal dryness and pain during intercourse [104]. Some non-commercial products used as lubricants, including olive oil, vegetable oil, and saliva, have been demonstrated to negatively impact sperm function. Most commercial lubricants have been shown to significantly decrease sperm motility after 30 minutes of contact with semen, while some also significantly increase sperm chromatin damage in comparison to the control medium [102, 104].

Preventive Care

While contraceptives are often associated with preventing pregnancy, several studies have demonstrated that condoms and oral contraceptives can preserve fertility in women as well [34, 105]. Contraceptives reduce the chances of contracting a sexually transmitted infection, thus reducing infertility. Contraceptives may also decrease time to conception. In one study, condom users had shorter time to conception compared to oral contraceptive users; oral contraceptive users in turn had shorter time to conception than those women not using any contraceptives [106]. Oral contraceptives were demonstrated to have positive effects on the prevention and management of endometriosis and pelvic inflammatory disease [106]. Scheduling regular doctor appointments may be beneficial for fertility. For women, visiting the gynecologist to receive an annual pap smear has been associated with being protective of fertility [105].

Coping Mechanisms and Interventions

Lifestyle Changes

The pre-conception period provides a good opportunity to encourage lifestyle modifications, since women are especially receptive to lifestyle advice at this time. One lifestyle intervention program targeted healthy diet, increased physical activity, and behavioral modification. The program included formulating individualized goals embedded in a "patient contract" with goal evaluation, feedback, and modifications [107]. Another study provided comprehensive behavioral weight loss counseling over eight years and produced clinically meaningful weight loss (≥5 percent) at year eight in 50 percent of patients with type-2 diabetes [108].

A novel online smartphone application delivering a personalized lifestyle coaching system to offer an effective, low-burden, and low-cost method of delivering periconceptional lifestyle advice has been described [109]. Tailored pre-conception counseling on lifestyle behaviors in subfertile couples was shown to reduce prevalence of harmful behaviors in the short-term [110]. Structured programs combining education counseling, support, and access to specialist health professionals should be available to facilitate appropriate lifestyle changes [111]. This will improve couples' chances of becoming pregnant and minimize the need for costly and invasive infertility treatment [112].

Resilience Training

Resilience is defined as the ability to rebound from tragedy, frustration, failure, and even from positive events [92]. Resilient patients possess high levels of self-esteem, self-efficacy, and optimism, and can use problem-solving skills to effectively cope with stress. Resilience can reduce infertile women's perceived psychological distress, which is conducive to maintaining their physical, mental, and social well-being. A dynamic process should be encouraged to build resilience in infertile patients. These patients should have their psychologic status evaluated, be provided with psychological counseling, and have advocates both from family and from within the healthcare system [113]. Other research also suggests that psychosocial interventions, particularly CBT, for couples in infertility treatment could be efficacious in both reducing psychological distress and improving clinical pregnancy rates [114].

Low-Resource Settings

Social Network Interventions

In low-resource countries, social network mechanisms have been proposed to improve maternal, neonatal, and child health outcomes. Specifically, intervention programs that focus on the peer influences that modify the social network of a target individual have been shown to be successful [115]. Social accountability approaches, which emphasize mutual responsibility and accountability by community members, healthcare workers, and local health officials have been implemented for improving health outcomes in the community. In a study from Malawi, facilitating the relationship between community members, healthcare providers, and local government officials contributed to important improvements in reproductive health-related outcomes such as contraceptive use, access to care, and overall service satisfaction. Further, the program ensured that solutions to problems were locally relevant and supported [116].

Activating Women's Empowerment

Gender equality is the state that affords women and men equal enjoyment of human rights, socially valued goods, opportunities, and resources. Interventions that do not recognize how gender dynamics affect behavioral outcomes are classified as gender-blind. Gender-aware interventions actively seek to identify and integrate activities that address the role of gender dynamics to achieve better behavioral and health outcomes.

Women's empowerment has been defined as the ability to make strategic life choices in a context where this ability was previously denied [117]. A systematic review demonstrated that gender-transformation interventions that empowered women in communities with participatory action groups experienced significantly reduced maternal mortality (37 percent) and reduced neonatal mortality (23 percent). Women's empowerment activities included gathering women for education, solidarity, planning actions, and advocacy [118]. Another review of 60 studies confirmed positive associations between women's empowerment and lower fertility, longer birth intervals, and lower rates of unintended pregnancy, with some variation in results [117].

Gynecological Wellness Using Complementary and Alternative Therapy Safely

Premenstrual Syndrome

Premenstrual syndrome (PMS) is a constellation of psychological, behavioral, and physical symptoms in the absence of organic or underlying psychiatric disease, which regularly recurs during the luteal phase of the menstrual cycle and disappears or significantly regresses with menstruation bleeding [119]. Up to 25 percent of menstruating women report moderate-to-severe premenstrual symptoms and about 5 percent have severe symptoms [120]. Suggested etiologies of PMS include abnormal neurotransmitter responses to normal ovarian functions, hormonal imbalances, sodium retention, or nutritional deficiencies [120]. Lifestyle factors such as stress, cigarette smoking, alcohol consumption, exercise, dietary habits, and BMI are associated with PMS, menstrual pain, and irregular menstrual cycles [121].

To treat PMS, non-pharmaceutical approaches including dietary changes, exercise, CBT, and complementary and alternative medicine (CAM) can be offered as first-line options [119]. Stress-reducing measures such as relaxation responses, yoga, aerobic exercise, acupuncture and acupressure, and cognitive therapy have been found to be effective in alleviating premenstrual symptoms [120, 121–126].

Menopause

Menopause is the cessation of menstrual periods or the final menstrual period, confirmed when a woman has been without a menstrual period for 12 consecutive months. The average age of menopause is 52 years but can vary from 40 to 58 years. As a result of aging, there is reduced ovarian function, which leads to lower levels of estrogen, androgens, and progestogens. Decreased hormone levels result in vasomotor symptoms consisting of hot flushes (or flashes) and night sweats. Non-vasomotor symptoms of menopause include anxiety, depression, difficulty concentrating, headaches, insomnia, irritability, loss of libido, and vaginal dryness. Hormone therapy (HT) with estrogens alone or with progestins is the most effective treatment for menopausal symptoms [127]. However, the results of the Women's Health Initiative revealed that treatment of menopausal symptoms with prescription hormones was associated with significant adverse effects such as coronary events, deep vein thromboembolisms, stroke, and breast cancer, which has resulted in women seeking alternative sources of treatment for menopausal symptoms [128]. Women looking for more natural or safer means to treat hot flushes, night sweats, and other menopausal symptoms have turned to mind and body practices such as exercise and yoga, and herbal products/dietary supplements such as soy and isoflavone products, valerian, and black cohosh. A recent review concluded that, of CAM treatments for menopausal symptoms, soy and soy isoflavones have the strongest evidence for being effective in reducing the frequency and severity of hot flushes. However, evidence for effectiveness and safety of CAM therapies in treatment of menopausal symptoms is limited [129].

Cancer Survivors

In women with breast cancer, modern treatment modalities, including surgery, targeted therapy, and chemotherapy, have allowed patients to survive longer. More than 60 percent of survivors develop climacteric syndrome, which includes hot flushes and menopause-related sleep disturbances. These symptoms can be clinically significant, negatively impact quality of life, and limit daily activities. Hormone therapy is unsuitable in these survivors because exposure to estrogen increases the risk of breast cancer recurrence and cardiovascular disease. Accordingly, many breast cancer patients with climacteric syndrome seek CAM to relieve their symptoms [130].

A recent meta-analysis which examined 844 breast cancer patients from 13 RCTs showed that acupuncture significantly alleviated menopause symptoms as described by the Kupperman index, which evaluates hot flush, sleeping disturbance, paresthesia, depression, joint pain, palpitation, headache, tingling, dizziness, and irritability. Therefore, breast cancer patients concerned about the adverse effects of hormone therapy may be interested in acupuncture treatment [131].

Primary Dysmenorrhea

Primary dysmenorrhea is defined as cramping pain in the lower abdomen that occurs just before or during menstruation without identifiable pelvic pathology [132]. A survey of 1266 female university students revealed a prevalence of primary dysmenorrhea of 88 percent, with 45 percent having regular painful menstruation and another 43 percent having some painful menstrual periods [133]. The pain and cramps in primary dysmenorrhea are due to hypercontractility of the uterus, leading to uterine hypoxia and ischemia as a result of the excessive production and release of prostaglandins during menstruation by the endometrium. Alternative interventions proposed for primary dysmenorrhea include acupuncture and acupressure, biofeedback, heat treatments, transcutaneous electrical nerve stimulation (TENS), and relaxation techniques [134].

Other interventions include lifestyle and dietary pattern changes, such as decreasing the consumption of salt and animal fat, increasing the intake of complex carbohydrates and fiber, increasing physical activity, reducing stressors, and receiving psychological support.

References

1. S Mcdonald, C Thompson *Women's Health.* London, Elsevier; 2005; 90–121.

2. Women's Preventive Services Guidelines. www.womenspreventivehealth.org (accessed March 1, 2019).

3. US Department of Health and Human Services, Office of Minority Health. National Partnership for Action to End Health Disparities. The National Plan for Action Draft as of February 17, 2010. Chapter 1: Introduction. www.minorityhealth.hhs.gov/npa/templates/browse.aspx?&lvl=2&lvlid=34 (accessed March 1, 2019).

4. US Department of Health and Human Services. The Secretary's Advisory Committee on National Health Promotion and Disease Prevention Objectives for 2020. Phase I report: Recommendations for the framework and format of Healthy People 2020. Section IV: Advisory Committee findings and recommendations. 2010. www.healthypeople.gov/sites/default/files/PhaseI_0.pdf (accessed March 1, 2019).

5. AA Creanga, CJ Berg, K Syverson et al. Pregnancy-related mortality in the United States, 2006–2010. *Obstet Gynecol* 2015; **125**: 5–12.

6. MF MacDorman, E Declercq, H Cabral, C Morton. Recent increases in the U.S. maternal mortality rate: disentangling trends from measurement issues. *Obstet Gynecol* 2016; **128**: 447–455.

7. MC Hogan, KJ Foreman, M Naghavi, et al., Maternal mortality ratios in selected countries over the past 30 years. *Lancet* 2010; **375**: 1609–1623.

8. SE Geller, D Rosenberg, SM Cox, et al. The continuum of maternal morbidity and mortality: factors associated with severity. *Am J Obstet Gynecol* 2004; **191**: 939–944.

9. Alliance for Innovation on maternal health (AIM). https://safehealthcareforeverywoman.org/aim-program (accessed March 1, 2019).

10. Maternal Safety Bundles. https://safehealthcareforeverywoman.org/patient-safety-bundles/#tab-maternal (accessed March 1, 2019).

11. W Grobman, E Howell. Presentation of reduction of peripartum racial/ethnic disparities bundle. https://safehealthcareforeverywoman.org/event/presentation-of-reduction-of-peripartum-racialethnic-disparities-bundle-2 (accessed March 1, 2019).

12. ME Coussons-Read, M Lobel, JC Carey, et al. The occurrence of preterm delivery is linked to pregnancy-specific distress and

elevated inflammatory markers across gestation. *Brain Behav Immun* 2012; **26**: 650–659.

13. CL Howerton, TL Bale. Prenatal programing: at the intersection of maternal stress and immune activation. *Horm Behav* 2012; **62**: 237–242.

14. PD Wadhwa, JF Culhane, V Rauh, SS Barve. Stress and preterm birth: neuroendocrine, immune/inflammatory, and vascular mechanisms. *Matern Child Health J* 2001; **5**: 119–125.

15. ME Coussons-Read, ML Okun, MP Schmitt, S Giese. Prenatal stress alters cytokine levels in a manner that may endanger human pregnancy. *Psychosom Med* 67: 625–631.

16. VJ Parker, AJ Douglas. Stress in early pregnancy: maternal neuro-endocrine-immune responses and effects. *J Reprod Immunol* 2010; **85**: 86–92.

17. J Kabat-Zinn. Mindfulness-based interventions in context: past, present, and future. *Clin Psychol Sci Pract* 2003; **10**(2): 144–156.

18. NI Gavin, BN Gaynes, KN Lohr, et al. Perinatal depression: a systematic review of prevalence and incidence. *Obstet Gynecol* 2005; **106**: 1071–1083.

19. O Vesga-Lopez, C Blanco, K Keyes, et al. Psychiatric disorders in pregnant and postpartum women in the United States. *Arch Gen Psychiatr* 2008; **65**: 805–815.

20. N Grote, J Bridge, A Gavin, et al. A meta-analysis of depression during pregnancy and the risk of preterm birth, low birth weight, and intrauterine growth restriction. *Arch Gen Psychiatr* 2010; **67** (10): 1012–1024.

21. CL Battle, AL Salisbury, CA Schofield, S Ortiz-Hernandez. Perinatal antidepressant use: understanding women's preferences and concerns. *J Psychiatr Pract* 2013; **19**(6): 443–453.

22. B Lever Taylor, K Cavanagh, C Strauss. The effectiveness of mindfulness-based interventions in the perinatal period: a systematic review and meta-analysis. *PLoS One* 2016; **11**(5): e0155720.

23. LE Sockol. A systematic review of the efficacy of cognitive behavioral therapy for treating and preventing perinatal depression. *J Affect Disord* 2015; **177**: 7–21.

24. KA Yonkers, A Forray, HB Howell, et al. Motivational enhancement therapy coupled with cognitive behavioral therapy versus brief advice: a randomized trial for treatment of hazardous substance use in pregnancy and after delivery. *Gen Hosp Psychiatr* 2012; **34**: 439–449.

25. X Xu, KA Yonkers, JP Ruger. Costs of a motivational enhancement therapy coupled with cognitive behavioral therapy versus brief advice for pregnant substance users *PLoS One* 2014; **9**(4): e95264.

26. ACOG. Safe prevention of the primary cesarean delivery obstetrics consensus No 1. *Obstet Gynecol* 2014; **123**: 693–711.

27. ACOG Committee. Opinion No 766: approaches to limit interventions during labor and birth. *Obstet Gynecol* 2019; **133**: e164–e173.

28. V Berghalla, JK Baxter, SP Chauhan. Evidence-based labor and delivery management. *Am J Obstet Gynecol* 2008; **199**(5): 445–454.

29. S Abdolahian, F Ghavi, S Abdollahifard, F Sheikhan. Effect of dance labor on the management of active phase labor pain & clients' satisfaction: a randomized controlled trial study. *Glob J Health Sci* 2014; **6**(3): 219–226.

30. KB Kozhimanil, PJ Johnson, LB Attanasio, et al. Use of non-medical methods of labor induction and pain management among U.S. women. *Birth* 2013; **40**(4). DOI:10.1111/birt.12064.

31. TK Jensen, AM Andersson, N Jorgensen, et al. Body mass index in relation to semen quality and reproductive hormones among 1,558 Danish men. *Fertil Steril* 2004; **82**: 863–870.

32. AO Hammoud, N Wilde, M Gibson, et al. Male obesity and alteration in sperm parameters. *Fertil Steril* 2008; **90**: 2222–2225.

33. R Sharma, KR Biedenharn, JM Fedor, A Agarwal. Lifestyle factors and

reproductive health: taking control of your fertility. *Reprod Biol Endocrinol* 2013; **11**: 66.

34. MA Mutsaerts, H Groen, HG Huiting, et al. The influence of maternal and paternal factors on time to pregnancy: a Dutch population-based birth-cohort study – the GECKO Drenthe study. *Hum Reprod* 2012; **27**: 583–593.

35. L Kimberly, A Case, AP Cheung, et al. Advanced reproductive age and fertility: no. 269, November 2011. *Int J Gynaecol Obstet* 2012; **117**: 95–102.

36. AF Stewart, ED Kim. Fertility concerns for the aging male. *Urology* 2011; **78**: 496–499.

37. DB Dunson, DD Baird, B Colombo. Increased infertility with age in men and women. *Obstet Gynecol* 2004; **103**: 51–56.

38. J Varshini, BS Srinag, G Kalthur, et al. Poor sperm quality and advancing age are associated with increased sperm DNA damage in infertile men. *Andrologia* 2012; **44**(Suppl. 1): 642–649.

39. JE Chavarro, JW Rich Edwards, BA Rosner, WC Willett. Diet and lifestyle in the prevention of ovulatory disorder infertility. *Obstet Gynecol* 2007; **110**: 1050–1058.

40. J Mendiola, AM Torres-Cantero, JM Vioque, et al. A low intake of antioxidant nutrients is associated with poor semen quality in patients attending fertility clinics. *Fertil Steril* 2010; **93**: 1128–1133.

41. WY Wong, GA Zielhuis, CM Thomas, HM Merkus, RP Steegers-Theunissen. New evidence of the influence of exogenous and endogenous factors on sperm count in man. *Eur J Obstet Gynecol Reprod Biol* 2003; **110**: 49–54.

42. MG Showell, J Brown, A Yazdani, MT Stankiewicz, RJ Hart. Antioxidants for male subfertility. *Cochrane Database Syst Rev* 2011; **1**: CD007411.

43. Healthy People 2010. Reduce the proportion of adults who are obese. www.healthypeople.gov/2010/document/html/objectives/19-02.htm (accessed March 1, 2019).

44. CL Ogden, MD Carroll, BK Kit, KM Flegal. Prevalence of obesity in the United States, 2009–2010. *NCHS Data Brief* 2012; **82**: 1–8.

45. AM Clark, B Thornley, L Tomlinson, C Galletley, RJ Norman. Weight loss in obese infertile women results in improvement in reproductive outcome for all forms of fertility treatment. *Hum Reprod* 1998; **13**: 1502–1505.

46. AC Martini, A Tissera, D Estofán, et al. Overweight and seminal quality: a study of 794 patients. *Fertil Steril* 2010; **94**: 1739–1743.

47. JE Chavarro, TL Toth, DL Wright, JD Meeker, R Hauser. Body mass index in relation to semen quality, sperm DNA integrity, and serum reproductive hormone levels among men attending an infertility clinic. *Fertil Steril* 2010; **93**: 2222–2231.

48. HI Kort, JB Massey, CW Elsner, et al. Impact of body mass index values on sperm quantity and quality. *J Androl* 2006; **27**: 450–452.

49. G Corona, E Mannucci, C Schulman, et al. Psychobiologic correlates of the metabolic syndrome and associated sexual dysfunction. *Eur Urol* 2006; **50**: 595; discussion 604.

50. D Vaamonde, ME Da Silva-Grigoletto, JM Garcia-Manso, et al. Response of semen parameters to three training modalities. *Fertil Steril* 2009; **92**: 1941–1946.

51. LM Redman. Physical activity and its effects on reproduction. *Reprod Biomed Online* 2006; **12**: 579–586.

52. MP Warren, NE Perlroth. The effects of intense exercise on the female reproductive system. *J Endocrinol* 2001; **170**: 3–11.

53. SL Gudmundsdottir, WD Flanders, LB Augestad. Physical activity and fertility in women: the North-Trøndelag health study. *Hum Reprod* 2009; **24**: 3196–3204.

54. K Anderson, V Niesenblat, R Norman. Lifestyle factors in people seeking infertility treatment: a review. *Aust N Z J Obstet Gynaecol* 2010; **50**: 8–20.

55. F Terzioglu. Investigation into effectiveness of counseling on assisted reproductive techniques in turkey. *J Psychosom Obstet Gynecol* 2001; **22**: 133–141.

56. H Klonoff-Cohen, E Chu, L Natarajan, W Sieber. A prospective study of stress among women undergoing in vitro fertilization or gamete intrafallopian transfer. *Fertil Steril* 2001; **76**: 675–687.

57. AL Gollenberg, F Liu, C Brazil, et al. Semen quality in fertile men in relation to psychosocial stress. *Fertil Steril* 2010; **93**: 1104–1111.

58. U Schweiger, M Deuschle, B Weber, et al. Testosterone, gonadotropin, and cortisol secretion in male patients with major depression. *Psychosom Med* 1999, **61**: 292–296.

59. M Pook, B Tuschen-Caffier, J Kubek, W Schill, W Krause. Personality, coping and sperm count. *Andrologia* 2005; **37**: 29–35.

60. B Zorn, J Auger, V Velikonja, M Kolbezen, H Meden-Vrtovec. Psychological factors in male partners of infertile couples: Relationship with semen quality and early miscarriage. *Int J Androl* 2008; **31**: 557–564.

61. C Augood, K Duckitt, AA Templeton. Smoking and female infertility: a systematic review and meta-analysis. *Hum Reprod* 1998; **13**: 1532–1539.

62. P Talbot, K Riveles. Smoking and reproduction: the oviduct as a target of cigarette smoke. *Reprod Biol Endocrinol* 2005; **3**: 52.

63. Y Li, H Lin, Y Li, J Cao. Association between socio-psycho-behavioral factors and male semen quality: systematic review and meta-analyses. *Fertil Steril* 2011; **95**: 116–123.

64. A Calogero, R Polosa, A Perdichizzi, et al. Cigarette smoke extract immobilizes human spermatozoa and induces sperm apoptosis. *Reprod Biomed Online* 2009; **19**: 564–571.

65. A Mitra, B Chakraborty, D Mukhopadhay, et al. Effect of smoking on semen quality, FSH, testosterone level, and CAG repeat length in androgen receptor gene of infertile men in an Indian city. *Syst Biol Reprod Med* 2012; **58**: 255–262.

66. SR Soares, MA Melo. Cigarette smoking and reproductive function. *Curr Opin Obstet Gynecol* 2008; **20**: 281–291.

67. N Battista, N Pasquariello, M Di Tommaso, M Maccarrone. Interplay between endocannabinoids, steroids and cytokines in the control of human reproduction. *J Neuroendocrinol* 2008; **20**(Suppl. 1): 82–89.

68. B Park, JM McPartland, M Glass. Cannabis, cannabinoids and reproduction. *Prostaglandins Leukot Essent Fatty Acids* 2004; **70**: 189–197.

69. BA Mueller, JR Daling, NS Weiss, DE Moore. Recreational drug use and the risk of primary infertility. *Epidemiology* 1990; **1**: 195–200.

70. M Rossato, C Pagano, R Vettor. The cannabinoid system and male reproductive functions. *J Neuroendocrinol* 2008; **20** (Suppl. 1): 90–93.

71. MS Gold. Cocaine and crack: clinical aspects. In: JH Lowinson, ed., *Substance Abuse: A Comprehensive Textbook* (3rd ed.) Baltimore, MD, Williams & Wilkins; 1997; 218–263.

72. VK George, H Li, C Teloken, et al. Effects of long-term cocaine exposure on spermatogenesis and fertility in peripubertal male rats. *J Urol* 1996; **155**: 327–331.

73. AC Thyer, TS King, AC Moreno, et al. Cocaine impairs ovarian response to exogenous gonadotropins in nonhuman primates. *J Soc Gynecol Investig* 2001; **8**: 358–362.

74. J Peugh, S Belenko. Alcohol, drugs and sexual function: a review. *J Psychoactive Drugs* 2001; **33**: 223–232.

75. C Wang, V Chan, RT Yeung. The effect of heroin addiction on pituitary testicular function. *Clin Endocrinol (Oxf)* 1978; **9**: 455–461.

76. G Ragni, L de Lauretis, O Bestetti, D Sghedoni, VGA Aro. Gonadal function in male heroin and methadone addicts. *Int J Androl* 1988; **11**: 93–100.

77. G Ragni, L De Lauretis, V Gambaro, et al. Semen evaluation in heroin and methadone addicts. *Acta Eur Fertil* 1985; **16**: 245–249.

78. M Revonta, J Raitanen, S Sihvo, et al. Health and life style among infertile men

and women. *Sex Reprod Health* 2010; **1**: 91–198.

79. RB Hakim, RH Gray, H Zacur. Alcohol and caffeine consumption and decreased fertility. *Fertil Steril* 1998; **70**: 632–637.

80. V Rasch. Cigarette, alcohol, and caffeine consumption: Risk factors for spontaneous abortion. *Acta Obstet Gynecol Scand* 2003; **82**: 182–188.

81. GC Windham, L Fenster, SH Swan. Moderate maternal and paternal alcohol consumption and the risk of spontaneous abortion. *Epidemiology* 1992; **3**: 364–370.

82. J Gill. The effects of moderate alcohol consumption on female hormone levels and reproductive function. *Alcohol Alcohol* 2000; **35**: 417–423.

83. KR Muthusami, P Chinnaswamy. Effect of chronic alcoholism on male fertility hormones and semen quality. *Fertil Steril* 2005; **84**: 919–924.

84. GP Donnelly, N McClure, MS Kennedy, SE Lewis. Direct effect of alcohol on the motility and morphology of human spermatozoa. *Andrologia* 1999; **31**: 43–47.

85. J Olsen, F Bolumar, J Boldsen, L Bisanti. Does moderate alcohol intake reduce fecundability? A European multicenter study on infertility and subfecundity. *Alcohol Clin Exp Res* 1997; **21**: 206–212.

86. DS Gaur, MS Talekar, VP Pathak. Alcohol intake and cigarette smoking: impact of two major lifestyle factors on male fertility. *Indian J Pathol Microbiol* 2010; **53**: 35–40.

87. BH Bech, EA Nohr, M Vaeth, TB Henriksen, J Olsen. Coffee and fetal death: a cohort study with prospective data. *Am J Epidemiol* 2005; **162**: 983–990.

88. PS Weathersbee, JR Lodge. Caffeine: its direct and indirect influence on reproduction. *J Reprod Med* 1977; **19**: 55–63.

89. JL Brazier, J Ritter, M Berland, et al. Pharmacokinetics of caffeine during and after pregnancy. *Dev Pharmacol Ther* 1983; **6**: 315–322.

90. K Wisborg, U Kesmodel, BH Bech, M Hedegaard, TB Henriksen. Maternal consumption of coffee during pregnancy and stillbirth and infant death in first year of life: prospective study. *BMJ* 2003; **326**: 420.

91. S Chalupka, AN Chalupka. The impact of environmental and occupational exposures on reproductive health. *JOGNN* 2010; **39**: 84–102.

92. Y Li, X Xin Zhang, M Shi, S Guo, L Wang. Resilience acts as a moderator in the relationship between infertility-related stress and fertility quality of life among women with infertility: a cross-sectional study. *Health Qual Life Outcomes* 2019; **17**: 38.

93. SC Sikka, R Wang. Endocrine disruptors and estrogenic effects on male reproductive axis. *Asian J Androl* 2008; **10**: 134–145.

94. SH Swan, RL Kruse, F Liu, et al. The Study for Future Families Research Group: semen quality in relation to biomarkers of pesticide exposure. *Environ Health Perspect* 2003; **111**: 1478–1484.

95. SH Swan. Semen quality in fertile US men in relation to geographical area and pesticide exposure. *Int J Androl* 2006; **29**: 62–68. discussion 105–108.

96. A Oliva, A Spira, L Multigner. Contribution of environmental factors to the risk of male infertility. *Hum Reprod* 2001; **16**: 1768–1776.

97. A Abell, E Ernst, JP Bonde. Semen quality and sexual hormones in greenhouse workers. *Scand J Work Environ Health* 2000; **26**: 492–500.

98. D Meirow, H Biederman, RA Anderson, WH Wallace. Toxicity of chemotherapy and radiation on female reproduction. *Clin Obstet Gynecol* 2010; **53**: 727–739.

99. A Agarwal, F Deepinder, RK Sharma, G Ranga, J Li. Effect of cell phone usage on semen analysis in men attending infertility clinic: an observational study. *Fertil Steril* 2008; **89**: 124–128.

100. A Agarwal, NR Desai, K Makker, et al. Effects of radiofrequency electromagnetic waves (RF-EMW) from cellular phones on human ejaculated semen: an in vitro pilot study. *Fertil Steril* 2009; **92**: 1318–1325.

101. A Agarwal, A Singh, A Hamada, K Kesari. Cell phones and male infertility: a review of recent innovations in technology and consequences. *Int Braz J Urol* 2011; **37**: 432–454.

102. F Deepinder, K Makker, A Agarwal. Cell phones and male infertility: dissecting the relationship. *Reprod Biomed Online* 2007; **15**: 266–270.

103. A Agarwal, F Deepinder, M Cocuzza, RA Short, DP Evenson. Effect of vaginal lubricants on sperm motility and chromatin integrity: a prospective comparative study. *Fertil Steril* 2008; **89**: 375–379.

104. S Kelly-Weeder, CL Cox. The impact of lifestyle risk factors on female infertility. *Women Health* 2006; **44**: 1–23.

105. M Revonta, J Raitanen, S Sihvo, et al. Health and life style among infertile men and women. *Sex Reprod Health* 2010; **1**: 91–98.

106. L van Dammen, V Wekker, AM van Oers, et al. Effect of a lifestyle intervention in obese infertile women on cardiometabolic health and quality of life: a randomized controlled trial. *PLoS One* 2018; **13**(1): e0190662.

107. Eight-year weight losses with an intensive lifestyle intervention: the look AHEAD study. *Obesity* 2014; **22**(1): 5–13.

108. KY Ng, S Wellstead, Y Cheong, N Macklon. A randomized controlled trial of a personalized lifestyle coaching application in modifying periconceptional behaviors in women suffering from reproductive failures (iPLAN trial). *BMC Women's Health* 2018; **18**: 196: doi:10.1186/s12905-018-0689-7.

109. F Hammiche, JS Laven, N van Mil, et al. Tailored preconceptional dietary and lifestyle counselling in a tertiary outpatient clinic in the Netherlands. *Hum Reprod* 2011; **26**(9): 2432–2441.

110. GF Homan, M Davies, R Norman. The impact of lifestyle factors on reproductive performance in the general population and those undergoing infertility treatment: a review. *Hum Reprod Update* 2007; **13**(3): 209–223.

111. E Britt, SM Hudson, NM Blampied. Motivational interviewing in health settings: a review. *Patient Educ Couns* 2004; **53**: 147–155.

112. CM Youssef-Morgan, F Luthans. Psychological capital and well-being. *Stress Health* 2015; **31**(3): 180–188.

113. D Herrmann, H Scherg, R Verres, et al. Resilience in infertile couples acts as a protective factor against infertility specific distress and impaired quality of life. *J Assist Reprod Genet* 2011; **28**(11): 1111–1117.

114. HB Shakya, D Stafford, DA Hughes, et al. Exploiting social influence to magnify population-level behaviour change in maternal and child health: study protocol for a randomized controlled trial of network targeting algorithms in rural Honduras. *BMJ Open* 2017; **7**: e012996.

115. S Gullo, C Galavotti, A Sebert Kuhlmann, et al. Effects of a social accountability approach, CARE's Community Score Card, on reproductive health-related outcomes in Malawi: a cluster-randomized controlled evaluation. *PLoS One* 2017; **12**(2): e0171316.

116. UD Upadhyaya, JD Gipson, M Withers, et al. Women's empowerment and fertility: a review of the literature. *Soc Sci Med* 2014; **115**: 111–120.

117. JM Kraft, KG Wilkins, GJ Morales, M Widyono, SE Middlestadt. Evidence review of gender-integrated interventions in reproductive and maternal-child health. *J Health Commun* 2014; **19**: 122–141.

118. S-Y Kim, H-J Park, H Lee, H Lee. Acupuncture for premenstrual syndrome: a systematic review and meta-analysis of randomized controlled trials. *BJOG* 2011; **118**: 899–915.

119. AH Jang, D Kim, M Choi. Effects and treatment methods of acupuncture and herbal medicine for premenstrual syndrome/premenstrual dysphoric disorder: systematic review. *BMC Complement Altern Med* 2014; **14**(11). www.biomedcentral.com/1472-6882/14/11.

120. KA Yonkers, MK Simoni. Premenstrual disorders. *Am J Obstet Gynecol* 2018; **218** (1): 68–74.

121. SY Tsai. Effect of yoga exercise on premenstrual symptoms among female employees in Taiwan. *Int J Environ Res Public Health* 2016; **13**(7): 721.

122. F Blake, P Salkovskis, D Gath, A Day, A Garrod. Cognitive therapy for premenstrual syndrome: a controlled trial. *J Psychosom Res* **45**: 307–318.

123. AM Maged, AH Abbassy, HRS Sakr, et al. Effect of swimming exercise on premenstrual syndrome. *Arch Gynecol Obstet* 2018; **297**(4): 951–959.

124. IL Goodale, AD Domar, H Benson. Alleviation of premenstrual syndrome symptoms with the relaxation response. *Obstet Gynecol* 1990; **75**: 649–655.

125. M Armour, CC Ee, J Hao, et al. Acupuncture and acupressure for premenstrual syndrome. *Cochrane Database Syst Rev* 2018; **8**: CD005290.

126. MD Grant, AT Marbella, AT Wang, et al. *AHRQ Comparative Effectiveness Reviews. Menopausal Symptoms: Comparative Effectiveness of Therapies.* Rockville, MD: Agency for Healthcare Research and Quality (US); 2015.

127. A Lethaby, J Marjoribanks, F Kronenberg, et al. Phytoestrogens for menopausal vasomotor symptoms. *Cochrane Database Syst Rev* 2013; **12**: CD001395.

128. A Gentry-Maharaja, C Karpinskyj, C Glazera, et al. Prevalence and predictors of complementary and alternative medicine/non-pharmacological interventions use for menopausal symptoms within the UK Collaborative Trial of Ovarian Cancer Screening. *CLIMACTERIC* 2017; **20**(3): 240–247.

129. HA Philp. Hot flashes: a review of the literature on alternative and complementary treatment approaches. *Altern Med Rev* 2003; **8**(3): 284–302.

130. T-J Chien, C-H Hsu, C-Y Liu, C-J Fang. Effect of acupuncture on hot flush and menopause symptoms in breast cancer: a systematic review and meta-analysis. *PLoS One* 2017; **12**(8): e0180918.

131. P Kannan, LS Claydon. Some physiotherapy treatments may relieve menstrual pain in women with primary dysmenorrhea: a systematic review. *J Physiother* 2014; **60**: 13–21.

132. A Polat, H Celik, B Gurates, et al. Prevalence of primary dysmenorrhea in young adult female university students. *Arch Gynecol Obstet* 2009; **279**: 527–532.

133. C Fisher, J Adams, L Hickman, D Sibbritt. The use of complementary and alternative medicine by 7427 Australian women with cyclic perimenstrual pain and discomfort: a cross-sectional study. *BMC Complement Altern Med* 2016; **16**: 129.

134. DA Bavil, M Dolatian, Z Mahmoodi, AA Baghban. Comparison of lifestyles of young women with and without primary dysmenorrhea. *Electron Physician* 2016; **8** (3): 2107–2114.

Allergic, Infectious, and Immunological Processes

Ossama Riaz, Sylvester Orimaye, Thabit Al-Khateeb, Patrick Sodeke, Adeola Awujoola, and Karl Goodkin

I'm not sick, but I'm not well.
Harvey Danger, "Flagpole Sitta"

The construct of "wellness" as it pertains to this chapter derives from an understanding of the interactions among psychosocial factors and behavioral changes, neuroendocrine responses, immune system changes, and inflammatory responses, and the impact of these relationships on physical health status. Mental and physical health and wellness are direct outcomes of the life stressor–social support–coping strategies (SSC) model, which addresses "mind–body medicine" (behavioral medicine) and the development of interventions centered on emotional, mental, physical, and spiritual well-being [1, 2]. Understanding the dynamic between these different facets of health will involve the psychosocial context of the person. This context predicts outcomes of disease prevention and positive wellness.

The SSC model emphasizes the role of life stressors, social support, and coping strategies in the regulation of mood, psychological distress, emotions, and anxiety, in order to improve overall health and wellness. This model has been used to educate medical providers about treatment modalities and wellness interventions that can complement the traditional standard of care in order to reduce disease burden, allow patients to feel more in control of their personal health, and encourage a positive outlook on life. The discussion of the allergic, infectious, and immunological processes through the prism of the SSC model is aimed at advocating that medical professionals become more receptive to and educated about the role of psychosocial factors and resilience techniques to improve patient wellness.

Wellness medicine encompasses an integrative approach toward physical and psychological health by making an individual an active participant in his or her own wellness. This integrative approach is also at the core of psychoneuroimmunology (PNI), which establishes a biological basis for mind–body relationships that can be focused toward personalized wellness-based medicine. As a multidisciplinary field, PNI studies bidirectional pathways involving emotional states and behaviors, the central and peripheral nervous systems, and the endocrine and immune systems. The construct of the biopsychosocial model has become a focal point in understanding disease processes by helping us decipher the interactions between psychosocial and biological factors and what roles they play in the etiology of human diseases. By understanding immune dysregulation as a mediator of the output of the SSC model through its connections to psychological distress and the neuroendocrine system, integrative wellness-oriented interventions involving psychological and pharmaceutical modalities can be designed to moderate life stressor impacts and promote well-being. Resilience therapies aimed at improving wellness engaging cognitive, expressive, physical, and sensory approaches that can be utilized in understanding life's obstacles and correspondingly help in developing social support and coping strategies to deal with these life stressors [1].

"Stress," according to Lazarus and Folkman, involves the interaction between personal, social-environmental, and illness-related stressor factors that influenced personal cognitive appraisals (perceived stressors) and coping patterns [3]. Psychoneuroimmunology, as discussed here, will encompass the outcome dynamics between different life stressors and the moderating roles of social support and coping strategies. This will be followed by a consideration of the cascade of adaptive outcomes mediated by positive mood state and the neuroendocrine–immune interaction promoting biological adaptation and overall physical health and wellness.

Psychoneuroimmunology and the SSC model outcomes cascade applied to disease highlights psychological states and sociobehavioral aspects that are classified as negative affect, or psychological distress (e.g., depressed mood, grief, loss of personal control, and illness-related uncertainty), having similar immunosuppressive effects as physically noxious or threatening stimuli. When exposed to powerful psychic life stressors or emotionally threatening stimuli, the SSC model outcomes cascade predicts transitions from psychological distress to deleterious neuroendocrine responses as life stressors manifesting with psychological distress activate the hypothalamic–pituitary–adrenocortical (HPA) axis and the sympathetic-adrenomedullary (SAM) system, thereby inducing immunosuppression. The HPA axis is highly relevant to PNI. Psychological stimuli are first perceived and evaluated by the limbic system. If the psychological stimuli are interpreted as being threatening, the hypothalamus is activated, which induces secretion of stress hormones, with the pituitary secreting adrenocorticotropic hormone (ACTH), which stimulates the adrenal cortex to release cortisol into circulation. With the HPA hormonal cascade initiated, the hypothalamus, responding to the threatening stimulus, simultaneously triggers the SAM system where the fight-or-flight response stimulates the adrenal medulla to secrete epinephrine [1].

The immunological and inflammatory response highlighted in the SSC model outcomes cascade addresses the bidirectional relationship between the neuroendocrine and immune systems. One of these bidirectional pathways involves the direct sympathetic innervation of lymphoid organs, such as the lymph nodes, thymus, and the spleen. Fibers connect the central nervous system (CNS) to the lymphoid organs, allowing instant communication from the brain to the immune system. The hormones produced by the endocrine glands also have receptors in the CNS and, hence, allow the brain to interact with the thyroid, adrenal glands, or the reproductive organs – and vice versa. Ligands attached to receptors on various types of brain cells influence our behavior, as illustrated by what is now described as "sickness behavior," which emphasizes the actions of immune products on the brain. Proinflammatory cytokines secreted by immune cells can induce a person to call in sick to work, develop fever, lose appetite, and suffer fatigue and hypersomnia, which may appear as a distressing adaptation – but at the same time a necessary one – designed to help us overcome illness. Inappropriate secretion of the same cytokines, however, leads to chronic fatigue and is associated with chronic fatigue syndrome. Lymphocytes are capable of manufacturing certain hormones, cytokines, and chemokines produced by the brain and nervous system – serving as a unifying network of nerve fibers that connect the different components of the neuroendocrine and immune systems and interlink them with the SSC model outcomes cascade [1].

Hence, PNI provides a scientific conceptual framework from which to understand and predict physiological associations contributing to the development of systematic psychobehavioral wellness interventions designed to moderate life stressors, provide social support, and offer coping strategies, with the ultimate goal of interfacing them with physical health status and quality of life [1].

The SSC Model

This chapter seeks to contextualize the impact of wellness on allergic and infectious diseases with the immune system as a mediator. Allergic and infectious diseases are naturally distinguished by external versus internal sources of antigens and by over- versus under-reaction of the immune system. Each disease type will be analyzed through the SSC model, which predicts both the disease in question as well as wellness and resilience strategies that reflect the tenets of PNI. The SSC model, originally proposed by Goodkin and colleagues (Figure 12.1), explains the psychosocial context as it pertains to the progression of immune-modulated diseases. The model involves two spheres: (1) an external sphere composed of life stressors and social support; and (2) an internal sphere composed of coping strategies [1].

Goodkin et al. posited that in the external sphere when stressful life events are unpredictable, uncontrollable, and chronic, and social support is unavailable, unsatisfactory, or insufficient, psychological distress will ensue. They also posited that if – in the internal sphere – there were predominantly passive, maladaptive coping strategies associated with social alienation, outward lack of emotional expression, pessimism, hopelessness, and fearfulness, that higher levels of psychological distress associated with increased disease progression will also ensue [1].

Alternatively, Goodkin et al. posited that if external sphere stressful life events are predictable, controllable, and acute, and social support is available, satisfactory, and sufficient, there is less tendency toward psychological distress and a greater tendency toward wellness. Within the internal sphere, a person could develop adaptive coping skills reflecting a psyche that is forceful, sensitive, connected to others, outwardly expressive, optimistic, hopeful, and without undue fears. The individual therefore learns active coping strategies to deal with problems, reflecting lower psychological distress and increased likelihood of stabilization or regression of disease [1].

In applying the SSC model to the allergic, infectious, and immunologic systems, this chapter will first assign their antigenic source and respective level of immune activity. It will then examine the role of life stressors, social support, and coping skills in establishing specific wellness interventions focused on the principles of PNI. The SSC model as it relates to this chapter will be meant to predict the SSC model outcome cascade. The most proximal outcome predictor in the SSC model outcome cascade would be psychological distress, which will include depressed, fatigued, and anxious mood, and that's where there would be the most variance accounted for by the SSC model components. The second outcome in the cascade of the SSC model will involve the neuroendocrine dynamic altered due to stress as a mediating factor, particularly the HPA axis and the SAM system. It is true to say that next to negative mood states, the neuroendocrine responses would be the most easily predicted outcomes of the SSC model. The next step down the cascade, and yet less easily predicted due to having less variance accounted for by SSC model predictors, would be the immune

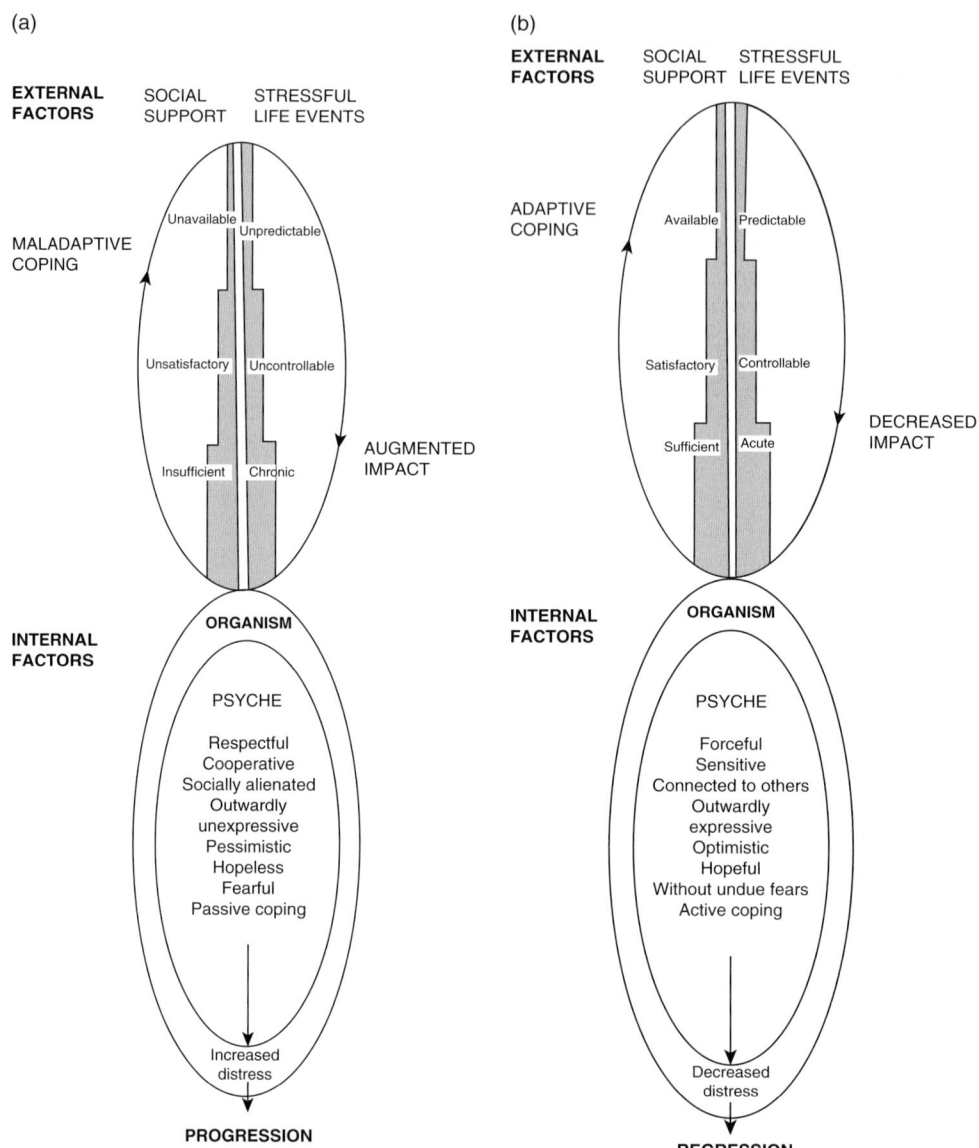

Figure 12.1 SSC model of disease regression versus progression.

system and inflammatory responses. Here, we note that the SSC model has a decreased penetration potential, as we become more distant from the psychosocial context of the SSC model predictors. Moreover, the SSC model can predict some, but not all, immune and inflammatory responses, which is a caution applicable to the model. The SSC model dictates immune system and inflammatory responses, but what is at issue here is how those immune system and inflammatory responses relate to the diseases in question. The outcome step, physical health status, has the smallest percentage of variance accounted for by SSC model predictors. While this chapter is entitled "Allergic, Infectious, and Immunological

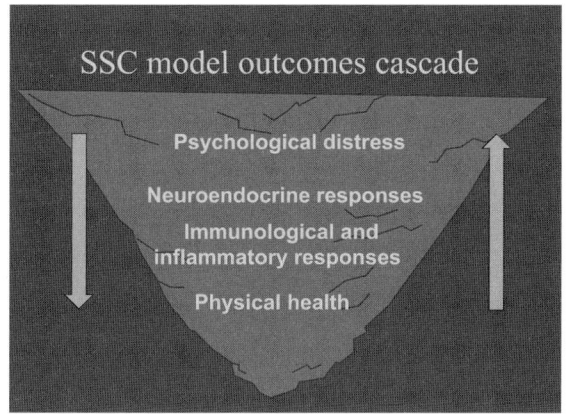

Figure 12.2 SSC model outcomes cascade.

Processes," the SSC model is not specific only to these outcomes. The model uses the immune system and inflammatory responses as mediators of physical health. Physical health embraces signs and symptoms that cause a patient to seek a doctor for treatment for any reason. Therefore, infectious diseases, allergic diseases, and autoimmune diseases are focused upon here but are viewed as part of the outcome domain of physical health that is predicted by the SSC model in its cascade of outcomes (Figure 12.2) [4–8].

Infectious Diseases

Infectious diseases are caused by external sources of antigens associated with a low reactivity of the immune system, implying that downregulation of the immune system leads to an increased risk for these diseases. Research has shown that an important role exists for life stressors in increasing the susceptibility to infectious diseases in humans. Cohen and Williamson found that participants were more likely to get a cold when exposed to a controlled dose of rhinovirus if they had a history of serious psychosocial stressors the previous month than were those with no such stress history [8]. Similarly, Stone et al. found that a higher number of major stressful life events over the course of a year was correlated with the development of colds after viral exposure, compared to those who did not develop infection [9]. Psychosocial stressors have also been implicated in Epstein–Barr virus and herpes simplex virus infections mediated through the mechanism of reactivation of latent viral infection and increases in subsequent antibody titers. In sum, these studies highlight how compromised immune system function caused by reactions to life stressors leads to an increased risk of infectious diseases [1, 10, 11].

There is difficulty in demonstrating evidence-based associations across the outcomes cascade of the SSC model from psychological distress (the most proximal outcome to the SSC model predictors) on to neuroendocrine system response, immune system response and inflammatory changes and, finally, on to clinical, physical health status – as it relates to infectious diseases, across types. Observed changes in the immune system in response to the negative impact of stressful life events are not necessarily associated with changes in clinical, physical health status due to limitations pertaining to the research, such as limited statistical power associated with small sample sizes, small and temporary changes in immune function, or selection of suboptimal immune or physical health markers proving to be related to one another. This section of the chapter will specifically focus on the SSC model relationships that have been observed and reported in human immunodeficiency virus (HIV) infection [12].

Goodkin et al., in investigating HIV infection, proposed that the psychosocial domains of the SSC model (life stressors, social support, and coping strategies) generate a multivariate vector predicting deleterious outcomes on psychological distress, the neuroendocrine system, the immune system, and inflammatory response, and on physical health. They posited that life stressors, especially when uncontrollable, unpredictable, and/or chronic, were associated with phenotypic (e.g., CD4 cell count) and functional (e.g., T cell proliferative responses) immune changes associated with disease progression. Further, they posited that passive, maladaptive coping strategies associated with attitudes of pessimism, hopelessness, and somatic anxiety, as well as unavailable, unsatisfactory, and/or insufficient social support, increase the deleterious impact of life stressors. This, in turn, leads to increased psychological distress, which leads to neuroendocrine system changes that mediate decreased cellular immune function resulting in more rapid HIV disease progression [13]. In *The Guidebook of Sexual Medicine* Dr. Waguih IsHak states that sexual dysfunction due to HIV infection can also be viewed as a major life stressor [14]. As HIV infection is chronic, Dr. IsHak suggests that it decreases a person's energy and forces that person to adapt or make adjustments that have lifelong implications, which can then become a severe source of distress and anxiety.

The Life Stressor Domain in HIV Infection

A diagnosis of HIV infection is associated with a multitude of life stressors. Those diagnosed with the infection face changes in health status that might impact their employment, health insurance, and cost of medical care, and lead to deterioration of their ability to take care of themselves. Prior to the current era of effective antiretroviral therapy (ART) in 1996, many experienced losses of their partners or loved ones to HIV. Men who have sex with men (MSMs) with HIV infection must further carry the burden of dealing with the stigma associated with the disease perpetrated by homophobic responses from friends and family, leading to a further sense of social isolation. This is also an issue for those experiencing the stigma against injecting substance use. Persons living with HIV experience high levels of anxiety, most prevalent during the asymptomatic stage, and depressed mood as symptoms of disease progression appear. Bereavement, as a particularly potent life stressor in HIV infection, has been shown to negatively influence immune system measures, such as natural killer cell cytotoxicity, CD8+ T lymphocyte counts, natural killer cytotoxicity (NKCC), and T cell proliferation [6].

The life stressor domain of the SSC model relates the occurrence of life stressors with a negative impact on HIV disease progression. Stigmatization, notification of HIV-positive status, the financial burden imposed by HIV infection, stress of symptoms referable to HIV, maintaining adherence to ART regimens, and laboratory reports related to HIV disease progression (plasma viral load; CD4 cell count) are among the primary life stressors experienced by persons living with HIV [1].

The Social Support Domain in HIV Infection

The SSC model posits a positive role for social support as it relates to HIV infection, with studies showing a positive impact of social support on the health of persons living with HIV, particularly for those with lower CD4 cell counts – except in cases of noxious social support. Studies have shown that large social support network sizes predict longevity among persons living with HIV, and that low social support was related to development of symptoms in those with low CD4 cell counts. A study evaluating the effects of three psychosocial variables – life stressors, depressive symptoms, and social support – in a prospective, five-year design with repeated (six-month) assessments found more rapid progression to AIDS associated with higher cumulative stressful life events, more cumulative depressive symptoms, and less cumulative social support. At 5.5 years, the probability of getting AIDS was 2–3 times higher among those above the median for life stressors or below the median for social support. Even two moderate life stressors increased the risk for progression to AIDS twofold, compared to those with no life stressors [1].

Researchers investigating disclosure found that MSMs who hid their sexual orientation had a more rapid course of HIV infection by 1.5–2 years. Higher emotional expression was also shown to be a positive predictor of survival in those with AIDS, when compared to those prior to AIDS. Moreover, emotionally hardy individuals and those with a sense of commitment and control and the ability to see adversity as a challenge were more likely to be alive at follow-up than less hardy individuals. The social support generated by healthcare connectedness, as well as healthy self-care, maintaining perspective, and life involvement, were discovered to relate to longer survival time among persons living with HIV. Increased survival time was associated with more collaborative relationships with doctors. The social support of being partnered, as well as high life involvement and emotional expression, were associated with less hopelessness [1]. Negative expectancies were found to interact with the loss of social support occurring with bereavement to show that those persons living with HIV having negative expectancies and multiple losses had the most marked declines in CD4 cell counts. In sum, wellness is associated with the social support domain of the SSC model and predicts a positive impact for socially supportive interpersonal interactions on physical health status. Disclosure of one's status, connecting with family and loved ones, maintaining an open and honest doctor–patient relationship, and down-modulating negative expectancies are some of the factors promoting social support interventions as an integral component of wellness interventions for persons living with HIV [12].

The Coping Strategies Domain in HIV Infection

To combat the distress many persons living with HIV feel, many have suggested that stress management interventions would be beneficial. These interventions may also be considered wellness interventions when they represent efforts toward secondary prevention and helping to prevent further deterioration and to enhance the quality of life. Such behavioral interventions highlight the impact of the SSC model by enhancing the sense of personal controllability and predictability over one's exposure to life stressors, increasing the recruitment of available social support, and encouraging the use of active, adaptive coping strategies to reduce the deleterious consequences of life stressors on psychological distress. It has been reported that cognitive-behavioral stress management (CBSM) enhances psychological resilience in individuals exposed to life stressors by:

- modifying the appraisal of life stressors;
- changing maladaptive cognitive distortions;
- decreasing hopeless thoughts;
- increasing the availability and utilization of adaptive coping responses; and
- increasing the availability and utilization of social support networks.

One specific CBSM intervention was tailored to address the issues of loss of personal control, coping demands, social isolation, and depressed mood. This type of intervention serves to enhance well-being across affective, cognitive, and social spheres of functioning and arms participants with several prophylactic "stress buffers" [13]. Dr. IsHak calls for a biopsychosocial evaluation plan and treatment for sexual dysfunction due to HIV infection to help those impacted to be supported [14]. The biopsychosocial plan detailed by Dr. IsHak aims at patient wellness by thoroughly investigating all biologic and psychosocial elements that might be causing the sexual dysfunction and involving the patient in their treatment plan [14].

As explained earlier, stressors and negative affective states lead to SAM system arousal and activation of the HPA axis, which in turn leads to downregulation of the immune system and to more rapid clinical disease progression. Hence, these interventions can be used to normalize sympathetic and HPA axis activation in this stressed population, as well as to attenuate neuroendocrine system-induced immunosuppression. Therefore, such inventions would lead to decreases in depressed mood and psychological distress overall. In line with the SSC model outcomes cascade, they would also reduce urinary cortisol and catecholamine levels and, possibly, normalize immunologic system impairment and increased inflammatory responses associated with depression.

Goodkin et al. studied a cohort of 118 persons living with HIV and 54 MSMs negative for HIV infection over 42 months, with assessments at six-month intervals. They found significant relationships between the SSC model, representing the three theoretical psychosocial predictor domains – life stressor burden, social support availability, and coping strategies – and the four SSC model outcome cascade domains of psychological distress, neuroendocrine system changes, immune system function and inflammatory responses, and physical health status. The study indicated life stressor levels, social support availability, and coping strategies to be associated with psychological distress in this patient population. In the early symptomatic stage of HIV infection, social support availability became more important, with stressor levels less crucial in relation to psychological distress [5].

The immune system and inflammatory response outcome domain has been found to be affected particularly by the life stressor and coping strategy SSC model predictor domains. Bereavement, a potent and frequent stressor in the cohort, demonstrated significant immunologic associations with both natural killer cell cytotoxicity and lymphocyte proliferative response in persons living with HIV. An active coping strategy was found to predict NK cell cytotoxicity inside and outside the setting of bereavement. Active coping strategies were also associated with lymphocyte proliferative response and with two laboratory progression markers of HIV infection – the CD4 cell count and the beta2-microglobulin level. In terms of the physical health SSC model outcome domain, research showed a negative role for life stressors and a salutary role for active coping strategies, with the latter becoming more clinically relevant in the early symptomatic stage of HIV infection [5].

This study adds credence to the role of behavioral interventions in the treatment of individuals with this infection. In targeting the outcome of psychological distress, prophylactic behavioral interventions would be prioritized for persons living with HIV with high levels of life stressors, low levels of social support availability, and low use of active coping strategies and/or high levels of passive, maladaptive coping strategies. The SSC model is prescriptive for behavioral interventions by each of its three domains. Those with a profile predominated by high life stressor burden would be targeted to receive stressor management techniques, e.g., deep muscular relaxation training, mental imagery, self-hypnosis,

		Immune system activity level	
		HIGH	**LOW**
Source of antigen	**INTERNAL**	Autoimmune	Cancer
	EXTERNAL	Allergies	Infections

Figure 12.3 Immune system activity versus source of antigen.

CBSM, meditation, and biofeedback techniques. Those with a profile predominated by low social support and/or suffering from losses due to HIV would be targeted to receive supportive group therapy and/or complicated grief therapy. Those with a profile predominated by low use of active coping strategies and/or high use of passive, maladaptive coping strategies would be targeted to receive coping skills enhancement training. These behavioral interventions have been shown to complement treatment modalities used in primary care settings for persons living with HIV [15].

Wellness as it pertains to HIV infection going forward calls for SSC model-based behavioral interventions aimed at enhancing positive mental and physical health outcomes rather than reducing or eliminating negative outcomes. They focus on positive affect and mood, a stable neuroendrocrine system balance, enhanced immunologic, phenotypic, and functional measures and salutary cytokine levels, and achieving a positive physical sense of well-being. This allows for optimizing positive mental and physical health for the person seen in an integrative care setting. It emphasizes the role of the patient as an active participant and collaborator in directing the "doctor–patient relationship," as well as incorporating the most current advances in primary medical care for persons living with HIV. Such a comprehensive care plan, built on mutual "person–doctor" participation, represents a true wellness-oriented approach as per the SSC model of health and disease in HIV. The multi-systems nature of HIV infection and care sets a strong precedent for utilization of the SSC model for a host of other medical illnesses with lower degrees of multi-system impacts (Figure 12.3).

Allergic Diseases

The immunoregulatory dysfunction present in allergic diseases is similar to that noted in populations exposed to high life stressor burdens. The history of allergic diseases as "psychosomatic disorders" dates back centuries. Asthma was referred to as "asthma nervosa," and atopic dermatitis was termed "neurodermatitis" in earlier medical texts. This section of the chapter focuses on the relationships among life stressor burden, social support, and coping strategy repertoires with allergic disease mediators and outcomes. It will also embrace wellness-promoting interventions and explain how these approaches apply to wellness sustainability and disease prevention vis-à-vis allergic diseases.

The SSC model will be utilized to show how life stressor burden, social support, and coping strategy psychosocial domains converge into a single, composite vector toward or away from allergic diseases. The SSC model will also be used to specify wellness-promoting interventions tailored to a person's psychosocial context in order to achieve the most salutary psychosocial outcomes possible. Allergic diseases involve external sources of antigens (allergens) stimulating and interacting with high immune system reactivity. The term "allergy" encompasses a group of related clinical diseases that impact one-third of the world's population. The underlying mechanism of the allergic process involves exposure to an allergen (e.g., drugs, dander, food, insect stings, pollen, and mold spores) that results in the production of allergen-specific immunoglobulin-E (IgE). This IgE then binds to mast cells, setting off a cascade of molecular and cellular events that result in clinical asthma attacks and symptomatic rhinitis. Both of these diseases involve the respiratory tract and may be associated with dermatitis and urticarial skin involvement, as well as with full-blown anaphylactic reactions [16].

Life Stressor Domain

Life stressors as viewed through the lens of the SSC model pertain to allergic diseases that have been shown in numerous studies to be regulated by mood and the occurrence of life stressors. Using final examinations as a chronic life stressor for students, multiple studies have shown stress-induced dysregulated cytokine production favoring a Th2 response. One study of sputum from bronchial samples of persons with asthma showed increases in Th2 cytokines and eosinophil counts after bronchial provocation tests [17]. Life stressors and the associated outcome of psychological distress have been shown to cause bronchoconstriction and reductions in pulmonary flow rates in children with asthma. Life stressors, such as performing mental arithmetic tasks, watching emotionally charged movies, and listening to stressful interpersonal interactions, have evoked increased bronchoconstriction in persons with asthma [18]. Children with asthma developing psychological distress find it more difficult to manage their symptoms. They require treatment with higher doses of corticosteroids and more frequent hospitalizations with longer-than-average lengths of stay. They also suffer from decreased functional status and an increased frequency of disability. Moreover, medication adherence becomes a concern, as most persons with asthma – as with HIV infection – must rely on self-management to gauge their life stressor burden and symptoms of psychological distress. The SSC model emphasizes the importance of how an individual is specifically impacted by life stressors and the stressor triggers of uncontrollability, unpredictability, and chronicity. Most persons with allergic diseases experience a sense of disconnectedness from their surroundings and develop learned helplessness coping strategies that distort their perception of self-efficacy and diminish their sense of wellness. Life stressors, such as financial strain and micro-aggression due to racial stigma, also play a role in asthma morbidity – as a disproportionate number of persons with asthma reside in inner-city neighborhoods. Children exposed to interpersonal violence – more frequent in such neighborhoods – have increased occurrences of asthma attacks and wheezing symptoms, and more frequently require prescriptions for bronchodilators [18].

Life stressors can aggravate and trigger other allergic diseases, such as atopic dermatitis (AD) – an inflammatory skin condition. Children with AD report reduced quality of life, irritability, mood changes, lower self-esteem, and higher levels of behavioral and emotional problems that increase with disease severity [19]. Children with AD also report increased social isolation compounded by bullying and teasing, further instigating emotional and behavioral problems. In AD, the person affected suffers from a severe urge to scratch oneself, which becomes a stressor itself – as the act of scratching worsens the dermatitis and creates a greater urge to scratch oneself. This "itch–scratch cycle" perpetuates a high sense of anxiety for the person suffering with the disease and further decreases quality of life [20]. Allergic rhinitis is another disease that is similarly associated with emotional lability – as well as impaired cognitive function and reduced quality of life [17, 21].

In allergic diseases, the role of the mother has been postulated to be vital, as maternal psychological distress can hamper the perinatal process, which can then influence the *in utero* environment leading to postnatal physiological and fetal developmental processes that increase the susceptibility to allergic diseases. Prenatal maternal psychological distress raises maternal and fetal stress hormone levels [22]. Wright et al. reported that increased life stressors in early childhood resulted in an atopic immune profile. They showed that infant perception of maternal distress in the first 2–3 months of life was associated with increases in IgE expression and concluded that early exposure to life stressors could produce immune reactivity among children, enhancing the Th2-type cytokine response [17]. Studies have found that chronic maternal stressors leading to prolonged and excessive cortisol excretion decrease the Th1/Th2 cytokine ratio in the fetus and the newborn, enhancing the suscept-ibility to allergic diseases [22]. Caregiver stressor burden is also a concern, as caregiver distress can increase the incidence of childhood wheezing, compounding prior psychologi-cal distress and leading to the development of clinical allergic diseases such as asthma and AD [23].

Food allergy has dramatically increased in recent years, with a doubling of related hospital admissions, including anaphylaxis. Food allergy and food hypersensitivity also have an impact on psychological distress and quality of life of children, adolescents, adults, and their families. Studies have shown that food allergies result in children living in a constant state of fear of stressful life events and anxiety pertaining to eating. This has a significant impact on their daily family lives as it relates to meal preparation and family social activities [24, 25].

Children allergic to foods have a higher rate of school absences and suffer from a greater burden of disease reflected in physical complaints, hospitalizations, use of medications, school and leisure activities, and friendships. Another issue is the association of one allergic disease with another. Comorbid allergies are found in about 46 percent of persons suffering with food allergies. They are frequently associated with asthma, hay fever, and atopic eczema. Families with children with comorbid allergic diseases suffer from poorer percep-tions of general health and greater limitations on family activities. Studies have found that atopic eczema and asthma have the most significant health-related impacts on quality of life. The areas of physical functioning, social timetables, somatic pain, and general health are most impacted by coexisting atopic disorders [24, 25].

Iio et al. found life stressors specific to school-age children with allergic diseases and reasoned that due to the "allergy match," defined as the progression of allergic diseases beginning in infancy, allergic diseases from food allergies and AD to asthma and rhinitis need to be considered collectively [21]. The allergic disease-specific life stressors they categorized involved the physical and mental influence on skin symptoms associated with itchiness, exacerbation of skin symptoms, and difficulty in refraining from scratching an itch. With asthma, the children were concerned about effects on school life of hospitaliza-tion; being unable to have pets with hair was also a concern. Visibility of the disease was also a major stressor, as misunderstanding of skin symptoms, having one's skin condition pointed out, and the futility and tiresomeness of explaining it to others is disconcerting. Further, the stressor of dining out and having a restrictive diet at events, parties, and gatherings was distressing, with the most impactful life stressor involving anxiety about self-coping for sudden anaphylaxis and asthma exacerbations [23].

Social Support Domain

The social support arm of the SSC model with respect to allergies emphasizes providing emotional, informational, instrumental, and affirmational assistance to the patient and highlights the important impact these have on the disease state. One study found stressful family factors such as parent separation/divorce, economic problems, and unemployment were associated with an inferior clinical response post specific sublingual immunotherapy against domestic dust mites. Another study showed that negative life events in childhood and adolescence, as well as a lack of social support to help cope with life stressors, were associated with increased rates of hospital admissions due to asthma. Social support in asthma management helps facilitate the asthma status and reduces the disruptive impact of environmental stressors, as shown by programs such as the Neighborhood Asthma Coalition (NAC), which helps to promote community support and encouragement of asthma management. Data from the NAC helped highlight that children of socially isolated parents reported more frequent asthma symptoms, limited activity, poorer asthma management practices, and more ER visits than those of non-isolated parents/caregivers. Hence, the NAC has instituted social support interventions emphasizing community support to aid asthmatic families that have resulted in reductions in acute care for asthmatic children. These organizations highlight the need to diversify one's social networks and educate those around us to understand the influence of social support in this field [25].

Allergic diseases such as AD involve the sufferer feeling embarrassed, socially isolated, stigmatized, and restricted in their abilities to own pets and play sports, leading to diminished quality of life for children. Maternal prenatal stressful life events such as divorce, death of a loved one, unemployment, and financial concerns were associated with AD in 3–14-year-old age groups. Depressed mothers postpartum were found to fail to respond appropriately to infant cues and alleviate infant stress, and were generally less sensitive and responsive toward their infants, which was predictive of increased rates of AD in childhood and adolescence. Maternal overprotection and control were also associated with AD as these mothers were more rejecting and less encouraging of the child's autonomy. Hence the role of social support for the mother is crucial as it provides a buffer to stressful life events, enhances the mother's self-esteem and self-efficacy, and aids in a smoother transition into motherhood, consequently promoting healthy child development. Without appropriate social support during this period, the transition can be cumbersome, negatively influencing the mother's psychological state and her ability to take care of the child. Lack of social support is strongly correlated with maternal depressive symptoms and highlights the protective role of social support for the mother [20].

Lind et al., in studying allergy and asthma, found social support to help alleviate the distress associated with allergic processes. They emphasized that social support can be divided into emotional, instrumental, and informative support in solving the problem posed by life stressors. The study showed that emotional support in the form of more understanding was more important than instrumental or informational support. The most support, the study concluded, was received from one's partner and family members, followed by healthcare systems, friends, and then coworkers. They found the higher the social support, the lower the frequency of asthma/allergy exacerbation [23].

With regard to food allergy, social support again was shown to play a role in patient wellness. Social support stressors for families here included the predominant fear of risk to life, fear following diagnosis, and fear for the present and future of the child's wellness. Mothers felt inadequately supported in bearing the responsibility of care for their child with a food allergy, which increased their levels of anxiety. Children with food allergies suffered increased disruption of their daily activities and impairment in the familial–social dynamic, which increased parental distress and resulted in limiting family activities. Parents more-over became overly protective and socially isolated in the process by avoiding family activities altogether, and by preventing their children from attending children's parties and school trips. Children themselves reported anxiety regarding going on holiday, attend-ing public events, and using public transport [25].

Everyday activities such as shopping and eating out can be life-threatening and hence frightening for children with food allergies. Parents find it difficult to separate themselves from their children and end up accompanying them in social situations beyond the age at which non-allergic children are accompanied. Food-allergic young adults, with overprotec-tiveness imposed during the early developmental years, experienced more anaphylactic reactions than those food-allergic adults who did not have overprotective parents. Mothers often end up burdened with the primary responsibility of dealing with their child's food allergy and lack of spousal support can increase the stress of living with a child's food allergy. This lack of help can create tension leading to breakdowns in support systems and can damage relationships. Hence, both parents must be equally involved in looking after the child to help increase the social support element that is important in buffering against emotional dysfunction [25].

Coping Strategies Domain

People with allergic diseases require coping strategies to engage life stressors and enhance wellness. Lind et al. discuss coping to help solve problems, impact emotions, and have one's personal coping style positively reflect a wellness-predictive technique. They discuss emotion-focused and problem-focused coping where the former includes expressing emotions to counter the unpredictable, uncontrollable, and unchangeable traits of the negative stressor sphere of the SSC model to avoid depression, with the latter reducing or eliminating life stressors in response to situations perceived to be threatening but susceptible to change [25]. Given the stressor of underlying atopic mechanisms, coping can be relayed to the various allergic processes. The study showed that the most viable coping options for allergies were avoiding certain environments, seeking healthcare, accepting the situation, and not thinking about the allergic situation. Accepting the situation allows the patients to be socially con-nected and acknowledge and understand their disease state, and consequently deal with the resulting emotions better. Another study found denial in asthma and categorized it as an adaptive strategy used by persons living with asthma that protected them from psychological distress. Denial as a coping mechanism in the allergic process allows the patient to modify the way they think about life stressors as opposed to modifying the stressor itself. Acceptance as coping in allergies allows patients to mold the emotions associated with the stressor and hence skew the perception of disease into a positive frame. It is the most commonly used emotion-focused strategy and helps in decreasing disease severity [23–26].

In the treatment of allergic diseases, unmet psychosocial needs must be identified. One study found that 70 percent of caretakers of children with food allergy reported asking for more mental health support due to current services provided being inadequate [25]. Additionally, chronic allergic disease management requires extensive psychoeducation regarding allergen avoidance and emergency preparedness, and many parents feel either insufficient information is being provided or, when provided, it is found to be overwhelming. Studies have called for a multidisciplinary approach involving different behavioral health providers working in unison to develop comprehensive psychoeducational materials in a patient-friendly format addressing coping, safety, and emotional concerns. Patients have expressed a preference for educational interventions followed by relaxation interventions.

In AD, educational interventions have been associated with improved disease severity and parental quality of life. Group-centered programs for AD were associated with reduced patient social anxiety, depression, catastrophizing cognitions, scratching behaviors, and improved parental disease management. Furthermore, educational interventions have allowed patients and their parental caregivers to be better able to differentiate between anaphylactic and anxiety symptoms and hence better respond accordingly. Parents at Boston's Children's Hospital were found to be assured and more confident in dealing with their child's allergic disease when educated about food allergies. Educational resources pertaining to how to read food labels, eating at restaurants, or being in public establishments are useful in overcoming the social anxiety and stress associated with the worry of what to do about food allergic triggers when outside the confines of the home setting. Medical care providers, in taking the time to educate and equip the food allergy sufferer and their family, can provide assurance by the simple act of writing a prescription for an auto-epinephrine pen. Letourneau et al. found that caregivers who were emotionally engaged and supportive of their children during infancy were better equipped to prevent poor infant immunological development, reducing the likelihood of childhood AD and asthma [16]. Other clinical studies have shown that psychotherapy and relaxation techniques can be beneficial in asthmatics and can improve respiration. With food allergies, coping management involved avoidance of food items, as well as emergency treatment of symptoms caused by accidental ingestion. Maternal adjustment to the food-allergic child was found to be beneficial and improved psychological distress [20].

Family-focused interventions are also important in allergies as they can provide families with the appropriate support and education to help normalize their experience of these stressors and to reduce anxiety, help them feel more competent, and improve their problem-solving skills to reduce the burden associated with having children with food allergies. School and workplace interventions are essential as educators and employers lack the knowledge and willingness to support the needs of sufferers. A well-coordinated effort involving schools encouraging implementation of appropriate accommodations and special educational classes if needed can help alleviate caregiver burden, better monitor treatment progress, promote adherence, facilitate peer acceptance and interactions, discourage bullying, and improve overall wellness. Adults can be aided at workplaces by being accommodated through having flexible workspaces, scheduling, and assistive technologies to help ease work burden and assist in achieving overall wellness. Public health interventions employed by the government can help in assisting the public on a larger scale. Measures such as food labeling and packaging can be emphasized, food retail establishments can modify menus and train staff to be more vigilant in pointing out allergens and detecting reactions when they occur, and help in reducing the risk of customer food allergic reactions [25].

Resilience in Allergic Diseases

Resilience in allergy as reflected in the SSC model involves understanding an individual's capacity to respond positively to adverse stimuli even when the risk of harm to self is great. Resilience involves protective factors that tie in with the SSC model in promoting wellness. Optimism, positive mood, self-esteem, self-care, independence, social support, and reduced psychological distress are all factors that promote wellness and encompass the SSC model. The correlation between low socioeconomic status (SES) and the development of asthma has been alluded to previously. However, not all children from lower SES backgrounds develop asthma, and instead some exhibit good asthma control despite living in an adverse environment. Chen et al. posit that children who cope well with asthma symptoms despite similar environments to those who do not develop resilience use a shift-and-persist approach to dealing with the stressors of low-SES life. This approach entails both shifting – adjusting to stressors through trying to find the positive in them – and engaging in persistence, which involves staying optimistic about the future and pursuing future goals [18].

People of low SES will be less likely to display negative psychological responses and, in turn, will reduce physiological activation of the HPA axis and SAM system in response to stressors. Over time, reduced exposure to stress hormones from these symptoms leads to pathogenic processes such as inflammation being diminished, and ultimately reduces the risk of associated diseases. Studying the shift-and-persist approach to dealing with stress highlighted how low-SES children displayed better asthma profiles through developing resilience. The study found lower-SES children with asthma who worked to reinterpret stressors in a more positive light while remaining optimistic about their future had less asthma inflammation and impairment. This was the first study of its kind that showed a health-protective effect, biologically and clinically, of a wellness-oriented coping method involving resilience [18].

The SSC model looks at life stressors in allergic diseases causing extremes of psychological distress leading to neuroendocrine system activation that secretes catecholamines and cortisol, which influence the immune system in shifting the Th1/Th2 cytokine balance in favor of Th2 action. The SSC model outcomes cascade emphasizes chronic rather than acute stressors, leading to allergic reactions and complicating subsequent control over them. The secretion of catecholamines and corticoids secondary to sustained, chronic stressors induces activation of the neuroendocrine system to produce a Th1/Th2 imbalance in favor of a Th2-mediated response favoring an "allergic" inflammatory response. Brain-derived neurotropic factor (BDNF) further increases production of specific IgE and reduces the Th1 cytokine profile, shifting the balance additionally in favor of a Th2-mediated response. Therefore, the SSC model profile lessens psychological distress, regulates the neuroendocrine response elicited by stress, and prevents overstimulation of the allergic inflammatory response, allowing the patient to achieve wellness [1].

Autoimmune Diseases

The immunologic system as it pertains to autoimmune processes will be the focus of this section of the chapter. Autoimmunity involves an internal source of antigen in response to which there is an overly high reactivity of the immune system, resulting in the etiology of autoimmune diseases. The etiology of autoimmune disease is multifactorial; yet, the onset of

50 percent of these diseases is attributed to "unknown trigger factors" [26]. Our SSC model investigates how life stressors, social support, and coping strategies jointly create a composite vector toward wellness versus distress, associated neuroendocrine, and, in turn, immune system responses that manifest with changes in physical health, which in this case represents the symptoms of autoimmune diseases. Studies have elucidated how psychological distress triggers life stressor-related hormonal responses that – with a lack of social support and with maladaptive coping strategies – could cause and/or exacerbate autoimmune diseases. Hence, we incorporate the tenets of the SSC model in treating autoimmune diseases so that behavioral interventions are included, and focus on optimal management of life stressors to alleviate psychological distress and restore neuroendocrine and immunologic balance, and, in turn, enhance resilience against autoimmune diseases and achieve true wellness [26, 27].

Life Stressor Domain

The pathogenesis of life stressor-related autoimmune diseases involves repeated acute and/ or chronic negatively impactful stressful life events inducing a type of "acute phase response" that subsequently may lead to chronic inflammation if left unchecked. This chronic inflammatory response with sustained or repetitive life stressors generates a milieu characterized by decreases in CD8 cell counts or less functional CD8 cells (in particular, the subset of CD8 cells known as "suppressor cells"). Chronic, sustained, and severe stressors are also associated with lower (rather than higher) plasma cortisol levels. Lower cortisol level is expected to be associated with less-than-normal immunosuppressive effects of cortisol, and lower levels of immunoglobulin-M (IgM). Life stressor changes may be associated with a hyperreactive immune response characteristic of autoimmune diseases [26]. Stressors not only act as a precipitating factor for autoimmune disease, but the disease itself causes significant psychological distress, potentially causing a recursive cycling of distress, increased inflammation, and worsened autoimmune disease clinical status. This milieu perpetuates an SSC model-induced profile of unpredictable, uncontrollable, and chronic stressful life events, coupled with unavailable, unsatisfactory, and insufficient social support, as well as maladaptive coping strategy use that leads to psychological distress, stressor-induced neuroendocrine changes, dysregulated suppressor CD8 cell numbers, and functional responses, and, finally, on to the etiology of autoimmune disease and the promotion of its severity.

Stojanovic studied patients with systemic lupus erythematosus (SLE), rheumatoid arthritis (RA), and primary antiphospholipid syndrome (PAPS) and reported that life stressors, such as bereavement, financial burdens, unemployment, and political destabilization, contribute to high levels of psychological distress among these patients. It was found that the perception of autoimmune disease chronicity by these patients, especially when compounded by maladaptive coping strategies such as smoking, were associated with prolonged anxiety. That is, one or several factors outside of a person's control, many of them persisting for long periods of time, were reported in the perception of auto-immune disease patients to be more likely to be considered as causes of their disease. A meta-analysis study focusing on the life stressor domain of the SSC model and addressing its impact on development of autoimmune diseases showed a significant, direct relationship of life stressors, particularly in the immediate pre-diagnostic period. This study showed that life stressors played a major role as an etiological agent of autoimmune diseases – regardless of the type of disease – as no significant differences in this relationship were observed between organ-specific and systemic disease pathologies [26].

Dube et al. investigated cumulative childhood life stressors (adverse childhood experiences or ACEs) leading to autoimmune diseases in adulthood [22]. They found that the number of traumatic life stressors experienced during childhood was associated with increased hospitalizations and Th1, Th2, and Th2-rheumatic changes, and that 21 types of autoimmune disease increased. Major childhood life stressors, such as physical, emotional, and/or sexual abuse, witnessing domestic violence, growing up with substance-use disorder or other mental disorders in the household, parental divorce, and/or an incarcerated family member were correlated with the development of autoimmune diseases as an adult. The relationship between ACEs and hospitalization was particularly high among the younger adult population. It has also been shown that persons living with autoimmune diseases suffer from more aversive symptomatology, disability, dysfunction, pain, and physical discomfort than the general population. Further, greater "illness intrusiveness" led to higher psychological distress due to valued activities by the sufferers no longer being gratifying. This gave the person suffering with autoimmune disease the sense of less personal control for achieving positive outcomes and avoiding negative ones in her/his life. Persons with autoimmune diseases also experienced financial stressors, including increased rates of unemployment, disability, costs of complex medical procedures, and dependence on expensive medical technology and personnel.

Major negative life event stressors combined with the impact of daily life hassles (minor stressors) have also been examined in studies conducted worldwide predicting the onset of Graves' disease. The cumulative results of the studies examined by Mizokami et al. found major negative life events in the preceding 12 months and daily hassles in the preceding six months to be predictive of Graves' disease onset. They also found the severity of the negative life events and hassles to be associated with increased severity of Graves' disease autoimmunity, once developed [27]. Of note, a prospective study focusing on patients with RA showed that those experiencing life stressors in the preceding six months had significantly increased pain, with another study showing traumatic life events leading to significantly higher rates of disease exacerbation in RA. Here, minor life stressors around interpersonal relationships, work, and finances were found to have more of a deleterious impact on disease states than major stressors in RA. It has also been reported that minor stressors were associated with high joint tenderness and pain in RA patients – with those experiencing highly stressful weeks suffering from higher disease activity, as measured with HLA-DR (a marker for chronic immune activation), CD3 (a marker for T lymphocytes) cells, and soluble IL-2 receptor levels. Higher levels of daily stressors have also been associated with high joint swelling and erosions, which worsened over time. Workplace and financial stressors have also been found to predict arthritic symptoms and pain in RA patients [28–30].

In RA and SLE, disrupted HPA axis and SAM system responses to life stressors have been demonstrated when compared to healthy persons. These results have been linked to altered neuroendocrine–immune interactions. The chronicity of autoimmune disorders may amplify the impact of even daily life stressors and typically adversely affects the patient, as the perception of chronic illness compounds disease-induced fatigue and other symptoms. Causal relationships between life stressor exposure and symptom onset, exacerbation, as well as relapse, have been studied in other autoimmune diseases as well, including psoriasis and inflammatory bowel disease (IBD). Similarly to RA and SLE, the life stressor response in these diseases has been tied to neuroendocrine–immune mediators that can promote psychological distress related to the condition (including anxiety, depression, denial, guilt, anger, and fear) [31–33]. Life stressors have long been recognized as triggers for clinical flare-ups in psoriasis. This has led to the utilization of stress reduction techniques in psoriasis for the reduction of the clinical symptoms. Psoriasis can virtually impose social isolation on the person experiencing it. It is the series of interactions among the external (life stressors and social support) and internal (coping strategy) psychosocial predictor domains with the psychosocial (psychological distress) and biological internal outcome domains (the neuroendocrine system, the immune and inflammatory response systems, and clinical disease status) that form the basis for understanding the scope of the SSC model as a whole. Psychological distress manifesting as the most proximal outcome of the SSC psychosocial model predictors in IBD may also act as a stressor in its own right when perceived by the patient to perpetuate high, subsequent psychological distress levels (e.g., depression and anxiety promoting clinical disease flare-ups in psoriasis and IBDs, such as ulcerative colitis and Crohn's disease).

Li et al. studied the disease severity as an uncontrollable stressor in its own right in order to examine "illness uncertainty" as a life stressor [31]. They expected that illness uncertainty would decrease the accuracy of discernment of changes in clinical disease status. This results in decreases in accurate attributions of disease-related clinical events and assessments of their significance – resulting in reduced predictability of disease progression. Educational level, social support, instrumental (utilitarian) support, and coping strategies – in line with the SSC model – were investigated to determine whether illness uncertainty influenced psychological distress, social support adaptations, treatment adherence, and wellness. It was concluded that lower educational level and income were associated with higher illness uncertainty. This would be expected to lead to increased psychological distress associated with hospitalizations in persons living with SLE. Illness uncertainty was associated with avoiding the implications of the disease and yielding to negative disease outcomes. This led to decreased effective adaptation to the disease, quality of life, hope levels, and capacity for resilience – thereby impeding wellness [31–34].

Social Support Domain

The health of persons living with chronic diseases, whether physical or psychological, is influenced by those around them, some of whom constitute the social support network for that person. Social support – as defined within the SSC model – comprises emotional, informational/instrumental, and appraisal resources required during a patient's time of need. Conversely, social constraints represent feelings of inadequate social support leading a patient to feel unsupported and negatively influencing the patient's wellness. Social support enhances a patient's overall wellness by allowing the individual to better process, contemplate, and communicate their experiences, emotions, and thoughts, allowing maintenance of a positive sense of self and overall wellness. In comparing the role of social support portrayed by the SSC model leading to either disease progression or regression, a cross-sectional survey described the balance between social support and social constraint.

Patients with autoimmune diseases reported spouse, family, and friendship interactions provided more social support than social constraint. In studying regression models, it was found that constraints from spouses, families, and friends were associated with worse patient psychological adjustment. Spousal support was found to be the most important factor in providing social support as a three-way interaction analysis found that patients with low spousal support had worse psychological adjustment as levels of family and friend support increased (Figure 12.4). In contrast, patients displayed better psychological adjustment when high levels of spousal support were provided with increasing family and friend support. Spousal support for chronic disease patients was found to be most important as

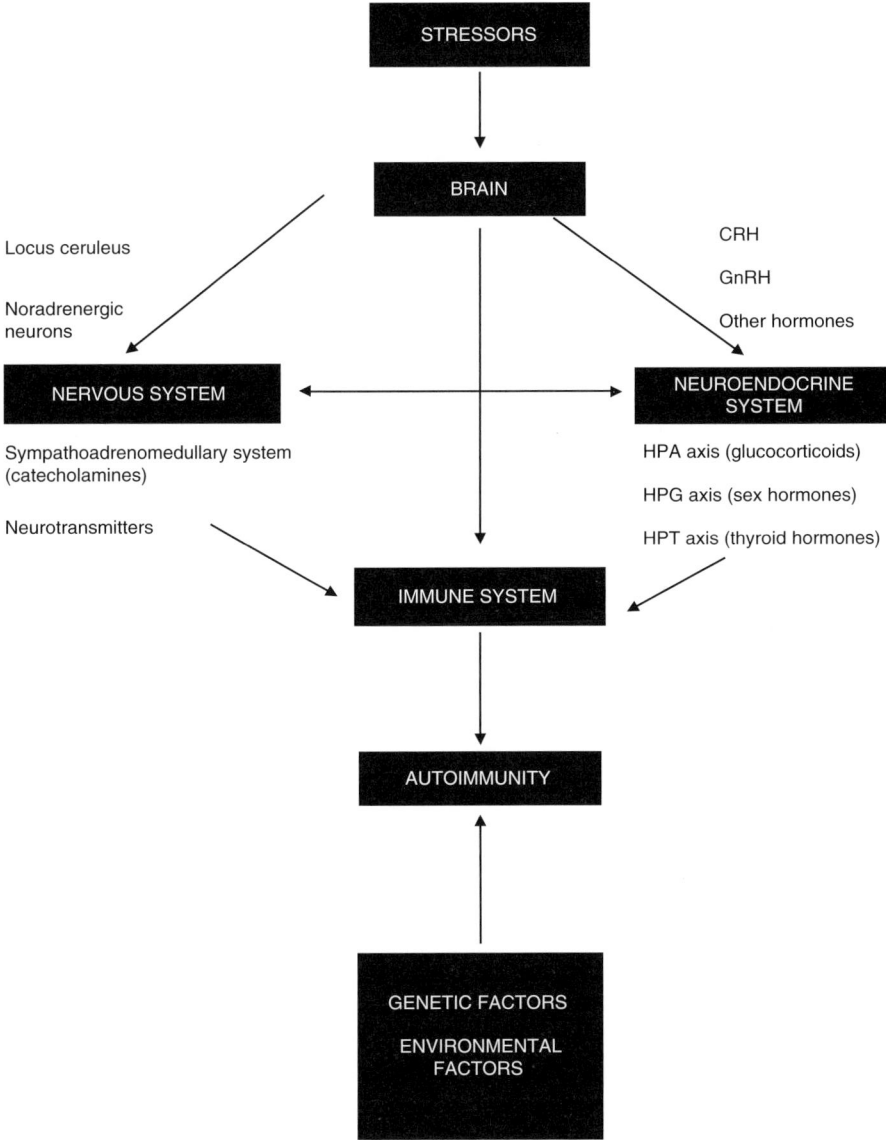

Figure 12.4 Stress and autoimmunity. Adapted from T Mizokami, AW Li, S El-Kaissi, JR Wall. Stress and thyroid autoimmunity. *Thyroid*, 2004; 14(12): 1047–1055.

married patients consistently demonstrated better illness coping skills, adherence to treatment regimens, motivation, and fewer episodes of depression and engagement in risky behavior. In contrast, spouses were also found to be sources of social constraint when they made supportive attempts that were not desired or did not match the patients' needs, negatively influencing the patients' psychological adjustment and disease outcomes, such as pain. Social constraints from spouses were also found to increase anxiety and depressive symptoms and lower patient adherence to self-care activities [34].

Utilizing various evaluation lists, scales, questionnaires, and qualitative methods to measure social support valuation in SLE, a literature review found that individuals living with SLE had to learn to live with a variety of unpredictable symptoms, making consistent support and information vital for daily illness management. Dissatisfaction was found to be higher among SLE patients in terms of the social support they received especially as it related to healthcare. Unsatisfactory contact with doctors pertaining to miscommunication and lack of information about the disease relayed to the patient ranked high among patient dissatisfaction. Increased disease activity in SLE patients was correlated with less social support, contrasted with more social support, sense of belonging, and positive self-esteem being related to lessened disease severity. Social support positively influenced the physical and mental health component when examining quality of life. Increased social support was found to be associated with lower occurrences of mood disturbance and fatigue. SLE patients who maintained interpersonal relationships through family, friends, or social support groups – as highlighted in an eight-week group psychoeducational course – showed improved verbal learning ability, self-reported memory functioning, and reduced depression. Moreover, programs such as the "Chronic Disease Self-Management Program" encourage low-income SLE patients to participate, yielding significant physical and cognitive improvements post-intervention. This is important, as mood disorders and psychiatric illnesses rank higher among SLE patients than any other autoimmune disease, and addressing life stressors and mood disturbances such as depression is paramount, as they are linked with suboptimal adherence to medications and increased risk of cardiovascular disease in this patient population [31–34].

Li and colleagues noted that social support has been shown to be crucial in influencing the course of SLE disease progression in persons hospitalized with SLE. These persons are known to suffer from high levels of illness uncertainty. Research results in SLE call for medical staff to pay attention to illness uncertainty. Persons living with SLE need clinical interventions to maximize their effective use of social support and to guide them in deterring their focus of attention away from their ongoing illness uncertainty (a special aspect of the psychological distress that they experience). Such interventions deter the promotion of disease, promote resilient responses in the face of disease, and enhance true positive wellness [34].

Coping Strategies Domain

The SSC model proposes implementing behavioral interventions to manage life stressor-induced psychological distress, neuroendocrine system activation, immune system dysfunction and inflammatory dysregulation, and clinical disease onset or exacerbation. Cognitive-behavioral stress management is prescribed by the SSC model when life stressor burden is particularly high, assuming equilibrium in the social support and coping strategies domains. Social support groups are prescribed by the SSC model when social support availability, sufficiency, and/or satisfaction is particularly low, assuming equilibrium in the life stressor burden and coping strategies domains. Social support has direct, salutary effects on physical health as well as a salutary, indirect effect buffering against the burden of negative life stressors. Finally, coping skills enhancement training is prescribed by the SSC model when passive, maladaptive coping strategies (such as denial, avoidance, and substance use) predominate over the impact of the life stressor and social support domains. Direct physical health interventions addressing weight management, diet, and maintaining a healthy home environment are also important to the prevention of clinical flare-ups of autoimmune diseases and to deterring the longer-term progression of autoimmune diseases.

Lifestyle and environmental factors can be modified to improve the SSC model profile in response to autoimmune diseases. "Resilience," as mentioned earlier, is an important construct in this regard. It arises as a prediction of the SSC model when a person successfully minimizes the negative impact of life stressors; improves social support availability, sufficiency, and satisfaction; and utilizes active and adaptive – as opposed to passive, maladaptive – coping strategies. Resilient responses can become entrained to the point that they are spontaneously used in response to life stressors that a person experiences. They then actively aid in protecting the person with autoimmune diseases by creating a "built-in" disposition against the risk for a high impact of negative life stressors.

Resilience in response to autoimmune diseases calls for an individual to deal with the autoimmune disease by acceptance coping (accepting his/her limitations), active behavioral coping (adhering to the prescribed treatment regimen), and planning (a strategy for coping by adjusting and adapting to adverse situations). Faria et al. studied resilience and treatment adherence in patients with SLE and argued that poor wellness outcomes occurred with suboptimal adherence to the treatment regimen; lack of education about the disease; lack of acknowledgment of one's own limitations; and lack of self-care (smoking; avoiding sunlight; and not controlling heart disease risk factors). Moreover, these factors all contributed to the more deleterious life stressor burden profile faced by the person with SLE. These authors also reported that persons with SLE showing high resilience helped other persons to overcome their life stressor burden and helped maintain their functional status in activities of daily living, despite their SLE diagnosis. In line with this, functioning was higher, adaptation improved to situations that previously were triggers, and protection was promoted by allowing persons with SLE to adhere to their treatment regimens. Persons with SLE were less forgetful in taking their medications, were more engaged in better understanding and educating themselves about their disease, were more likely to follow their medical recommendations, and more frequently became aware of the importance of treatment adherence in this setting. Further, persons with SLE reported high overall wellness, high quality of life, low symptom burden, and good physical health status. Hence, resilience in autoimmune diseases incorporates the impacts of external/social and internal/psychological factors. The goal of promoting resilience and true wellness requires effectiveness of medication delivery, better access to consultations and examinations, and accessible educational resources for persons with autoimmune diseases (particularly for the subgroup who are the most susceptible to non-adherence) [35–37].

Faria and colleagues call for public health services to be more proactive in promoting school programs and educative initiatives to create more awareness to help the population better understand SLE and to be more engaged in promoting self-care. Their approach focuses on enhancing the social support domain – by implementing friendly assistance services, by improving ways of caring and treatment, and by tailoring treatment to the educational and socioeconomic needs of persons living with SLE. They also promote the use of the coping strategies domain by advocating for persons with SLE themselves to embrace resilient processes by active behavioral coping (and learned self-efficacy), coping by maintaining a sense of humor, and active cognitive coping (developing insight). The literature also alludes to persons with SLE achieving resilience through spiritual/religious coping – a coping strategy capable of promoting resilience and achieving wellness [32, 33].

Resilience was also studied by Rojas et al. in autoimmune rheumatic diseases, as these diseases have long been associated with high life stressor burdens for the persons living with them [37]. As autoimmune diseases are chronic conditions, they involve an increased "allostatic load" defined as physiological consequences accumulated over time operating in conjunction with aging and cumulative life stressor exposure, resulting in deleterious psychological and physical health consequences. The profile of psychosocial context created by the SSC model refers to various potentially deleterious situations that can nevertheless be responded to with resilience. Per Rojas and colleagues, such resilience may be influenced by years of formal education, gender, and SES. They reported that women who were low in educational level and resided in resource-poor environments were more susceptible to psychological distress and poor physical health – with an increased incidence of autoimmunity. As a result, they proposed instituting behavioral training programs in resilience promotion in order to improve the quality of life; decrease pain levels; promote active coping strategies; and achieve overall wellness. It was concluded that women with rheumatic autoimmune diseases could become more resilient and less vulnerable to the deleterious consequences of autoimmune diseases.

Flachenecker discussed the use of rehabilitation as a coping strategy for promoting wellness in RA and multiple sclerosis (MS), the autoimmune diseases with the most extensive research literature in the area of psychosocial context [30]. The focus of rehabilitation enlists all three predictor domains of the SSC model in dictating the achievement of optimal psychological and physical wellness outcomes. Thereby, rehabilitation integrates the person suffering from autoimmune disease into their environment. An aim of rehabilitation is to improve patient independence and quality of life using, for example, a moderate-to-high intensity of physical exercise. Such exercise levels have been reported to be effective for persons with SLE to increase their aerobic capacity and physical functioning levels while reducing psychological distress and fatigue levels. Both of the latter may become disabling to a person with autoimmune disease. With respect to RA, short-term aerobic capacity training, non-aerobic, muscle strength training, and water-based aerobic training were each found to be effective in improving functional abilities of persons living with RA. These interventions also improved overall wellness through the prevention of secondary de-conditioning due to reduced physical activity levels [30]. With respect to MS, physiotherapy has been demonstrated across numerous studies to be effective in decreasing motor dysfunction, gait instability, and fatigue, while enhancing ambulation, physical fitness, and endurance. Further, a systematic review reported that psychotherapy offered by personnel trained in psychological and cognitive difficulties experienced by persons living with MS was beneficial to those with moderate to severe disability in reducing depressive distress and in improving the adjustment to and coping strategies for MS. Flachenecker developed a three-week coping program delivered during inpatient rehabilitation that focused upon individualized and deficit goal-oriented rehabilitation techniques [30]. Through individual therapy, group therapy, lectures, and discussions relevant to MS, persons living with MS improved their ability to overcome challenges and their fatigue and depressive distress. Long-lasting effects were also observed in health-related quality of life and wellness.

The SSC model focuses upon and predicts the role of the life stressor domain as it pertains to autoimmune diseases and how this domain maps to induce psychological distress as the "most proximal" outcome. The SSC model outcomes cascade outlines how repeated exposure to acute or chronic life stressors, when insufficiently mitigated by the social support and coping strategies domains, predicts psychological distress and increased cortisol release, which, in turn, increases the levels of proinflammatory cytokines (particularly TNF-α, IL-1, and IL-6) that may persist with chronic inflammation. The SSC model is prescriptive for specific distress-alleviating and wellness-enhancing interventions that are expected to downregulate chronic inflammatory responses and to increase the count of and improve the function of the suppressor subset of CD8+ T lymphocytes, which may be hypoactive in autoimmune diseases.

Summary

In summary, the study of the relationship between psychosocial factors and immunological and inflammatory indices requires an intensive investigative approach in order to elucidate the actual risk factors and effective intervention strategies that will reduce psychological distress and enhance true wellness. In addition, new research explicitly employing the SSC model is needed in order to properly delineate how it operates in determining clinical outcomes in specific diseases (infectious diseases; allergic diseases; and autoimmune diseases) as well as how its use might promote true wellness in the general population. It is especially relevant to focus on how the SSC model might generate specific predictions about on decreasing morbidity, disability, and mortality. Beyond the person suffering with a disease, the SSC model can be used to assess the risk and the most promising interventions for the psychological distress and physical illnesses experienced by the caregiver of the person suffering from a disease (perhaps most notably Alzheimer's disease). The SSC model (comprising its life stressor, social support, and coping strategy domain predictors) can be used as part of a measurement-based care approach to assess its association with overall functional and physical health outcomes in persons seeking general clinical care as part of the future of integrative medicine.

References

1. K Goodkin, A Visser. *Psychoneuroimmunology: Stress, Mental Disorders, and Health.* Washington, DC, American Psychiatric Press; 2001.

2. N McCain, D Gray, J Walter, J Robins. Implementing a comprehensive approach to the study of health dynamics using the psychoneuroimmunology paradigm. *Adv Nurs Sci* 2005; 28(4): 320–332.

3. RS Lazarus, S Folkman. *Stress, Appraisal, and Coping.* New York, Springer; 1984.

4. K Goodkin, I Fuchs, D Feaster, et al. Life stressors and coping style are associated with immune measures in HIV-1 infection: a preliminary report. *Int J Psychiatr Med* 1992; 22: 155–172.

5. K Goodkin, R Tuttle, NT Blaney, et al. A bereavement support group intervention is associated with immunological changes in HIV-1þ and HIV-1- homosexual men: paper presented at the annual meeting of the American Psychosomatic Society Williamsburg, VA. *Psychosom Med* 1996; 58 (1): 83–84.

6. K Goodkin, D Feaster, D Asthana, et al. A bereavement support group intervention is longitudinally associated with salutary effects on the CD4 cell count and number of physician visits. *Clin Diagn Lab Immunol* 1998: 382–391.

7. K Goodkin, NT Blaney, DJ Feaster, et al. A randomized controlled clinical trial of

a bereavement support group intervention in human immunodeficiency virus type 1-seropositive and-seronegative homosexual men. *Arch Gen Psychiatr* 1999; **56**: 52–59.

8. S Cohen, GM Williamson. Stress and infectious disease in humans. *Psychol Bull* 1991; **109**(1): 5–24.

9. AA Stone, DH Bovbjerg, A Napoli, et al. Development of common cold symptoms following experimental rhinovirus infection is related to prior stressful life events. *Behav Med* 1992; **18**(3): 115–120.

10. J Sheridan, C Dobbs, D Brown, B Zwilling. Psychoneuroimmunology: stress effects on pathogenesis and immunity during infection. *Clin Microbiol Rev* 1994; **7**(2): 200–212.

11. M Kemeny, M Schedlowski. Understanding the interaction between psychosocial stress and immune-related diseases: a stepwise progression. *Brain Behav Immunity* 2007; **21**(8): 1009–1018.

12. S Lutgendorf, MH Antoni, G Ironson, et al. Changes in cognitive coping skills and social support during cognitive behavioral stress management intervention and distress outcomes in symptomatic human immunodeficiency virus (HIV)-seropositive gay men. *Psychosom Med* 1998; **60**(2): 204–214.

13. K Goodkin, CL Mulder, NT Blaney, et al. Psychoneuroimmunology and human immunodeficiency virus type 1 infection revisited. *Arch Gen Psychiatry* 1994; **51**(3): 246–248.

14. WW IsHak. *The Guidebook of Sexual Medicine*. Beverly Hills, CA, A&W Publishing; 2008.

15. A Carrico, M Antoni. Effects of psychological interventions on neuroendocrine hormone regulation and immune status in HIV-positive persons: a review of randomized controlled trials. *Psychosom Med* 2008; **70**(5): 575–584.

16. GD Marshall, SR Roy. Stress and allergic diseases. *Psychoneuroimmunology* 2007; **31**: 799–824.

17. RJ Wright, M Rodriguez, S Cohen. Review of psychosocial stress and asthma: an integrated biopsychosocial approach. *Thorax* 1998; **53**(12): 1066–1074.

18. E Chen, R Strunk, A Trethewey, et al. Resilience in low-socioeconomic-status children with asthma: adaptations to stress. *J Allerg Clin Immunol* 2011; **128**(5): 970–976.

19. M Steinhoff, A Suárez, J Feramisco, J Koo. Psychoneuroimmunology of psychological stress and atopic dermatitis: pathophysiologic and therapeutic updates. *Acta Dermato Venereologica* 2012; **92**(1): 7–15.

20. NL Letourneau, AL Kozyrskyj, N Cosic, et al. Maternal sensitivity and social support protect against childhood atopic dermatitis. *Allerg Asthma Clin Immunol* 2017; **13**(1). DOI:10.1186/s13223-017-0199-4.

21. M Iio, M Hamaguchi, M Nagata, K Yoshida. Stressors of school-age children with allergic diseases: a qualitative study. *J Pediatr Nurs* 2018; **42**: e73-e78.

22. S Dube, D Fairweather, W Pearson, et al. Cumulative childhood stress and autoimmune diseases in adults. *Psychosom Med* 2009; **71**(2): 243–250.

23. N Lind, M Nordin, E Palmquist, et al. Coping and social support in asthma and allergy: the Västerbotten Environmental Health Study. *J Asthma* 2014; **52**(6): 622–629.

24. JS Lebovidge, H Strauch, LA Kalish, LC Schneider. Assessment of psychological distress among children and adolescents with food allergy. *J Allerg Clin Immunol* 2009; **124**(6): 1282–1288.

25. J Cummings, RC Knibb, RM King, JS Lucas. The psychosocial impact of food allergy and food hypersensitivity in children, adolescents and their families: a review. *Allergy* 2010; **65**(8): 933–945.

26. B Porcelli, A Pozza, N Bizzaro, et al. Association between stressful life events and autoimmune diseases: a systematic review and meta-analysis of retrospective case–control studies. *Autoimmun Rev* 2016; **15**(4): 325–334 .

27. T Mizokami, AW Li, S El-Kaissi, JR Wall. Stress and thyroid autoimmunity. *Thyroid* 2004; **14**(12): 1047–1055.

28. L Stojanovich. Stress and autoimmunity. *Autoimmun Rev* 2010; **9**(5). DOI:10.1016/j .autrev.2009.11.014.

29. GM Devins. Using the Illness Intrusiveness Ratings Scale to understand health-related quality of life in chronic disease. *J Psychosom Res* 2010; **68**(6): 591–602.

30. P Flachenecker. Autoimmune diseases and rehabilitation. *Autoimmun Rev* 2012; **11** (3): 219–225.

31. X Li, L He, J Wang, M Wang. Illness uncertainty, social support, and coping mode in hospitalized patients with systemic lupus erythematosus in a hospital in Shaanxi, China. *PLoS One* 2019; **14**(2): e0211313.

32. DAP Faria, LS Revoredo, MJ Vilar, EMC Maia. Resilience and treatment adhesion in patients with systemic lupus erythematosus. *Open Rheumatol J* 2014; **8**: 1–8.

33. DAP Faria, J Goncalves, R Dias. Neuropsychiatric systemic lupus erythematosus involvement: towards a tailored approach to our patients? *Rambam Maimonides Med J* 2017; **8**(1): e001.

34. D Mazzoni, E Cicognani. Social support and health in patients with systemic lupus erythematosus: a literature review. *Lupus* 2011; **20**(11): 1117–1125.

35. DM Carpenter, CT Thorpe, DS Alexander, et al. The relationship between social support, social constraint, and psychological adjustment for patients with rare autoimmune disease. *Curr Rheumatol Rev* 2016; **12**(3): 232–238.

36. CJ McCray, SK Agarwal. Stress and autoimmunity. *Immunol Allerg Clin North Am* 2011; **31**(1): 1–18.

37. M Rojas, Y Rodriguez, Y Pacheco, et al. Resilience in women with autoimmune rheumatic diseases. *Joint Bone Spine* 2018; **85**(6): 715–720.

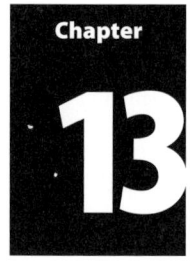

Wellness in Endocrine and Metabolic Disorders

Steven Clevenger, Lidia Eskander, Tiffany Lin, and Waguih William IsHak

Introduction

Wellness is a term encompassing many aspects of the human experience, including physical health. Much of the regulation and maintenance of the human body occurs via hormonal expression. The human endocrine organs include the pituitary, adrenals, thyroid, testes, and ovaries, and produce many of the hormones responsible for maintaining homeostasis and optimal cellular function [1]. Many factors can alter hormonal expression, including aging, environmental toxins, disease, nutrition, and even stress [1]. Hormonal imbalances often lead to poorer health outcomes and decreased wellness in the long run. This chapter will give an overview of the most common endocrine disorders, how they impact wellness, and what has been done to improve patient quality of life (QOL).

Adrenal Gland

Cushing Syndrome

Cushing syndrome (CS) is a relatively rare but serious condition that results from chronic hypercortisolism [2]. Exogenous CS is most commonly caused by glucocorticoid administration, while endogenous CS is further divided into adrenocorticotropic hormone (ACTH) dependent and independent. Cortisol is a glucocorticoid steroid hormone produced in the adrenal cortex that is important in regulating the body in response to stressors. In the hypothalamic–pituitary–adrenal (HPA) axis of the endocrine system, physical and psychological stress stimulates the hypothalamus to release corticotropin-releasing hormone (CRH), which in turns stimulates ACTH release. In turn ACTH directly stimulates the adrenal cortex to release cortisol, which negatively regulates CRH release. Cushing syndrome causes significant morbidity and mortality due to cardiovascular, metabolic, and psychiatric sequelae [3]. Features of CS include fatigue, weight gain, central obesity, facial plethora, muscle wasting, weakness, thinned skin, depression, emotional lability, and cognitive impairment [4]. Due to its variable symptoms, CS is often difficult to diagnose, resulting in a prolonged disease course.

Patients with CS exhibit significantly decrease health-related quality of life (HRQOL) due to symptoms and sequelae of the disease, including metabolic syndrome, bone loss and fractures, opportunistic infections, neuropsychiatric dysfunction, and cognitive impairment [5]. Though HRQOL improves after surgical treatment, it continues to be lower compared to gender- and age-matched controls [6]. Unfortunately, many effects of hypercortisolism do not fully resolve even after surgical cure, and there appears to be a correlation between the chronicity of hypercortisolism and the irreversibility of its effects [6]. Studies

160

have showed that patients with CS had an overall lower HRQOL, with lower body image perception and higher levels of depression compared to healthy controls, particularly if disease is persistent despite surgery [7]. They continued to experience problems in multiple domains of life after being cured; patients perceived themselves as more depressed, anxious, fatigued, and having poorer physical health, environment, and social adjustment [8]. Regarding impact on functioning, one study found 34 percent of patients with mild, 26 percent with moderate, 29 percent with severe, and 11 percent with very severe psychiatric disability [9].

Early diagnosis of hypercortisolism aids in the process of normalizing excessive cortisol levels, thus preventing or lessening the severity of symptoms in CS patients. Because CS is often difficult to diagnose, the chronicity of the disease often results in physical and neuropsychiatric sequelae that take much longer to resolve. In cases where neuropsychiatric symptoms such as depression and anxiety persist, treatment using antidepressants and psychotherapy may be considered [10]. Other alternative therapies also exist that may help improve QOL. Nutritionally, CS patients should consume greater amounts of calcium to prevent bone loss, increase sodium intake to reduce weight gain, and increase protein intake to reduce muscle loss [11]. Regular exercise has also been shown to reduce or prevent glucocorticoid-induced muscle atrophy that is common in CS [12]. Carelson et al. noted that mindfulness-based stress reduction (MSBR) improved the function of the HPA axis, leading to decreased salivary cortisol [13]. Similarly, yoga has long been touted as a stress-relieving exercise routine leading to reductions in cortisol and improved symptoms of depression [14]. Cushing syndrome remains a condition that can severely degrade QOL; prompt treatment of the cause is the best way to ensure optimal clinical outcomes, and healthy habits can lead to improvement or prevention of some of these deleterious effects.

Adrenal Insufficiency

Adrenal insufficiency can either be primary (Addison's disease) or secondary (ACTH deficiency). In either scenario, adrenal insufficiency occurs, leading to deficient production of glucocorticoids, mineralocorticoids, and androgens [15]. Symptoms include fatigue, syncope, nausea, vomiting, diarrhea, mood changes, hyperpigmentation, and even death in an adrenal crisis [16]. Hyperpigmentation is only found in primary adrenal insufficiency as it is secondary to ACTH hypersecretion [17]. Treatment requires replacement of the absent hormones via oral corticosteroids and fludrocortisone [18]. Quality of life can be greatly impacted by adrenal insufficiency. Using the Addison's disease-specific quality of life questionnaire (AddiQoL), Meyer attempted to ascertain what predicted decreased HRQOL in 200 Addison's disease patients. Factors associated with significantly reduced HRQOL included age of manifestation ($p < 0.001$), autoimmune comorbidities ($p = 0.01$), female gender ($p < 0.001$), and, most significantly, latency of first diagnosis ($p < 0.001$) [15]. Dehydroepiandrosterone (DHEA) is also deficient in adrenal insufficiency and not normally replaced. Hunt et al., in a study of 39 patients, found that 50 mg oral DHEA daily significantly improved self-esteem, mood, and fatigue [19].

Although serious, adrenal insufficiency is a treatable condition. Ufferman et al., in a study of dogs with adrenalectomies, showed that renal diluting capacity can be preserved on a high-sodium diet, independent of mineralocorticoid replacement [20]. Although this study was done on nonhumans, dog physiology is similar enough to suggest increasing sodium intake could improve kidney urine production in post-adrenalectomy patients.

Adrenal fatigue is a similar condition to adrenal insufficiency, in which there is a derangement in the production and regulation of adrenal hormones [21]. In a review article by Anderson, numerous dietary recommendations were made to optimize adrenal gland function. Generally it was recommended that a diet consist of 45 percent complex carbohydrates, 30 percent protein, and 25 percent fats [21]. Several herbal supplements also showed improvement in adrenal function. *Ocinum sanctum* fed to rats was shown to improve corticosterone response in acutely and chronically fatigued rats. Similarly *Cordyceps sinensis* reduced adrenal weight, which could prevent adrenal exhaustion [21]. Ronzio et al. made recommendations to supplement with important vitamins in adrenal steroid hormone synthesis, including B complex vitamins and vitamins A and C [22]. In order to maximize wellness in these patients, early detection and optimal treatment are recommended in adrenal gland pathologies.

Estrogen and Progesterone

Estrogen is the primary hormone in female-specific physiology and comes in three forms: estradiol, estriol, and estrone [1]. Estradiol is the most potent and is secreted by follicles of the ovaries; estrone is secreted by fat cells and ovaries; and estriol is the weakest and is secreted by the placenta during pregnancy [1, 23]. Estrogen is important in maintaining female health and wellness. Estrogen levels generally peak during the reproductive years and fall off sharply after menopause. Contrary to this, estrone levels tend to rise after menopause due to their synthesis from androgens in fat cells [1]. Progesterone, synthesized in the corpus luteum, acts as an antagonist to estrogen in order to maintain hormonal homeostasis and prevent adverse effects of excess estrogen, such as endometrial and breast tissue hyperplasia [24].

Hormone replacement therapy (HRT) utilizing estrogen, progesterone, or an admixture of the two has been used for decades to mediate the physiologic changes of menopause. It can reduce menopause symptoms including hot flashes, vaginal atrophy, skin aging, vaginal dryness, bone loss, decreased muscle mass, and sexual dysfunction [25]. Williams et al. used the Menopause-Specific Quality of Life Questionnaire (MENQOL) on 2703 postmenopausal women and found that vasomotor symptoms such as hot flashes had the biggest impact on daily activities [26]. The two primary classes of hormone medications are bioidentical and nonidentical formularies. Bioidentical hormones have identical structures to those in humans, while nonidentical hormones differ, causing these two classes to have differing effects on the human body [1, 24].

Early in the history of HRT a link between endometrial and breast carcinoma was noted, particularly for nonidentical synthetic conjugated estrogens [27, 28]. Later, the Women's Health Initiative (WHI) study – a long-term, large-scale study – was abruptly ended in 2002 due to increased incidence of malignancy, myocardial infarction (MI), and stroke in the conjugated estrogen and synthetic progestin study groups [29]. While these results caused widespread questioning of HRT, studies have not been universal in the finding of adverse side effects. In a large prospective French cohort study of 98,997 women, it was found that micronized (versus synthetic) progestins were associated with significantly lower breast cancer risk; additionally, consistent HRT usage was lower risk than intermittent use [30]. The Danish Nurse Cohort Study followed 19,898 women age 45 and above and found that estrogen combined with synthetic progestin exhibited the highest risk of cancer [31]. Nelson evaluated use of conjugated estrogen versus estradiol and found similar efficacy in relieving menopausal symptoms; however, conjugated estrogen was associated with increased incidence of breast cancer, stroke, and MI [32]. Given the mixed results of the research on HRT, more studies should be done to stratify the risks associated with bioidentical versus nonidentical hormones.

There are still other methods that individuals may use before, during, and after menopause in order to improve QOL. Vitamin D intake is of vital importance for older women experiencing menopause. Adequate vitamin D intake is associated with improved bone health and has even been associated with a 17 percent decreased risk of early menopause [33, 34]. Sleep disturbances are commonly reported in and around menopause. Supplementing the diet with resveratrol, tryptophanum, glycine, and vitamin E may help to promote optimal sleep [35]. In a study on postmenopausal Native American women, flaxseed consumption at 30 g per day significantly reduced low-density lipoprotein cholesterol (LDL-C) by 10 percent, which could help mitigate risk for adverse cardiac events [36]. Hot flashes are often experienced during menopause and can detract from QOL. Kroenke et al. performed a weight loss study on 17,473 women and found that those who lost a large amount of weight (>10 percent) were significantly more likely to see resolution of their hot flashes [37]. Yoga exercises have also been shown to be helpful in alleviating menopause-related sleep disturbances [38].

Growth Hormone

Growth hormone (GH) is secreted by the pituitary gland. This is an important hormone in cell growth, cell reproduction, and cell regeneration. Additionally, it stimulates the release of IGF-1 [39]. Growth hormone deficiency can occur pathologically in adults and children. In adults the most common cause is pituitary adenoma [40]. Growth hormone deficiency results in growth failure and delayed sexual maturation in children; osteoclastic activity is upregulated and there is osteoporosis in adults [41]. Growth hormone deficiency can cause decreased QOL and it is thought to be an important hormone in mental and emotional well-being. Prodam et al. found that adults with GH deficiency suffered higher rates of depression; Nyberg and Hallberg noted that GH administration improves cognitive function [42, 43]. Growth hormone replacement therapy (GRT) has also been noted to improve cardiac function, immunity, blood pressure, strength, and energy [1]. Due to the pulsatile nature of GH and risks associated with stimulation tests, IGF-1 is generally used to test GH levels in age-related GH deficiency [1]. Growth hormone replacement therapy is controversial, with known side effects of water retention, joint pain, reduced insulin sensitivity, and a purported link to cancer [44, 45]. Conflicting data exists regarding a relationship between IGF-1 levels and breast and colorectal cancers [46, 47]. However, studies of more than 19,000 pediatric and 100 adult patients undergoing GH replacement therapy found no evidence of recurrent or *de novo* malignancies associated with the treatment [48, 49]. Patients treated with GH dosages that keep IGF-1 levels within physiologic range have shown a plethora of benefits; however, other options exist to boost GH endogenously. Vigorous exercise has been shown to increase GH. Godfrey et al. showed that exercise above the lactate threshold and for greater than 10 minutes is maximally beneficial for GH secretion [50]. Obesity itself could lead to diminished GH levels via excessive insulin. Lanzi et al. compared GH releasing hormone (GHRH) induced GH levels in obese and non-obese patients. The response from non-obese patients was found to be significant ($p < 0.01$) [51]. Thus, exercise may promote GH release in the short term with appropriate intensity and in the long term via fat loss. Nutritional supplementation with amino acids may also prove beneficial. One study of 16 subjects dosed with 1500 mg L-arginine and 1500 mg L-lysine immediately before exercise showed significantly greater amounts of GH release than the non-supplemented exercise control group [52]. Kerndt et al. studied fasting and its effects on various hormones; they found a progressive rise in GH levels peaking at day 26 of fasting [53].

Excessive GH production can occur at any age, most commonly due to a pituitary tumor composed of somatotroph cells [54]. GH-secreting tumors in adults result in a condition called acromegaly, characterized by excessive growth of the jaw, fingers, and toes, muscle weakness, and insulin resistance [55]. First-line treatment for GH excess is surgical removal of the tumor, focused radiation, or pharmacotherapy with pegvisomant [56]. Subsequent pharmacotherapy with somatostatin analogs (octreotide/lanreotide) and dopamine agonists (cabergoline) is utilized [56]. Acromegaly can result in significant decreases in QOL. Rowles et al. developed the Acromegaly Quality of Life Questionnaire (AcroQOL) and surveyed 80 patients with acromegaly. Severe impairment in QOL was found in acromegaly patients; vitality and general health categories were the most impaired [57]. Likewise, SF-36 questionnaire scores are significantly lower for acromegaly patients in the domain of physical function [58]. Treatment of acromegaly appears to yield mixed results in wellness scores. Studies using the AcroQOL have consistently observed higher scores in treated patients, whereas the generic questionnaire (PGWBS) observed a persistently low QOL, especially in areas of general health and vitality [57, 59]. The literature is sparse regarding alternative therapies to ease symptoms of gigantism and acromegaly, likely due to their rarity. However, measures taken to improve the most common comorbidities, such as diabetes, hypertension, and arthritis, would likely be effective. Early detection and treatment is ideal for promoting wellness in patients with GH excess.

Insulin and Diabetes

Diabetes is a metabolic and endocrine disorder characterized by high blood sugar secondary to insulin resistance (type-2) or insulin absence (type-1) in the body. Type-2 diabetes (T2D) chief risk factors include obesity and poor diet, both of which lead to development of insulin resistance [60]. Type 1 diabetes (T1D) results from autoimmune destruction of insulin-producing pancreatic beta cells [61]. Symptoms include polydipsia, polyuria, increased hunger, and fatigue. Long-term health consequences of poorly managed diabetes include cardiovascular disease (CVD), chronic kidney disease (CKD), foot ulcers, neuropathy, and blindness [60]. Diabetes presents a high level of disease burden and thus negatively impacts psychological well-being. Depression is three times more common in diabetics and is associated with poorer glycemic control, self-care, and medication adherence [60, 62]. Despite the heavy burden on QOL that diabetes presents, studies have shown numerous methods for improving outcomes. Toumpanakis et al. performed a systemic review of the effects of a plant-based diet on T2D [60]. The review found that plant-based diets were associated with significant improvements in QOL ($p < 0.05$), emotional well-being, physical well-being ($p < 0.001$), HbA1C ($p = 0.002$), and LDL ($p < 0.001$). Wellness programs encompassing full lifestyle changes have also been designed to improve and prevent diabetes. The Diabetes Prevention Program (DPP) is an intensive lifestyle intervention program designed to reduce new cases of diabetes. One YMCA study utilizing the DPP achieved a 5.7 kg average weight loss; prior trials of DPP had shown that just 5 kg of weight loss was associated with 58 percent fewer new cases of T2D [63]. Some workplace programs use financial incentives to motivate their employees to change; however, these programs have met with little success. Furthermore, they have been cited as cost shifting to less healthy employees as benefits tend to accrue to the healthier workers [64]. Health coaching from medical professionals is another avenue that has yielded positive results. Pinto et al. explored the benefits of pharmacist-provided medication therapy management (MTM), whereby patients had regularly scheduled consultations with pharmacists about their medications. At one year the average HbA1C dropped by 0.27 and patient knowledge of their disease improved [65]. Mindfulness-based programs have also met with some success, with the MBSR program being the most prominent example. A randomized controlled trial (RCT) on students using this program found significant decreases in overall stress ($p = 0.2$), uncontrolled eating ($p = 0.02$), and emotional eating ($p = 0.02$) [66]. While far less common, children can also suffer from diabetes mellitus and see markedly decreased wellness as a result. In a small study of children with T1D, a humor-based wellness program resulted in a significant decrease in behavioral problems and increase in resiliency [67]. Diabetes can severely detract from patient QOL. Fortunately, there has been ample research to suggest that interventions targeted at improving lifestyle, medication adherence, and disease knowledge help improve patient wellness.

Obesity

Obesity is an increasingly common metabolic disorder that is most often secondary to chronic excess caloric intake. Adipocytes are the central cell involved in fat synthesis and storage, acting as endocrine cells in their own right [68]. Two hormones synthesized and secreted by adipose cells and involved in or affected by obesity are leptin and adiponectin [69, 70]. Leptin regulates energy balance by suppressing hunger and is present in increased quantities in obese patients [69]. Adiponectin regulates metabolic processes involved in glucose regulation and fatty acid oxidation [70, 71]. Both hormones have been studied as possible therapeutic agents. Heymsfield et al. tested exogenous leptin administration on 127 lean and obese human subjects; the therapy lasted 20 weeks and resulted in the greatest weight loss at a dose of 0.1 mg/kg at four weeks, with a loss of 1.9 kg, and at 0.3 mg/kg at 20 weeks with a loss of 7.1 kg [69]. When leptin was combined with adiponectin, additional benefits were noted. In a mouse study, Yamauchi et al. documented the reversal of insulin resistance in lopatrophic mice when dosing with physiologic doses of leptin and adiponectin [70]. The clinical applications of leptin and adiponectin therapy appear promising and should be investigated further.

More traditional approaches to obesity have been through nutrition and exercise. There are many varieties of diets and exercise routines available of differing efficacy. One common controversy regarding exercise is whether aerobic training (AT) or resistance training (RT) offers superior benefits. Lee et al. tested resistance training versus aerobic training versus no exercise in an RCT with 45 obese boys on a normal diet. At the end of the study both AT and RT prevented weight gain seen in the control group; RT had the added benefit of insulin sensitivity in 27 percent [72]. Banz et al. designed a similar study evaluating cardiac risk factors and the effects of RT versus AT. At the end of 10 weeks, RT had decreased body fat while AT increased HDL cholesterol [73]. While these studies offer insights into the benefits of both training regimens, they are often done in tandem with calorie-restricted diets when fat loss is the goal. Bryner et al. studied the effects of a very low calorie diet (VLCD) plus either RT or AT on lean body mass and resting metabolic rate (RMR). The VLCD + RT group showed no decrease in lean body mass and had an increase in RMR (2.6 to 3.1 O_2 ml/kg/min) while AT + VLCD showed significantly more decrease in body mass and lean body mass ($p < 0.01$) and a significantly lower 24-hour RMR ($p < 0.05$) [74].

Diet is another area of debate – namely the balance of the major energy macromolecules: proteins, fats, and carbohydrates. Two studies compared high-protein + low-fat and high-carb + low-fat calorie-restricted diets. Brinkworth et al. found the results to be statistically similar, but the high-protein diet gave greater weight loss (4.1 kg versus 2.9 kg) [75]. Skov et al. found that high-protein diets were significantly better ($p = 0.001$) than high-carb diets, producing an average weight loss of 8.9 kg versus 5.1 kg [76]. The Atkins diet is composed of high-fat, high-protein, and low-carb proportions. Foster et al. tested this diet against a standard low-calorie high-carb, low-fat diet. At three months the Atkins diet showed superior results; however, by 12 months the results were equivocal [77]. One possible explanation for the efficacy of high-protein diets is that protein is more satiating than either carbohydrates or fats [78]. Some concern has been expressed over the safety of high-protein diets, but the Institute of Medicine has found no clear evidence that they increase the risk of renal stones, osteoporosis, cancer, or CVD, and recommends that protein intake of 10–35 percent of total caloric intake could be safe [78].

There is also great interest in supplements that help with weight loss. Hasani-Ranjbar et al. reviewed 77 studies utilizing herbal supplementation for weight loss. The supplements were classified into three broad categories by their mechanism of action on fat loss: increasing metabolism, appetite suppression, and impeding digestion [79]. Effective appetite suppressants included *Agave tequilana*, *Dasylirion* spp., pomegranate leaf, Korean red ginseng, tree peony and *Gyeongshang angjeehwan*, parasitic loranthus, and *Panax* ginseng berry [79]. Ma Huang or ephedra-containing plants acted primarily by boosting metabolism, but had the secondary effect of appetite suppression, particularly when combined with caffeine. Dosages of 40 mg ephedra per day and 100 mg caffeine per day were found to be most effective in longer-term use. However, caution should be exercised with use of ephedra due to rare but serious side effects being documented [79]. Two other broadly studied and effective supplements included several varieties of ginseng and *Cissus quadrangularis* [79]. As with all supplement use, caution should be exercised and the user should see their primary care physician before incorporating them into a weight loss plan.

Parathyroid Hormone

Parathyroid hormone (PTH) is secreted by the parathyroid glands, located adjacent to the thyroid gland. This hormone plays a key role in bone remodeling; it is stimulated by low blood calcium and acts to activate osteoclasts, releasing calcium [80]. It also acts to increase calcium reabsorption in the kidney and indirectly in the GI system via vitamin D (calcitriol) synthesis [81].

Hypoparathyroidism can have a variety of causes, with the most common being surgical or traumatic removal of the parathyroid [82]. Symptoms of hypoparathyroidism secondary to hypocalcemia include paresthesia, muscle cramps and spasms, and peri-oral tingling [83]. Long-term treatment for hypoparathyroidism is use of vitamin D analogs, calcium supplementation, and PTH analogs [84]. Hypoparathyroidism can lead to significantly decreased QOL. In two separate studies, Cusano et al. evaluated hypoparathyroidism patients' QOL scores before and after treatment with PTH(1-84). When using the RAND 36-item health survey, pretreatment patients were significantly lower than normative baseline in all domains ($p < 0.001$); treatment scores significantly improved in the mental and physical components and total score at one year ($p = 0.001$) [85]. In a second study utilizing the short form (SF-36), similar significant improvements in QOL were observed at five years ($p = 0.001$) [85]. Astor et al. noted significantly lower scores on SF-36 and Hospital Anxiety and Depression scales compared to the normative baseline population in patients treated with vitamin D and calcium [54]. In addition to calcium supplementation, it is recommended that foods high in calcium be consumed, including almonds, legumes, dark leafy greens, and oats [86]. Hypoparathyroidism lowers QOL; prompt treatment appears to improve patient wellness to a significant extent.

Hyperparathyroidism comes in three forms, primary hyperparathyroidism, secondary hyperparathyroidism, and tertiary hyperparathyroidism [87]. Primary hyperparathyroidism is generally cause by a parathyroid adenoma; secondary hyperparathyroidism stems from a variety of causes that induce hypocalcemia [87, 88]. Clinical symptoms of primary hyperparathyroidism can include fatigue, bone pain, nausea, vomiting, polyuria, polydipsia, cognitive impairment, osteopenia, osteoporosis, and kidney stones [89]. Secondary hyperparathyroidism can present similarly or differently, depending on the etiology. Treatments can vary depending on the variety and source of hyperparathyroidism. Surgical parathyroidectomy is appropriate for symptomatic primary hyperparathyroidism [90]. Secondary hyperparathyroidism treatment should be directed at the cause of elevated PTH. Calcimimetics are useful for patients who are symptomatic and unable to undergo surgery or are on dialysis [91]. Quality of life can be severely impaired in both physical and mental categories of well-being. With severe hyperparathyroidism, parathyroidectomies have been shown to improve QOL. Edwards et al., in a study of 100 parathyroidectomy patients, noted a sustained improvement at one-year post-op in HRQOL using the Health Outcomes Institute Health Status Questionnaire (HSQ). Improvements were noted in areas of muscle strength, health, endurance, anxiety, and overall health ($p = 0.001$) [92]. Similar improvements were seen in a 66-patient study on parathyroidectomy patients using SF-12, HADS, and PHQ-9 [93]. Cunningham et al. showed that cinacalcet therapy was useful in improving HRQOL in patients with secondary hyperparathyroidism. Use of cinacalcet significantly reduced parathyroidectomies (RR = 0.07), fractures (RR = 0.46), and cardiovascular hospitalizations (RR = 0.61), and improved the physical component summary score and general health perception in the SF-36 survey [94]. Supplementing with chaste tree 20–40 mg before breakfast may help to promote optimal bone growth in hyperparathyroid patients [95]. The Mayo Clinic has made several useful recommendations in promoting wellness in hyperparathyroidism. Adequate vitamin D and calcium is important, even though hypercalcemia can be a component of the disease. Additionally, adequate hydration prevents kidney stones; not smoking and engaging in exercise helps to strengthen bones [96]. Vaidya et al., in a prospective cohort study with 69,621 subjects, showed that low physical activity and low calcium consumption were associated with a 2.37-fold (CI 1.60–3.51) increased risk for developing primary hyperparathyroidism. This indicated that intense exercise regimens could prevent hyperparathyroidism [97]. When approaching the issue of wellness in hyperparathyroidism, treatment of symptomatic hyperparathyroidism appears to significantly improve HRQOL, clinical outcomes, and mental wellness.

Testosterone

Testosterone plays in an integral role in both male and female physiology. Testosterone is produced in the testes of males, while in females is it synthesized in the adrenal glands and ovaries [1]. While not the driving factor in female physiology, testosterone is thought to play a role in female sexual libido. Additionally, in men and women testosterone has a role in pain tolerance, subjective well-being, mood, bone density, and muscle mass [1, 98, 99].

Female testosterone concentrations vary pre- and post-menopause, with lower total levels occurring after menopause. Few studies have been done utilizing testosterone replacement therapy (TRT) in normal healthy aging female populations; despite this, some benefits of TRT have been noted in females. When added with conjugated estrogen, testosterone helped increase fat-free body mass [100]. Similarly, an increase in thigh muscle mass was observed using CT scan in a double-blind RCT involving 51 androgen-deficient women [101]. Testosterone has also been implicated in female libido. One randomized study of 75 women post-oophorectomy and hysterectomy noted a two- to threefold increase in sexual desire, masturbation, and sexual intercourse when given high-dose transdermal testosterone [102]. Testosterone replacement therapy is not without risks in female patients. The Framingham Heart study showed menopausal and postmenopausal women were at increased risk of coronary heart disease (CHD) and mortality associated with it, possibly due to relatively higher androgen levels [103]. Androgen therapy in females holds promise; however, more research needs to be done to assess side effects.

Testosterone is a major factor in many physiologic processes within the male body, including muscle strength, bone mass, libido, spermatogenesis, and maturation during puberty [1]. Androgen deficiency occurs through primary testicular failure, hypogonadotropic hypogonadism, or normal aging [104]. Symptoms of androgen deficiency in males include reduced muscle mass, increased body fat, decreased libido, erectile dysfunction, infertility, and depression [1, 104]. Studies on TRT in males have shown improvements in several aspects of male health and wellness. Cardiovascular benefits are several-fold, with one UK placebo-controlled double-blind study of 46 men with stable angina finding that 5 mg testosterone patch therapy led to a 22 percent improvement in exercise before ST-depression onset [105]. Other cardiovascular benefits include reduced insulin resistance and adiposity [106]. Low libido also has the potential for improvement with TRT, with several studies showing improved erectile duration and sexual function [106, 107]. Testosterone replacement therapy is not without risks for men either. The well-reported link between androgens and prostate cancer was first discovered by Huggins and Hodges, who observed that castration led to prostate cancer regression [108]. However, a 2008 meta-analysis of 3886 men with prostate cancer and 6438 controls found no relationship between androgen levels and prostate cancer [109]. Myocardial infarction and heart disease occur with greater frequency in men who supplement with testosterone either for hypogonadism or for athletic enhancement, possibly due to supra-physiologic doses [98]. Testosterone replacement therapy shows promise in treating numerous conditions; however, risks associated with TRT should not be ignored.

Non-pharmacologic methods do exist for increasing endogenous testosterone. Trials of exercise in elderly [110] and obese [111] individuals have shown significant increases in testosterone after several weeks of consistent workouts. Vitamin D, if not being consumed in high enough doses, could also aid in boosting testosterone, as found by a 165-subject study [112]. Nutrition plays an important role in testosterone synthesis, with diets rich in protein, fats, and fish oil seeming to promote increased testosterone production [113–115]. Testosterone is an important hormone for men and women, and many options exist to alleviate low testosterone.

Thyroid Hormone

Thyroid hormone is an integral part of body homeostasis, acting on nearly every cell. It regulates everything from basal metabolic rate to protein synthesis [116]. Two forms of thyroid hormone are released from the thyroid gland, T3 and T4; T3 is the active form and is more potent than the more plentiful T4 [116]. Both hypo- and hyperthyroidism are medical issues that afflict many people and reduce QOL.

Hypothyroidism presents with a variety of symptoms, including fatigue, weakness, constipation, weight gain, cold intolerance, muscle aches, depression, and hair loss [1]. The leading cause of hypothyroidism globally is iodine deficiency; in developed countries it is autoimmune thyroiditis [117]. There is also decreased thyroid dysfunction with age that is often difficult to detect with lab values, yet still presents with clinical symptoms [118]. Mild thyroid failure (MTF) is associated with increased risk of morbidity and mortality [119]. Mild thyroid failure significantly increased the risk for arthrosclerosis (OR = 1.9) and MI (OR = 3.1) in the Rotterdam study of 1149 postmenopausal women [120]. Additionally, Walsh and colleagues found subclinical hypothyroidism to be associated with a 2.2-fold increase in coronary artery disease (CAD) and 1.5-fold increase in cardiovascular mortality [121]. There is little evidence to suggest that thyroid hormone supplementation improves QOL in MTF. Villar et al., in a review of 12 RCTs with a total of 350 patients with subclinical hypothyroidism, found no improvement in HRQOL in intervention groups [122]. Nutrition recommendations to increase thyroid function include the consumption of sufficient selenium and zinc [123, 124]. Selenium, when kept at physiologic levels through administration of 100 µg/day, prevented thyroid pathologies such as cancer and promoted improved thyroid functionality in Graves' disease [123]. Zinc supplementation of 26.4 mg/day to two college students with hyperthyroidism showed increased T3 concentrations [124]. In a review article, one study of 490,000 subjects noted significant reduction in thyroid cancer (RR = 0.57) with consumption of one or more alcoholic drinks per day, particularly in papillary thyroid cancer (RR = 0.58) [125]. Bansal et al., in a study of 20 treated hypothyroid patients, found that regular exercise significantly reduced TSH ($p < 0.001$) and significantly raised T3 and T4 ($p = 0.007$, $p < 0.001$ respectively) when compared to sedentary patients [126]. Many pharmacologic and non-pharmacologic opportunities for improving hypothyroidism exist; individuals should choose the options that work best for their clinical situation.

Hyperthyroidism is a condition of excessive thyroid hormone. Symptoms of hyperthyroidism can include irritability, muscle weakness, sleeping problems, tachycardia, heat intolerance, and weight loss [127]. The most common cause of hyperthyroidism in the USA is Graves' disease [127]. Quality of life is significantly affected along multiple dimensions in patients suffering hyperthyroidism. Suwalska et al. surveyed 58 patients with the World Health Organization Quality of Life questionnaire (WHOQOL) and found a significant decrease in perceived QOL, with a high prevalence of depressive symptoms [128]. Thyroid eye disease (TED) is also a source of significant decreases in wellness among hyperthyroid patients. In a review of 20 original studies, Estcourt et al. noted a decrease in QOL and psychosocial function in TED patients, likely secondary to substandard care [129]. Treatment of excess thyroid hormone production can involve the use of antithyroid hormone drugs, radio-iodide ablation, or thyroid resection. Beta-blockers are frequently used to decrease symptoms of hypertension, tachycardia, tremors, and anxiety [130]. High iodine content foods should be avoided by patients with autoimmune hyperthyroidism [131]. Thyroid cancer can lead to hyperthyroidism; in a study of nitrates in the drinking water of Iowa, concentrations exceeding 5 mg/l nitrate-N were associated with a RR = 2.6 increase in the risk of thyroid cancer [132].

For those already suffering hyperthyroidism, yoga may be useful. Gupta et al. studied eight hyperthyroid patients and found yoga decreased anxiety in patients with hyperthyroidism; however, the effect did not reach statistical significance [133]. *Lawsonia inermis* (henna leaf) may help dampen the hyper-production of thyroid hormone in Graves' disease via its oxidant effect, lowering H^+ within thyroid cells and inhibiting thyroid hormone. Zumrutdal et al. studied hyperthyroid mice given a placebo or *L. inermis*; mice given the herbal supplement showed consistently lower T4 scores than the control group [134]. Many options exist for treatment of hyperthyroidism, even beyond first-line clinical recommendations. Maximizing QOL in hyperthyroidism should focus on providing optimal clinical care and follow-up.

Conclusion

The endocrine system serves an important function in regulating nearly all aspects of homeostasis, development, and reproduction. Wellness broadly defined encompasses all aspects of good physical and mental health. Endocrine wellness is an integral part of overall health; derangements in hormonal function can have drastic and long-lasting impacts on overall wellness. Endocrine disorders commonly involve the HPA axis, pituitary gland, thyroid gland, reproductive organs, and even the pancreas with diabetes. Diabetes mellitus, with around 425 million cases worldwide, is one of the most common endocrine disorders and has been shown to severely decrease QOL and life expectancy. Decreases in endocrine wellness also occur as a normal part of the aging process. Declines in testosterone in andropause and estrogen in menopause can cause decreased QOL in the elderly. Many treatment approaches have been researched and are available to improve endocrine dysfunction.

References

1. ET Schwartz, K Holtorf. Hormones in wellness and disease prevention: common practices, current state of the evidence, and questions for the future. *Prim Care* 2008;**35**(4): 669–705.

2. A Santos, E Resmini, C Pascual, et al. Psychiatric symptoms in patients with Cushing's syndrome: prevalence, diagnosis and management. *Drugs* 2017; **77**: 829–842.

3. G Arnaldi, A Angeli, AB Atkinson, et al. Diagnosis and complications of Cushing's syndrome: a consensus statement. *J Clin Endocrinol Metab* 2003; **88**: 5593–5602.

4. LK Nieman. Cushing's syndrome: update on signs, symptoms and biochemical screening. *Eur J Endocrinol* 2015; **173**: M33–M38.

5. A Santos, I Crespo, A Aulinas, et al. Quality of life in Cushing's syndrome. *Pituitary* 2016; **18**(2): 95–200.

6. R Pivonello, MC De Martino, M De Leo, et al. Cushing's disease: the burden of illness. *Endocrine* 2017; **56**: 10.

7. N Alcala, S Ozkan, P Kadioglu, et al. Evaluation of depression, quality of life and body image in patients with Cushing's disease. *Pituitary* 2013; **16**: 333–340.

8. AH Heald, S Ghosh, S Bray, et al. Long-term negative impact on quality of life in patients with successfully treated Cushing's disease. *Clin Endocrinol (Oxf)* 2004; **61**: 458–465.

9. MN Starkman, DE Schteingart. Neuropsychiatric manifestations of patients with Cushing's syndrome: relationship to cortisol and adrenocorticotropic hormone levels. *Arch Intern Med* 1981; **141**: 215–219.

10. N Sonino, GA Fava. Psychiatric disorders associated with Cushing's syndrome: epidemiology, pathophysiology and treatment. *CNS Drugs* 2001; **15**: 361–373.

11. 4 Lifestyle Tips for Cushing's Syndrome. 2016 www.endocrineweb.com/conditions/cushings-syndrome/4-lifestyle-tips-cushings-syndrome (accessed July 9, 2019).

12. RC Hickson, JR Marone. Exercise and inhibition of glucocorticoid-induced muscle atrophy. *Exerc Sport Sci Rev* 1993; **21**(1): 135–168.

13. LE Carlson, M Speca, KD Patel, et al. Mindfulness-based stress reduction in relation to quality of life, mood, symptoms of stress and levels of cortisol, dehydroepiandrosterone sulfate (DHEAS) and melatonin in breast and prostate cancer outpatients. *Psychoneuroendocrinology* 2004; **29**: 448–474.

14. J Thirthalli, GH Naveen, MG Rao, et al. Cortisol and antidepressant effects of yoga. *Indian J Psychiatry* 2013; **55**(3): S405.

15. G Meyer. What affects the quality of life in autoimmune Addison's disease? *Horm Metab Res* 2013; **45**(2): 92–95.

16. S Ten, M New, N Maclaren. Clinical review 130: Addison's disease. *J Clin Endocrinol Metab* 2001; **86**(7): 2909–2922.

17. WW De Herder, AJ van der Lely. Addisonian crisis and relative adrenal failure. *Rev Endocr Metab Disord* 2003; **4**(2): 143–147.

18. A Michels, N Michels. Addison disease: early detection and treatment principles. *Am Fam Physician* 2014; **89**(7): 563–568.

19. PJ Hunt, EM Gurnell, FA Huppert, et al. Improvement in mood and fatigue after dehydroepiandrosterone replacement in Addison's disease in a randomized, double blind trial. *J Clin Endocrinol Metab* 2000; **85**(12): 4650–4656.

20. RC Ufferman, RW Schrier. Importance of sodium intake and mineralocorticoid hormone in the impaired water excretion in adrenal insufficiency. *J Clin Invest* 1972; **51**(7): 1639–1646.

21. DC Anderson. Assessment and nutraceutical management of stress-induced adrenal dysfunction. *Intregrat Med* 2008; **7**: 5.

22. RA Ronzio. Nutritional support for adrenal function. *Am J Nat Med* 1998; **5**(5): 12–17.

23. CJ Saldanha, L Remage-Healey, BA Schlinger. Synaptocrine signaling: steroid synthesis and action at the synapse. *Endocr Rev* 2011; **32**(4): 532–549.

24. A Schindler, C Campagnoli, R Druckman, et al. Classification and pharmacology of progestins. *Maturitas* 2003; **46**: S7–16.

25. CA Stuenkel, SR Davis, A Gompel, et al. Treatment of symptoms of the menopause: an Endocrine Society clinical practice guideline. *J Clin Endocrinol Metab* 2015; **100**(11): 3975–4011.

26. RE Williams, KB Levine, L Kalilani. Menopause-specific questionnaire assessment in US population-based study shows negative impact on health-related quality of life. *Maturitas* 2009; **62**(2): 153–159.

27. D Tourgeman, E Gentzchein, F Stanczyk, et al. Serum and tissue hormone levels of vaginally and orally administered estradiol. *Am J Obstet Gynecol* 1999; **180**(6): 1480–1483.

28. H Ziel, W Finkle. Increased risk of endometrial carcinoma among users of conjugated estrogens. *N Engl J Med* 1975; **293**(23): 1167–1170.

29. J Rossow, G Anderson, R Prentice, et al. Writing group for the Women's Health Initiative: risks and benefits of estrogen plus progestin in healthy postmenopausal women. *JAMA* 2002; **288**(3): 321–333.

30. A Fournier, F Berrino, F Clavel-Chapelon. Unequal risks for breast cancer associated with different hormone replacement therapies: results from the E3 N cohort study. *Breast Cancer Res Treat* 2008; **107** (1): 103–111.

31. C Stahlberg, A Pedersen, E Lynge, et al. Increased risk of breast cancer following different regimens of hormone replacement therapy frequently used in Europe. *Int J Cancer* 2004; **109**: 721–727.

32. HD Nelson. Commonly used types of postmenopausal estrogen for treatment of hot flashes. *JAMA* 2004; **291**(13): 1610–1620.

33. C Durosier-Izart, E Biver, F Merminod, et al. Peripheral skeleton bone strength is positively correlated with total and dairy protein intakes in healthy postmenopausal women. *Am J Clin Nutr* 2017; **105**(2): 513–525.

34. AC Purdue-Smithe, BW Whitcomb, KL Szegda, et al. Vitamin D and calcium intake and risk of early menopause. *Am J Clin Nutr* 2017; **105**(6): 1493–1501.

35. F Parazzini. Resveratrol, tryptophanum, glycine and vitamin E: a nutraceutical approach to sleep disturbance and irritability in peri-and post-menopause. *Minerva Ginecologica* 2015; **67**(1): 1–5.

36. A Patade, L Devareddy, EA Lucas, et al. Flaxseed reduces total and LDL cholesterol concentrations in Native American postmenopausal women. *J Women's Health(Larchmt)* 2008; **17**(3): 355–366.

37. CH Kroenke, BJ Caan, ML Stefanick, et al. Effects of a dietary intervention and weight change on vasomotor symptoms in the Women's Health Initiative. *Menopause* 2012; **19**(9): 980.

38. N Vaze, S Joshi. Yoga and menopausal transition. *J Midlife Health* 2010; **1**(2): 56.

39. S Ranabir, K Reetu. Stress and hormones. *Indian J Endocrinol Metab* 2011; **15**(1): 18–22.

40. ME Molitch, DR Clemmons, S Malozowski, et al. Evaluation and treatment of adult growth hormone deficiency: an Endocrine Society clinical practice guideline. *J Clin Endocrinol Metab* 2006; **91**(5): 1621–1634.

41. D Ignatavicius, L Workman. *Medical-Surgical Nursing: Patient-Centered Collaborative Care*. Philadelphia, PA, WB Saunders; 2016.

42. F Prodam, M Caputo, S Belcastro, et al. Quality of life, mood disturbances and psychological parameters in adult patients with GH deficiency. *Panminerva Medica* 2012; **54**(4): 323–331.

43. F Nyberg, M Hallberg. Growth hormone and cognitive function. *Nature Rev. Endocrinol* 2013; **9**(6): 357–365.

44. C Wuster, U Melchinger, T Eversmann, et al. Reduced incidence of side-effects of growth hormone substitution in 404 patients with hypophyseal insufficiency: results of a multicenter indications study. *Med Klin* 1998; **93**(10): 585–591.

45. K Chihara, E Koledova, A Shimatsu, et al. An individualized GH dose regimen for long-term GH treatment in Japanese patients with adult GH deficiency. *Eur J Endocrinol* 2005; **153**(1): 57–65.

46. SE Hankinson, WC Willett, GA Colditz, et al. Circulating concentrations of insulin-like growth factor-1 and risk of breast cancer. *Lancet* 1998; **351**(9113); 1393–1398.

47. R Palmqvist, G Hallmans, S Rinaldi, et al. Plasma insulin-like growth factor 1, insulin-like growth factor binding protein 3, and risk of colorectal cancer: a prospective study in northern Sweden. *Gut* 2002; **50**: 642–646.

48. SL Blethen, DB Allen, D Graves, et al. Safety of recombinant deoxyribonucleic acid-derived growth hormone: the National Cooperative Growth Study experience. *J Clin Endocrinol Metab* 1996; **81**: 1704–1710.

49. G Frajese, WM Drake, RA Loureiro, et al. Hypothalamopituitary surveillance imaging in hypopituitary patients receiving long-term GH replacement therapy. *J Clin Endocrinol Metab* 2001; **86**(11): 5572–5575.

50. RJ Godfrey, Z Madgwick, GP Whyte. The exercise-induced growth hormone

response in athletes. *Sports Med* 2003; **33** (6): 599–613.

51. R Lanzi, L Luzi, A Caumo, et al. Elevated insulin levels contribute to the reduced growth hormone (GH) response to GH-releasing hormone in obese subjects. *Metabolism* 1999; **48**(9): 1152–1156.

52. RR Suminski, RJ Robertson, FL Goss. Acute effect of amino acid ingestion and resistance exercise on plasma growth hormone concentration in young men. *Int J Sport Nutr* 1997; **7**(1): 48–60.

53. PR Kerndt, JL Naughton, CE Driscoll, et al. Fasting: the history, pathophysiology and complications. *West J Med* 1982; **137**: 379–399.

54. MC Astor, K Lovas, A Debowska. Epidemiology and health-related quality of life in hypoparathyroidism in Norway. *J Clin Endocrinol Metab* 2016; **101**(8): 3045–3053.

55. A Ben-shlomo, S Melmed. Acromegaly. *Endocrinol Metab Clin North Am* 2008; **37** (1): 101–122.

56. A Giustina, P Chanson, D Kleinberg, et al. Expert consensus document: a consensus on the medical treatment of acromegaly. *Nat Rev* 2014; **10**: 243–248.

57. SV Rowles, L Prieto, X Badia, et al. Quality of life (QOL) in patients with acromegaly is severely impaired: use of novel measure of QOL – acromegaly quality of life questionnaire. *J Clin Endocrinol Metab* 2005; **90**(6): 3337–3341.

58. MD Johnson, CJ Woodburn, ML Vanle. Quality of life in patients with a pituitary adenoma. *Pituitary* 2003; **6**(2): 81–87.

59. SM Webb, X Badia, NL Surinach, et al. Validity and clinical applicability of the acromegaly quality of life questionnaire, AcroQoL: a 6-month prospective study. *Eur J Endocrinol* 2006; **155**(2): 269–277.

60. A Toumpanakis, T Turnbull, I Alba-barba. Effectiveness of plant-based diets in promoting well-being in the management of type 2 diabetes: a systemic review. *BMJ Open Diabetes Res Care* 2018; **6**(1): e000534.

61. B Roep. The role of T-cells in the pathogenesis of type 1 diabetes: from cause to cure. *Diabetologia* 2003; **46**(3): 305–321.

62. EH Lin, W Katon, M Von Korff, et al. Relationship of depression and diabetes self-care, medication adherence, and preventive care. *Diabetes Care* 2004; **27**: 2154–2160.

63. R Ackerman, E Finch, E Brizendine, et al. Translating the Diabetes Prevention Program into the community: the DEPLOY pilot study. *Am J Prev Med* 2008; **35**(4): 357–363.

64. JR Horwitz, BD Kelly, JE DiNardo. Wellness incentives in the workplace: cost savings through cost shifting to unhealthy workers. *Health Aff (Millwood)* 2013; **32**(3): 468–476.

65. SL Pinto, K Kumar, G Partha, et al. Pharmacist-provided medication therapy management (MTM) program impacts outcomes for employees with diabetes. *Popul Health Manag* 2014; **17**(1): 21–27.

66. LN Lyzwinski, L Caffery, M Bambling, S Edirippulige. The Mindfulness App trial for weight, weight-related behaviors, and stress in university students: randomized controlled trial. *JMIR Mhealth Uhealth* 2019; **7**(4): e12210.

67. IO Sim. Humor intervention program for children with chronic diseases. *Appl Nurs Res* 2015; **28**(4): 404–412.

68. S Sidhu, T Parikh, K Burman. *Endocrine Changes in Obesity*. South Dartmouth, MA, MDText.com; 2000.

69. SB Heymsfield, AS Greenberg, K Fujioka, et al. Recombinant leptin for weight loss in obese and lean adults: a randomized, controlled, dose-escalation trial. *JAMA* 1999; **282**(16): 1568–1575.

70. T Yamauchi, J Kamon, H Waki, et al. The fat-derived hormone adiponectin reverses insulin resistance associated with both lipoatrophy and obesity. *Nat Med* 2001; **7** (8): 941–946.

71. K Ohashi, S Kihara, N Ouchi, et al. Adiponectin replenishment ameliorates obesity-related hypertension. *Hypertension* 2006; **47**(6): 1108–1116.

72. S Lee, F Bacha, T Hannon, et al. Effects of aerobic versus resistance exercise without caloric restriction on abdominal fat, intrahepatic lipid, and insulin sensitivity in obese adolescent boys: a randomized, controlled trial. *Diabetes* 2012; **61**(11): 2787–2795.

73. WJ Banz, MA Maher, WG Thompson. Effects of resistance versus aerobic training on coronary artery disease risk factors. *Exp Biol Med(Maywood)* 2003; **228**(4): 434–440.

74. RW Bryner, IH Ullrich, J Sauers. Effects of resistance vs. aerobic training combined with an 800 calorie liquid diet on lean body mass and resting metabolic rate. *J Am Coll Nutr* 1999; **18**(2): 115–121.

75. GD Brinkworth, M Noakes, JB Keogh. Long-term effects of a high-protein, low-carbohydrate diet on weight control and cardiovascular risk markers in obese hyperinsulinemic subjects. *Int J Obes Relat Metab Disord* 2004; **28**(5): 661–670.

76. AR Skov, S Toubro, B Ronn, et al. Randomized trial on protein vs carbohydrate in ad libitum fat reduced diet for the treatment of obesity. *Int J Obes Relat Metab Disord* 1999; **23**(5): 528–536.

77. GD Foster, HR Wyatt, JO Hill, et al. A randomized trial of a low-carbohydrate diet for obesity. *N Engl J Med* 2003; **348** (21): 2082–2090.

78. A Astrup. The satiating power of protein: a key to obesity prevention. *Am J Clin Nutr* 2005; **82**(1): 1–2.

79. S Hasani-Ranjbar, N Nayebi, B Larijani, et al. A systemic review of the efficacy and safety of herbal medicines used in the treatment of obesity. *World J Gasotroenterol* 2009; **15**(25): 3073–3085.

80. SS Khan. *Physiology, Parathyroid Hormone (PTH)*. Treasure Island, FL, StatPearls Publishing; 2019.

81. L Stryer. *Biochemistry*. New York, W.H. Freeman and Company; 1995.

82. JP Bilezikian, A Khan, JT Potts, et al. Hypoparathyroidism in the adult: epidemiology, diagnosis, pathophysiology, target-organ involvement, treatment, and challenges for future research. *J Bone Miner Res* 2011; **26**(10): 2317–2337.

83. JT Potts Jr. *Diseases of the Parathyroid Gland: Harrison's Principles of Internal Medicine*. New York, McGraw-Hill; 2005.

84. KK Winer, B Zhang, J Shrader, et al. Synthetic human parathyroid hormone 1-34 replacement therapy: a randomized crossover trial comparing pump versus injections in the treatment of chronic hypoparathyroidism. *J Clin Endocrinol Metab* 2012; **97**(2): 391–399.

85. NE Cusano, MR Rubin, DJ McMahon, et al. The effects of PTH(1-84) on quality of life in hypoparathyroidism. *J Clin Endocrinol Metab* 2013; **98**(6): 2356–2361.

86. Hypothyroidism. 2016. http://pennstate hershey.adam.com/content.aspx?productId =107&pid=33&gid=000093 (accessed July 9, 2019).

87. WD Fraser. Hyperparathyroidism. *Lancet* 2009; **374**(9684):145–158.

88. J Cunningham, F Locatelli, M Rodriguez. Secondary hyperparathyroidism: pathogensis, disease, progression, and therapeutic options. *Clin J Am Soc Nephrol* 2011; **6**(4): 913–921.

89. AK Chan, QY Duh, MH Katz, et al. Clinical manifestations of primary hyperparathyroidism before and after parathyroidectomy. A case-control study. *Ann Surg* 1995; **222**(3): 402–414.

90. JP Bilezikian, SJ Silverberg. Clinical practice: asymptomatic primary hyperparathyroidism. *N Engl J Med* 2004; **350**(17): 1746–1751.

91. AE Ballinger, SC Palmer, I Nistor, et al. Calcimimetics for secondary hyperparathyroidism in chronic kidney disease patients. *Cochrane Database Syst Rev* 2014; **12**: CD006254.

92. ME Edwards, A Rotramel, T Beyer, et al. Improvement in the health-related quality-of-life symptoms of hyperparathyroidism is durable on long-term follow-up. *Surgery* 2006; **140**(4): 655–663.

93. T Weber, M Keller, I Hense, et al. Effect of parathyroidectomy on quality of life and

neuropsychological symptoms in primary hyperparathyroidism. *World J Surg* 2007; **31**(6): 1202–1209.

94. J Cunningham, M Danese, K Olson, et al. Effects of the calcimimetic cinacalcet HCL on cardiovascular disease, fracture, and health-related quality of life in secondary hyperparathyroidism. *Kidney Int* 2005; **68** (4): 1793–1800.

95. W Wuttke, JV Christoffel, SD Seidolva-Wuttke. Chaste tree (*Vitex agnus-castus*): pharmacology and clinical indications. *Phytomedicine* 2003; 10(4): 348–357.

96. Hyperparathyroidism. 2019. www .mayoclinic.org/diseases-conditions/hype rparathyroidism/symptoms-causes/syc-2 0356194 (accessed July 9, 2019).

97. GC Vaidya, JM Curhan, M Paik, et al. Physical activity and the risk of primary hyperparathyroidism. *J Clin Endocrinol Metab* 2016; **101**(4): 1590–1597.

98. V Tyagi, M Scordo, RS Yoon, et al. Revisiting the role of testosterone: are we missing something? *Rev Urol* 2017; **19**(1): 16–24.

99. S Roux, P Orcel. Bone loss: factors that regulate osteoclast differentiation – an update. *Arthritis Res* 2000; **2**(6): 451–456.

100. S Davis, K Walker. Effects of estradiol with and without testosterone on body composition and relationship with lipids in postmenopausal women. *Menopause* 2000; 7: 395–401.

101. K Miller, B Biller, C Beauregard. Effects of testosterone replacement in androgen-deficient women with hypopituitarism: a randomized, double-blind placebo-controlled study. *J Clin Endocrinol Metab* 2006; **91**: 1683–1690.

102. J Shifren, G Braunstein, J Simon. Transdermal testosterone treatment in women with impaired sexual function after oophorectomy. *NEJM* 2000; **343**: 682–688.

103. T Gordon, WB Kannel, MC Hjortland, et al. Menopause and coronary heart disease: the Framingham Study. *Ann Intern Med* 1978; **89**(2): 157–161.

104. J Winters. Current status of testosterone replacement therapy in men. *Arch Fam Med* 1999; **8**: 257–263.

105. KM English, RP Steeds, HT Jones, et al. Low-dose transdermal therapy improves angina threshold in men with chronic stable angina: a randomized, double-blind placebo-controlled study. *Circulation* 2000; **102**: 1906–1911.

106. F Saad, L Gooren, A Haider, et al. Effects of testosterone gel followed by parenteral testosterone undecanoate on sexual dysfunction and on features of the metabolic syndrome. *Andrologia* 2008; **40**: 44–48.

107. R Shabsigh, J Kaufman, C Steidle, et al. Randomized study of testosterone gel as adjunctive therapy to sildenafil in hypogonadal men with erectile dysfunction who do not respond to sildenafil alone. *J Urol* 2008; **179**(5): S97–S102.

108. ML Eisenberg. Testosterone replacement therapy and prostate cancer incidence. *World J Mens Health* 2015; **33**(3): 125–129.

109. Endogenous Hormones and Prostate Cancer Collaborative Group, AW Roddam, NE Allen, et al. Endogenous sex hormones and prostate cancer: a collaborative analysis of 18 prospective studies. *J Natl Cancer Inst* 2008; **100**: 170–183.

110. D Vaamonde, ME Da Silva-Grigoletto, JM García-Manso, et al. Physically active men show better semen parameters and hormone values than sedentary men. *Eur J Appl Physiol* 2012; **112**(9): 3267–3273.

111. H Kumagai, A Zempo-Miyaki, T Yoshikawa, et al. Increased physical activity has a greater effect than reduced energy intake on lifestyle modification-induced increases in testosterone. *J Clin Biochem Nutr* 2016; **58** (1): 84–89.

112. S Pilz, S Frisch, H Koertke et al. Effects of vitamin D supplementation on testosterone levels in men. *Horm Metab Res* 2011; **43**(3): 223–225.

113. DT Bishop, AW Melkle, ML Slattery, et al. The effects of nutritional factors on sex

hormone levels in male twins. *Genet Epidemiol* 1995; **5**(1): 43–59.

114. A Belanger, A Locong, C Noel, et al. Influence of diet on plasma steroids and sex hormone-binding globulin levels in adult men. *J Steroid Biochem* 1969; **32**(6): 829–833.

115. J Delarue, O Matzinger, C Binnert. Fish oil prevents the adrenal activation elicited by mental stress in healthy men. *Diabetes Metab* 2003; **29**(3): 289–295.

116. R Mullur, YY Liu, GA Brent. Thyroid hormone regulation of metabolism. *Physiol Rev* 2014; **94**(2): 355–382.

117. AJ Chakera, SH Pearce, B Vaidya. Treatment for primary hypothyroidism: current approaches and future possibilities. *Drug Des Devel Ther* 2012; **6**: 1–11.

118. GJ Canaris, NR Manowitz, G Mayor, et al. The Colorado thyroid disease prevalence study. *Arch Intern Med* 2000; **160**: 526–534.

119. MT McDermott, C Ridgway. Subclinical hypothyroidism is mild thyroid failure and should be treated. *J Clin Endocrinol Met* 2001; **86**(10): 4585–4590.

120. EA Hak, HA Pols, TJ Visser, et al. Subclinical hypothyroidism is an independent risk factor for atherosclerosis and myocardial infarction in elderly women: the Rotterdam study. *Ann Intern Med* 2000; **4**: 270–278.

121. JP Walsh, AP Bremner, MK Bulsara, et al. Subclinical thyroid dysfunction as a risk factor for cardiovascular disease. *Arch Intern Med* 2005; **165**(21): 2467–2472.

122. HC Villar, H Saconato, O Valente, et al. Thyroid hormone replacement for subclinical hypothyroidism. *Cochrane Database Syst Rev* 2007; **3**: CD003419.

123. M Ventura, M Melo, F Carrilho. Selenium and thyroid disease: from pathophysiology to treatment. *Int J Endocrinol* 2017; 2017: 1297658.

124. C Maxwell, SL Volpe. Effects of zinc supplementation on thyroid hormone function. *Ann Nutr Metab* 2007; **51**: 188–194.

125. YP Balhara, KS Deb. Impact of alcohol use on thyroid function. *Indian J Endocrinol Metab* 2013; **17**(4): 580–587.

126. A Bansal, A Kaushik, CM Singh, et al. The effect of regular physical exercise on the thyroid function of treated hypothyroid patients: an interventional study at a tertiary care center in Bastar region of India. *Arch Med Health Sci* 2015; **3**(2): 244.

127. GA Brent. Clinical practice: Graves' disease. *New Eng J Med* 2008; **358** (24): 2594–2605.

128. A Suwalska, K Lacka, D Lojko, et al. Quality of life, depressive symptoms and anxiety in hyperthyroid patients. *Rocz Akad Med Bialymst* 2005; **50**(1): 61–63.

129. S Estcourt, AG Quinn, B Vaidya. Quality of life in thyroid eye disease: impact of quality of care. *Eur J Endocrinol* 2011; **164**: 649–655.

130. DL Geffner, JM Hershman. Beta-adrenergic blockade for the treatment of hyperthyroidism. *Am J Med* 1992; **93**(1): 61–68.

131. S De Leo, SY Lee, LE Braverman. Hyperthyroidism. *Lancet* 2016; **388** (10047): 906–918.

132. MH Ward, BA Kilfoy, PJ Weyer et al. Nitrate intake and the risk of thyroid cancer and thyroid disease. *Epidemiology* 2010; **21**(3): 389–395.

133. N Gupta, S Khera, RP Vempati et al. Effect of yoga based lifestyle intervention on state and trait anxiety. *Indian J Physiol Pharmacol* 2006; **50**(1): 41–47.

134. E Zumrutdal, F Karateke, K Daglioglu, et al. *Lawsonia inermis*: an alternative treatment for hyperthyroidism? *Bratisl Lek Listy* 2014; **115**(2): 66–69.

Chapter 14

Wellness Interventions in Patients Living with Chronic Medical Conditions

Alexander J. Steiner, Leslie Aguilar-Hernandez, Demetria R. Pizano, Julieta Dascal, and Waguih William IsHak

Introduction

Clinicians are consistently presented with the arduous task of characterizing, identifying, classifying, and evaluating response-to-intervention when treating or examining a broad array of patient populations. The primary aim of this chapter is to outline and define wellness among patients living with chronic medical conditions (PLW-CMC). An operational definition of a chronic medical condition is one requiring ongoing management and treatment over extended periods of time, often comprised of a broad constellation of conditions including heart disease, stroke, cancer, chronic respiratory diseases, infectious diseases, metabolic/endocrine disorders, genetic disorders, and disorders resulting in disability/impairment [1]. The number of persons living with one or more chronic medical conditions continues to increase, both nationally and internationally. Thus, the need for literature pertaining to interventions that optimize a patient's quality of life (QOL) is pertinent, as health status is known to be associated with an individual's perception or appraisal of wellness, life satisfaction, happiness, and overall well-being [2].

A concise synthesis of theoretical models will be discussed, followed by the latest evidence-based assessment techniques and interventions that aim to promote optimal wellness among PLW-CMC. Although existing intervention techniques have been proven effective for a variation of chronic medical illnesses, it has remained difficult to identify the mechanism(s) that are most effective across differing patient populations with chronic illness. Many PLW-CMC have multiple chronic conditions, and thus evolved approaches and research efforts may be the best way to move forward, rather than the current methods of focusing on isolated treatment for each disease. Therefore, clear examples will be reviewed in great detail in this chapter, and in particular the aim will be to discuss the subtle nuances between various patient populations and commonalities across all patient groups [3–5]. Regardless of the specific etiology or pathophysiology of respective chronic medical conditions, a number of common universal patient experiences and challenges have been identified in the scientific literature and will be reviewed in greater detail in the sections that follow. Nonetheless, optimal care for PLW-CMC lies with each individual clinician and researcher as they look to the future in uncovering, identifying, and maintaining awareness of the variability across this diverse patient population.

Defining Wellness

It is beyond the scope of this chapter to define the construct of wellness and means of assessing and measuring its factors (the reader is encouraged to review Chapters 1, 2, and 4 in the present volume). However, it should be noted that wellness has generally been thought of as a quality or state of being, as it relates to the health of one's body and mind, and deliberate pursuit of preventing illness. Common factors associated with wellness include well-being, life satisfaction, and QOL. The traditional Western medicine model's focus on symptom reduction and treatment of diseases is beginning to shift. Now, there is an emerging interest in and consideration of wellness as a primary goal in delivering patient care, in conjunction with an acknowledgment that medicine should focus on the treatment of each individual from a biopsychosocial paradigm (as reviewed in Chapter 3), while further prioritizing prevention.

From a global health perspective, the primary aim is to focus on developing valid and reliable assessment tools, forms of interventions, and preventive measures for chronic medical conditions. Conversely, the treatment paradigm from an individual's perspective would suggest that the main objective is to enhance one's wellness and QOL [1, 6]. Unfortunately, there are various factors that have been identified to negatively impact constructs that can positively influence wellness on an individual and global level. Such factors are known to impede and diminish one's sense of wellness, and intervention techniques will be discussed in the intervention section in this chapter.

Differentiating Chronic Medical Conditions from "Acute" or "Terminal" Illness

The present chapter is concerned with wellness within patients experiencing chronic medical conditions. The term "chronic" is best defined as an illness or medical disorder that is persistent, of a long duration (often lifelong), with high chance of recurrence and marked difficulty in fully "eradicating" or "curing." Chronic medical conditions encompass a different set of philosophical, spiritual, medical, psychological, social, and economic conundrums, many of which serve as impediments and barriers to self-care and treatment adherence [6]. Many chronic medical conditions can present as stable, while other conditions have variable patterns of symptom onset, duration, severity, frequency, and periods of temporary remission (e.g., multiple sclerosis). With that said, the term "chronic" infers that full resolution of illness is, by definition, unlikely. Information reviewed in the sections that follow will be specific to conditions, disorders, and illnesses that are "chronic" in nature, rather than conditions that are better characterized as either "acute" (e.g., pain disorders; see Chapter 17) or "terminal" (see Chapters 18 and 19).

In contrast to treating patients with acute or terminal illness, the treatment of chronic conditions requires each member of the treatment team, as well as the patient, to appreciate and understand that a "cure" is not the primary goal of treatment, and that daily attention to the management of chronic conditions is frequently required [6]. In relation to this, the primary focus of the information reviewed in the sections that follow will apply to adult patient populations rather than to pediatric or older adult populations (reviewed in Chapters 15 and 16). There is a common misconception that chronic diseases or medical conditions occur mainly among older adults. However, nearly half of deaths related to chronic medical conditions occur prematurely in persons under 70 years of age, while nearly one-quarter of deaths related to chronic diseases occur in persons under the age of 60, and the average adult is statistically more likely to suffer as a PLW-CMC [1]. It is known that health, functioning, and disability among older adults is a dynamic process, as the confluence of issues that emerge throughout the aging process can compromise optimal wellness [7].

Suboptimal Wellness in Chronic Medical Conditions

Countless studies have identified the inverse relationship between chronic medical conditions and optimal wellness, QOL, well-being, life satisfaction, psychiatric illness, and functional abilities. It would be difficult to summarize the ever-growing body of scientific literature related to suboptimal wellness, QOL, and related constructs among PLW-CMC. Further complicating our understanding of the association between wellness and chronic medical conditions is the reality that many meta-analytic and systematic review studies lack homogeneity. Specifically, they often group rather distinct chronic diseases, conditions, and illnesses together, making the generalizability of incidence/prevalence rates and response-to -intervention difficult to elucidate. Select chronic medical conditions (i.e., chronic obstructive pulmonary disease, chronic kidney disease) have received adequate attention from previous scientific investigators, while other chronic conditions, including many that are quite common, are underrepresented in the literature. Thus, specificity is lacking with respect to our understanding of wellness and available treatments for PLW-CMC, both between and within different patient populations.

In short, what remains clear is that patients living with multimorbidity are reported to be at increased risk of worse wellness and QOL, relative to healthy controls or patients living with one chronic medical condition [5]. Relatedly, depression is 2–3 times more likely to occur in people with multimorbidity compared to people without multimorbidity or those without a chronic condition; 45 percent greater odds of having a depressive disorder with each additional chronic condition has been reported, compared to the odds of having a depressive disorder without a chronic physical condition [8].

Above and beyond clinicians' careful examination of the number of chronic medical conditions present, it is important to understand that the presence of a chronic medical condition can serve as a risk factor for poor wellness and QOL, with some research indicating that it may depend on the characteristics of the specific condition [2, 5, 9]. For example, a comprehensive study by Megari investigated wellness and QOL among PLW-CMC, as well as identifying factors associated with health, wellness, and QOL through the method of stratifying this heterogeneous group into categories based on distinct organic/pathological medical conditions, including cancer, heart diseases and/or stroke, diabetes, hepatitis C, HIV, bowel disease, renal disease, multiple sclerosis, and transplant patients [10].

Theoretical Framework for Conceptualizing Wellness in Chronic Medical Conditions

The clinician's approach to conceptualizing wellness in PLW-CMC should be grounded in a deep understanding of existing theoretical models that have been applied to this heterogeneous population. It goes without saying that existing theoretical propositions that apply to non-clinical populations retain their usefulness in being applied to PLW-CMC. Abraham Maslow's famous *Hierarchy of Needs* theory, initially proposed in 1943, assumed that humans intrinsically partake in behavioral motivation, but that motivation is organized hierarchically, such that the more basic levels of need, including "physiological" or "safety" needs, are necessarily required to be met prior to one's ability to be motivated by higher-level needs, famously termed "self-actualization" [11]. This theoretical model proposed that seeking happiness occurred at the latter stage of needs, namely "self-actualization." In consequence, this general theory is applicable to all clinicians interested in promoting wellness within their patients' lives, as basic needs not being met can serve as barriers to wellness. Integrating this theoretical framework into clinical practice means considering whether or not the basic needs of each patient are being met, prior to delivering interventions that promote self-efficacy.

It is important to ask why a patient might not be complying with standing treatment recommendations for their respective chronic medical condition(s). Often, without careful consideration of structural and systemic factors in our patients' lives, non-compliance with treatment can manifest as resistance, when in reality there might be other precipitating conditions associated with treatment non-compliance. For example, a patient living with comorbid diabetes and chronic kidney disease may be perceived as non-compliant, with inconsistent attendance at scheduled medical appointments due to resistance, while other factors may also be at play. Possible factors could include lack of transportation means (either due to physical immobility or lack of financial recourses to cover travel costs), or lack of insurance to cover necessary treatments (e.g., medications, hemodialysis). What if a patient is monolingual and cannot access a provider proficient in their native language? What if spiritual or religious values and beliefs are mitigating a patient's appraisal of the consequences of non-compliance with treatment? These commonly occurring scenarios are likely to be encountered routinely, and such factors should be considered prior to assuming that treatment resistance or issues related to self-efficacy are responsible.

The Biopsychosocial Paradigm

The biopsychosocial assessment is reviewed in greater detail elsewhere in this text (see Chapter 3). With that said, clinicians are encouraged to become familiar with the general biopsychosocial paradigm, particularly as it relates to PLW-CMC. Expanding upon this paradigm, Bayliss and colleagues [3] invited a number of experts to the Patient-Centered Outcomes Research Institute and were able to synthesize and outline a number of important key factors across multiple contextual levels that exist with respect to PLW-CMC; findings from this impressive undertaking have numerous clinical, academic, and policy implications [3] (Figure 14.1).

The Chronic Care Model

As described above, treating PLW-CMC presents rather distinct challenges, many of which differ from treating other patient populations. Given the protracted course of disease/illness, structural interventions and frameworks tailored to populations with distinct needs have been proposed. A current intervention used is the chronic care model (CCM), which has been developed to improve care for PLW-CMC. This model emphasizes interactions between patients and their respective healthcare providers. The concentrated domains and interactive factors related to healthcare include the community, health system, self-management techniques, delivery system design, and clinical information systems, all of which encompass a larger social ecological perspective [6, 12].

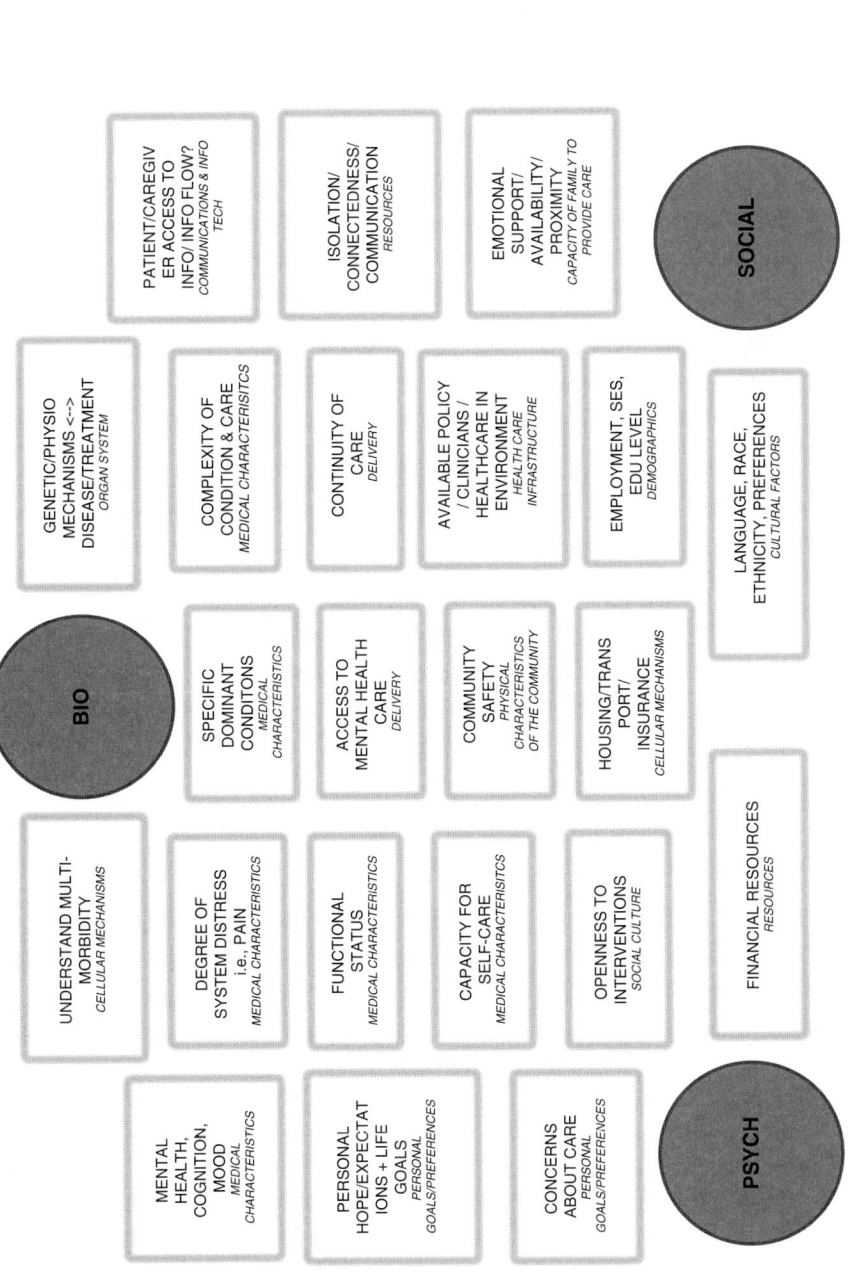

Figure 14.1 Multiple levels and examples of key contextual factors. Adapted from Bayliss EA, Bonds DE, Boyd CM, et al. Understanding the context of health for persons with multiple chronic conditions: moving from what is the matter to what matters. *Ann Fam Med* 2014;12: 260–269.

Evidence-Based Approach to Assessment, Measurement, and Evaluation of Wellness in Chronic Medical Conditions

The validity and reliability of several promising measures/instruments specifically developed for screening for, quantifying, and characterizing wellness and associated constructs for both broad PLW-CMC populations and chronic condition-specific measures continues to grow at a rapid pace. One of the most crucial considerations necessary is ensuring clinicians and researchers gain familiarity with the psychometric, statistical, and application properties of measures assessing wellness, well-being, QOL, life satisfaction, functioning, disability, and psychiatric symptomatology. The aim of such measures should also be examined for their clinical utility and applicability to a clinician's patient population (e.g., pediatric patients) [13].

Many opinions exist with respect to the "gold standard" of assessing wellness across PLW-CMC. Several questions come to mind. Is it appropriate to use a general measure of wellness or an associated construct with a PLW-CMC if no measures have been validated for that population? What if a patient has several chronic medical conditions? What should clinicians or researchers do in cases where "abnormal norms," or in other words, normative data developed on a given patient population, do not exist? In the last example, an inherent problem that could arise is that a cutoff value may inherently become more "lenient" or "stringent," resulting in the unintentional consequence of losing sensitivity/specificity, and positive or negative predictive value, to accurately classifying an individual as having a given trait. For example, should a standard cutoff value be applied when a patient diagnosed with more than one chronic medical condition shares symptoms that overlap with depression, consequently inflating functional disability or artificially reducing QOL? The reality is that the answer to this important clinical dilemma is not straightforward. Instead, healthcare providers attempting to characterize and assess patient-reported outcomes, such as wellness, should be familiar with the properties of each measure and any confounding conditions that could inflate or reduce the respective trait being assessed.

With all the standards of practice and measurement previously reviewed, it is important to acknowledge the impressive body of empirical literature that has validated population-specific measures to assess wellness and associated constructs, increasingly through the use of advanced methodological and statistical techniques (e.g., item response theory). For example, to address the need for a brief, reliable, and valid measure of assessing QOL in clinical research settings among patients living with neurologic conditions, the Neuro-QOL measurement system was developed, which includes 13 brief measures assessing distinct patient-reported QOL domains [14]. Alongside the topic of wellness, out of the larger Neuro-QOL measurement system, one of the brief measures developed was the positive affect and well-being scale [15].

Self-Care and Barriers to Treatment

When evaluating and treating PLW-CMC, clinicians should first identify and examine the patient's ability to engage in adequate self-care. Often, self-care is comprised of more than what the individual is able to provide for themselves, as a number of stakeholders are involved. Such individuals include the individual patient, their families, and the greater communities to which they belong. Principal components of self-care can include one's ability to promote health and active prevention, self-monitor their specific needs, manage their medication regimen independently and adhere to recommended treatment plans, and willingness to proactively seek necessary support [6]. An emerging concept within the scientific literature pertaining to PLW-CMC is self-management, which is one's ability to "self-manage" the pervasive symptoms and consequences associated with living with a chronic condition [6, 12, 16]. Initial evaluation of each PLW-CMC should include a review of the patient's ability to practice self-care, and, consequentially, engage in self-management. By establishing collaborative partnerships with patients, healthcare providers can increase the likelihood of favorable outcomes.

Discrepancies often exist between the treating healthcare professionals' beliefs of what the barriers to self-care are and those of their patients. Clinicians should strive to work in a collaborative partnership with their patients, as it is the patient's unique perception of what constitutes barriers to self-care that should hold the highest value. Certainly, a number of exceptions can exist, such as when a patient's capacity for medical decision-making is compromised or in question; in these circumstances, while clinicians should strive for respecting the patient's dignity and autonomy, it may be necessary to help identify and guide treatment recommendations with the consideration that the patient may lack the capacity to appreciate the consequences of failing to identify such barriers.

As a general guideline, previous research has operationalized barriers to the self-management of chronic conditions into five distinct categories, including physical, psychological, cognitive, economic, and social/cultural [6]. Therefore, research recommends that healthcare providers engaging in the delivery of services to PLW-CMC evaluate the respective role of these five areas and how they can serve as obstructions to a patient's ability to practice self-management. A provider's consideration of these five areas is of critical importance, as their knowledge of independent risk factors for non-compliance with medical treatment will help clinicians routinely consider whether such risk factors are present. This will then mitigate the probability that such a factor would continue to result in treatment non-compliance. To illustrate this crucial point, it is well-established that depressed patients are more likely to be non-compliant with medical treatment recommendations compared to non-depressed patients. A meta-analytic study reported that the odds of treatment non-compliance are three times greater among depressed patients [17].

Evidence-Based Treatments and Interventions for Wellness in Chronic Medical Conditions

Part IV of the present volume includes numerous chapters detailing a broad array of wellness interventions. In the sections that follow, evidence-based interventions reviewed will be those specifically developed, validated, adapted, or applicable for PLW-CMC.

Biological, Pharmacological, and Physical Interventions

The breadth of biological and pharmacological interventions restricted to chronic medical conditions and their effects on wellness are covered in Part II of the current volume, which reviews chronic medical conditions by organ system. Additional interventions (e.g., nutrition-based, exercise-based, sleep-based, holistic) are reviewed in Part IV. Nonetheless, all treatment providers are encouraged to routinely examine PLW-CMC and their compliance with recommended treatment plans, as non-adherence with biological and pharmacological treatments could be disastrous and dramatically decrease the likelihood of subjective wellness. For a review of empirically validated interventions used to improve medication adherence in PLW-CMC, or self-management interventions for PLW-CMC, the reader is referred elsewhere [12, 18].

Exercise training programs have proven to be effective in significantly reducing depressive symptom severity among PLW-CMC [19]. Likewise, a meta-analytic study reported that physical activity interventions retain efficacy among PLW-CMC, in slightly improving both biological markers of favorable health outcomes (e.g., HbA1C) and functional status; surprisingly it also suggested that patients potentially perceived enhanced mastery over their chronic medical condition [4]. In contrast, another meta-analytic study examining the efficacy of exercise interventions in both clinical and healthy populations found that psychological QOL improved significantly less among the disease management group relative to controls, a finding that persisted for over one year [20]. Thus, healthcare providers are encouraged to consider the potential neutral, or, of greater concern, deleterious effects of physical exercise on QOL and wellness for select PLW-CMC.

Psychotherapeutic Interventions

In 2019, various psychotherapeutic techniques were developed for PLW-CMC, including individual/group therapy interventions, interventions from a wide array of healthcare providers, self-help social support groups, and technology-based self-help therapeutic interventions. While beyond the scope of this chapter, a number of empirical studies have examined the treatment efficacy of internet-based self-help therapeutic interventions to increase wellness and decrease psychiatric symptom severity associated with chronic health conditions. The reader is encouraged to review the work of Beatty and Lambert, and their comprehensive systematic review of internet-based interventions with PLW-CMC [21]. Still, findings from their systematic review did reveal consistent evidence of treatment efficacy to improve disease-related symptoms across health conditions, with the exception of diabetes, while identifying mixed findings for the efficacy of these internet-based interventions on reducing distress-related outcomes [21].

A number of other psychotherapeutic techniques have been validated as effective in helping patients overcome barriers to self-care, including motivational interviewing, assessing a given patient's cultural beliefs, interventions aimed at enhancing self-efficacy, and a number of self-help and peer-facilitated support groups [6]. Another evidence-based intervention, acceptance and commitment therapy (ACT), has been proposed to be effective for improving outcomes and wellness among PLW-CMC. Generalizations about ACT's clinical efficacy in improving levels of wellness, QOL, and symptom control among PLW-CMC have been variable; with questionably low quality and few randomized clinical trials executed, the results remain preliminary, but promising data supporting the application of ACT within select patient populations (e.g., epilepsy, HIV, cancer, disease self-management in PLW-CMC) has been reported [22].

In addition to the psychotherapeutic intervention modalities discussed, it is becoming increasingly recognized that a number of mindfulness-based meditation techniques are effective in treating PLW-CMC, yet findings in the literature have been variable. Several meta-analytic studies reported that across eight randomized studies with inclusion of a control group for comparison (prior research groups conducting meta-analytic studies have failed to exclude non-randomized studies or studies without a control condition), mindfulness-based stress reduction (MBSR) interventions have relatively small effect sizes on depression, anxiety, and psychological distress among PLW-CMC [23]. Collaborative care interventions have been demonstrated to improve depression and QOL among PLW-CMC being treated in primary care settings [9].

Psychosocial Interventions

In addition to benefits of patient–provider interaction, peer-support groups, and other treatment modalities, the influence of social relationships on mental health and well-being is gaining increasing attention, particularly in persons with disabilities [24]. Yet, the integration of persons with disabilities into social networks alone may be insufficient; healthcare providers and professionals working in unison to ensure the provision of high-quality relationships and tailored support is more likely to lead to favorable outcomes [24].

Real-World Clinical Applications and Future Directions for Research in Chronic Medical Conditions

Acknowledging that the etiologies of chronic medical conditions are countless, all treating providers must consider whether or not the observed presentation of suboptimal wellness, poor QOL, or psychiatric symptom severity is related to psychosocial stressors surrounding a patient's given condition, or if the presentation of such factors is a pathognomonic feature of the chronic medical condition. This is an important distinction in clinical practice, because understanding the mechanistic or pathological origin of such symptom presentation can have differing treatment implications. For example, depression is common in patients living with HIV. However, subjective report of depression could be related to the psychosocial stressors/stigma associated with HIV serostatus, or it could be the result of central nervous system compromise due to subcortical insult, chronic neuroinflammation, opportunistic infection, neurotoxicity secondary to highly active antiretroviral therapy (HAART), or the indirect consequence of HAART, which could result in a HAART-related metabolic syndrome that manifests as subjective depression [25].

We provide this vignette to convey our shared sentiment that when a clinician is effectively examining wellness and appropriate treatment strategies among PLW-CMC, the duty to develop an appropriate treatment plan falls on the shoulders of the respective healthcare provider. Being aware of the symptoms associated with each chronic medical condition, as well as secondary or indirect effects of associated treatments (e.g., disrupted sleep, metabolic disturbance), and their subsequent negative effect on wellness, is a complex and enduring process to work through with each new patient treated. Nonetheless, this high level of clinical conceptualization can make all the difference in the lives and subsequent wellness of our patients.

Conclusion

Patients living with chronic medical conditions are at increased risk of suboptimal wellness, QOL, well-being, and life satisfaction, and are also at increased risk of disability, psychiatric illness, and functional compromise. Effective treatment of PLW-CMC requires healthcare providers to examine their patients from a biopsychosocial perspective, with further consideration of potential systemic or situational factors that may be mitigating favorable outcomes. All researchers and clinicians working with PLW-CMC are guided to be mindful of a patient's ability to access appropriate resources and treatments under the restrictions of limited language proficiency, remote habitation, financial status, disability status, and spiritual beliefs or values; this list is certainly not all-inclusive. Given the persistent and often lifelong nature of chronic medical conditions, multidisciplinary treatment teams with strong working relationships and collaborative efforts to bolster and foster patients' sense of self-efficacy and ability to self-manage their respective chronic conditions are critical.

References

1. World Health Organization and Public Health Agency of Canada. *Preventing Chronic Diseases: A Vital Investment*. Washington, DC, World Health Organization; 2005.

2. KH Ngamaba, M Panagioti, CJ Armitage. How strongly related are health status and subjective well-being? Systematic review and meta-analysis. *Eur J Public Health* 2017; **27**: 879–885.

3. EA Bayliss, DE Bonds, CM Boyd, et al. Understanding the context of health for persons with multiple chronic conditions: moving from what is the matter to what matters. *Ann Fam Med* 2014; **12**: 260–269.

4. VS Conn, AR Hafdahl, LM Brown. Meta-analysis of quality-of-life outcomes from physical activity interventions. *Nurs Res* 2009; **58**: 175–183.

5. RE Mujica-Mota, M Roberts, G Abel, et al. Common patterns of morbidity and multi-morbidity and their impact on health-related quality of life: evidence from a national survey. *Qual Life Res* 2015; **24**: 909–918.

6. LC Baumann, TT Dang. Helping patients with chronic conditions overcome barriers to self-care. *Nurse Pract* 2012; **37** : 32–38.

7. S Chatterji, J Byles, D Cutler, T Seeman, E Verdes. Health, functioning, and disability in older adults: present status and future implications. *Lancet* 2015; **385**: 563–575.

8. JR Read, L Sharpe, M Modini, BF Dear. Multimorbidity and depression: a systematic review and meta-analysis. *J Affect Disord* 2017; **221**: 36–46.

9. LC Watson, HR Amick, BN Gaynes, et al. Practice-based interventions addressing concomitant depression and chronic medical conditions in the primary care setting: a systematic review and meta-analysis. *J Prim Care Community Health* 2013; **4**: 294–306.

10. K Megari. Quality of life in chronic disease patients. *Health Psychol Res* 2013; **1**: 141–148.

11. AH Maslow. A theory of human motivation. *Psychol Rev* 1943; **50**: 370.

12. S Newman, L Steed, K Mulligan. Self-management interventions for chronic illness. *Lancet* 2004; **364**: 1523–1537.

13. C Eiser, R Morse. A review of measures of quality of life for children with chronic illness. *Arch Dis Child* 2001; **84**: 205–211.

14. D Cella, JS Lai, CJ Nowinski, et al. Neuro-QOL: brief measures of health-related quality of life for clinical research in neurology. *Neurology* 2012; **78**: 1860–1867.

15. JM Salsman, D Victorson, SW Choi, et al. Development and validation of the positive affect and well-being scale for the neurology quality of life (Neuro-QOL) measurement system. *Qual Life Res* 2013; **22**: 2569–2580.

16. PA Grady, LL Gough. Self-management: a comprehensive approach to management of chronic conditions. *Am J Public Health* 2014; **104**: e25–e31.

17. MR DiMatteo, HS Lepper, TW Croghan. Depression is a risk factor for noncompliance with medical treatment: meta-analysis of the effects of anxiety and depression on patient adherence. *Arch Intern Med* 2000; **160**: 2101–2107.

18. S Kripalani, X Yao, RB Haynes. Interventions to enhance medication adherence in chronic medical conditions: a systematic review. *Arch Intern Med* 2007; **167**: 540–550.

19. MP Herring, TW Puetz, PJ O'Connor, RK Dishman. Effect of exercise training on depressive symptoms among patients with a chronic illness: a systematic review and meta-analysis of randomized controlled trials. *Arch Intern Med* 2012; **172**: 101–111.

20. FB Gillison, SM Skevington, A Sato, M Standage, S Evangelidou. The effects of exercise interventions on quality of life in clinical and healthy populations; a meta-analysis. *Soc Sci Med* 2009; **68**: 1700–1710.

21. L Beatty, S Lambert. A systematic review of internet-based self-help therapeutic interventions to improve distress and disease-control among adults with chronic health conditions. *Clin Psychol Rev* 2013; **33**: 609–622.

22. CD Graham, J Gouick, C Krahe, D Gillanders. A systematic review of the use of acceptance and commitment therapy (ACT) in chronic disease and long-term conditions. *Clin Psychol Rev* 2016; **46**: 46–58.

23. E Bohlmeijer, R Prenger, E Taal, P Cuijpers. The effects of mindfulness-based stress reduction therapy on mental health of adults with a chronic medical disease: a meta-analysis. *J Psychosom Res* 2010; **68**: 539–544.

24. H Tough, J Siegrist, C Fekete. Social relationships, mental health and wellbeing in physical disability: a systematic review. *BMC Public Health* 2017; **17**: 414.

25. AA Williams, LJ Sitole, D Meyer. HIV/HAART-associated oxidative stress is detectable by metabonomics. *Mol Biosyst* 2017; **24** : 2202–2217.

Wellness in Older Individuals

Allison M. Mays, Elizabeth Whiteman, and Sonja Rosen

Introduction

Given the increase in life expectancy and increased number of older people, larger numbers of older people will develop more comorbidities and functional impairments. Wellness in older individuals includes the continuum of primary and secondary prevention toward healthy aging, to both help prevent and screen for these comorbidities and functional impairments. This chapter reviews primary and secondary prevention, with a focus on healthcare maintenance, social isolation, physical activity in older adults, and nutrition. The first section reviews United States Preventive Services Task Force (USPSTF), Centers for Disease Control and Prevention (CDC), Advisory Committee on Immunization Practices (ACIP), and American Cancer Society (ACS) recommendations for immunizations and appropriate screening tools for age, as well as comprehensive geriatric assessment. Regarding physical activity in older adults, there is an extensive review of evidence-based recommendations for patients, including guidelines and tools providers may use. The international epidemic of social isolation is reviewed, along with the importance of screening for it and its associated morbidity and mortality. Finally, screening, risk factors, and interventions for nutritional problems in older persons are reviewed.

Healthcare Maintenance

Americans have had an increase in life expectancy from 47.3 years in 1900 to 77.2 years in 2001. By 2030 the population over 65 will more than double compared to the year 2000. In the United States in 2000, 35 million people were over the age of 65; in 2030, there will be over 70 million persons over that age [1]. Given the increase in life expectancy and increased number of older people, larger numbers of older people will develop more comorbidities and functional impairments. Therefore, a key aspect of wellness is healthcare maintenance, which includes the continuum of primary, secondary, and tertiary prevention. Primary prevention aims to prevent disease before it occurs. Secondary prevention aims to reduce the impact of disease that has already occurred. Finally, tertiary prevention aims are to decrease the effect of illness that has lasting effects. In this section, we review this continuum of healthcare maintenance in primary and secondary prevention to help ensure optimal wellness in our older population.

Primary Prevention

Primary prevention in older persons includes immunization, exercise, social engagement, and optimal nutrition. Immunization will be reviewed here; exercise, social engagement, and optimal nutrition are reviewed in subsequent sections. The recommendations for immunization are based on the CDC ACIP [2].

Flu Vaccine

All adults need a seasonal flu vaccine every year. People 65 and older are at higher risk for flu-related complications. Vaccination should be offered by the end of October. Fluzone High-Dose is also available and recommended for people over 65 years of age, but no preference is expressed for any one vaccine type at this time.

Pneumonia Vaccine

The CDC recommends immunocompetent adults 65 years of age and older receive both pneumococcal polysaccharide vaccine (Pneumovax 23) and pneumococcal conjugate (Prevnar 13) as part of a two-vaccine sequential regimen. For pneumococcal vaccine-naïve persons ≥65 years, Prevnar 13 should be administered first and then Pneumovax 23 administered at least one year later. For those who previously received Pneumovax 23 at age ≥65 years, then Prevnar13 should be administered at least one year later. People who previously received Pneumovax 23 before age 65 years, and who are now ≥65 years, should receive Prevnar 13 at least one year later, at or after the age of 65.

TDAP Vaccine

The ACIP recommends routine vaccination for tetanus, diphtheria, and pertussis. Older adults are recommended to receive a booster tetanus and diphtheria toxoids (Tdap) vaccine every 10 years to ensure ongoing protection against tetanus and diphtheria and acellular pertussis.

Shingles Vaccine

A new shingles vaccine called Shingrix was licensed by the US Food and Drug Administration (FDA) in 2017. The CDC recommends that healthy adults 50 years and older get two doses of Shingrix, 2–6 months apart. Shingrix provides strong protection against shingles and post-herpetic neuralgia, and is the preferred vaccine over Zostavax.

Secondary Prevention

Secondary prevention aims to reduce the impact of disease that has already occurred. Here, the focus is on finding disease early so that interventions can be implemented earlier and eliminate disease. Secondary prevention involves screening for diseases. The recommendations cited here are based on the USPSTF [3], as well as the American Cancer Society (ACS) [4] recommendations. Walter and Covinsky recommend a framework for decision-making in a hallmark review, taking into account the patient's life expectancy when determining appropriate screening tests for older adults [5]. Patients with life expectancies less than five years are unlikely to derive any survival benefit from cancer screening.

Breast Cancer Screening

Breast cancer increases with age, and in fact, other than being a woman, aging is the single most important risk factor in developing breast cancer [6]. The ACS recommends that women 55 and older should switch to mammograms every two years or continue yearly screening, and that screening should continue as long as a woman is in good health and is expected to live 10 more years or longer. The USPSTF recommends yearly screening for those 49–75 years of age. After age 75, the USPSTF concludes that the current evidence is insufficient to assess benefits and harms of screening mammography. The importance of life expectancy and informed decision-making with patients is key to patient-centered planning that is in line with the patient's goals of care.

Colon Cancer Screening

The USPSTF and ACS recommend screening for colorectal cancer starting at age 50 years and continuing until age 75 years. Between the ages of 75 and 85, the recommendation for colon cancer screening is individualized. Adults in this age group who have never been screened for colorectal cancer are more likely to benefit. Screening is most appropriate among adults who are healthy enough to undergo treatment if colorectal cancer is detected and who do not have comorbid conditions that would significantly limit their life expectancy. There are various screening tests at different intervals that are now accepted, with the focus being encouragement for some screening rather than only the gold standard of colonoscopy [7].

Cervical Cancer Screening

Both the ACS and USPSTF recommend that women over age 65 who have had regular cervical cancer testing in the past 10 years with normal results should not be tested for cervical cancer. Women with a history of a serious cervical pre-cancer should continue to be tested for at least 20 years after that diagnosis, even if testing goes past age 65.

Prostate Cancer Screening

There remains controversy regarding the benefit of current screening strategies in reducing the morbidity and mortality associated with prostate cancer, and the research in this area is continuing to evolve. The ACS recommends that men make an informed decision with a healthcare provider about whether to be tested for prostate cancer, and those with a life expectancy <10 years not be tested [8]. The USPSTF currently recommends against routine screening for prostate cancer in men >75 years of age, and that the evidence is indeterminate in those <75 [9]. Again, overall health and life expectancy and informed decision-making are key.

Osteoporosis Screening

The USPSTF recommends screening for osteoporosis in women aged 65 years and older [10]. There is a lack of evidence regarding optimal screening intervals or justification for repeat screening. Due to limitations in the precision of testing, a minimum of two years may be needed to reliably measure a change in bone mineral density. There is insufficient evidence to recommend routine screening for osteoporosis in men.

Comprehensive Geriatric Assessment

Comprehensive geriatric assessment (CGA) by the individual clinician extends beyond the above screening measures, and includes an assessment of cognitive, affective, functional, social, environmental, spiritual domains, and discussion of patient preferences. A patient's risk for falls, presence of cognitive impairment, or social isolation, for example, can be found within geriatric assessment screening tools. To date, there are no easily administered criteria to determine which older people will benefit from CGA in different settings [11]. Most CGA programs exclude patients with terminal illness, complete functional dependence, or nursing home placement, or patients that are "too healthy" to benefit. Geriatric assessment has been adapted into different models of care, and this continues to develop in healthcare systems today. The Medicare Annual Wellness Visit is an example of this type of health risk assessment that incorporates geriatric assessment, including screening for cognitive impairment and fall risk, in a recommended annual visit for patients over 65 [12].

Physical Activity in Older Adults

Older adults in the USA report high levels of inactivity, with 26.9 percent of those aged 65–74 and 35.3 percent of those older than 75 reporting no physical activity in the past month [13], notwithstanding clear guidelines for exercise recommendations for older adults [14] and robust evidence that physical activity delays chronic disease and decreases mortality [15]. Both the CDC [16] and leaders within healthcare [17] advocate for increasing efforts for physical activity promotion within healthcare, yet the best way to promote physical activity in community-dwelling older adults remains unclear [18, 19]. While the USPSTF determined that for adults there is inconclusive evidence that counseling by primary care clinicians is an effective method of increasing physical activity [20, 21], studies focusing on older adults [22–24] have found counseling to be an effective approach.

Given restrictions on time and resources in the primary care setting, it is particularly important to understand the impact of brief counseling interventions on the uptake of physical activity. A broad range of interventions have been tested in clinical trials, but many are resource- or time-intensive, and not practical in terms of broad adoption into routine clinical practice [25]. While participants in Martinson et al.'s intervention saw a significant increase in adherence to exercise guidelines – by 10 percent compared to controls – participants were engaged in four lectures, one group orientation, 23 phone calls, lending library materials, and three motivational contests. Brief interventions, taking 3–5 minutes, remain the most practical, low-cost intervention; however, as stated previously, their effectiveness remains unclear [26].

We recommend a counseling approach based on an adaptation of Donabedian's Quality of Care Model that identifies links between the health system factors or structure, processes of care, and their associated health outcomes [27]. In this conceptual framework, the use of health system factors, including maintenance of community partnerships and the use of the electronic medical record to structure exercise recommendations and provide written materials for patients and providers, will in turn facilitate a streamlined process of care.

For the counseling itself we are utilizing a patient-centered model that incorporates elements of the transtheoretical model [28] and patient-centered elements of counseling, which focus on identifying cognitive, attitudinal, instrumental, behavioral, and social factors that may influence the patient's ability and willingness to overcome barriers and utilize resources. The transtheoretical model integrates a patient's readiness to change into physician recommendations. For physical activity, the stages of change as outlined by Pinto et al. are listed in Table 15.1.

This approach has been described as "The 5 As" (Address the Agenda, Assess, Advise, Assist, and Arrange follow-up) and is adapted from tobacco cessation counseling to

Table 15.1 Stages of change for physical activity

Precontemplation	No physical activity and does not intend to start.
Contemplation	No physical activity but intends to start.
Preparation	Irregular physical activity.
Action	Regular physical activity (≥3 times/week) for < 6 months.
Maintenance	Regular physical activity (≥3 times/week) for ≥ 6 months.

incorporate the patient-centered and transtheoretical models as outlined by Pinto et al. It has been evaluated as an approach to exercise counseling and been found to be able to mediate motivational readiness for physical activity in older adults [29]. It is also recommended by the USPSTF as an evidence-based approach for behavioral counseling [30].

A script for exercise counseling using the 5 As approach is:

1. Agenda: "I'd like to talk to you about your level of physical activity."
2. Assess: current level of activity; feelings about changing activity level; prior experience with physical activity; barriers to physical activity.
3. Advise: benefits of physical activity; encourage change.
4. Assist: negotiate intervention plan, matched to readiness to change.
5. Arrange follow-up: "I'd like to hear about your progress" – electronic message, telephone, or future visit; or referral to community exercise programs.

A sample of information to be included in patient after-visit instructions could be as follows:

Benefits of exercise:

- improved conditioning, strength, flexibility, overall physical fitness;
- improved mobility and reduced risk of falls;
- reduced risk of heart disease, stroke, high blood pressure, diabetes, osteoporosis, obesity, colon cancer, breast cancer, anxiety, depression, and memory loss.

Some Physical Activity Is Better than None

It's never too late to become physically active – even if you have been sedentary, studies show that if you start exercising you'll still get significant benefit.

Physical activity guidelines recommend a **minimum** 30 minutes of aerobic exercise on five or more days of the week. Recommendations from the AHA and American College of Sports Medicine (ACSM) include:

1. Aerobic exercise:
   a. use of large muscle groups, sustained for >10 minutes, e.g., brisk walking, jogging, swimming, dancing, cycling, cardio equipment;
   b. minimum of 30 minutes of moderate-intensity 5×/week or 20 minutes of vigorous-intensity 3×/week – the more the better;
   c. note these are in **addition** to regular self-care activities including cleaning, bathing, walking to the car, running errands;
   d. activities can be spread throughout the day in smaller allotments.

2. Muscle strengthening
   a. weight training, weight-bearing calisthenics, resistance training;
   b. progressive and requires gradual increases over time;
   c. minimum of two non-consecutive days of the week, target 8–10 major muscle groups.

3. Flexibility/balance:
   a. necessary to perform activities such as putting on shoes, reaching for objects overhead, turning around when driving a car;
   b. flexibility exercises should be performed twice a week for >10 minutes;
   c. group classes such as Tai Chi improve balance.

Additionally, addressing social and environmental supports for exercise and focusing on enjoyment of exercise, especially in a group setting, have been found to be effective in increasing adherence to physical activity, as well as yielding additional benefits to well-being [18, 31]. A study of Silver Sneakers membership – in which Medicare recipients receive free access to exercise classes and facilities – found a decrease in social isolation and loneliness after enrollment into the program [32]. Based on these studies we highly recommend referring older adults to community-based exercise programs. Through federal funding via the US Administration for Community Living (ACL) distributed through local Area Agencies on Aging as outlined in the Older Americans Act, several evidence-based community health programs, including exercise classes, are offered to assist older adults in aging in place, throughout the USA.

Social Isolation and Connectedness in Older Adults

According to an AARP Foundation study, approximately 48 percent of adults aged 62–91 report feeling some degree of loneliness. Lonely individuals are more likely to be unmarried, to live alone, to have lower household incomes, and to have more physical limitations [33]. Up to 17 percent of older adults may be socially isolated [34]. In a meta-analysis, Holt-Lunstad et al. found that greater social connection is associated with a 50 percent reduced risk of early death [35]. There has also been an association seen between social connection and cognitive decline [36]. Socially isolated older adults in an analysis by the AARP Public Policy Institute were also found to have increased Medicare expenditures mediated through increased length of hospital stays and increased likelihood of skilled nursing home admission, resulting in fewer days at home for socially isolated individuals [37]. Therefore, in addition to the improved well-being that comes with social connections, there are likely morbidity, mortality, and quality-of-life benefits as well.

We recommend screening for social isolation and loneliness in routine clinical care of the older adult, as there are significant health as well as psychosocial consequences from the absence of social connection. In our practice we refer socially isolated individuals to community-based programming as well as a consultation with a clinic social worker.

Nutrition and Healthy Aging

Nutrition and maintaining a healthy weight are important for health in older adults. Multiple medical issues may make it more difficult to maintain a healthy diet as people get older. Making healthy food choices and maintaining adequate nutrition as the body changes are important for good health. Appetite loss in older people is common and is associated with undernutrition, immunosuppression, and sarcopenia, which can lead to frailty and higher rates of morbidity and mortality [38, 39]. It is important to monitor diet and screen for malnutrition in older adults.

Screening instruments for nutrition may vary; many screening tools have been developed to screen for nutrition in community-dwelling older adults as well as hospitalized and nursing-home patients. Screening tools vary in sensitivity and specificity and not all have been adequately validated [40]. The Mini Nutritional Assessment tool (MNA) is an accurate assessment tool for nutritional problems; however, it was not validated for all populations. A multidisciplinary approach and a CGA can help clinicians monitor and assess those at risk. In community-dwelling older adults, risk factors include involuntary weight loss (e.g., >2 percent in one month, >10 lb in six months, >4 percent in one year), BMI < 22 kg/m^2, hypoalbuminemia, sarcopenia, loss of subcutaneous fat, and fluid accumulation (edema) [41]. Currently 16 percent of those >65 years and 2 percent of those >85 years are classed as malnourished [40].

Contributing risk factors for weight loss can include medical, psychological, and social issues. Often, risk for malnutrition is multifactorial and ongoing assessment is necessary. Maintaining a nutrient-dense diet is critically important for older adults because of the impact of food intake on health. Years of research have demonstrated that diet quality has a huge effect on physical condition, cognitive condition, bone health, eye health, vascular function, and the immune system. This can be challenging to achieve for several reasons [42]. Social isolation, difficulty chewing or swallowing, changes in taste and smell, poor calorie intake due to financial or functional limitations, and decreased physical activity can lead to poor oral intake. Medical conditions such as glucose intolerance, gastric reflux, congestive heart failure, chronic pulmonary disease, renal insufficiency, coronary artery disease, and malignancies may lead to dietary restrictions and recommendations that make food less palatable and put patients at risk for weight loss. Depression and dementia may be factors playing a role in appetite decline. Dementia patients often forget to eat or are limited in their ability to shop and cook. Nutrition may be limited by medication interactions or side effects. Dental or swallowing problems may add to poor nutrition. Those living in facilities may have limited food choices and limited meal schedules. Financial limitations or the inability to access healthy meals, as well as physical decline, may limit food options [43, 44]. It is important to have a high variety of foods and continued access to food to maintain good health.

Interventions to improve nutrition include education for choosing healthy foods, adding exercise, and considering meal adjustments such as flavor enhancements, increasing variety, adding supplements, or medications [45]. Making meals social, such as meals at community centers, senior activity groups, or family activities can be additional resources for patients. Education on high protein and variety of food choices is important to avoid muscle loss. Clinicians can also recommend exercise to help boost energy and increase metabolism.

Maintaining a healthy weight should include consultation with the physician to review medications and lifestyle. Unnecessary medications should be discontinued and the full physical exam review of active and new medical issues should include weight loss, dental, and social limitations as one ages. Choosing healthy meals should include making eating a social event, drinking plenty of fluids, knowing how much to eat, and understanding the nutrient facts label [46].

Vitamins and minerals are usually not recommended for older people unless a specific deficiency is indicated. Too much of certain vitamin supplements can be harmful, such as the fat-soluble vitamins A, D, E, and K. Patients may often take additional supplements they don't need. A thorough review of medications in older patients should also include any vitamins or supplements. Each patient should be individualized for vitamin needs and screening for risk factors like osteoporosis, malabsorption, or anemia may require some vitamin supplementation. Protein supplements in older adults with malnutrition risk can have beneficial effects on weight gain and mortality. According to the PROT-AGE Study Group a daily intake in the range of at least 1.0–1.2 g protein per kilogram of body weight is required to reduce the loss of muscle mass and strength, and to prevent the development of frailty [47]. Supplements should be given between meals rather than with meals to encourage eating at meal time [46, 48]. Patients should be encouraged to continue with regular meals and if early satiety occurs they can try multiple small meals spread throughout the day to increase calorie intake.

For patients with anorexia of aging or anorexia due to medical conditions there are currently no FDA-approved medications for weight gain. Several medications have been examined to stimulate appetite in older adults, but none of them is recommended in routine clinical practice. Appetite-stimulating medications (e.g., megestrol acetate, tetrahydrocannabinol, dronabinol, or cyproheptadine) have been associated with numerous side effects, including delirium, fluid retention, and abdominal symptoms. For these reasons, they are of limited benefit in clinical practice [49–51]. Other medications including growth hormone, testosterone in men, and corticosteroids show no improved outcomes and, due to the high side-effect risk, should be avoided. One of the leading causes of weight loss is depression. Patients with depression should be treated with appropriate antidepressants. Although not FDA-approved for appetite, mirtazapine (Remeron) has been shown to increase appetite and promote weight gain while also treating the underlying depression.

Anorexia of aging can negatively impact quality of life, morbidity, and mortality. Despite its high prevalence, it is rarely recognized or treated. This represents one of the major challenges of geriatric medicine. Anorexia needs to be considered an important indicator of significant disorder of energy metabolism during the aging process. One of the most important aims in the care of older adults is the enhancement of their nutritional status. The first step is the identification of people who are at risk of anorexia of aging by using geriatric assessment tools. Then, potentially reversible factors that promote loss of appetite and diminish food intake should be evaluated. Specific individualized care plans should be implemented to help provide adequate amounts of food and limit weight loss. Finally, multi-stimulus interventions and specific strategies, including food texture adjustments, flavor enhancements, and protein supplements, may be effective in the management of nutrition in older people.

References

1. www.census.gov/newsroom.press-releases/2018/cb18-41-population-projections.html (accessed March 15, 2019).

2. www.cdc.gov/vaccines/adults/rec-vac/index.html (accessed March 15, 2019).

3. www.uspreventiveservicestaskforce.org/BrowseRec/Index (accessed March 15, 2019).

4. www.cancer.org/healthy/find-cancer-early/cancer-screening-guidelines/american-cancer-society-guidelines-for-the-early-detection-of-cancer.html (accessed March 15, 2019).

5. LC Walter, KE Covinsky. Cancer screening in elderly patients: a framework for

individualized decision making. *JAMA* 2001; **285**: 2750–2756.

6. S Rosen, N Weintraub. The efficacy of performing screening mammograms in the frail elderly population. *J Am Med Dir Assoc* 2006; **7**: 230–233.

7. www.uspreventiveservicestaskforce.org/Page/Document/RecommendationStatementFinal/colorectal-cancer-screening2#tab (accessed March 18, 2019).

8. www.cancer.org/cancer/prostate-cancer.html (accessed March 18, 2019).

9. www.uspreventiveservicestaskforce.org/Page/Document/UpdateSummaryFinal/prostate-cancer-screening-2008 (accessed March 18, 2019).

10. www.uspreventiveservicestaskforce.org/Page/Document/RecommendationStatementFinal/osteoporosis-screening (accessed March 18, 2019).

11. DB Reuben, S Rosen, H Schickendanz. Principles of geriatric assessment. In: *Hazzard's Principles of Geriatric Medicine and Gerontology* (7th ed.). New York, McGraw Hill; 2017.

12. www.cms.gov/Outreach-and-Education/Medicare-Learning-Network-MLN/MLNProducts/MLN-Publications-Items/CMS1246474.html (accessed March 20, 2019).

13. KB Watson, SA Carlson, JP Gunn, et al. Physical inactivity among adults aged 50 years and older: United States, 2014. *MMWR Morb Mortal Wkly Rep* 2016; **65**: 954–958.

14. US Department of Health and Human Services. *Physical Activity Guidelines for Americans*. Washington, DC, US Department of Health and Human Services; 2008.

15. D Taylor. Physical activity is medicine for older adults. *Postgrad Med J* 2014; **90**: 26–32.

16. Centers for Disease Control and Prevention. *The State of Aging and Health in America*. Atlanta, GA, Centers for Disease Control and Prevention; 2013.

17. IM Vuori, CJ Lavie, SN Blair. Physical activity promotion in the health care system. *Mayo Clin Proc* 2013; **88**(12): 1446–1461.

18. A Zubala, S MacGillivray, H Frost, et al. Promotion of physical activity interventions for community dwelling older adults: a systematic review of reviews. *PloS One* 2017; **12**(7): e0180902.

19. G Orrow, A-L Kinmonth, S Sanderson, S Sutton. Effectiveness of physical activity promotion based in primary care: systematic review and meta-analysis of randomized controlled trials. *BMJ* 2012; **344**: e1389.

20. KB Eden, CT Orleans, CD Mulrow, NJ Pender, SM Teutsch. Does counseling by clinicians improve physical activity? A summary of the evidence for the US Preventive Services Task Force. *Ann Intern Med* 2002; **137**(3): 208–215.

21. DA Lawlor, B Hanratty. The effect of physical activity advice given in routine primary care consultations: a systematic review. *J Public Health Med* 2001; **3**: 219–226.

22. N Kerse, CR Elley, E Robinson, B Arroll. Is physical activity counseling effective for older people? A cluster randomized, controlled trial in primary care. *J Am Geriatr Soc* 2005; **53**(1): 1951–1956.

23. GS Kolt, GM Schofield, N Kerse, N Garrett, M Oliver. Effect of telephone counseling on physical activity for low-active older people in primary care: a randomized, controlled trial. *J Am Geriatr Soc* 2007; **55**(7): 986–992.

24. O Olanrewaju, S Kelly, A Cowan, C Brayne, L Lafortune. Physical activity in community dwelling older people: a systematic review of reviews of interventions and context. *PLoS One* 2016;**11**: e0168614.

25. BC Martinson, AL Crain, NE Sherwood, et al. Maintaining physical activity among older adults: six-month outcomes of the Keep Active Minnesota randomized controlled trial. *Prevent Med* 2008: **46**: 111–119.

26. S Pears, M Bijker, K Morton, et al. A randomized controlled trial of three very brief interventions for physical activity in primary care. *BMC Pub Health* 2016; **16**: 1033.

27. A Donabedian. The quality of care: how can it be assessed? *JAMA* 1988; **260**: 1743–1748.

28. BM Pinto, MG Goldstein, BH Marcus. Activity counseling by primary care physicians. *Prevent Med* 1998: 506–513.

29. BM Pinto, H Lynn, BH Marcus, J DePue, MG Goldstein. Physician-based activity counseling: intervention effects on mediators of motivational readiness for physical activity. *Ann Behav Med* 2001; **23**: 2–10.

30. EP Whitlock, CT Orleans, N Pender, J Allan. Evaluating primary care behavioral counseling interventions: an evidence-based approach. *Am J Prevent Med* 2002; **22**: 267–284.

31. C Martín-Borràs, M Giné-Garriga, A Puig-Ribera, et al. A new model of exercise referral scheme in primary care: is the effect on adherence to physical activity sustainable in the long term? A 15-month randomized controlled trial. *BMJ Open* 2018; **8**: e017211.

32. S Brady, LA D'Ambrosio, A Felts, et al. Reducing isolation and loneliness through membership in a fitness program for older adults: implications for health. *J Appl Gerontol* 2018; **39**: 0733464818807820.

33. LC Hawkley, M Kozloski, J Wong. A profile of social connectedness in older adults. AARP; 2017.

34. H Ortiz. Crossing new frontiers: benefits access among isolated seniors. National Center for Benefits Outreach and Enrollment (NCBOE); 2011.

35. J Holt-Lunstad, T Smith, JB Layton. Social relationships and mortality risk: a meta-analytic review. *PLoS Med* 2010. DOI:10.1371/journal.pmed.1000316.

36. JT Cacioppo, S Cacioppo. Older adults reporting social isolation or loneliness show poorer cognitive function 4 years later. *Evid Based Nurs* 2014; **75**: 59–60.

37. L Flowers. Medicare spends more on socially isolated older adults. *Insight Issues* 2017; **125**.

38. BS Van Der Meij, AH Wijnhoven, JS Lee, et al. Poor appetite and dietary intake in community dwelling adults *J Am Geriatr Soc* 2017; **65**: 2190–2197.

39. F Landi, R Calvani, M Tosato, et al. Anorexia of aging risk factors, consequences, and potential treatments. *Nutrients* 2016; **8**: 69.

40. P Soysal, AT Isik, F Arik, et al. Validity of the mini-nutritional assessment scale for evaluating frailty status in older adults. *J Am Med Dir Assoc* 2019; **20**(2): 183–187.

41. V Malafarina, F Uriz-Otano, L Gil-Guerrero, R Iniesta. The anorexia of aging: physiopathology, prevalence, associated comorbidity and mortality, a systematic review. *Maturitas* 2013; **74**: 293–302.

42. Providing Healthy and Safe Foods as We Age: Workshop Summary, Nutrition Concerns for Aging Populations. The National Academy, Institute of Medicine (US) Food Forum.

43. F Landi, F Lattanzio, G Dell'Aquilla, et al. Prevalence and potentially reversible factors associated with anorexia among older nursing home residents: results from the Ulisse Project. *J Am Med Dir Assoc* 2013; **14**: 119.

44. MA Bernstein, KL Tucker, ND Ryan, et al. Higher dietary variety is associated with better nutritional status in frail elderly people. *J Am Dietetic Assoc* 2002; **102**: 1096–1124.

45. NJ Cox, K Ibrahim, AA Sayer, SM Robinson, H Roberts. Assessment and treatment of the anorexia of aging: a systematic review. *Nutrients* 2019; **11**: 144.

46. National Institute on Aging, Choosing healthy meals as you get older. www.nia.nih.gov/health/choosing-healthy-meals-you-get-older (accessed April 21, 2020).

47. J Bauer, G Biolo, T Cederholm, et al. Evidence-based recommendations for optimal dietary protein intake in older people: a position paper from the PROT-AGE Study Group. *J Am Med Dir Assoc* 2013; **14**: 542–559.

48. V Pouyssegur, P Brocker, SM Schneider, et al. An innovative solid oral nutritional supplement to fight weight loss and anorexia: open randomized controlled trial of efficacy in institutionalized, malnourished older adults. *Age Ageing* 2015; **44**: 245–251.

49. DB Reuben, SH Hirsch, K Zhou, GA Greendale. The effects of megestrol acetate suspension for elderly patients with reduced appetite after hospitalization: a phase II randomized clinical trial. *J Am Geriatr Soc* 2005; **53**: 970–975.

50. F Landi, R Calvani, M Tosato, et al. Anorexia of aging: risk factors, consequences, and potential treatments. *Nutrients* 2016; **27**: 69.

51. JE Morley. Anorexia of aging: physiologic and pathologic. *Am J Clin Nutr* 1997; **66**: 760–773.

Wellness in Children and Adolescents

Cassidy Zanko and Margaret L. Stuber

Introduction

Healthcare providers working with children and adolescents spend much of their training becoming experts in assessment, diagnosis, and treatment of disordered states, focusing on what has or may go wrong. Providers dedicate little time to understanding how to assess positive signs of wellness, such as happiness, life satisfaction, and internal strengths. This is partially because the study of youth wellness is recent, having emerged in the past 10–15 years. In that time, we have also witnessed significant advances in neuroscience, which have furthered our understanding of vital factors that influence youth wellness and development. Consequently, evidence-based wellness interventions are emerging. In contrast to wellness interventions with adult patients, most data-driven recommendations for youth currently require involvement of caregivers and/or are delivered through school-based programs.

As with adults, wellness medicine in youth includes physical, psychological, social, emotional, and spiritual health, with the critical addition of family and caregiver health. This chapter provides an overview of these areas, addressing assessment and practical interventions through empirical research that can be recommended by providers in collaboration with children and their caregivers. Following a summary of general youth wellness domains will be a brief survey of nutraceutical and pharmaceutical considerations.

Family and Caregiver Health

The most fundamental and foundational aspect of a youth's well-being is family health. This includes the dynamics of the family system, caregiver style(s), and caregiver mental health and well-being. Healthcare providers must carefully evaluate each of these factors due to their impact on attachment, bonding, and positive development. Assessment may be through direct observation in family therapy and/or caregiver self-report questionnaires aimed at identifying emotional–behavioral issues. These issues may be impacting the family unit and, once identified, can be targeted. Evidence-based family approaches, such as family-focused therapy (FFT) for bipolar disorder, emphasize skills exemplified by authoritative parenting, a caregiver style with robust evidence. These skills include communication techniques, praise and warmth, reinforcement of positive behaviors, appropriate limit setting, and shared problem-solving. When utilized, approaches like FFT benefit the well-being and trajectory of the entire family [1].

In addition to strengthening the family dynamics and caregiver–child relationship, supporting a caregiver's health is vital to optimal learning and implementation of wellness strategies in order to create a loving, predictable home so that both caregiver and child thrive. Significant evidence exists describing the negative impact of caregiver psychopathology on a child's wellness, resulting in child behavioral challenges and risk for subsequent development of psychopathology [2]. Fortunately, with timely treatment these risks can be reduced [2]. For example, a 2008 review presented evidence that reduction or remission of parental depressive symptoms was related to a maintained reduction in the child's symptoms [2]. Therefore, encouraging caregivers to identify their own need to seek treatment and cultivate their own wellness is essential to successful implementation of a wellness plan for children.

Positive Relationships

Positive relationships between family members are building blocks to positive relationships outside of the home. As children enter adolescence and explore their identities outside of the nuclear family, their relationships with non-family members become increasingly integral to their psychosocial development. This includes relationships with peers, coaches, mentors, and teachers. As adolescents explore their peer relationships and emulate behaviors that diverge from their nuclear family, unnecessary concern in their caregiver may result. For example, when youth want to alter their hair or clothing to reflect their peers, caregivers are encouraged to allow identity exploration while remaining involved and assessing for safety or mood changes. Concern is better focused on youth who are isolating from friendships, activities, and family relationships.

If isolation or lack of outside relationships is identified, a psychological assessment is recommended. Intervention(s) will then depend on the cause of the isolating behavior. Interventions include social skills groups and/or treatment of mental health conditions that can impair a youth's desire for social engagement, such as depression, anxiety, psychosis, or autism spectrum disorder.

Physical Wellness

Areas of physical wellness, which impact both physical and mental health outcomes, include nutrition, physical activity, yoga, screen media use, and sleep.

Nutrition

With the rise of childhood obesity, nutrition and dietary quality are increasingly scrutinized for their impact on physical health, as well as optimal psychological functioning [3, 4]. The impact of dietary quality on a child's mental health begins with a mother's diet during gestation, and continues into early childhood [5]. Specifically, the data suggests that young children who consume a diet high in sugar, processed foods, and saturated fats and/or a diet low in nutrient-dense foods such as vegetables and fruits display behaviors consistent with mental health problems [4]. This pattern continues, with poor dietary quality contributing to risk for common mental illnesses such as depression and anxiety in both adolescents and adults [4]. In addition to inquiring about diet quality when discussing nutrition with families, evaluating for healthy eating habits is important. This includes assessing for nutritional breakfast consumption and discussing the value of family meals for connection and communication.

While working with families to promote healthy eating and dining habits, mindfully avoid a weight-focused approach. Focus on weight may increase the risk of eating disorders and excessive exercise, and has *not* been shown to improve the obesity epidemic [5]. Instead, the American Academy of Nutrition and Dietetics is in favor of evidence-based youth programs that use child-friendly concepts [6]. These programs include information about acceptance and diversity of body types, thus promoting a sense of self-worth [6]. One such example is the *Healthy Bodies: Teaching Kids What They Need to Know Curriculum*, published by the National Eating Disorders Association [5].

Controversy remains about what defines a "healthy diet." Data supporting the Mediterranean diet appears promising for prevention of childhood obesity as well as other common pediatric ailments, but requires larger-scale, long-term studies [6]. "Functional foods" are also being investigated. For example, the ketogenic diet may target refractory and severe seizure control in some children, comparable to antiepileptic drugs, and certain elimination diets may benefit attention deficit hyperactivity disorder (ADHD) or autism spectrum disorder [6]. However, there is a lack of evidence supporting standard use and a potential risk of nutrient deficiencies [6]. While more research is being conducted on these diets, use the *2015–2020 Dietary Guidelines for Americans* (www .choosemyplate.gov) to help families choose a healthy, nutritionally adequate and balanced diet that benefits the entire family's physical and mental health.

Physical Activity

The Centers for Disease Control (CDC) reports that "the evidence is clear – physical activity fosters normal growth and development, can reduce the risk of various chronic diseases, and can make people feel better, function better, and sleep better" [7]. The US Department of Health and Human Services (HHS) goes on to explain that physically active youth have higher levels of cardiorespiratory fitness, lower body fat, and stronger muscles and bones [8]. Physical activity (PA) also contributes to psychological and social health benefits, such as reduced symptoms of depression and anxiety, higher self-esteem, improved social skills, and greater levels of connectedness [8, 9]. Cognitively, moderate-to-vigorous physical activity improves areas of functioning involved in ADHD, such as memory, executive function, processing speed, attention, and academic performance [8]. Finally, PA provides access to positive role models and important life skills.

To optimize all of these benefits, the HHS guidelines recommend that preschool-aged children (ages 3–5) engage in active play and structured activities for about three hours per day of mixed intensities, and school-aged youth (ages 6–17) be involved in at least 60 minutes of moderate-to-vigorous daily physical activity [8]. Additionally, twin studies illustrate how healthcare can positively promote physical activity by working together with caregivers [10]. These studies show that from early childhood through mid-adolescence, family environment and parenting behaviors have greater effect than genetics on influencing exercise behavior; in late adolescence this switches [10]. It is therefore important to assess the caregiver's attitudes regarding PA. It is also important to understand that participation becomes more challenging as children age into an "elite" sports culture that selects players based on ability [3]. Providers can help support families by preparing them and encouraging continued physical activity through methods in line with the youth's strengths.

Yoga

Yoga has become increasingly popular in Western nations, and its benefits are emerging in childhood and adolescence [6]. Research in youth has shown a positive effect on psychological functioning, physical health, and cognitive performance, with improvement in the core symptoms of ADHD [6]. Additionally, prenatal yoga may reduce maternal anxiety and depression and improve the *in utero* environment [6]. Therefore, incorporating yoga into pregnancy wellness when appropriate may also positively impact the infant's wellness and development.

Screen Media Use

US society is saturated with technologies, exposing youth to an environment in which an increasing amount of their time is spent facing a screen [11]. This immersion with screens has positive and negative effects on physical health, mental health, and well-being [11]. Positive effects include meaningful connections between distant family members through video-chatting, increased ease of support-seeking, and smartphone applications targeting healthy behaviors and habits [11]. However, the negative effects in youth are concerning, particularly in adolescent high-users (7+ h/day) [11]. Negative effects may include depression and anxiety, obesity, and disconnection [12]. In addition, it may lead to impaired sleep and lower ability to self-regulate [11].

The American Academy of Pediatrics (AAP) has released specific recommendations, including screen media time restrictions and resources to help families maintain a healthy media diet [12]. Age limits include no use under 18 months; co-viewing and discussion of high-quality programs at age 18–24 months; co-viewing and limiting to no more than 1 h/day of high-quality programs at age 2–5 years; and consistent limits on time spent and types of media used for age 6 and older, with close monitoring [12]. Screens should not replace sleep, physical activity, or other behaviors essential to health [12]. An interactive, online tool that families can use to create a personal family media use plan can be accessed at www.healthychildren.org.

Clinically, healthcare providers can encourage caregivers to learn about social media sites and applications used by their children (a helpful site for caregiver education is www.commonsensemedia.org). Providers can discuss the value of creating digital curfews and unplugged time/spaces, and encourage playtime, particularly for at-risk adolescents [12]. The AAP recommends caregivers treat media as they would any other environment, with appropriate limit setting (e.g., knowing their child's friends online and offline), as well as caregiver modeling and engaging with screen media together [12]. When working with adolescents, providers can inquire about the quantity, content, and psychological impact of their digital use. Recommendations for health-promoting phone applications can also be made, which are linked to wellness interventions such as mindfulness meditation. Finally, providers can discuss the importance of screen-replacement activities such as sports, music, art, and reading [12].

Sleep

Establishing good sleep practices is a vital component of wellness. Unfortunately, an estimated 25–40 percent of children suffer from a sleep problem [13]. In youth, the amount and quality of sleep impacts school performance, mental health, suicidal thoughts, reckless behavior, substance-use, and weight gain [13, 14]. Working memory is particularly influenced by poor sleep, which may contribute to risky decision-making [13].

When assessing sleep habits, a thorough work-up of non-behavioral etiologies of insomnia, such as obstructive sleep apnea and restless leg syndrome, must be ruled out.

One imperative assessment area is if there is a screen in the bedroom, as these devices decrease sleep duration due to arousing content and light exposure [15]. It is also important to understand the developmental changes occurring in adolescence that impact their sleep [15]. These include reduction in slow-wave sleep and changes to their circadian rhythm, which delay sleep initiation and make waking up for early school starts challenging [15].

As in adults, treatment of insomnia is moving away from medication management and toward cognitive-behavioral therapy for insomnia (CBT-I) [15]. This has shown benefits including decreased somatic complaints, anxiety, oppositional behavior, and ADHD symptoms [15]. Access to this treatment is limited, so group-based CBT-I and validated internet-based CBT-I can be used as effective alternatives [15].

Psychological, Social, and Emotional Wellness

The wellness areas and interventions in these next sections positively influence youth social–emotional development, psychopathology prevention, coping skills, and optimal functioning. The National Alliance on Mental Illness (www.nami.org/Learn-More/Mental-Health-Conditions) explains: "half of mental health conditions begin by age 14, and 75% of mental health conditions develop by age 24," so early assessment and preventive interventions are imperative.

Resilience, Social-Emotional Learning, and Adverse Childhood Experiences

Adverse childhood experiences (ACEs) and early exposure to poverty contribute to child toxic stress [16]. Toxic stress is believed to permanently affect brain architecture and make children vulnerable to stress-related diseases [16]. Adverse childhood experiences can be assessed through direct questions about challenging life events that families have endured. Fortunately, children's responses to toxic stress can improve with psychosocial interventions that promote resilience [16].

Resilience – referred to as the ability to withstand, adapt to, and recover from adversity – mitigates the effects of toxic stress and ACEs [16]. Resilience results from a complex interplay between the child's genetics, temperament, coping skills, past experiences, social supports, and societal resources. A recent review in *Pediatrics* identified five modifiable resilience factors that can be incorporated into pediatric clinical care. They are: (1) encouraging caregiver positive appraisal and good executive function; (2) nurturing parenting; (3) maternal mental health; (4) good self-care skills and consistent household routines; and (5) an understanding of trauma [16]. This same review includes recommendations that incorporate resilience factors into clinical care settings for providers working with youth. These factors include training in trauma-informed care and in a wide range of assessment and resilience tools, such as appropriate screening techniques for youth ACEs, maternal psychopathology/ACEs, family functional capacity, and family violence [16].

Resilience is also being addressed in strength-based school programs, which reduce anxiety and depression, improve school performance, and increase optimism [17]. Penn Resiliency Program (PRP) is one of the most widely researched programs designed to prevent depression in youth [18]. It is a school-based program that teaches cognitive reframing, relaxation, coping skills, and creative brainstorming. Over the past 20 years, 17 studies (including randomized controlled trials) have been conducted with PRP, including

2000 8–15-year-old students [18]. These studies demonstrated reduced symptoms of depression and anxiety with significant, long-lasting effects on well-being [17, 18].

Other school-based initiatives are being developed to assess students' subjective well-being and to cultivate social and emotional health. Examples include the Well-Being Promotion Program and the Collaborative for Academic, Social and Emotional Learning (CASEL) [19]. These programs include approaches discussed below, such as positive psychology, mindfulness-based interventions (MBIs), and cognitive-behavioral therapy (CBT).

Positive Psychology

Martin Seligman, an American psychologist and prior president of the American Psychological Association (1998), influenced the scientific community with his theories of positive psychology and well-being [19]. The three pillars of positive psychology are positive emotions and experiences (e.g., happiness), positive individual traits (e.g., character strengths), and positive institutions (e.g., healthy, supportive schools and families) [19]. In 2011, Seligman shifted focus from what had been termed *authentic happiness* to *well-being theory* [19]. The shift essentially deemphasized life satisfaction as the primary outcome and broadened well-being to include five elements: positive emotions, engagement, relationships, meaning, and accomplishments (PERMA) [19].

The Well-Being Promotion Program is an example of how positive psychology is being utilized with youth. The program was developed and implemented by Shannon Suldo and colleagues, and contributes to improvements in sixth graders' life satisfaction [17, 19]. Activities focused on gratitude and kindness are relevant aspects of this program that can be utilized by healthcare providers to enhance wellness.

Gratitude and Acts of Kindness

Suldo's Well-Being Promotion Program includes exercises such as gratitude and acts of kindness [19]. Gratitude activities that show positive effects on subjective well-being among adolescents include "counting blessings," also known as "gratitude journaling," and expressing gratitude through writing and delivering a letter of thanks, termed a *gratitude visit* [19]. Increased happiness has been demonstrated among middle-school and college students who have completed both a gratitude visit and gratitude journaling [19].

Another example in Suldo's program is "acts of kindness" [19]. These are actions that benefit others at the cost of one's own personal time or effort. In just one week, children who performed three acts of kindness experienced gains in subjective well-being [19]. These exercises meaningfully improve students' perceived quality of life, which subsequently enhances academic performance [19]. Clinically, these are typically short, simple exercises that can be easily carried out during visits with youth [17].

Mindfulness-Based Interventions

Jon Kabat-Zinn, creator of mindfulness-based stress reduction (MBSR), defines mindfulness as "awareness that arises through paying attention, on purpose, in the present moment, non-judgmentally in the service of self-understanding and wisdom." Research in adults suggests that MBIs have positive effects on both mental and physical health [20]. Given that self-regulation and executive functioning develop markedly across childhood and adolescence, MBIs may be particularly valuable for this population [20].

A recent meta-analysis provided support for MBIs through data from randomized controlled trials looking at improvement in mental health, behavior, and cognition of people aged 18 years or younger [20]. Mindfulness-based interventions had significant effects on executive function, attention, measures of depression, anxiety/stress, and negative behaviors [20]. Age and duration of treatment were significant modifiers, with longer duration having more impact on negative behaviors, and older adolescents (14–18 years old) exhibiting the greatest benefits [20]. This effect in adolescents may be due to heightened brain plasticity and self-reflection during this time [20]. While the research on mindfulness interventions in children and adolescents is at an early stage, findings thus far support the benefits of incorporating these techniques.

Cognitive-Behavioral Therapy

Cognitive-behavioral therapy, pioneered by Aaron T. Beck, is a form of psychotherapy that highlights the important role of maladaptive cognitions in our emotional and behavioral responses [21]. Cognitive-behavioral strategies aim to change these maladaptive cognitions and eventually lead to reduction in emotional distress and problematic behaviors [21].

In youth, CBT has received preferential support in treating symptoms of anxiety disorders such as obsessive-compulsive disorder, and, to a lesser degree, depression [21]. It appears to work equally well as other psychotherapies, and in some cases is superior to medications, due to reduced side effects and greater cost-effectiveness [21]. The effects are more mixed for disruptive classroom behaviors and aggressive/antisocial behaviors, demonstrating less efficacy than pharmacological approaches [21]. Similarly for ADHD, CBT shows some efficacy but not superior to medications [21]. This is also true for smoking and substance-use, with small to medium efficacy but not more than other psychotherapies [21].

Music/Art

The developmental benefits of playing a musical instrument have been increasingly evaluated. Findings from the National Institutes of Health show increased development of the brain's cortex during adolescence in those who receive musical training compared with youth who do not [22]. This cortical thickness maturation was found in frontoparietal areas, regions implicated in attention control and behavioral inhibition, and was associated with not only the pathophysiology of ADHD but also with subclinical inattention and hyperactivity in healthy youths [22]. Other artistic pursuits, such as writing, painting, and singing, provide training in commitment and practice as well as personal outlets for creativity and confidence building.

Community, Spiritual, and Religious Wellness

Feeling a connection to a community is a core human need. For many, family provides this connection and, for some, religious or spiritual groups provide this community. There is evidence that religion and spirituality buffer some youth against mental health problems, negative and/or risky health behaviors, and delinquency [23]. The relationship between organized religion, spirituality, and youth well-being is a complex topic with inconsistent findings requiring more longitudinal studies [23]. Regardless of youth or family involvement in organized religious or spiritual groups, it is important for providers and caregivers to assess where and with whom youth feel a meaningful sense of belonging. This is to ensure it is a safe, supportive environment that promotes compassion and encourages personal moral development and empathy.

Nutraceutical and Pharmaceutical Considerations in Children and Adolescents

The interventions discussed have been largely preventive or early interventions and entirely non-pharmaceutical options. However, just as we now understand most of psychiatric illnesses along a spectrum, we must also appreciate the spectrum of wellness and when it declines to the point of illness [3]. Once a youth's wellness is compromised to the degree of poor functioning, it is important to consider all interventions available, including nutraceutical and pharmaceutical options.

Nutraceuticals are defined as "foodstuff" (fortified food or dietary supplement) that is thought to provide health or medical benefits in addition to its basic nutritional value. Unlike pharmaceuticals, they are not monitored by the FDA but instead monitored as "dietary supplements" according to the Dietary Supplement, Health and Education Act (DSCHEA) of 1994. Examples of dietary supplements commonly used in children include fish oil and melatonin [6]. Fish oil is one of the most commonly used natural products in children according to the 2012 National Health Interview Survey (NHIS) and has been associated with improvement of some neuropsychiatric disorders, such as ADHD, with minimal adverse effects noted [6]. However, efficacy of pharmaceutical treatment for ADHD remains superior [24]. Melatonin is also widely used in children to decrease sleep latency; however, long-term studies on the safety and efficacy are lacking [6, 15].

When is it appropriate to opt for pharmaceutical options in youth? This is a complex and sensitive question for providers and families. While functional impairment is a good indication that pharmaceuticals may be necessary, a more emergent indication is when the wellness–illness spectrum shifts to safety concerns including risk of self-harm or harm to others. For example, if a child expresses suicidal or homicidal thoughts, referral and evaluation by a child and adolescent psychiatrist is critically recommended. At that time, both pharmaceutical options and therapeutic counseling would likely be considered. The referring provider can assist by offering the family psychoeducation and normalizing the referral by reminding them that as physical health sometimes requires pharmaceuticals, the same is true for mental health.

Summary

Healthcare providers working with youth and seeking to understand the full spectrum of their health from illness to wellness are encouraged to consider all of the areas discussed in order to personalize a family's wellness treatment plan. As the first section on family and caregiver health details, this treatment plan must be thoughtful and targeted to the entire family, not just to the child or adolescent. This is vital because the family health has a significant impact directly on the child's wellness, and the caregiver controls implementation of many of the interventions. Additionally, an important aspect of wellness planning for youth is partnering with schools to support the delivery of these evidence-based approaches. Finally, the future direction of wellness treatment planning is incorporating all of the key components discussed above into daily healthcare practice. One such example is the Vermont Family Based Approach (VFBA) developed by the child psychiatry director

Jim Hudziak [3, 25]. This approach thoroughly assesses the degree to which a family is able to integrate wellness elements into the child's life and thereafter offers monitoring and guidance as treatment continues through the use of Family Wellness Coaches, Focused Family Coaches, Family-Based Psychiatrists, primary care providers, and community partners [3, 25]. It will take time until this is a practical reality for all outpatient youth care centers, but there is recent evidence to support its feasibility [25].

Until this is a reality, finding simple approaches to capture each of the above domains is recommended. For example, providers can utilize pre-visit questionnaires, reminders to address specific aspects at each visit, and/or templated treatment guidance to summarize each session. Devoting time to diligently assess and target disordered *and* well states ensures that youth and families reach their potential of wellness and ultimately thrive.

References

1. DJ Miklowitz. Family-focused therapy for bipolar disorder: reflections on 30 years of research. *Family Process* 2016; **55**: 483–499.

2. ML Gunlicks, MM Weissman. Change in child psychopathology with improvement in parental depression: a systemic review. *J Am Acad Child Adolesc Psychiatry* 2008; **47**: 379–389.

3. DC Rettew. Positive child psychiatry. In: BW Palmer, DV Jeste, eds., *Positive Psychiatry: A Clinical Handbook*. Washington, DC, American Psychiatric Publishing; 2015; 285–304.

4. FN Jacka, E Ystrom, AL Brantsaeter, et al. Maternal and early postnatal nutrition and mental health of offspring by age 5 years: a prospective cohort study. *J Am Acad Child Adolesc Psychiatry* 2013; **52**: 1038–1047.

5. J Saul, RF Rodgers. Wellness, not weight: changing the focus in child and adolescents. *J Am Acad Child Adolesc Psychiatry* 2016; **55**: 7–9.

6. H McClafferty, S Vohra, M Bailey, et al. Pediatric integrative medicine. *Pediatrics* 2017; **140**: e20171961.

7. Centers for Disease Control and Prevention (CDC). Physical activity basics. 2018. www.cdc.gov/physicalactivity/basics/index.htm (accessed February 20, 2019).

8. US Department of Health and Human Services. *Physical Activity Guidelines for Americans* (2nd ed.). Washington, DC, US Department of Health and Human Services; 2018. https://health.gov/paguidelines/second-edition/pdf/Physical_Activity_Guidelines_2nd_edition.pdf (accessed February 16, 2019).

9. RM Eime, JA Young, JT Harvey, et al. A systematic review of the psychological and social benefits of participation in sport for child and adolescents: informing development of a conceptual model of health through sport. *Int J Behav Nutr Phys Act* 2013; **10**: 1–21.

10. C Huppertz, M Bartels, CEM Van Beijsterveldt, et al. The impact of shared environmental factors on exercise behavior from age 7 to 12. *Med Sci Sports Exerc* 2012; **44**: 2025–2032.

11. J Radesky, D Christakis, Council on Communications and Media. Media and young minds. *Pediatrics* 2016; **138**: e2016-e2591.

12. American Academy of Pediatrics. American Academy of Pediatrics announces new recommendations for children's media use. 2016. www.aap.org/en-us/about-the-aap/aap-press-room/Pages/American-Academy-of-Pediatrics-Announces-New-Recommendations-for-Childrens-Media-Use.aspx (accessed January 15, 2019).

13. AG Thomas, KC Monahan, AF Lukowski, et al. Sleep problems across development: a pathway to adolescent risk taking through working memory. *J Youth Adolesc* 2015; **44**: 447–464.

14. KM Keyes, J Maslowsky, A Hamilton, et al. The great sleep recession: changes in sleep duration among US adolescents, 1991–2012. *Pediatrics* 2015; **135**: 460–468.

15. I Donskoy, D Loghmanee. Insomnia in adolescence. *Med Sci* 2018; **6**: E72.

16. F Traub, R Boynton-Jarrett. Modifiable resilience factors to childhood adversity for clinical pediatric practice. *Pediatrics* 2017; **139**: e2016–e2569.

17. DC Rettew, I Satz, SV Joshi. Teaching well-being from kindergarten to child psychiatry fellowship programs. *Child Adolesc Psychiatric Clin N Am* 2019; **28**; 267–280.

18. MEP Seligman, RM Ernst, J Gillham, et al. Positive education: positive psychology and classroom interventions. *Oxford Rev Educ* 2009; **35**: 293–311.

19. SM Suldo. *Promoting Student Happiness. Positive Psychology Interventions in Schools.* New York, The Guilford Press; 2016.

20. S Zoogman, SB Goldberg, WT Hoyt, et al. Mindfulness interventions with youth: a meta-analysis. *Mindfulness* 2015; **6**: 290–302.

21. SG Hofman, A Asnaani, IJJ Vonk, et al. The efficacy of cognitive behavioral therapy: a review of meta-analyses. *Cogn Ther Res* 2012; **36**: 427–440.

22. JJ Hudziak, MD Albaugh, S Ducharme, et al. Cortical thickness maturation and duration of music training: health-promoting activities shape brain development. *J Am Acad Child Adolesc Psychiatry* 2014; **53**: 1153–1161.

23. GW Holden, PA Williamson. Religion and child well-being. In: A Ben-Arieh, F Casas I Frones, JE Korbin, eds., *Handbook of Child Well-Being*. New York, Springer; 2014; 1137–1169.

24. MH Bloch, A Qawasmi. Omega-3 fatty acid supplementation for the treatment of children with attention-deficit/hyperactivity disorder symptomatology: systematic review and meta-analysis. *J Am Acad Child Adolesc Psychiatry* 2011; **50**: 991–1000.

25. MY Ivanova, L Dewey, P Swift, et al. Health promotion in primary care pediatrics: initial results of a randomized clinical trial of the Vermont Family Based Approach. *Child Adolesc Psychiatric Clin N Am* 2019; **28**: 237–246.

Chapter 17

Wellness in Pain Disorders

Charles Louy, Chona Sweet, Gabriel Pollock, Catherine de Zagon, Zara Louy, Jeanne M. Weiss, and Dermot P. Maher

Introduction

Pain is the most common complaint in primary care medicine, with approximately one-third of the world's population currently experiencing some type of chronic pain [1]. It's not always a bad thing; pain serves an evolutionary purpose of warning us of unwellness. But when this signal persists, changes within the peripheral and central nervous systems perpetuate the process, leading to chronic pain (defined as experiencing pain for longer than 3–6 months) [1]. Thus, chronic pain is not merely a symptom of an underlying condition; it is a disease in itself and must be treated as such.

Opioid therapy has been the mainstay treatment for chronic pain. However, effective treatment of chronic pain is rarely achieved with a single modality and, more frequently, requires the use of several different treatment modalities – a "multimodal approach" – including pharmacological and interventional therapies in addition to other evidence-based treatment strategies. These techniques are particularly attractive, given the recent opioid crisis and guidelines from the US Centers for Disease Control and Prevention (CDC) indicating that non-opioid therapy is the preferred method for the treatment of chronic pain [2]. Broadly, when choosing any strategy to manage pain, including pharmacologic agents and interventional procedures, consideration must be given to balancing a given modality's safety profile against efficacy. By the end of this chapter, readers should be convinced that a wellness approach to pain that encapsulates the whole person is essential to treating it effectively, and that the discussed modalities are not only useful adjuncts but also are used as first-line pain management therapies.

Pain Assessment

Focusing on unidimensional pain scores may be an insufficient assessment tool. Because "the chronic pain experience is shaped by a myriad of biomedical, psychosocial, and behavioural factors ... assessing each of these three domains through a comprehensive evaluation of the person with chronic pain is essential for treatment decisions and to facilitate optimal outcomes" [3]. Table 17.1 provides a comprehensive list of related assessment tools for chronic pain patients.

Pharmacologic Management Strategies

Opioids

For chronic pain, there is strong evidence to support short-term analgesic efficacy of opioids, but no convincing evidence of long-term analgesic efficacy, and strong evidence

Table 17.1 Pain assessment tools

Measure	Number of items	Domain assessed
Unidimensional pain measures		
Numerical Rating Scale (NRS)	1	Pain intensity using a numbered scale (e.g., 0–10, 0–100)
Verbal Rating Scale (VRS)	1	Pain intensity using verbal descriptors (e.g., mild, moderate, severe)
Visual Analog Scale (VAS)	1	Pain intensity using 10 or 100 mm line, anchored by no pain and worst possible pain
Facial Pain Scale (FPS)	1	Pain intensity using a range of facial expressions
Pain thermometer	1	Pain intensity using a depicted thermometer to rate pain
Pain quality and location		
McGill Pain Questionnaire (MPQ)	20	Pain quality, location, exacerbating and ameliorating factors
Short-form-McGill Pain Questionnaire-2 (SF-MPQ-2)	22	Pain quality, location, exacerbating and ameliorating factors
Neuropathic Pain Scale (NPS)	10	Neuropathic pain qualities
Regional Pain Scale (RPS)	19 sites	Extent of body pain
Pain interference and function: general		
Pain Disability Index (PDI)	7	Pain disability and interference of pain in functional, family, and social domains
Brief Pain Inventory (BPI)	32	Pain intensity and interference of pain with functional activities
PROMIS pain interference and pain behaviors item banks	Interference bank = 41; Behaviors bank = 39	Pain interference and behaviors related to the impact of pain
Functional Independence Measure	18	Physical and cognitive ability, burden of care
Pain interference and function: disease-specific		
Western Ontario MacMaster Osteoarthritis Index (WOMAC)	24	Pain and function in people with osteoarthritis
Fibromyalgia Impact Questionnaire (FIQ)	20	Health status for people with fibromyalgia
Roland–Morris Disability Questionnaire (RDQ)	24	Pain and disability for people with back pain

Table 17.1 (cont.)

Measure	Number of items	Domain assessed
HRQOL*		
Medical Outcomes Study Short Form Health Survey (SF-36)	36	Mental and physical health
West Haven–Yale Multidimensional Pain Inventory (MPI)	60	Pain severity, interference, mood, activities, sense of control, support, quality of life
EuroQOL (EQ-5D)	5	Health status, pain, and mood
Sickness Impact Profile (SIP)	136	Physical and psychosocial dysfunction
Psychosocial measures		
Beck Depression Inventory (BDI)	21	Depressive mood
Profile of Mood States (POMS)	65	Mood and emotional functioning
Symptom Checklist-90 Revised (SCL-90 R)	90	Multiple domains of psychological functioning
Pain Catastrophizing Scale (PCS)	13	Catastrophic thoughts related to pain
Coping Strategies Questionnaire (CSQ)	10	Coping strategies for chronic pain
Observational pain assessment		
Pain Behavior Checklist (PBC)	16 categories	Observational measure to assess patient's pain behaviors
Real-time assessment of pain behavior	5 categories	Real-time assessment of pain behaviors integrated with a standardized assessment

* HRQOL = health-related quality of life.
From EJ Dansie, DC Turk. Assessment of patients with chronic pain. *Br J Anaesth* 2013; **111**(1): 19–25, with permission

of harm, especially at high doses of >100 mg oral morphine equivalents per day [4]. Additionally, high doses administered on a scheduled basis lead to negative outcomes, both physiologically (respiratory depression, sedation, pruritus, urinary retention, immunosuppression, constipation, androgen suppression) and behaviorally [4]; preliminary evidence supports that intermittent use provides equivalent or better analgesia and is preferred by patients [4]. However, the data indicate that opioids' effectiveness may be lost over time due to several commonly observed phenomena, such as opioid tolerance, wherein a higher dose is required to achieve the same effect, or opioid-induced hyperalgesia, wherein escalating doses can actually increase sensitivity to continued painful stimuli.

The general rule for initiating opioid therapy is to initiate a low dose with titration until the lowest effective dose has been reached. The use of long-acting formulations of opioids, such as methadone, is appropriate for chronic unrelenting pain such as that from cancer. The use of mixed agonist–antagonists, such as buprenorphine, may present a viable alternative for the treatment of pain in high-risk individuals. The co-prescription of stool softeners and home-use naloxone is often recommended in almost all populations.

Non-Steroidal Anti-Inflammatory Drugs

Non-steroidal anti-inflammatory drugs (NSAIDs) are a commonly used class of medications that inhibit the function of cyclooxygenase (COX), an enzyme responsible for the production of prostaglandins (PGs) and other inflammatory mediators. Prostaglandins sensitize peripheral nociceptors to the effect of several neurotransmitters involved in pain modulation and transmission, resulting in a hyperalgesic state often associated with inflammation. As such, NSAIDs are often considered first-line therapy for pain associated with arthritis and many forms of mild pain. NSAIDs have demonstrated efficacy for use in many different types of pain, including low back pain [5]. Several medications have been developed that primarily inhibit an isoform of COX that is usually found in inflamed tissue, COX-2.

The inhibition of PG formation is also responsible for a number of side effects associated with NSAID use. Prostaglandins are responsible for the development and maintenance of the gastric mucosal layer secreted by foveolar cells and for reducing acid secreted by gastric chief cells. The use of NSAIDs has been associated with the development of gastric ulcers, but not the worsening of gastroesophageal reflux disease. Concomitant use of a gastroprotective agent, such as omeprazole, or prescribing a COX-2 inhibitor, has been demonstrated to reduce these risks. There was a previously held belief that non-covalently binding NSAIDs (i.e., all except aspirin) had the potential to cause platelet inhibition and coagulopathy, but this has largely been disproven. Additionally, the risk of a major cardiovascular event was previously thought to be greater with COX-2 medications as a class, but this seems to be more a function of individual agents, such as rofecoxib. All types of NSAIDs can induce renal damage.

Unlike opioids, NSAIDs also have what is known as an analgesic ceiling effect in which escalating doses will produce increased side effects but not increased analgesia. Several NSAIDs are available over the counter. However, stronger NSAIDs with greater COX selectivity, such as the COX-2 selective agent celecoxib or higher ceiling, are available by prescription (Table 17.2).

Neuropathic Pain Medications

Neuropathic pain manifests due to damage to, irritation of, or mediation by the somatosensory nervous system and includes diagnoses such as diabetic neuropathy, radiculopathy, trigeminal neuralgia, and post-herpetic neuralgia (PHN). Many forms of chronic pain stem from non-neuropathic sources of pain such as arthritis, and develop neuropathic features such as allodynia, hyperalgesia, or paroxysmal expression phenotypes. Many of the medications that have been identified to treat this sort of pain were initially used to treat other non-painful conditions but transitioned to have pain-relieving indications at low doses following clinical observation or further understanding of pain pathogenesis (Table 17.3).

Table 17.2 Commonly used NSAIDs

Generic name	Trade names	Dosage range (mg/day)	Half-life (hours)
Aspirin	Many	600–1500 mg QID PO	2–3
Naproxen	Aleve, Naprosyn	250–500 mg BID PO	14
Ibuprofen	Advil, Motrin	200–800 mg QID PO or 400–800 mg IV QID	6 for PO; 2 for IV
Diclofenac	Voltaren, Flector, Pennsaid, Cataflam	50–75 mg BID–QID PO or 2–4 g QID gel or 180 mg patch	1 for PO; 12 for 1 percent gel or 1.3 percent patch
Etodolac	Lodine	200–300 mg BID–QID	7
Indomethacin	Indocin	25–75 mg BID PO	4
Nabumetone	Relafen	500–750 mg BID	20–24
Meloxicam	Mobic	7.5–15 mg daily	15–20
Celecoxib	Celebrex	100–200 mg QD - BID	6–12
Acetaminophen	Tylenol, others	325–1000 mg QID	2–3

Anticonvulsants, such as gabapentin and pregabalin, are approved for the treatment of neuropathic pain and act by decreasing neurotransmitter release from presynaptic neurons. Both have been studied and found to be at least partially effective treatment for myriad pain conditions, including neuropathic pain and fibromyalgia (FM). They are minimally metabolized and are primarily renally excreted. Both may precipitate weight gain, dizziness, somnolence, and nausea, but their side effect and safety profiles are vastly superior to opioids. In general, an initial low dose is followed by a gradual upward titration. Evidence suggests that it may take several weeks at reasonable doses in order to achieve clinically meaningful benefits. A number of anticonvulsant medications are effective for certain forms of pain, such as carbamazepine and oxcarbazepine used for the treatment of trigeminal neuralgia. In general, these medications require close monitoring for side effects and gradual dose escalation and de-escalation.

A number of antidepressants have found new use as treatment for pain. The tricyclic antidepressants (TCAs) are a related group of medications that promiscuously bind to several different receptor families and have an unclear mechanism of action. Tricyclic antidepressants have been found to be effective for the treatment of several pain conditions such as neuropathic pain and a prophylactic measure against certain migraines. While still effective for pain, TCAs have largely been replaced for the treatment of depression by serotonin–norepinephrine reuptake inhibitors (SNRIs) and selective serotonin reuptake inhibitors (SSRIs). Selective serotonin reuptake inhibitors are largely devoid of pain properties, while SNRIs have been found to be effective for the treatment of several forms of pain.

Several newer medications are also emerging or are finding new use for the treatment of pain, such as ketamine [6], which has been shown to be most effective for complex regional pain syndrome (CRPS) [7].

Table 17.4 summarizes the pharmacological interventions by chronic pain disorders [8].

Table 17.3 Commonly used neuropathic pain medications

Generic name	Trade names	Dosage range (mg/day)	Maximum dose (mg/day)	Half-life (hours)
Tricyclic antidepressants				
Amitriptyline	Elavil, Levate	10–150 mg	300 mg	9–27
Doxepin	Sinequan, Deptran	10–150 mg	300 mg	15; N-desmethyldoxepin 31
Desipramine	Norpramin, Pertofrane	10–150 mg	300 mg	10–30
Nortriptyline	Pamelor, Allegron, Sensoval	10–150 mg	200 mg	20–55
Serotonin–norepinephrine reuptake inhibitors				
Venlafaxine	Effexor	150–225 mg/day	225 mg/day	3–7
Duloxetine	Cymbalta	30–60 mg/day	120 mg/day	8–17
Milnacipran	Savella	12.5–50 mg BID	100 mg BiD	8–10
Desvenlafaxine	Pristiq	25–50 mg/day	50 mg/day	11
Anticonvulsants				
Gabapentin	Neurontin, Horizant	600–1200 mg TID	1200 mg TID	5–7 hours
Pregabalin	Lyrica	150–600 mg/day	600 mg/day	5.5–6.7 hours

Table 17.4 Effectiveness of non-opioid medications on various chronic pain disorders

		CLBP	MPS	FM	PHN	PDN	RP	CRPS
NSAIDs	**US trade names**							
Naproxen	Aleve, Naprosyn, Anaprox	+						
Celecoxib	Celebrex	+						
Piroxicam	Feldene	+						
Indomethacin	Indocin	+					+	
Diclofenac	Voltaren	+						
Diclofenac TPI			+					
Tricyclic antidepressants								
Amitryptiline	Elavil			+	+	+	+	
Doxepin	Sinequan	+						
Desipramine	Norpramin	+			+	+		
Nortryptiline	Pamelor	+			+		+	
Imipramine	Tofranil					+		
Tetracyclic antidepressant								
Maprotiline	Ludiomil	+						
SNRIs								
Venlafaxine	Effexor					+		
Duloxetine	Cymbalta	+		+		+	+	
Milnacipran	Savella			+				
SSRIs								
Fluoxetine	Prozac			+	+			
Paroxetine	Paxil					+		
Paroxetine CR	Paxil CR			+				
Anticonvulsants								
Gabapentin (NMDA antagonist)	Neurontin, Horizant			+	+	+		+
Pregabalin (NMDA antagonist)	Lyrica			+	+	+		
Topiramate	Topamax	+				+		
Levetiracetam	Keppra				+			
Lamotrigine	Lamictal					+		
Oxcarbazepine	Trileptal					+		
Zonisamide	Zonegran					+		
Other NMDA antagonists								
Maemantine	Namenda			+				
Dextromethorphan						+		

Table 17.4 (cont.)

		CLBP	MPS	FM	PHN	PDN	RP	CRPS
Opioid antagonists								
Low-dose naltrexone	Revia			+				
Muscle relaxants								
Carisoprodol	Soma	+						
Cyclobenzaprine	Flexeril	+		+				
Diazepam	Valium	+						
Methocarbamol	Robaxin		+					
Mixed SNRI/opioid								
Tramadol	Ultram	+			+	+		
Tramadol/ acetaminophen	Utracet	+		+				
Tapentadol	Nucynta	+						
Tapentadol ER	Nucynta ER					+		
Local anesthetics								
Mexilitene	Mexitil					+		
Cannabinoids								
Inhaled cannabis						+		
Nabilone	Cesamet			+		+		
Bisphosphonates								
Alendronate	Fosamax							+
Pamidronate (IV)	Aredia							+
Neridronate (IV)								+
Clodronate (IV)	Bonefos							+
IV Ketamine								+
IVIG								+
DMSO								+
Calcitonin	Fortical, Miacalcin							?
Topical								
Clonidine (cream, patch)						+		
Capsaicin (cream, patch)		+			+	+		
Diclofenac sodium patch	Flector Patch			+				
Lidocaine patch	Lidoderm			+	+			
BoNT-A	Botox	+	+		+	+		
Tanezumab		+						

Table 17.4 (cont.)

	CLBP	MPS	FM	PHN	PDN	RP	CRPS
TPIs with							
Diclofenac		+					
Bupivacaine		+					

+, positive significant result; ?, unclear result.

CLBP, chronic low back pain; MPS, myofascial pain syndrome; FM, fibromyalgia; PHN, post-herpetic neuralgia; PDN, painful diabetic neuropathy; RP, radicular pain; CRPS, complex regional pain syndrome; TPI, trigger point injection; SNRI, serotonin–norepinephrine reuptake inhibitor; SSRI, selective serotonin reuptake inhibitor; NMDA, N-methyl-D-aspartate; IVIG, intravenous immunoglobulin; DMSO, dimethyl sulfoxide; BoNT-A, botulinum toxin type A.

Abstracted from AL Nicol, RW Hurley, HT Benzon. Alternatives to opioids in the pharmacologic management of chronic pain syndromes: a narrative review of randomized, controlled, and blinded clinical trials. *Anesth Analg* 2017; **125**(5): 1682–1703

Interventional Management Strategies

The efficacy of many interventional procedures for treatment of chronic pain is either firmly established or the subject of ongoing research. In general, chronically inflamed tissue is registered by the nervous system as a recurrent, acutely painful process. It logically follows that administration of a potent anti-inflammatory in a targeted manner to an inflamed region of the body will afford the greatest regional concentration of medication in an area while minimizing systemic side effects, resulting in decreased pain [9]. A major caveat in determining whether interventional therapy will be effective is the proficiency of the physician performing the intervention.

Epidural Blocks

Transforaminal, interlaminar, and caudal epidural steroid injections have been found to provide durable analgesia for the treatment of radicular pain emanating from herniated intervertebral discs [10]. However, there is less encouraging data for their use in other forms of painful pathology, such as nonradicular axial back pain, spinal stenosis, or postsurgical pain. In general, the lowest dose of steroid should be used, such as 40 mg methylprednisolone or 30 mg triamcinolone [10].

Radiofrequency Ablation

For the treatment of axial back pain, radiofrequency ablation (RFA) of the zygapophyseal, or facet, joint is frequently performed [11]. Evidence suggests that ablating the medial branches of the posterior ramus which innervates the painful facet joints, as determined by diagnostic injections, results in long-lasting reduction in pain for an interval between one month and two years. Once again, operating skill and experience are essential to a meaningful outcome [11].

Other Somatic Interventions

A number of other injections have been described and evaluated over the years, with many being deemed as efficacious, including sacroiliac joint blocks, trigger point injections, vertebral augmentation (kyphoplasty and vertebroplasty), intra-articular joint injections, bursa injections, and peripheral nerve blocks.

Sympathetic Blocks

Sympathetic blockade has been used to treat sympathetically mediated pain components of chronic conditions including CRPS, other neuropathic conditions such as post-herpetic neuralgia (PHN), and vascular and visceral pain. In addition to treating painful conditions, sympathetic blockade has been used to improve perfusion, treat angina, and even suppress symptoms of posttraumatic stress disorder (PTSD). Since there are limited randomized controlled trials (RCTs) available regarding its efficacy, the interventional pain management community relies on case series [12]. The most common sympathetic blocks are stellate ganglion blocks for pain and circulatory disorders of the upper extremities and angina pectoris; celiac plexus and splanchnic nerve blocks for chronic upper abdominal pain, including cancer pain; lumbar sympathetic blocks for various sympathetically mediated pain conditions of the lower extremities; superior hypogastric plexus block for pelvic pain; and ganglion impar block for pain originating from the perineum, distal rectum, and the distal thirds of the urethra and vagina [12].

Neuromodulation

Therapeutic neuromodulation refers to a broad range of targeted interventions that alter neuronal activity, often through electrical stimulation [13]. Proposed indications for neuromodulation range from neurologic disorders such as Parkinson's disease to chronic pain from a variety of causes. Likewise, the invasiveness of these therapies varies greatly from noninvasive devices which provide transcutaneous stimulation, to devices which are implanted surgically.

In the field of chronic pain management, one of the most studied neuromodulation therapies is spinal cord stimulation (SCS) through an implanted spinal cord stimulator. These devices are often recommended for chronic pain secondary to neuropathic or ischemic pain such as CRPS, or radicular low back pain that persists after surgical intervention. Since neuromodulation is typically reserved for patients who have failed conservative medical management, few studies have directly compared these two approaches. However, several studies have shown that SCS reduces the opioid requirements in patients with conditions such as CRPS and failed back surgery syndrome (FBSS) [13]. Early prescription and high dosage of opioids used to treat back pain have been associated with increased disability and poor functional outcome. Therefore, neuromodulation should be considered prior to initiating patients on high-dose opioid therapy [13]. This approach can be particularly useful in patients with lumbar radicular pain that is persistent or recurrent following surgical intervention. For this population, SCS has demonstrated improved pain scores, improved patient satisfaction, and lower opioid requirements compared to reoperation on the lumbar spine [13].

Transcranial magnetic stimulation (TMS), another form of neuromodulation, has shown variable results in the treatment of chronic pain, in part due to the lack of standardization of protocols. When studied in the population affected by comorbid pain and depressive symptoms, repetitive TMS (rTMS), a subset of TMS, has demonstrated reduction in pain in patients with FM as an add-on treatment, PHN, trauma-related headache, and neuropathic pain [14].

Another area of emerging research is the use of neuromodulation in the treatment of primary headache disorders by targeting the vagus nerve or the sphenopalatine ganglion. Recent studies have examined the effect of noninvasive transcutaneous vagus nerve stimulation on pain, targeting headaches that may be related to the autonomic nervous system, such as migraine headaches and trigeminal autonomic cephalgias [15]. In these studies, vagus nerve stimulation has been more effective at terminating migraines than at prevention [15]. Similarly, the sphenopalatine ganglion drew interest in the treatment of migraines when the administration of nasal lidocaine was observed to reduce pain during migraine headaches [15]. Since this observation, a neuromodulation device that targets the sphenopalatine ganglion has been developed and found to be useful in the acute treatment of cluster headache attacks, with decreased frequency of recurrence as a secondary long-term benefit [15]. While further research is needed, this may be a useful bedside tool in the treatment of patients with refractory migraines, cluster headaches, and trigeminal neuralgia.

Acupuncture

Acupuncture has been practiced in traditional Chinese medicine for thousands of years. It is safe, effective, and carries low risk of adverse effects. Current literature provides stronger evidence for the benefit of acupuncture compared to other complementary therapies. As a treatment for acute and chronic pain, it has been shown to reduce opioid use and opioid-induced side effects [2, 16]. Strong positive evidence supports acupuncture's role in short- and long-term treatment of knee osteoarthritis (OA), chronic low back pain (CLBP), chronic neck and shoulder pain, and peripheral neuropathies related to diabetes mellitus, Bell's palsy, carpal tunnel syndrome, and HIV [2, 16]. Acupuncture plus physical therapy was found to be superior to either modality separately for chronic upper body pain. Hip OA, tension headache, cancer-related pain such as side effects of radiation therapy or chemotherapy-induced neuropathy, and myofascial pain – but not FM – all are known to benefit from acupuncture [17]. Symptoms and signs of rheumatoid arthritis (RA) are improved with acupuncture; however, its role in treating RA needs further study in large RCTs [18]. Finally, acupuncture is recommended for functional dyspepsia when prokinetic agents are contraindicated, and for dysmenorrhea when NSAIDs are contraindicated [2].

Physical Therapy and Exercise

Physical therapy and exercise have shown benefit in chronic pain, and are recommended in most guidelines. They are the common modalities for many conditions against which other modalities are compared [2, 16–18].

Manual Therapy

Manual therapy has been found effective for a range of conditions, especially when combined with exercise and/or multimodal therapy [2].

Massage therapy techniques have largely been studied in chronic pain syndromes of the musculoskeletal system, such as neck pain, non-radicular low back pain, and OA. Both the American College of Physicians (ACP) Clinical Practice Guidelines and the Agency for Healthcare Research and Quality (AHRQ) find massage therapy to be a beneficial intervention for CLBP [2]. While these techniques have demonstrated moderate improvement in pain control and mobility, the benefits are largely short in duration. Massage therapy is a low-risk intervention when provided by a trained practitioner [2]; it has demonstrated preliminary positive evidence for its use in chronic pain [16].

Osteopathic manipulation, including spinal manipulation therapy (SMT), has primarily focused on the treatment of CLBP [16]. It is endorsed by the ACP Clinical Practice Guidelines for CLBP and was shown to be an effective intervention by AHRQ for the same condition [2, 16]. While complementary medicine techniques are typically known to have few adverse effects, cervical spinal manipulation can be associated with rare vertebral artery dissection even in controlled clinical settings [16]. Overall, spinal manipulation has demonstrated preliminary positive evidence for its use in chronic back pain [16], with benefits maintained for up to six weeks [16].

Psychological Interventions

Rather than focusing on pain itself, psychotherapy offers an opportunity to address the cognitive, emotional, social, and behavioral factors that both contribute to and result from pain-related distress and dysfunction [19]. Operant-behavioral therapy, cognitive-behavioral therapy (CBT), mindfulness-based stress reduction, and acceptance and commitment therapy (ACT), the main psychological interventions that play important roles in augmenting self-efficacy in chronic pain patients [19], are listed in Table 17.5, along with corresponding pain disorders known to benefit from each.

Mind–Body and Relaxation Therapies

Relaxation therapies target the regulation of sympathetic–parasympathetic balance to mitigate the sympathetic arousal seen in chronic pain patients [2], providing a variety of benefits such as increased pain relief through the enhancement of endogenous opioids, less

Table 17.5 Psychological interventions in pain disorders

Therapeutic modality	Pain disorders
Operant-behavioral therapy	Complex regional pain syndromes, lower back pain, mixed chronic pain, whiplash-associated disorders
Cognitive-behavioral therapy	Cancer, chronic lower back pain, chronic headaches, chronic migraines, chronic orofacial pain, complex regional pain syndromes, fibromyalgia, HIV/AIDS, irritable bowel syndrome, mixed chronic pain, nonspecific heart pain, multiple sclerosis, nonspecific musculoskeletal pain, osteoarthritis, rheumatoid arthritis, spinal cord injury, systemic lupus erythematosus, whiplash-associated disorders
Mindfulness-based stress reduction	Arthritis, cancer, chronic lower back pain, chronic headache, chronic migraine, complex regional pain syndromes, fibromyalgia, irritable bowel syndrome, rheumatoid arthritis, chronic neck pain
Acceptance and commitment therapy	Musculoskeletal pain (full-body, lower back, lower limb, neck, upper limb), whiplash-associated disorders

JA Sturgeon. Psychological therapies for the management of chronic pain. *Psychol Res Behav Manag* 2014; **7**: 115–124.

muscle tension, and modulated pain awareness. Neuroimaging studies have confirmed these techniques are relevant for chronic pain patients [18]. The most studied relaxation intervention which incorporates daily meditation and mindfulness practice is mindfulness-based stress reduction (see Table 17.5 for additional information on specific pain populations). Other meditation techniques that have been investigated for the treatment of chronic pain include transcendental, Zen, and Jyoti [18]. Research has illustrated that meditation "modulated the contextual evaluation of pain and lowers pain sensitivity" dynamically with time and experience [18]. As such, meditation may affect how pain is perceived by the individual rather than the cause of the pain [18]. Additional non-movement oriented relaxation therapies include guided imagery (specific positive evidence for FM), hypnosis, and biofeedback (specific positive evidence for CLBP, tension headache, and FM) [2]. Research shows that these relaxation interventions are safe and well-tolerated across pain populations [2].

Movement-based relaxation therapies may lead to similar positive effects as they utilize similar pathways to the relaxation response [18]. The practice of yoga has been suggested, based on weak positive evidence, for the treatment of many chronic pain conditions including low back pain, OA, headaches, FM, endometriosis-related pelvic pain [16], RA, and chronic neck pain [18]. It was found to have positive effects for pain and associated disability, even as a short-term intervention, across a variety of populations, according to a systematic review of the literature [2]. The potential benefit may be related to physical exercise or to increased GABA levels that have been demonstrated in experienced practitioners [16]. There was no advantage found in practicing a particular type of yoga; it is recommended that patients choose a style based on personal preference and availability [2]. Tai chi has also been found to have preliminary positive evidence for pain reduction for neck pain, RA, OA, CLBP, and FM [16, 18]. While both yoga and tai chi have demonstrated benefits in chronic pain management, it is difficult to differentiate their effects from the effects of physical exercise in general. Both were found to be as safe as usual care and exercise [2]. While there are fewer studies on these specific therapies, Alexander Technique, Pilates, and Feldenkrais Method have shown preliminary positive evidence for mitigating chronic pain with low risk of related adverse events [2].

Virtual Reality

Virtual reality (VR) therapy has been commonly found to be beneficial in the reduction of burn-induced pain and burn wound care, as well as potentially beneficial in inpatient cancer-related procedure pain [2]. While the main analgesic mechanism of VR has been attributed to distraction, preliminary studies are uncovering other mechanisms that explain beneficial long-term effects of VR in chronic pain disorders such as fibromyalgia [20].

Nutrition and Supplementation

Literature review of nutrition interventions has found a positive effect on the pain experience, but studies are of limited quality [21]. As chronic inflammation is associated with a variety of disorders, both mental and psychiatric, that can exacerbate pain, following an anti-inflammatory diet (e.g., the Mediterranean diet) may prove beneficial for chronic pain patients. It is thought that this kind of dietary regimen optimizes mitochondrial enzyme functioning through balancing tissue pH [2]. There is preliminary positive evidence for pain reduction in RA patients following the Mediterranean diet. Other nutritional interventions that have been studied in the management of chronic pain disorders include low-FODMAP, gluten-free [21], and plant-based diets, and fasting therapy [18]. There is little evidence to support particular dietary interventions in mitigating chronic back and neck pain and disability independently of weight reduction [18].

The microbiome has been deemed a major determinant of overall health; poor nutrition, as well as certain drugs (including NSAIDs), can adversely affect the gut [2, 22]. Thus, it is recommended that any digestive comorbidities, and the prioritization of gut health, be addressed in chronic pain patients.

Turmeric or its derivative curcumin is used for opioid- and NSAID-sparing effects in perioperative pain, a wide variety of inflammatory conditions, joint and musculoskeletal pain, and inflammatory bowel disease [2]. Ginger has also been studied for its effect on pain, including joint pain, as well as nausea. Neither ginger nor turmeric, as foods or supplements, shares the significant morbidity and mortality side-effect profile that NSAIDs carry [2]. Moreover, curcuminoids have been found to have moderate to high non-inferiority to NSAIDs in musculoskeletal pain and were equal to NSAIDs in terms of pain improvement [2]. Overall, the literature shows that curcuminoids should be considered as a viable oral medication option for chronic pain.

Supplementation of deficient nutrients is a topic of research for chronic pain as well as for overall health. Vitamin D deficiency is among the most studied of micronutrient deficiencies in chronic pain patients. It is correlated with delayed healing, muscle fatigue risk factors, and pain [2].

Another common micronutrient deficiency is magnesium deficiency, which has been associated with muscle spasm, neuropathic pain, and systemic inflammation [2]. Magnesium infusions are deployed for migraine, and this intervention is utilized in many emergency rooms [2]. Magnesium also shows promise for the treatment of neuropathic pain as it has been studied as an NMDA (N-methyl-D-aspartate) receptor blocker [2]. Moreover, based on animal studies, magnesium improves neuropathic pain by potentiating opioid analgesia as well as mitigating the development of hyperalgesia [2].

Omega-3 fatty acids found in some fish oils have been shown to reduce proinflammatory prostaglandins and reduce NSAID consumption in RA patients [2]. Given that the current standard American diet is high in the proinflammatory omega-6 fatty acids, nutrition counseling is key in maintaining wellness for chronic pain patients [2].

Vitamin B12 deficiency is widely recognized as an underlying cause of chronic neurological disorders, including neuropathic pain, though more research is needed in the context of chronic pain as researchers are only able to measure serum B12 levels, which may not accurately reflect the active B12 levels in tissues [2].

Amino acids in the form of collagen, carnitine, and theramine as studied in knee OA, joint pain, and back pain were found to have the most statistically significant positive results [21]. Specific supplements for the treatment of knee OA pain, such as glucosamine chondroitin, methylsulfonylmethane, and S-adenosylmethionine (SAMe) have been studied but show conflicting evidence for pain reduction; more research is needed in this realm [16, 17].

Botanicals

A variety of botanicals has been explored in the management of chronic pain conditions, including borage seed oil, blackcurrant seed oil, evening primrose oil, thunder god vine, curcumin (derived from turmeric), willow bark, rose hip, and boswellia; however, there is limited data from Western complementary medicine for their clinical efficacy [18]. Borage seed oil and curcumin/turmeric do have more evidence than other herbal interventions for RA specifically, and may be tried in treatment-resistant cases [18]. Moreover, some herbal interventions from traditional Chinese and Ayurvedic practices might be helpful in RA, but more information is needed in terms of safety [18]. For chronic back and neck pain, evidence for herbs is weak. Although herbal medications are generally well tolerated, with only minimal adverse effects when adequately dosed, some herbs do have profound pharmacologic effects and may interact with standard drugs, producing an increased risk of serious adverse effects [18].

Music Therapy

In a large meta-analysis, music therapy resulted in a reduction not only of acute and chronic pain, including cancer pain, but also of emotional distress due to pain, and in a small but significant decrease in analgesic use, both opioid and non-opioid. The Consortium Pain Task Force recommends music therapy as one of the non-pharmacologic therapies for acute and chronic pain [2].

Pet Therapy

There are many benefits of pet therapy, such as an increase in quality of life and well-being for older patients, addressing the emotional needs of patients receiving chemotherapy, and the reduction of cardiovascular risk [23]. An RCT study concluded that the use of therapy dogs has a positive effect on patients' pain level and satisfaction after total joint replacement [24]. However, no controlled study seems to have addressed the benefits of pet therapy specifically for chronic pain. Of note, two longitudinal studies with thousands of patients have not shown a zoonotic infection or adverse event from pet therapy [24].

Conclusion

Government leaders, the US Office of the Army Surgeon General Pain Management Task Force (PMTF) Report, the US Institute of Medicine (IOM) (now the National Academy of Medicine, NAM), the Interagency Pain Research Coordinating Committee's National Pain Strategy, and others have declared the opioid crisis a national emergency [2]. Their recommendations consistently promote a shift toward a more comprehensive, patient-centered, and health-focused approach to pain. In this model, collaborative care is team-based, interdisciplinary, and involves both pharmacologic and non-pharmacologic approaches. Individually tailored interdisciplinary pain clinics can significantly reduce costs by more than the cost of the intervention itself [2].

References

1. Institute of Medicine (US) Committee on Advancing Pain Research, Care, and Education. *Relieving Pain in America: A Blueprint for Transforming Prevention, Care, Education, and Research*. Washington, DC, National Academies Press (US); 2011.

2. H Tick, A Nielsen, KR Pelletier, et al. Evidence-based nonpharmacologic strategies for comprehensive pain care: the Consortium Pain Task Force white paper. *Explore (NY)* 2018; **14**(3): 177–211.

3. EJ Dansie, DC Turk. Assessment of patients with chronic pain. *Br J Anaesth* 2013; **111**(1): 19–25.

4. JC Ballantyne. Opioids for the treatment of chronic pain: mistakes made, lessons learned, and future directions. *Anesth Analg* 2017; **125**(5): 1769–1778.

5. WTM Enthoven, PDDM Roelofs, RA Deyo, MW van Tulder, BW Koes. Non-steroidal anti-inflammatory drugs for chronic low back pain. *Cochrane Database Syst Rev* 2016; **2**: CD012087.

6. WW IsHak, RY Wen, L Naghdechi, et al. Pain and depression: a systematic review. *Harv Rev Psychiatry* 2018; **26**(6): 352–363.

7. DP Maher, L Chen, J Mao. Intravenous ketamine infusions for neuropathic pain management: a promising therapy in need of optimization. *Anesth Analg* 2017; **124**(2): 661–674.

8. AL Nicol, RW Hurley, HT Benzon. Alternatives to opioids in the pharmacologic management of chronic pain syndromes: a narrative review of randomized, controlled, and blinded clinical trials. *Anesth Analg* 2017; **125**(5): 1682–1703.

9. DP Maher, SP Cohen. Opioid reduction following interventional procedures for chronic pain: a synthesis of the evidence. *Anesth Analg* 2017; **125**(5): 1658–1666.

10. SP Cohen, MC Bicket, D Jamison, I Wilkinson, JP Rathmell. Epidural steroids: a comprehensive, evidence-based review. *Reg Anesth Pain Med* 2013; **38**(3): 175–200.

11. SP Cohen, JHY Huang, C Brummett. Facet joint pain: advances in patient selection and treatment. *Nat Rev Rheumatol* 2013; **9**(2): 101–116.

12. S Baig, JY Moon, H Shankar. Review of sympathetic blocks: anatomy, sonoanatomy, evidence, and techniques. *Reg Anesth Pain Med* 2017; **42**(3): 377–391.

13. TR Deer, N Mekhail, D Provenzano, et al. The appropriate use of neurostimulation of the spinal cord and peripheral nervous system for the treatment of chronic pain and ischemic diseases: the Neuromodulation Appropriateness Consensus Committee. *Neuromodulation* 2014; **17**(6): 515–550; discussion 550.

14. JH Hsu, ZJ Daskalakis, DM Blumberger. An update on repetitive transcranial magnetic stimulation for the treatment of co-morbid pain and depressive symptoms. *Curr Pain Headache Rep* 2018; **22**(7): 51.

15. DY Wei, RH Jensen. Therapeutic approaches for the management of trigeminal autonomic cephalalgias. *Neurotherapeutics* 2018; **15**(2): 346–360.

16. Y-C Lin, L Wan, RN Jamison. Using integrative medicine in pain management: an evaluation of current evidence. *Anesth Analg* 2017; **125**(6): 2081–2093.

17. RL Nahin, R Boineau, PS Khalsa, BJ Stussman, WJ Weber. Evidence-based evaluation of complementary health approaches for pain management in the United States. *Mayo Clin Proc* 2016; **91**(9): 1292–1306.

18. L Chen, A Michalsen. Management of chronic pain using complementary and integrative medicine. *BMJ* 2017; **357**: j1284.

19. JA Sturgeon. Psychological therapies for the management of chronic pain. *Psychol Res Behav Manag* 2014; **7**: 115–124.

20. A Gupta, K Scott, M Dukewich. Innovative technology using virtual reality in the treatment of pain: does it reduce pain via distraction, or is there more to it? *Pain Med* 2018; **19**(1): 151–159.

21. K Brain, TL Burrows, ME Rollo, et al. A systematic review and meta-analysis of nutrition interventions for chronic noncancer pain. *J Hum Nutr Diet* 2019; **32**(2): 198–225.

22. H Tick. Nutrition and pain. *Phys Med Rehabil Clin N Am* 2015; **26**(2): 309–320.

23. ET Creagan, BA Bauer, BS Thomley, JM Borg. Animal-assisted therapy at Mayo Clinic: the time is now. *Complement Ther Clin Pract* 2015; **21**(2): 101–104.

24. CM Harper, Y Dong, TS Thornhill, et al. Can therapy dogs improve pain and satisfaction after total joint arthroplasty? A randomized controlled trial. *Clin Orthop Relat Res* 2015; **473**(1): 372–379.

18 Wellness in Cancer and Neoplastic Diseases

Luma Bashmi and Waguih William IsHak

Introduction

Cancer is the first or second leading cause of death before age 70 years in 91 of 172 countries, ranking third or fourth in an additional 22 countries [1]. It accounts for 1 in every 6 deaths worldwide – more than HIV/AIDS, tuberculosis, and malaria combined [1–3]. GLOBOCAN reported that an estimated 18.1 million cases of cancer were diagnosed around the world, with 9.6 million cancer deaths, in 2018. Approximately 70 percent of cancer deaths occur in low- and middle-income countries, where a majority of these countries lack the medical resources and health systems to support the disease burden. The current risk of developing the disease in a lifetime is 1 in 8 for men and 1 in 10 for women [1]. Additionally, the economic impact of cancer is significant and continues to increase; in 2010, the total annual cost was estimated at approximately $1.16 trillion [3].

The American Cancer Society (ACS) estimates that the global burden of the disease is expected to reach 27.5 million new cancer cases and 16.3 million cancer deaths by 2040, solely due to aging and growth of the world population. Lung cancer is the most commonly diagnosed cancer (11.6 percent of the total cases) and leading cause of cancer death (18.4 percent of the total cancer deaths) worldwide, closely followed by female breast cancer (11.6 percent), prostate cancer (7.1 percent), colorectal cancer (6.1 percent) for incidence, and colorectal cancer (9.2 percent), stomach cancer (8.2 percent), and liver cancer (8.2 percent) for mortality [1–3].

Defining Cancer and Neoplastic Diseases

The World Health Organization (WHO) defines cancer as a generic term used to refer to a group of related diseases in which abnormal body cells begin to divide without stopping and spread into surrounding tissues [3]. Cancer can occur almost anywhere in the human body and negatively impacts the orderly process of cell growth and death [4].

Like cancer, neoplastic diseases are diseases that involve the abnormal growth and proliferation of abnormal cells or an abnormal number of cells. They include various types of growths, including benign (non-cancerous) tumors, precancerous growths, carcinoma *in situ*, and malignant (cancerous) tumors. Unlike cancer, neoplastic growths do not metastasize or spread to other parts of the body. However, in some cases benign tumors still need to be monitored as they can cause symptoms or become malignant after a certain amount of time [5].

Cancer Risk Factors

Some of the major cancer risk factors include unhealthy behaviors and lifestyles associated with emerging economies or a *Western lifestyle*, such as tobacco and alcohol use, an unhealthy diet, and physical inactivity, as well as changes in reproductive patterns, like having fewer children or giving birth to the first child at a later age [1–3, 6]. Chronic carcinogenic infections such as *Helicobacter pylori*, human papillomavirus (HPV), hepatitis B virus, hepatitis C virus, and Epstein–Barr virus have also been associated with up to 15 percent of diagnosed cancers in 2012 [3].

Cancer and Wellness

Wellness among cancer patients is a crucial factor in successful treatment and long-term health. Wellness is a term that has been defined in various ways; however, there is a general consensus among health and wellness practitioners that health is the state of optimal *being* and not just the absence of disease, whereas wellness is a state of actively pursuing healthy *living*. The National Wellness Institute further defines wellness as comprising three tenets [7]:

1. "Wellness is a conscious, self-directed and evolving process of achieving full potential.
2. Wellness is multidimensional and holistic, encompassing lifestyle, mental and spiritual well-being, and the environment.
3. Wellness is positive and affirming."

As survival trends are generally increasing globally, even for typically lethal cancers, and the primary goal is to cure cancer and prolong life, wellness becomes essential in achieving this.

Cancer Survivorship

In 2008, the CONCORD program was established to provide global surveillance of cancer survival to measure the effectiveness of health systems, monitor trends in cancer survival, and inform global policy [8]. The CONCORD-3 is the third edition and largest, most up-to-date report globally covering two-thirds of the world population – 71 countries – and 37.5 million patients diagnosed with cancer in a 15-year period from 2000 to 2014. Findings demonstrated that survival trends are generally increasing, even for typically lethal cancers of the liver, pancreas, and lung. Countries with the highest five-year net survival include the USA, Canada, Australia, New Zealand, Finland, Iceland, Norway, and Sweden [8].

As of January 2019, the National Cancer Institute (NCI) estimates that there are 16.9 million cancer survivors (5 percent of the population) in the USA. The number of survivors in the USA is projected to increase to 26.1 million in 2040 [9]. The most commonly represented survivors are female breast (23 percent, 3.6 million), prostate (21 percent, 3.3 million), colorectal (9 percent, 1.5 million), gynecologic (8 percent, 1.3 million), and melanoma (8 percent, 1.2 million). With increased survivorship, the devastating impact of cancer diagnosis and its subsequent overwhelming treatment on a person's life and wellness is more evident, contributing to worse quality of life (QOL), morbidity, and mortality [10–12]. Despite this, significantly less effort has been made toward studies that identify and examine how cancer treatments affect health in the long term [13].

Posttreatment Symptoms and Long-Term Effects

Of the studies that exist, results have demonstrated that adjuvant cancer treatment is often associated with several long-term and latent effects, such as cancer-related fatigue, lymphedema, cardiotoxicity, neuropathy, cognitive dysfunction, bone health and musculoskeletal issues, premature menopause and infertility, sexual dysfunction, body image concerns, mental health issues, bowel dysfunction, bladder dysfunction, ostomy/stoma-related complications, neuromuscular dysfunction, sleep apnea, and others [10]. Psychosocial effects of survivorship can include anxiety, depression, and posttraumatic stress disorder (PTSD) [14].

Demographic and Clinical Variables Affecting Wellness in Cancer

Demographic and disease-related variables including age, race, employment, education, income, type and stage of cancer, duration of illness, duration of treatment, and potential progression of the disease can also have a significant impact on QOL and wellness [15, 16]. Furthermore, patients are often faced with both surgery and additional cancer treatment, such as adjuvant chemo- or chemoradiotherapy. This leads to a decrease in physical fitness, which has also been related to mortality and morbidity, respectively [17].

WHO estimates that 30–50 percent of cancers can be prevented, and survival rates can be increased with early detection, better diagnosis, avoiding or modifying risk factors, and engaging in interventions to address psychological distress and unhealthy lifestyle behaviors (e.g., healthier diet, more physical exercise, quitting tobacco use) associated with cancer, especially after completion of active treatment [3, 6, 11, 14, 17–25].

Assessment Methods to Enhance Wellness in Cancer Patients

Early Detection, Screening, and Risk Factor Modification

Screening through the use of simple tests is an important step for early detection and reducing mortality for cancers of the breast, colon, rectum, cervix, prostate, and lung (among current and heavy smokers). Global screening guidelines and best practices for regular testing and procedures at certain ages in certain populations (e.g., screening women yearly for breast cancer through mammograms starting from the age of 35) have been shown to significantly increase early detection and chances for successful treatment, reduce the need for advanced multiple adjuvant treatment, and increase survival rates. Further studies are being conducted to assess low-cost screening approaches for use in low-resource settings [1–3].

The ACS estimates that at least 42 percent of newly diagnosed cancers in the USA can be potentially avoided through education (e.g., increased awareness of risk factors and early signs of cancer), access to care, and modifying unhealthy behaviors. These include cancers that are caused by smoking (19 percent) and unhealthy lifestyle behaviors such as a combination of smoking, physical inactivity, excess alcohol consumption, poor nutrition, and excess body weight (18 percent of cancers) [2]. Cancers that are caused by infectious diseases can be avoided through vaccines or treatment of the infection. Melanoma can also be prevented through extra skin protection and less exposure of the skin to the sun and indoor tanning devices [2, 3].

Wellness Outcome Measures

The most frequently used and validated wellness measures in cancer research and their characteristics are included in Table 18.1. The measures included in this chapter cover the

Table 18.1 Characteristics of wellness measures validated in cancer populations measuring QOL, fatigue, pain, physical functioning, anxiety, depression, and sleep.

Measure(s)	Overview	Reliability	Populations / validity
QoL			
Functional Assessment of Chronic Illness Therapy (FACIT) Measurement System/Functional Assessment Cancer Therapy-General (FACT-G)	27-item measure divided into four primary QOL domains: physical, social/family, emotional, and functional well-being Administration: 5–10 minutes; self-report or via interview	Cronbach's alpha coefficients range from 0.61 to 0.90	FACT-G has been validated in diverse cancer populations and translated into over 45 languages FACIT has scales for different cancer types: breast (FACT-B), colorectal, head and neck, bladder, brain, and lung
EORTC Quality of Life Questionnaire Core 30 (EORTC QLQ-C30)	30-item core cancer questionnaire measuring HRQOL in cancer patients with five subscales relating to functioning: physical, role, emotional, cognitive, social; nine symptom subscales (fatigue, pain + nausea + vomiting, dyspnea, insomnia, appetite loss, constipation, diarrhea, financial impact), global health status, and one isolated item	Cronbach's alpha coefficients range from 0.69 to 0.87	Translated into more than 35 languages and used in over 1500 studies worldwide
Rotterdam Symptom Checklist (RSCL)	39-item self-report scale used to measure psychological distress, physical distress, activity level, and overall valuation of life based on symptoms Via self-report or interview	Cronbach's alpha coefficients range from 0.63 to 0.88	Validated in European populations and used in cancer patients undergoing treatment by different modalities (undergoing surgery, chemotherapy and radiotherapy): breast, prostate, ovarian, lung, colorectal, gastric, bladder, renal, head and neck, testicular cancer; early and advanced stages

Measure	Description	Reliability	Validation
Symptom Distress Scale (SDS)	13-item self-report scale assessing distress for 11 symptoms: nausea, appetite, insomnia, pain, fatigue, bowel pattern, concentration, appearance, outlook, breathing, and cough	Cronbach's alpha coefficients range from 0.67 to 0.88	Validated in various settings, countries, and cancer sites
The Quality of Life Index (QL-I)	33-item self-report questionnaire covering four domains: health + functioning, social + economic, psychological/spiritual, family	Cronbach's alpha coefficients range from 0.73 to 0.96	Validated in different cancer sites, settings, and general populations
Fatigue			
Brief Fatigue Inventory	Nine-item self-report measure of general, mental, and physical dimensions of fatigue, levels of motivation, and activity	Cronbach's alpha coefficient of >0.95	Validated in multiple languages, illnesses, and adults > 65 years
Brief FACT-Fatigue (FACT-F)	13-item scale that measures severity and presence of CRF and anemia-related concerns in cancer patients.	Cronbach's alpha coefficients range from 0.93 to 0.95	Validated in patients with a variety of diagnoses receiving various treatments, 45 languages
Pain			
Brief Pain Inventory-Short Form	11-item self-report scale measuring sensory and reactive pain with two subscales: (1) severity of pain and (2) extent to which pain interferes with life activities	Cronbach's alpha coefficients range from 0.77 to 0.95	Validated in different cancer sites, metastatic cancer, and multiple languages
Physical functioning			
Medical Outcomes Study Short-Form 36 (SF-36)	36-item self-report scale with eight sections: vitality, physical functioning, bodily pain, general health perceptions, physical role functioning, emotional role functioning, social role functioning, mental health	Cronbach's alpha coefficients range from 0.78 to 093	Validated in various illnesses, cancer sites, and sociodemographic backgrounds. The SF-36 does not measure sleep as a variable and is not widely validated in 65+ populations

Table 18.1 (cont.)

Measure(s)	Overview	Reliability	Populations / validity
Anxiety and depression			
Hospital Anxiety & Depression Scale (HADS)	14-item measure with two subscales: anxiety and depression	Cronbach's alpha coefficients range from 0.67 to 0.93	Validated in different cancer sites, patient care settings, multiple languages, and countries
The State-Trait Anxiety Scale (STAI)	20-item measure of anxiety with two subscales assessing frequency and intensity	Cronbach's alpha coefficient of 0.93	Validated in different cancer sites, patient care settings, multiple languages, and countries
Center for Epidemiologic Studies Depression Scale (CES-D)	20-item measure of depressive symptomatology with four subscales: depressive affect, somatic symptoms, well-being, and interpersonal relations	Cronbach's alpha coefficients range from 0.84 to 0.90	Validated in diverse populations but variations in the four-factor model have been demonstrated in different ethnic and socioeconomic groups
Profile of Mood States, Short Form (POMS-SF)	37-item scale measuring total mood disturbance and subscale scores for: fatigue-inertia, vigor-activity, tension-anxiety, depression-dejection, anger-hostility, and confusion-bewilderment.	Cronbach's alpha coefficients range from 0.80 to 0.91	Validated in different cancer sites, settings, languages, and diseases
Patient Health Questionnaire (PHQ-9)	Nine-item scale measuring depression in clinical settings	Cronbach's alpha coefficient of 0.84	Validated in patients with comorbid depression and cancer, multiple settings, languages, and diseases
Sleep			
Pittsburgh Sleep Quality Index	19-item self-report measure assessing sleep quality over one month: subjective sleep quality, sleep latency, sleep duration, habitual sleep efficiency, sleep disturbances, use of sleep medication, and daytime dysfunction	Cronbach's alpha coefficient of 0.70	Validated in different cancer sites, settings, languages, and diseases

following variables: QOL, fatigue, pain, physical functioning, anxiety, depression, and sleep. These variables were selected as appropriate wellness outcome measures for cancer patients due to their high correlation with wellness and related variables, frequency of use in cross-sectional and longitudinal studies of cancer, and high reliability and validity in diverse populations by cancer type, settings, ethnicity, and socioeconomic background worldwide [16, 26–31].

It is important to note that the list is limited to wellness measures applicable to cancer in general and does not necessarily cover measures specific to: one cancer site only, such as the supplementary Functional Assessment of Chronic Illness Therapy (FACIT) measures (e.g., FACT-B for breast cancer) other than the FACT-G; or a group within the larger cancer population such as the Long-Term Quality of Life (LTQL) instrument for long-term *female* cancer survivors.

Quality of Life and Health-Related QOL

Quality of life has become increasingly significant in determining wellness in cancer patients as it: (1) indicates groups of patients at risk for developing high levels of distress, and (2) allows for a comparison of the effectiveness of different treatments or care programs, supporting decision-making in clinical oncology [26]. Quality of life is a broad multidimensional concept defined as "an individual's or group's perceived physical and mental health over time" [27]. Its domains encompass physical, social/family, emotional, and functional well-being. Though used interchangeably, health-related QOL (HRQOL) more specifically looks at the impact of treatment on QOL [15, 16, 26, 29, 32, 33].

Cancer-Related Fatigue (CRF), Pain, and Reduced Physical Functioning

Cancer-related fatigue (CRF) is the most commonly reported symptom by cancer patients, especially after chemotherapy [22]. Defined as "a subjective feeling of the energy lack to commence or sustain any activity, a feeling that is not related to depression or decreased muscle power," high CRF levels have been associated with low QOL levels [12]. Cancer-related fatigue has been measured as a single item within several QOL and other measures listed in Table 18.1, including the EORTC QLQ-C30, RSCL, SDS, and SF-36. However, these scales treat CRF as unidimensional, measuring its presence or absence only, but rarely severity or related effects. Further investigation shows that CRF is multidimensional, affecting behavioral, cognitive, somatic, and affective domains of patient functioning. Additionally, CRF has demonstrated a positive correlation with both pain and reduced physical functioning, common cancer symptoms that also have a significant impact on patient wellness [12, 31].

Anxiety and Depression

Up to 50 percent of cancer patients report having a psychiatric disorder after diagnosis. Anxiety and depression are the most common; after cancer treatment, one in four cancer patients meet the criteria for depression, whereas anxiety in the cancer population ranges between 15 and 28 percent [22].

Sleep and Other Health-Related Behaviors

Between one-third and one-half of cancer patients experience sleep disorders, especially insomnia, poor sleep quality, and short sleep duration. Sleep difficulties in cancer patients are positively correlated with the illness itself and other wellness variables like pain, CRF, hospitalization, and specific medical treatments [12, 16, 21, 34].

Other health-related behaviors such as dietary intake, alcohol and tobacco use, and anthropometric measures including height, weight, and waist-to-hip ratio should be ideally measured via validated and reliable measures in cancer settings [34].

Methodological Issues in Measuring Wellness in Cancer

Wellness measures commonly used to identify levels of wellness in cancer patients tend to be self-report, leading to several weaknesses. For example, many researchers identify that certain wellness facets, such as anxiety and depression, cannot be determined through self-report only, and would need to be accompanied by individual clinical interviews, considered as the gold standard for diagnosing mental illnesses. However, both methods can lead to cognitive biases like confirmation or experimenter bias. Furthermore, mood-related states like fatigue, anxiety, and depression tend to overlap in symptoms, making it difficult to find validated measures with strong construct and discriminant validity [34, 32].

With QOL and HRQOL, using generic (measuring broader terms like physical, mental, and social health) versus specific (related to diseases) measures can cause difficulty in comparing results across studies. Unidimensional versus multidimensional measures of HRQOL are also problematic. For example, the EORTC QLQ-C30 and the FACT-G use only one item to measure HRQOL, which does not provide an accurate assessment of the variable [32].

RAND released a study suggesting that while the impact of treatment and care decisions are significant for a cancer patient's QOL and may improve patient–physician communication, QOL measures are only used in clinical trials and not widely used in cancer care, especially for brain cancer [33]. This suggests that emphasis needs to be placed on utilizing multidimensional, consistent QOL measures in clinical practice to improve health outcomes.

Interventions to Improve Wellness in Cancer

The US Institute of Medicine (IOM) published a report in 2005 on cancer survivorship. The report acknowledged that "after the completion of active treatment, cancer patients have important unmet needs; often, they feel lost as they transition back to the care of their primary care provider (PCP), lacking clear guidelines for ongoing care" [35]. In the following years, a series of publications focused on survivors, noting the gap in the literature and lack of organized and consistent survivorship care plans from clinicians [14].

The IOM, NCI, WHO, and ACS are now in consensus that cancer patients require a consistent and clear posttreatment care plan focused on monitoring for late effects of cancer and recurrence, incorporating interventions addressing illnesses post-cancer or due to treatment, and coordinating care between specialists and PCPs; these are referred to as Survivorship Care Plans (SCPs). Having SCPs with a multidimensional biopsychosocial approach to improve wellness during and after treatment will have a more positive impact [2, 3, 4, 14, 35].

Published Research Articles on Wellness Interventions

We conducted a literature search in April 2019 with no date, age, sex, or language limits using PubMed, OVID MEDLINE, and PsycINFO databases for articles using the following keywords: "Cancer" OR "Neoplastic diseases" AND "intervention" OR "plan" or "program" AND "wellness" OR "quality of life" OR "well-being." The search results gave 1,089,813 published research articles, which included: 502,948 on diet (including healthy eating), 397,992 on exercise (including physical exercise or physical fitness), 85,536 on social support, 35,011 on psychosocial interventions, 6455 on spirituality, 2271 on meditation or mindfulness-based stress reduction, 1527 on yoga, and 58,073 miscellaneous.

These interventions have focused on addressing several objectives to improve wellness, increase survivorship, and decrease recurrence. A combination of the following components were featured: (1) achieving and maintaining a healthy weight; (2) being physically active; (3) eating a healthy diet mainly composed of fruits, vegetables, and whole grains; (4) getting the recommended cancer screenings regularly; (5) creating a survivorship care plan with an experienced healthcare provider; and (6) taking care of emotional health through social support (e.g., family, friends, cancer support group) and/or spirituality (e.g., nature, meditation, prayer, art therapy, psychosocial therapy) [14, 17–25].

Survivorship Care Plans

In 2015, the Commission on Cancer of the American College of Surgeons proposed a new accreditation standard, making SCPs a requirement. An SCP should provide the following: (1) summary of cancer treatment; (2) a plan for surveillance and preventive care; and (3) a plan for rehabilitation care [22]. Despite the endorsement by accredited bodies and awareness of the need for SCPs in cancer care, a recent systematic review suggests that adoption is slow due to time and resources needed to develop and implement them; and there is little awareness and consistency of the benefits [36]. Jacobsen et al. conducted a comprehensive review of SCPs' impact on health outcomes and healthcare delivery in several forms of cancer. The majority of studies demonstrated statistically nonsignificant findings. Of the few significant findings, SCPs had a positive impact on depression, health worry, outlook on life, satisfaction with care, and amount of information received. The review suggested that more focus should be placed on enhancing the methodological quality of SCPs, with an emphasis on randomized studies, consistency of content, delivery, and comparable outcome measures (with differentiation between proximal and distal outcomes) [36].

Physical Exercise and Yoga

While there is limited evidence on SCPs improving health outcomes, other interventions like physical exercise suggest a more significant impact on health outcomes, specifically HRQOL, among cancer patients going through adjuvant treatment postsurgery [17]. At least four systematic reviews have reviewed the benefits of physical exercise and yoga on wellness, QOL, and CRF in cancer patients, including safety and feasibility. However, Loughney and colleagues' systematic review of exercise's impact on cancer patients noted that the featured studies had limited generalizability (14 of 17 studies were on female breast cancer patients), more RCTs were needed, and that no gold standard was established yet in regard to the program (aerobic versus resistance training), frequency, duration, intensity, setting, and type of exercise.

Psychosocial Interventions

Psychosocial interventions including therapeutic communication have been effective in minimizing stress, treating depression, improving QOL, and supporting cancer patients during diagnosis and recovery [11, 37]. A range of therapies including cognitive-behavioral therapy (CBT), problem-solving therapy, counseling, and mindfulness-based interventions (e.g., mindfulness-based stress reduction and mindfulness-based cognitive therapy) have shown effectiveness in improving wellness in cancer settings [11, 22, 24, 37]. For example, an acceptance-based CBT intervention for lung cancer patients demonstrated significant improvements in psychological (HADS, $ES = 0.182$) and cancer-specific distress ($ES = 0.056$), depression (CES-D, $ES = 0.621$), and health-related stigma (CLCSS, $ES = 0.139$); despite this, however, QOL declined (FACT-L, $ES = 0.023$) [21]. Similar studies focusing on self-forgiveness and acceptance among patients and caregivers provided comparable improvements in QOL, distress, and mood in mixed cancer types [11, 21].

Spirituality

Cancer's impact on wellness can go beyond physical and psychological distress; the illness can be a threat to a patient's meaning to life, causing multiple paradoxes such as feeling hopeful about being cured, but also fearful about recurrence [25]. Research has shown that spirituality or religion, including giving and receiving love and relating to God or a higher being, has helped patients cope with this experience [24, 25]. A systematic review found that the majority of studies (31 of 36) showed a positive association between spirituality and emotional well-being, but no major conclusions could be drawn due to shortcomings of some studies [25].

Conclusion

Developments in cancer research have helped save and extend survivors' lives. In order to fully benefit from these advances, more clinical research is needed to understand long-term effects of treatments, enabling physicians and survivors to manage symptoms, actively detect early signs of complications, and control therapy dosing. Providing SCPs using a biopsychosocial model to enhance wellness by targeting physical exercise, nutrition, and psychosocial support can significantly improve health outcomes and prolong lives. Further research should focus on utilizing wellness measures to empower patients to make decisions about their care after discharge, where treating people rather than the disease should be a priority.

References

1. F Bray, J Ferlay, I Soerjomataram, et al. Global cancer statistics 2018: GLOBOCAN estimates of incidence and mortality worldwide for 36 cancers in 185 countries. *CA Cancer J Clin* 2018; **68**(6): 394–424.

2. American Cancer Society. *Cancer Facts and Figures 2019*. Atlanta, GA, American Cancer Society; 2019. www.cancer.org/content/dam/cancer-org/research/cancer-facts-and-statistics/annual-cancer-facts-and-figures/2 019/cancer-facts-and-figures-2019.pdf (accessed March 31, 2019).

3. World Health Organization. Cancer key facts. September 18, 2018. www.who.int/news-room/fact-sheets/detail/cancer (accessed April 1, 2019).

4. National Cancer Institute. What is cancer? February 9, 2015. www.cancer.gov/about-cancer/understanding/what-is-cancer (accessed April 1, 2019).

5. Institute for Quality and Efficiency in Health Care. How do cancer cells grow and spread? September 21, 2016. www .ncbi.nlm.nih.gov/books/NBK279410 (accessed April 11, 2019).

6. F Bray, I Soerjomataram. The changing global burden of cancer: transitions in human development and implications for cancer prevention and control. *Cancer Dis Control Priorities* 2015; **3**(3): 23–44.

7. The National Wellness Institute. The six dimensions of wellness. 2019. www .nationalwellness.org/page/Six_Dimensions (accessed April 6, 2019).

8. C Allemani, T Matsuda, V Di Carlo, et al. Global surveillance of trends in cancer survival 2000–14 (CONCORD-3): analysis of individual records for 37,513,025 patients diagnosed with one of 18 cancers from 322 population-based registries in 71 countries. *Lancet* 2018; **391**: 1023–1075.

9. S Bluethmann, A Mariotto, J Rowland. Anticipating the "silver tsunami": prevalence trajectories and comorbidity burden among older cancer survivors in the United States. Cancer *Epidemiol Biomarkers Prev* 2016; **25**(7):1029–1036.

10. N Gegechkori, L Haines, JJ Lin. Long-term and latent side effects of specific cancer types. *Med Clin North Am* 2017; **101**(6): 1053–1073.

11. B Hoeck, L Ledderer, HP Hansen. Dealing with cancer: a meta-synthesis of patients' and relatives' experiences of participating in psychosocial interventions. *Eur J Cancer Care* 2017; **26**: e12652.

12. M Franc, B Michalski, I Kuczerawy, et al. Cancer related fatigue syndrome in neoplastic diseases. *Prz Neopazualny* 2014; **13**(6): 352–355.

13. Nature. Study cancer survivors. *Nature* 2019; **568**: 143.

14. M Rushton, R Morash, G Larocque, et al. Wellness Beyond Cancer Program: building an effective survivorship program. *Curr Oncol* 2015; **22**(6): 419.

15. MG Nayak, A George, MS Vidyasagar, et al. Quality of life among cancer patients. *Indian J Palliat Care* 2017; **23**(4): 445–450.

16. G Wyatt, A Sikorskii, D Tamkus, et al. Quality of life among advanced breast cancer patients with and without distant metastasis. *Eur J Cancer Care* 2013; **22**: 272–280.

17. L Loughney, MA West, GJ Kemp, et al. Exercise intervention in people with cancer undergoing adjuvant cancer treatment following surgery: a systematic review. *Eur J Surg Oncol* 2015; **41**(12): 1590–1602.

18. AF Heldens, BC Bongers, J de Vos-Geelen, et al. Feasibility and preliminary effectiveness of a physical exercise training program during neoadjuvant chemoradiotherapy in individual patients with rectal cancer prior to major elective surgery. *Eur J Surg Oncol* 2016; **42**(9): 1322–1330.

19. MT Knobf, AS Thompson, K Fennie, et al. The effect of a community-based exercise intervention on symptoms and quality of life. *Cancer Nurs* 2014; **37**: E43–E50.

20. A Navigante, PC Morgado. Does physical exercise improve quality of life of advanced cancer patients? *Curr Opin Support Palliat Care* 2016; **10**(4): 306–309.

21. SK Chambers, BA Morris, S Clutton, et al. Psychological wellness and health-related stigma: a pilot study of an acceptance-focused cognitive behavioral intervention for people with lung cancer. *Eur J Cancer Care* 2014; **24**(1): 60–70.

22. J Moye, M Langdon, JM Jones, et al. Managing health care after cancer treatment: a wellness plan. *Fed Pract* 2014; **31**(3): 27S–32S.

23. X Zhang, H Xiao, Y Chen. Effects of life review on mental health and well-being among cancer patients: a systematic review. *Int J Nurs Stud* 2017; **74**: 138–148.

24. EG Mistretta. Spirituality in young adults with end-stage cancer: a review of the literature and a call for research. *Ann Palliat Med* 2017; **6**(3): 279–283.

25. A Visser, B Garssen, A Vingerhoets. Spirituality and well-being in cancer patients: a review. *Psycho-Oncology* 2009; **19**(6): 565–572.

26. M Tamburini. Health-related quality of life measures in cancer. *Annals Oncol* 2001; **12** (3): S7–S10.

27. Center for Disease Control and Prevention. Health-related quality of life. October 31, 2018. www.cdc.gov/hrqol/concept.htm (accessed April 8, 2019).

28. K Webster, D Cella, K Yost. The Functional Assessment of Chronic Illness Therapy (FACIT) measurement systems: properties, applications, and interpretations. *Bio Med Central* 2003; **1**: 79.

29. W Spitzer, A Dobson, J Hall, et al. Measuring the quality of life of cancer patients. a concise QL-Index for use by physicians. *J Chron Dis* 1981; **34**: 585–597.

30. AK Gandhi, S Roy, A Thakar, et al. Symptom burden and quality of life in advanced head and neck cancer patients: AIIMS study of 100 patients. *Indian J Palliat Care* 2014; **20**: 189–193.

31. M Horneber, I Fischer, F Dimeo, et al. Cancer-related fatigue: epidemiology, pathogenesis, diagnosis, and treatment. *Dtsch Arztebl Int* 2012; **109**(9): 161–172.

32. X-J Lin, I-M Lin, S-Y Fan. Methodological issues in measuring health-related quality of life. *Tzu Chi Med J* 2013; **25**(1): 8–12.

33. S King, J Exley, S Parks, et al. The use and impact of quality of life assessment tools in clinical care settings for cancer patients, with a particular emphasis on brain cancer: insights from a systematic review and stakeholder consultations. *Nature* 2016; **25** (9): 2245–2256.

34. D Anderson, C Seib, D Tjondronegoro, et al. The women's wellness after cancer program: a multisite, single-blinded, randomised controlled trial protocol. *BMC Cancer* 2017; **17**(1). DOI:10.1186/s12885-017-3088-9.

35. M Hewitt, S Greenfield, E Stovall. *From Cancer Patient to Cancer Survivor: Lost in Transition*. Washington, DC, National Academies Press; 2005.

36. P Jacobsen, A DeRosa, T Henderson, et al. Systematic review of the impact of cancer survivorship care plans on health outcomes and health care delivery. *J Clin Oncol* 2018; **36**(20): 2088–2100.

37. B Raingruber. The effectiveness of psychosocial interventions with cancer patients: an integrative review of the literature (2006–2011). *ISRN Nurs* 2011; **2011**: DOI:10.5402/2011/638218.

Wellness in Terminal Illness

Monika Chaudhry, Alex Gordon, Emile Tadros, Carrian Sun, Gabriel Tobia, and Waguih William IsHak

Even if you have a terminal disease, you don't have to sit down and mope. Enjoy life and challenge the illness that you have.

Nelson Mandela

Introduction

In 2014, 2.6 million people died in the USA. Death is inevitable and can find someone in any number of ways, and most hope for a good death [1]. Terminal illness is an irreversible or incurable disease condition from which death is expected in the foreseeable future. Some often regulate this to a prognosis of the last 6–12 months of life; however, some live longer with a terminal illness in palliative or hospice care. Even with a terminal illness, many patients continue to receive treatment to reduce symptom burden, continue to keep fighting with experimental procedures (sometimes to give purpose), at times not to disappoint family members, and at other times it is part of their values [2]. The transition from a chronic illness to a terminal illness can be devastating for some patients, and navigating this change requires a significant amount of work from both the practitioner and the patient for a good quality of life [3].

Advances in modern medicine and improved access to care have led to an aging population, with many patients seeking ongoing treatment for terminal illnesses and improved access to care. Terminal illness often afflicts the elder population but can occur at any stage in life. The stressors patients face include major decisions about health, treatment-related issues, changes in social relation, anxiety about the future and death, dependency on others, limited physical functioning, and worsening of symptoms, especially pain [4]. A perceived threat to psychosocial or physical integrity leads to severe stress or suffering. It is important to complete an assessment of the suffering and offer relief to help cope through this transition. Psychological distress in terminal illness tends to be underdiagnosed and undertreated. It has been well documented that uncontrolled pain is a major risk factor for depression and suicide among terminally ill patients. Often, though, terminally ill patients are treated with pharmacologic agents to treat the illness and symptoms without promoting wellness and preventing any further damage. To promote wellness, health professionals must encourage active participation in one's life up until the very end of it, with the creation of meaning and connection through active participation in activities of daily living. The implementation of those concepts will have a positive impact on well-being and quality of life for the terminally ill patient.

Quality of life encompasses a holistic view of the patient, touching upon physiologic, psychological, social, and spiritual aspects of their life. This is driven by both patients and practitioners and takes into account patients' desires, values, cultural influences, and spiritualism. Throughout this process it is important for providers to touch upon end-of-life care, which focuses on the patient's wishes through an advanced directive, discussing their desire to die, and symptom management. Having a good quality of life is a goal. The term *wellness*, almost interchangeable with *quality of life*, further delineates an active process. In one study regarding health, wellness, and quality of life, several participants called it a "doing" process in one's dying. This would mean that in a wellness approach it is important that patients and their families engage in a continuation of various activities in their lives and continue to be productive. The study termed it "finishing business." Medical professionals should encourage connectedness in order to help their terminally ill patients realize their goals on a level beyond receipt of care. Terminally ill patients may be in a fragile state as they confront challenges and uncertainty at the ends of lives. Many faced with the diagnosis of a terminal illness must cope with anxiety, fear, and despair. This is why it is imperative to utilize a wide range of physical, pharmaceutical, nutraceutical, psychosocial, and spiritual solutions to promote wellness in terminally ill patients. The wellness philosophy for health does not take away from regular medical practice, but adds to it.

Wellness is a complex and multifaceted concept that incorporates into one's own self physical, mental, and emotional health and well-being. It touches upon one's resilience, self-awareness, self-care, and maintenance of values. To achieve wellness, one needs balance, social support, adequate rest, and regular physical activity, supplemented by a positive attitude, religious belief system, and fulfillment in life. These are all essential to any person regardless of where they are in life, personally, or professionally [5].

End-of-Life Care

Patients who have been suffering from chronic illnesses of cardiovascular disease, heart failure, neurologic complications (dementia, ALS, stroke, Parkinson's or Huntington's disease), cancer, chronic kidney disease, liver failure, or HIV/AIDS suffer from depression, anxiety, and demoralization, and find it hard to make the transition to end-of-life care. The transition entails an acceptance of impending death from the illness. End-of-life care requires complex decision-making about prolonging life. Transitioning to dying brings about fears of suffering, existential questions about what is beyond and the meaning of life, and burden of loss to other family members [6].

A study by Lewis et al. had three focus group discussions and six in-depth interviews with adults suffering from terminal conditions. They identified seven major themes: quality of life, sense of control, life on hold, need for health system support, being at home, talking about death, and competent and caring health professionals, with an underpinning priority of knowing and adhering to the patient's wishes [7]. End-of-life care is something that practitioners avoid talking about earlier in the course of a patient's chronic illness, for fear of losing hope, breaking rapport, and difficulty navigating challenging situations with the patient and family. However, earlier consideration may enable patients to make more informed decisions in line with their values, ensure improved coping/acceptance, give them a chance to navigate relationships or unresolved conflicts, and have a good death. Patient-centered care allows the patient to maintain a sense of control when their body or mind is failing them; it gives them a sense of dignity [8].

Palliative care has been around for almost 60 years [9]. The goals are relief of suffering, and over the last two decades or so referrals to palliative care have occurred during chronic illness rather than when the patient is transitioned to end-of-life care. A palliative care approach improves the quality of life of individuals and their families when they are facing problems associated with life-threatening illness, by preventing or relieving suffering. Earlier involvement of palliative care in chronic illness reduces stigma around loss of hope, giving up, and dying. Early identification of pain, nutrition, hydration, confusion, depression, anxiety, and social support has shown more positive outcomes. This is done by reducing symptom burden, actively addressing goals of care, and providing psychosocial support. Discussing goals of care and values requires deft communication to help patients maintain hope, have a sense of control, and not feel abandoned. Goals of care balance personal values, illness trajectory, leveraging social relationships, and adherence to spiritual/cultural/religious concepts of death, dying, and transition to the afterlife. The vast majority of terminally ill patients want to name someone to make decisions, know what to expect about their physical condition, have their financial affairs in order, know the doctor is comfortable talking about death and dying, feel that they and their families are prepared for their death, have funeral arrangements in place, and have treatment preferences in writing. These meaningful conversations about prognosis and patients' wishes will help drive discussions about code status, artificial nutrition, and acceptable level of burden, and help the physician balance level of pain, awareness, agitation, and perceived suffering. Palliative care is a collaborative team of physicians, nurses, chaplains, pharmacists, social workers, and psychiatrists who engage the patient and family to elicit the patient's wishes, make realistic expectations, relieve suffering, and provide support [9].

More people today are living with terminal illness who find it difficult to transition their care; they find it difficult to imagine that hospice care can give them quality of life, but also potentially a longer life. Reducing active medical treatments like chemotherapy lessens negative side effects or symptoms. Additionally, reducing doctor appointments and scans allows a patient to have more time for social activities and provides the ability to focus on other portions in their life, not only identifying with the disease or illness. This concept requires overcoming the notion of "giving up." The USA is starting to have decreased use of chemotherapy in the last 30 days of life, and patients increasingly prefer to die at home, relying less on hospitalization at the end of life. One study by Wright et al. surveyed patients who died with advanced lung or colorectal cancer. It concluded that patients who had been enrolled in at least three days of hospice care had a better quality of life near death and best alignment of care with their wishes [2].

Hospice care allows for ongoing treatment of symptoms, following through with the patient's wishes and goals of care, a peaceful transition to the last days to months of life – usually the last 6–12 months. Hospice care can help patients understand and continue to explore goals as they learn to accept this transition and confront the idea of death. Spiritual care addresses the meanings of life and death, helps with anxiety, and guides patients and practitioners with culturally sensitive rituals needed for transition. Hospice care allows patients the opportunity to feel in control, reduces patient visits and treatments with significant side effect profiles, focuses on quality over quantity, and prepares the patient. It also provides support to families through bereavement programs after death, which can be reassuring to the patient. Hospice care may not be for all patients if in their belief system they must continue fighting to the end and not withdraw from any care that is offered.

Physiologic Well-being

Patients suffering from chronic illnesses like coronary artery disease (CAD), congestive heart failure (CHF), chronic kidney disease (CKD), arthritis, chronic obstructive pulmonary disease

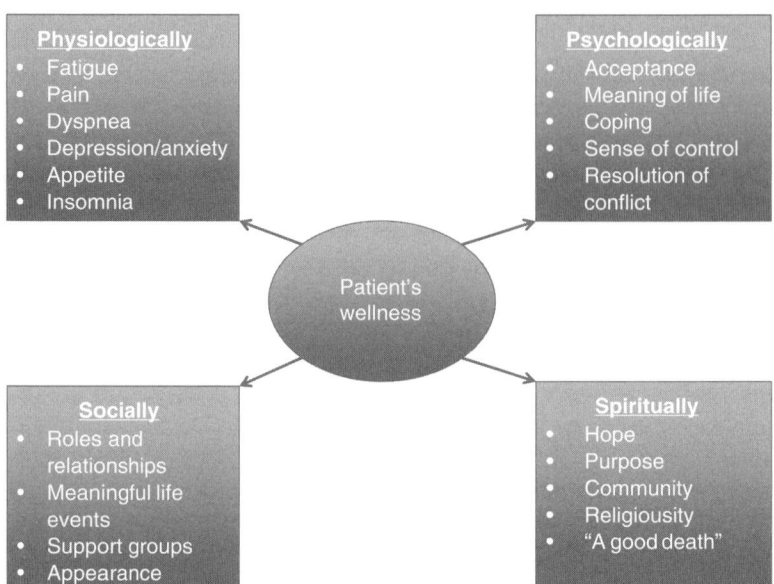

Figure 19.1 Biopsychosocial–spiritual components of wellness in terminal illness.

(COPD), and progressive neurologic diseases showed raised levels of depressed mood and impaired hedonic and eudemonic well-being [10]. Uncontrolled physical symptoms and impaired psychological well-being (fatigue, pain, dyspnea, depression, anxiety, and delirium) can hasten physical and psychological decline and place undue stress on caregivers [11] (Figure 19.1).

A number of underlying causes for fatigue include disease progression, cachexia, anemia, depression, anxiety, infection, hypoxia, autonomic dysfunction, immobility, and hypogonadism. Treatment modalities include pharmacologic use of steroids, megestrol, methylphenidate, modafinil, oxygen, and transfusions. Non-pharmacologic modalities include exercise, cognitive-behavioral therapy (CBT), physical therapy, and occupational therapy.

Pain can be viewed as physical, psychological, or spiritual; it is considered part of suffering and something that patients fear at the end of life. It can be distressing and disabling, impacting 70–90 percent of patients with advanced stage disease. There are many studies and evidence-based guidelines for pain assessment and non-pharmacologic, pharmacologic, and radiotherapy interventions. In terminal illness there is less concern for addiction, but more for hastening death. For use of NSAIDs – like ketorolac, celecoxib, or meloxicam – bleeding risk and kidney function should be monitored. Opioids are usually reserved for moderate to severe pain. Level of pain and route of administration will determine medication selected for basal pain control and breakthrough. Most often used for basal maintenance is morphine sulfate contin, fentanyl patch, or methadone. Breakthrough pain is typically managed with morphine, hydromorphone, and oxycodone. To avoid constipation and subsequent abdominal pain and nausea, a bowel regimen should be used. If switching classes of opioids, it is important to use 50–75 percent of the equianalgesic dose due to cross-reactivity and incomplete tolerance to respiratory and sedative effects. For neuropathic pain, anticonvulsants like gabapentin, carbamazepine, steroids of dexamethasone, prednisone, tricyclic antidepressants amitriptyline, nortriptyline, or alpha-2 agonist clonidine can be used, as well as methadone and ketamine. Additionally, palliative radiotherapy can be done on bone or tissue metastases that are causing significant pain, and there is a risk of pathologic fractures [9].

Unintended side effects of treating pain include excessive sedation, fatigue, and depressed mood, which can impact meaningful time with family and quality of life. A randomized double-blind placebo-controlled trial in 30 hospice patients who were dosed with 10–40 mg of methylphenidate showed improvement on the Visual Analogue Scale for Fatigue, Edmonton Symptom Assessment Scale, and Beck Depression Inventory [12].

Dyspnea or breathlessness is an uncomfortable sensation in breathing, which is experienced by nearly 90 percent in end-stage lung disease, 70 percent with cancer, 50 percent end-stage renal disease, and more than 60 percent with CKD [13]. Untreated dyspnea can increase fatigue, anxiety, and caregiver stress. Treatment options include lorazepam, morphine, or chlorpromazine [9]. If there are associated death rattle secretions, scopolamine or glycopyrrolate are used, and oxygen can be given for comfort.

Delirium occurs in 85 percent of dying patients [13] and can be worsened by severe somnolence or agitation, including insomnia, restlessness, irritability, poor attention, emotional labiality, hallucinations, and memory impairments. This can occur in patients with dementia and brain tumors/metastasis, or those undergoing whole-brain radiation or prolonged hospital stays. Treatment remains dealing with the underlying medical causes of pain, constipation, dehydration, or hypoxia, with benzodiazepines or antipsychotics reserved for severe symptoms. Medications used are, dependent on symptom cluster and goal of management (e.g., insomnia, hallucinations, agitation, or terminal sedation), lorazepam, trazodone, zolpidem, haloperidol, chlorpromazine, olanzapine, quetiapine, or risperidone [14].

Nausea can afflict 70 percent of cancer patients and 50 percent of patients with non-cancer diagnoses. The impact of nausea is severe, as oral gratification impacts psyche and nutrition is important for energy, mood, and anxiety, which if addressed adequately leads to improved well-being. Medications often used are lorazepam, metoclopramide, dexamethasone, or haloperidol [9, 14].

Depression and anxiety often occur as one approaches death. There is the difficulty with transition, anticipated loss, and feeling hopeless and helpless, compounded by physical change, nutritional deficiencies from therapies and poor appetite, insomnia, fatigue, guilt, and thoughts of suicide. It is important to screen patients and introduce treatments that can manage a variety of symptom clusters to reduce pill burden; for example, for insomnia, low mood, and low appetite one can use mirtazapine. If there are components of neuropathic pain, one can consider use of tricyclics. If looking to energize a patient, promote eating, and reduce nausea, neuropathic pain, and inflammation, one can consider corticosteroids. Traditionally, SSRIs or SNRIs have also been recommended, especially with concurrent anxiety, but may take time to work, and thus psychostimulants and benzodiazepines are recommended [14].

Psychological Well-being

When a patient becomes acutely aware they are dying, there is a struggle to cope and potential for depression and anxiety. This may increase the symptom burden, functional decline, and fear of death, i.e., intensify suffering. According to Chapman and Gavrin, "Suffering is a complex negative emotional and cognitive state characterized by perceived threat to the integrity of the self, perceived helplessness in the face of that threat, and exhaustion of psychosocial and personal resources for coping with that threat" [15]. At the heart of human adaptation is resilience, the ability to create a positive world for oneself often in the face of stressful life experience, and the ability to resist being overtaken by negative experiences when they seem to be overwhelming. As people adapt to illness, it can lead to lower levels of distress and impairment in the quality of life. Approaching death, one realizes that life is short and there are different approaches to facing the end: reevaluation of life, opportunity for growth, resignation/acceptance. It is important to control psychological symptoms with medications and promote a feeling of satisfaction in life, establishing end-of-life goals and facilitating good-quality communication between patients and their family.

Hope is a powerful concept that helps drive people to a better future. The demands of treatment take a toll on patients, both physically and psychologically. Some patients cope and pursue treatment to the end because any loss of hope would be devastating. It is important to develop new kinds of hope, reintegrating into activities and family life, emphasizing the importance of well-being. Hope for future activities can help the patient create meaning, impart wisdom, and share memories (e.g., videos, letters). This can be therapeutic in the form of a life review.

Depression and anxiety are the most common psychological symptoms that are focused on in therapy as a patient transitions to dying. Guilt is a powerful symptom that reflects internal conflicts a patient feels as they struggle with failure to themselves and life respon-sibilities, being a burden to their family, and worrying about family after they are gone. Strategies used to resolve these conflicts include interpersonal therapy for role change, psychodynamics to deal with perceived personal and family failures, and cognitive-behavioral therapy to reframe negative thoughts [16]. Acceptance is key to psychological well-being, but patients with poor coping mechanisms are often in denial and may turn to illicit substances, and use venting as a means of coping. Avoidance may not allow one to achieve life satisfaction, repair relationships, communicate with providers about their end-of-life care, and may cause increased risk of suffering at the end of life.

Adjustment to Loss

A patient who is terminal may struggle to accept and may be avoiding or in denial, but can react by trying to obtain a sense of control over the healthcare services as they cannot control their physical decline and perceived suffering [16]. The psychological response to an abrupt disruption in life is to attempt to regain a sense of control (self-preservation) as the patient is learning to cope with the loss of their life/future. Adjustment to the end of life requires comprehension, creative adaptation, and reintegration [17]. Trying to obtain a sense of control may include avoiding doctor's appointments or potentially falling out of treatment as they process this threat to their body integrity. These patients equate dignity in dying with being in control, and have a strong desire for self-determination in their end-of-life care [16]. This can help drive patients' end-of-life care in terms of interventions, resuscitation, where they want to die, and the ultimate locus of control of physician aid in dying. In Norway and Belgium, euthanasia exists and is a cultural norm. In the USA there are six states that allow patients in their last six months of life to request medication to end their lives. The patients must be able to take the medication on their own. Studies have shown that only 50 percent of the patients end up using the medication. This remains controversial because, on one hand, practitioners are to do no harm, but on the other, they must relieve suffering [1].

Life satisfaction is on a U-shaped curve, indicating that the young and the elderly are the happiest compared to those in middle age [11]. The young are often carefree, and explore with support from their family; the middle-aged are the balancing generation with professional careers; and the elderly are retired and focus on imparting wisdom to their family and community (spiritually). Socioemotional selectivity theory posits that as people age they accumulate emotional wisdom that leads to selection of more emotionally satisfying events, friendships, and experiences. Even with the death of loved ones, loss of status associated with retirement, deteriorating health, and reduced income, older people maintain and even have increased self-reported well-being. Life evaluation using the Cantril Ladder (Cantril's 1965 Self Anchoring Ladder of Life Satisfaction – patients imagine their lives in the best possible light and describe their hopes and wishes for the future, rating it on a 0–10 scale) allows one to think about the quality or goodness of one's life, overall satisfaction, or sometimes how happy one is with one's life [5].

Eriksonian Stages

Terminal illness can occur at any point in life. Looking at the Eriksonian development stage, a clinician can better understand psychologically at noted milestones the conflicts and impacts of not being at the same level as one's peers, and one's ability to process death. If a person does not have a fully structured ego or self-awareness, they remain stuck at a specific stage, which can lead to unresolved conflict on top of facing the idea of death. Often, these conflicts can manifest as fear, anxiety, hopelessness, depression, despair, spiritual distress, and suicidality [18].

Qualitative studies interviewing parents show that terminally ill children experience sadness, apathy, and anger toward their parents and the professionals due to being isolated from their natural environment, being uncertain about the future, and anticipating pain [19]. As a child, not only will coping strategies be limited, but any concept of death will be challenging to explain or resolve [20]. When observing a child, it is important to take into consideration behavioral changes through crying, facial expressions, aggression, and isolation, which can reflect sadness, anger, apathy, pain, and uncertainty. It is important to provide emotional support, assess the origin of pain, and understand social relationships and expectations of the child and parent.

A teenager or young adult would often struggle to understand their sense of self, loss of romantic relationships, loss of a professional career, or leaving a baby. In adulthood, one is focused on their career, raising children, and potentially caring for elderly parents. There will be anxiety around the meaning of loss to kids, and acceptance around death. In the elderly there is a crisis between ego and integrity, often finding meaning/purpose with a failing body and essentially acknowledging achievement and life satisfaction.

Life Review

Part of wellness in terminal illness would be psychologically working with the patient, often using techniques of life review, which will help elucidate developmental crises and attitudes toward death, and help to reorganize a patient's perspectives. This includes recall of past memories, finding meaning in life, and achieving emotional resolution. One narrates life experiences from the earliest memory to the present; unresolved conflicts and pleasurable experiences are evaluated and reframed to find meaning. Given this psychological space, the patient has the opportunity to express emotions, confirm life roles, reassess thoughts about death and adjust perspective on life. A life review gives the patient a chance to reorganize life events, restore coping, and create a positive view of life [18].

Spiritual Well-being

The role of spirituality in the dying patient is vital to well-being. Often, as patients experience physical decline, their cognition remains and they search for hope and struggle with questions about mortality and the meaning and purpose of life and transcendence. Studies show spiritual well-being reduces psychological distress (depression, hopelessness, desire for hastened death, and suicidal ideations). One can be spiritual but not adhere to a specific religion – the construct of a higher power can be universal; religion is a framework for organized behavior, socialization, and cultural value sets that can drive patients at the end of life. The Functional Assessment of Chronic Illness Therapy–Spiritual Well-Being Scale focuses on faith and meaning [21].

It is important for practitioners to understand that different religions, cultures, and ethnicities have different values, ways of handling the process of dying, and ways to seek care from providers. The variation includes the use of religious texts; looking for a paternalistic role in the provider versus autonomy versus shared decision-making; needing spiritual guidance to help transition to care; minimizing sedation at the end of life; maintaining integrity of the body; and, in some cases, certain religions do not allow withdrawal of care as it is an important part of the life-and-death process. Traversing the spectrum of values makes the experience for the patient and provider unique and thoughtful and promotes the goals of a good life and a good death. Approaching the patient early in the disease process allows for integration of culture, spirituality, religion, and personal value sets to better understand the patient's wishes for the end of life and support them through this transition by relieving suffering from physical, psychological, and spiritual pain [21].

Existential suffering reflects complex phenomena related to fear, pain, and spiritual experiences. Renz posits that the transition to dying initially is ego-based (pre-), then moves to an ego-distant perception/consciousness (post-), and that spiritual (transcendental) experiences occur in periods of calmness. In moments of ego-distant mode there is less or no fear/struggle/denial or loss of consciousness (transformation of perception) as death approaches. Patients with spiritual experiences (deathbed visions or end-of-life dreams) often have decreasing fear/pain/denial [22].

Death anxiety is the existential fear related to the basic knowledge that human life must end. Coping with this fear requires understanding of a patient's attachment style, ongoing life conflicts, and spiritual/cultural context of death. Denial as a defense mechanism allows one to live life freely and without bounds, but if not confronted can lead to a wide range of psychiatric symptoms. More so, patients fear suffering at the end of life, with concerns about life after death. Spiritualism or religion creates a framework to better understand death in the context of life. Additionally, using the psychological intervention of life review allows one to provide meaning and purpose in life, understand points of conflict that require resolution, and provide a positive context to life and eventually acceptance [23].

The construct of coping utilizes the interplay between psychological therapy and spiritual/religious awareness. Well-being is achieved through religion by being an integral part of everyday life influencing the patient's experiences and concepts of death and the afterlife. Religion's framework gives hope and allows one to live with ease as one regulates the parts of life to God's will. This concept is psychologically protective for some patients and allows them to find global meaning in the world and their role in it. As they process this, it can resolve internal struggles and conflicts with family, social relationships, and loss of their life, and help them achieve acceptance. It is imperative to ensure any underlying depression and anxiety are also treated, which will help the patient to cope. Religion/spiritualism has grown out of the human need to comprehend existence, framing the world via philosophical orientations and belief systems that allow one to traverse life. During life stressors one looks to God for meaning in regards to punishment, a test, or the belief that God would not give one something one could not handle, and that this is God's plan. Religion can be one tool to help one cope – sometimes patients find life events too traumatic and may cease to believe in the existence of God, being unable to find meaning. Religion allows for positive reappraisals of stressors, and over a lifetime creates growth and resilience [24].

Social Well-being

Social stressors impact patients' well-being. This includes finances and changes in roles and relationships. They may lose their role in the community, in the workplace, and in the family. Feelings of loss or burden arise and psychologically addressing these can help a patient to accept and to cope. Open dialog with caregivers and families may help alleviate these feelings. Patients value close personal relationships, and a relationship with God or a higher power. Depending on the patient's physical function, they may integrate back into their community, no longer pursue active treatment, and attend fewer physician appointments, which may allow them to have improved connection, social support, spiritual guidance, and purpose [25].

Conclusion

Wellness in patients with terminal illnesses requires a multifaceted approach (Figure 19.2). A healthcare provider must simultaneously maintain physiological well-being, psychological well-being, and spiritual well-being in a patient to achieve this goal. Physiological treatments involve taking care of physical pain and symptoms such as depression or anxiety with medications and other therapies. Psychological treatment involves understanding the patient's mindset and helping them mentally adjust to facing the end of their life and maintain hope and motivation. Spiritual care varies based on the patient's belief system and culture, but typically addresses the patient's feeling of meaning in this world and possibly a relationship to some higher power. Wellness in end-of-life situations is crucial to optimizing the experience of the final days.

References

1. H Bauchner, PB Fontanarosa. Death, dying, and end of life. *JAMA* 2016; **315**(3): 270–271.

2. A Gawande. Quantity and quality of life duties of care in life-limiting illness. *JAMA* 2016 **315**(3): 267–269.

3. S Rees, A Williams. Promoting and supporting self-management for adults living in the community with physical chronic illness: a systematic review of the effectiveness and meaningfulness of the

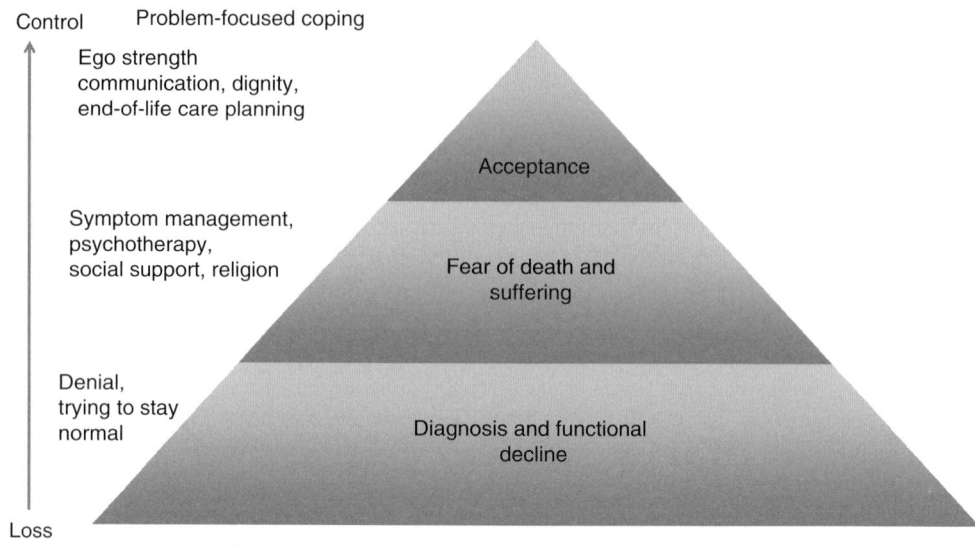

Figure 19.2 Psychological framework in terminal illness.

patient–practitioner encounter. *JBI Libr Syst Rev* 2009; 7(13): 492–582.

4. R Garg, V Chauhan, B Sabreen. Coping styles and life satisfaction in palliative care. *Indian J Palliat Care* 2018; 24(4): 491–495.

5. A Steptoe, A Deaton, AA Stone. Psychological wellbeing, health and ageing. *Lancet* 2015; 385(9968): 640–648.

6. B Hanratty, E Lowson, G Grande, et al. Transitions at the end of life for older adults: patient, carer and professional perspectives – a mixed-methods study. *Health Serv Deliv Res* 2014; 2(17).

7. ET Lewis, R Harrison, L Hanly, et al. End-of-life priorities of older adults with terminal illness and caregivers: a qualitative consultation. *Health Expect* 2019; 22: 405–414.

8. DE Threapleton, RY Chung, SYS Wong, et al. Care toward the end of life in older populations and its implementation facilitators and barriers: a scoping review. *JAMDA* 2017; 18: 1000e1009.

9. JL Abrahm. Update in palliative care and end of life care. *Annu Rev Med* 2003; 54: 53–72.

10. WJ Katon, EH Lin, MV Korff, et al. Collaborative care for patients with depression and chronic illnesses. *N Engl J Med* 2010; 363(27): 2611–2620.

11. P Frijters, T Beatton. The mystery of the U-shaped relationship between happiness and age. *J Econ Behav Organization* 2012; 82(102): 525–542.

12. CW Kerr, J Drake, RA Milch, et al. Effects of methylphenidate on fatigue and depression: a randomized, double-blind, placebo-controlled trial. *J Pain Symptom Manage* 2012; 43(1): 68–77.

13. JJ Strand, MM Kamdar, EC Carey. Top 10 things palliative care clinicians wished everyone knew about palliative care. *Mayo Clin Proc* 2013; 88(8): 859–865.

14. PA Riordan, J Briscoe, TJ Uritsky, et al. Top ten tips palliative care clinicians should know about psychopharmacology. *J Palliat Med* 2019; 22: 572–579.

15. CR Chapman, J Gavrin. Suffering and its relationship to pain. *J Palliat Care* 1993; 9: 5–13.

16. R Montoya-Juarez, MP Garcia-Caro, C Campos-Calderon, et al. Psychological

responses of terminally ill patients who are experiencing suffering: a qualitative study. *Int J Nurs Stud* 2013; **50**: 53–62.

17. SJ Knight, L Emanuel. Processes of adjustment to end-of-life losses: a reintegration model. *J Palliat Med* 2007; **10**(5): 1190–1198.

18. CWM Kwan, CWH Chan, KC Choi. The effectiveness of a nurse-led short-term life review intervention in enhancing the spiritual and psychological well-being of people receiving palliative care: a mixed method study. *Int J Nurs Stud* 2019; **91**: 134–143.

19. R Montoya-Juárez, MP García-Caro, J Schmidt-Rio-Valle, et al. Suffering indicators in terminally ill children from the parental perspective. *Eur J Oncol Nurs* 2013; **17**: 720e725.

20. RR Pravin, TEK Enrica, TA Moy. The portrait of a dying child. *Indian J Palliat Care* 2019; **25**(1): 156–160.

21. A Bovero, P Leombruni, M Miniotti, et al. Spirituality, quality of life, psychological adjustment in terminal cancer patients in hospice. *Eur J Cancer Care* 2016; **25**: 961–969.

22. M Renz, O Reichmuth, D Bueche, et al. Fear, pain, denial, and spiritual experiences in dying processes. *Am J Hosp Palliat Care* 2018; **35**(3): 478–491.

23. M Wnuk, JT Marcinkowski. Do existential variables mediate between religious-spiritual facets of functionality and psychological wellbeing? *J Relig Health* 2014; **53**: 56–67.

24. CL Park. Religion as a meaning-making framework in coping with life stress. *J Social Issues* 2005; **61**: 707–729.

25. M Prince-Paul. Understanding the meaning of social well-being at the end of life. *Oncol Nurs Forum* 2008; **35**(3): 365–371.

Wellness Interventions in the Workplace

Robert A. Chernoff

Introduction

In recent years, workplace wellness programs have become a popular and established feature of corporate life. Their aim is simple: to create opportunities for employees in the workplace to improve their health and well-being. At the modest end, wellness programs offer employees screenings to help them identify possible health risks. More intensive programs make services and resources available to employees to help them prevent or manage diseases associated with lifestyle habits, like poor nutrition, lack of exercise, or smoking. The payoff for employers is a healthier workforce, yielding higher productivity and lower healthcare costs [1].

In one survey, 69 percent of employers offered their employees a wellness program. Eighty percent of workplaces with more than 1000 employees had a wellness program, as did 90 percent of those with more than 50,000 employees. Some 75 percent of programs offered financial incentives to encourage participation [2]. In the USA, the Affordable Care Act created new incentives to encourage employers to promote employer wellness programs and encourage opportunities to support healthier workplaces [3].

But what do we really know about these programs? How did this approach to promoting health and wellness originate? What are the principles that guide the creation of such programs? Do they actually promote employee health and help employees prevent serious health risks? Do wellness programs in the workplace actually lead to lower healthcare costs for employers?

Historical Origins

The idea that health, disease, and the workplace are interconnected goes back centuries. The Italian physician Bernardino Ramazzini studied the health problems that workers developed over time from their trades. In 1700 and again in 1713, he published *De Morbis Artificum Diatriba*, or *Diseases of Workers*, linking specific work activities to particular medical conditions. Ramazzini was one of the first to suggest that prevention of work-related illness was preferable to treating such illnesses after the damage was done [4].

The English surgeon Percivall Pott drew a link between workplace and disease in 1775, when he observed the unusually high prevalence of scrotal cancer among London's chimney sweeps. Without the benefit of protective clothing, sweeps were constantly exposed to soot, which accumulated near their scrotums. It was one of the earliest linkages between a specific trade and an environmental carcinogen [5].

With the coming of the Industrial Revolution in the nineteenth and twentieth centuries, the connection between workplace hazards, injury, and illness had never been starker. New developments in machinery, mass production, and manufacturing processes brought with them hazardous and dangerous working conditions. Workers, many of them children, labored for long hours with few health and safety protections, risking injury, disease, and death. Over many decades, the public outcry over dangerous working conditions led governments to enact legislation and regulations to make the workplace healthier and safer [6].

In 1970, the landmark Occupational Safety and Health Act (OSHA) was enacted in the USA, acknowledging by law that the workplace could be harmful to the health of workers. A comprehensive, nationwide set of rules mandated employers to provide their employees with a safe working environment free of dangers and hazards [7].

Although OSHA made the workplace a safer environment for workers, they continued to face other health risks in the workplace. Many of the leading illnesses, like cardiovascular disease, stroke, diabetes, obesity, high blood pressure, pulmonary disease, and cancer, were often associated with the lifestyle habits of the modern world, like a sedentary lifestyle, insufficient physical activity, poor diet, smoking, and stress. It was widely recognized that many of the risk factors associated with poor health were present in workplace environments [8].

Increasingly, employers came to understand that an unhealthy workforce would have direct consequences for the workplace. Unhealthy workers were more likely to be absent from work, less productive, and eventually unable to work. Many employers came to believe that the health of their workers was not solely the responsibility of the employee, but was a shared responsibility between employee and employer. Employers therefore had a vested interest in helping to promote the good health and wellness of their employees in the workplace [9].

In the 1960s and 1970s, corporations like Rockwell, Goodyear, Xerox, and Pepsico began to implement corporate fitness programs. Around the same time, in the USA, the President's Council on Physical Fitness and Sports had already disseminated to managers of companies the concept that health-promotion programs would be beneficial to both employees and the company. The American Association of Fitness Directors in Business and Industry helped to push the distribution of promotional materials for physical fitness programs in the workplace. It was also around this time that the concept of "wellness" was becoming more widely known and accepted [9].

One of the most ambitious attempts to create a workplace wellness intervention was the "Live for Life" program launched in 1978 at the pharmaceutical and consumer product giant Johnson & Johnson. As the producer of healthcare products like Band-Aid adhesive bandages and Tylenol, the company wanted a program to enhance the health and safety of its employees. Unhealthy behaviors, like smoking, overeating, alcohol abuse, emotional stress, high blood pressure, and unsafe driving were perceived as factors that threatened the overall health of the workforce and drove up the company's healthcare costs. The Live for Life program sought to fully integrate health and wellness into the company's culture and operations by making health-promotion activities accessible to its employees with on-site programs and services.

Live for Life was a comprehensive multi-component program that focused on nutrition education, weight management, exercise, smoking cessation, stress management, and blood pressure control. Employee participation rates were voluntary and exceeded 50 percent. Data collected on the impact of the program showed positive health outcomes among workers, including improvements in weight, blood pressure, cholesterol, and smoking cessation. These outcomes led to an estimated reduction in healthcare costs of 3–5 percent. Hospitalization rates declined to one-third the rate of other companies without wellness programs, and absenteeism was reduced by 18 percent. Other positive impacts included higher employee morale, job satisfaction, and organizational commitment [10].

In the years that followed, wellness programs like Live for Life proliferated. The percentage of companies with 250 or more employees with formal organized fitness programs rose from 2.5 percent in 1979 to 32.4 percent in 1985. By the late 1980s, some 50,000 companies with 100 or more employees were estimated to provide some type of employer-sponsored health-promotion program focusing on disease prevention, increased awareness of personal health behaviors, and better quality of life [9]. By 2012, some 69 percent of employers were offering their employees a workplace wellness program, and larger employers were offering wellness programs at an even higher rate [2].

Conceptual Foundation of Workplace Wellness Programs

Individual/Organizational Interaction

Most workplace wellness programs are created for the pragmatic reason of promoting the health and well-being of workers and providing financial benefits to the employer. With some exceptions, few wellness programs are theory-based. Nevertheless, well-designed workplace wellness programs can be said to have certain conceptual features and characteristics in common. One of these is a model of health that posits a reciprocal interaction between the individual and the organization.

The health and well-being of employees is partly shaped by their personal resources, health practices, coping responses, knowledge, beliefs, attitudes, and genetic vulnerabilities. But their health is also affected by the environments in which they work. The physical conditions of the workplace matter. The psychosocial conditions of the workplace – the culture and the climate of the organization – make a difference. Management practices, like work overload, unscheduled overtime, arguments with supervisors, and deadlines, can all place a heavy burden on the health of employees. While the personal health practices of employees are immensely important, the interplay of environmental, social, and organizational factors with the personal health practices of employees will exert a major influence on workers' overall health and wellness [11].

The 1997 Luxembourg Declaration on Workplace Health Promotion in the European Union recognized that individual and organizational factors are interactive, and that any effective workplace wellness program must pay attention to both. Successful wellness programs will naturally focus on unhealthy behaviors like overeating, lack of physical activity, and smoking. They will also target organizational environments and consider how they can be modified to help promote the health of employees. Targets for organizational change might include having an on-site fitness center, creating a smoke-free work setting, making healthy foods available at cafeterias and vending machines, and providing breaks during the workday for walks, naps, yoga, or meditation [12].

Prevention

Most workplace wellness programs are predicated on the concept of preventing serious health problems from developing in the future. Programs with a primary prevention focus try to help generally healthy workers maintain their healthy habits. Primary prevention programs rely heavily on the use of screening assessments to detect early signs of potential health problems.

Secondary prevention interventions identify people at high risk for developing health problems. Smoking, overeating, heavy drinking, and physical inactivity are all potential targets of secondary prevention efforts, to help the employee avert the development of progressively worse health conditions. Employees who are obese, or who show abnormally high blood pressure, for example, are targeted for health promotion efforts to help them reduce their risk of developing diseases like diabetes or heart disease.

At the tertiary prevention level, health promotion programs reach out to workers diagnosed with such conditions as heart disease, diabetes, asthma, COPD, back pain, depression, or addiction. Programs of this type are engaged in disease management, helping employees have better medication compliance or adherence to clinical practice guidelines, like reducing salt in their diet, or connecting them to services like physical therapy, psychotherapy, or addiction treatment [1].

What Constitutes a High-Quality Workplace Wellness Program?

Workplace wellness programs can vary greatly in quality and intensity. Although there are no official or universal standards of accreditation, there have been efforts to define best practices for such programs. In its *Healthy People 2010* initiative, the Centers for Disease Control and Prevention defined the characteristics of a "comprehensive health promotion program." Such programs approach health promotion at the individual and organizational levels through multiple methods, embodying at least five characteristics:

1. *Health education*: They disseminate health information to increase awareness of healthy and unhealthy lifestyle choices, and help employees learn skills for making lifestyle behavior changes.
2. *Supportive social and physical work environment*: They create environments and policies in the workplace that support healthy behaviors and risk reduction.
3. *Integration*: They are fully integrated into the very fabric, culture, and climate of the organization.
4. *Linkage*: They link employees to related and necessary programs as needed.
5. *Worksite screening and education*: They screen employees for health conditions using health risk assessments and biometric screenings, provide feedback to employees about what the screenings mean, and provide referrals to appropriate services as needed [13].

High-quality workplace wellness programs tend to share other characteristics in common. The RAND Corporation conducted a case study analysis of high-quality programs and identified five factors associated with highly effective wellness programs:

1. *Leadership engagement*: Workplace wellness programs are more likely to succeed when they align with the organization's core values, norms, and goals. All levels of management share the goals of the program, help generate enthusiasm for it, and participate in it themselves.
2. *Effective communication*: Programs succeed when outreach, messaging, and internal marketing happen at all levels, both face-to-face and through broader message dissemination methods like email and website announcements.
3. *Opportunities for engagement*: Effective programs make wellness activities in the workplace convenient and accessible. Employees feel that they can fit the program into

their schedules without penalty and are encouraged to do so by all levels of the organization.

4. *Use of existing resources*: Programs are effective when the organization makes the best use of its internal resources and external relationships with outside partners, like health plans.
5. *Continuous evaluation*: The most successful programs engage in ongoing assessment and solicitation of feedback from employees and use the information to evaluate how well the program is meeting its goals and how it can be improved [8, 14].

How Programs Measures Success

Program success depends partly on the rate of employee participation. The best strategy for increasing participation is leadership support at all levels and effective communication about the program to employees. The next best strategy for increasing participation has been the use of financial incentives to foster enthusiasm and encourage employees to participate. Reward incentives can include cash payments, cash equivalents like merchandise or travel vouchers, gym memberships, and discounts on health plan costs, with the average annual value of incentives ranging from $100 to $500 [8]. Even with incentives, participation rates are often below 50 percent, making program success a challenge [2].

The most common method for evaluating the success of workplace wellness programs is of course better health outcomes among employees. Program success can be gauged by improvements in biological measures like weight, blood pressure, cholesterol, and blood glucose. Behavioral measures of success can include reductions in numbers of cigarettes smoked or alcohol consumed, as well as increases in self-reported exercise time, or higher intake of fruits and vegetables. Lower rates of hospitalization and healthcare utilization, as well as fewer cases of newly diagnosed illness, are other ways of measuring improvements in employee health.

Other measures of success include behaviors that benefit the worksite. Lower rates of absenteeism and number of sick days taken are an indication that a wellness program is having a positive impact. Lower turnover among employees, improvements in productivity and efficiency, and higher job satisfaction are additional ways of measuring success [1, 2].

Types of Programs

Physical Health: Fitness, Nutrition, and Smoking Cessation

By far the most common workplace wellness programs are those that help employees improve their physical health, usually by helping them to increase their level of physical activity, improve their dietary choices, or quit smoking. Such programs are often focused on fitness, nutrition, and weight loss, while others are framed more broadly as reducing cardiovascular risk or promoting a "healthy lifestyle" [14, 15].

Wellness program participants usually complete a comprehensive questionnaire about their health behaviors so that potential health risks can be detected. Employees also complete a series of biometric measures for weight, body mass index, blood pressure, lipids, cholesterol, and blood glucose. In the best wellness programs, employees are provided with feedback about their health risk assessment. The feedback may be generic information about health risks, or it may be more individualized and tailored to the employee, accompanied by some form of counseling in person, by phone, or online. The feedback is intended

to give employees information about their health and potentially motivate them to participate in more aspects of the wellness program so that they can either maintain their good
health if the results are positive, or explore ways of improving their health if they are at risk
for particular health problems [15].

Most workplace wellness programs that provide something more than health risk
screenings will provide health-promoting information, like the benefits of physical activity
and healthy eating or the dangers of smoking. Many programs offer tips on healthy
nutrition and recipes, make exercise videos available, or furnish advice on how to incorporate exercise into the workday. Health information may be offered via brochures, weekly
emails, e-newsletters, or website pages. In other cases it may be offered in one or more
educational modules in person or online. In programs that are mostly knowledge-based,
employees are expected to take health information and initiate behavior changes on
their own.

The more ambitious wellness programs go well beyond the mere provision of information and the assumption that knowledge is sufficient to result in behavior change. These
programs encourage behavior change through skill training and coaching. There is a greater
emphasis on using social support to help employees make and maintain behavior changes.
Professional health counselors or trained lay leaders are available to provide individualized
and tailored feedback to employees to help them set reasonable goals for healthy eating,
physical activity, weight loss, or smoking cessation.

Peer social support from fellow employees is another feature of more comprehensive
programs, whether the focus is weight loss, fitness, or smoking cessation. Social support is
available to help employees stay motivated and overcome obstacles to their goals. It can be
provided by in-person support groups, web chats, phone, email, or e-bulletin boards, for as
many times as needed. Physical activity can lend itself to being done in groups, like
structured physical exercise groups, group aerobics, group dancing, or group resistance
training. In programs in which social support is emphasized, it is an ongoing and continuous experience. The idea is to help employees stay motivated over the long run rather than
become discouraged.

As employees make changes to physical activity, nutrition, or smoking cessation, the
best wellness programs ask employees to monitor and track their ongoing behavior changes
in logs or e-diaries. Some programs ask their employees to measure their steps through the
use of pedometers. In other programs, employees can measure their blood pressure at home
and transmit their readings to a server so that they can track their progress through
a website. Self-monitoring and tracking are ongoing and continuous, so that employees
can see their progress, identify where they have problems, and remain motivated toward
achieving their goals.

In the best wellness programs, the organization supports what its employees are doing
and makes changes to the workplace to support the employees. The most important practice
the organization can institute is to communicate to employees that the employer is making
health promotion the highest priority. One way that employers can transmit this message is
to provide an on-site fitness center, or trails and pathways for employees to use during the
workday. If not feasible, organizations can make physical activity during the work shift
a priority, rather than expecting all physical activity to be done after hours. Employers can
encourage employees to take breaks for walking, or schedule "walking meetings." With food
and nutrition, employers can provide healthy and nutritious food in the cafeteria or vending
machines. Signs and flyers can emphasize the importance of good nutrition. Employers can

sponsor contests or challenges involving weight loss or fitness. Employers can encourage smoking cessation by creating smoke-free environments at the workplace [1, 14–17].

Psychological Health

Many business leaders have long understood that wellness in the workplace should include concepts like psychological health and emotional well-being. Employees can experience problems in their lives outside of work, like stress, anxiety, depression, family conflict, or substance abuse. Employees can experience stress and other emotional challenges on the job as well, especially as the workplace has increasingly become a place where employment security is not guaranteed. Obviously emotional problems can adversely affect a worker's job performance. Additionally, when work stress and other untreated emotional problems among employees lead to absenteeism, low productivity, tardiness, or turnover, the welfare of the entire business can be indirectly affected [18].

One of the oldest methods of addressing the emotional health and wellness of individual workers has been the employee assistance program (EAP). These usually provide counseling, advice, and assistance to employees or their families when they are experiencing psychological or behavioral problems in their lives. Employee assistance programs are designed to help employees address both work-related problems and personal problems outside of work that may have an adverse impact on job performance. It has been difficult to evaluate the effectiveness of EAP programs in any systematic, rigorous way, in part because EAPs can differ widely. But in some peer-reviewed evaluations of EAPs, they have been found to increase worker job satisfaction, job attendance, and quality of life [18].

The EAP approach usually involves referring the employee to outside resources. Other organizations have used in-house resources to provide support for employees undergoing stress, with stress management programs being one of the most common approaches. Worksite stress management programs are designed to help employees reduce or manage the symptoms of stress, or teach employees how to modify their appraisal of stressful situations. The techniques used in such workplace interventions have included muscle relaxation, meditation, biofeedback, cognitive-behavioral skill training, or a combination of these approaches [19]. In a meta-analysis of 36 studies of stress management interventions in the workplace, they were found to have a moderate effect size in reducing stress [20].

More recent workplace wellness programs have used mindfulness interventions to help workers address occupational and life stress. Mindfulness is an ancient practice found in cultures around the world, but the version of mindfulness associated with Buddhism is perhaps the best known among Western healthcare providers. Mindfulness, which means focusing attention and awareness on the present moment experience, in a non-evaluative, non-judgmental way, has formed the basis of such evidence-based interventions as mindfulness-based stress reduction. Some versions of mindfulness training have found their way into workplace wellness programs and have increasingly grown in popularity [21].

Mindfulness-based interventions for reducing stress have been presented in the workplace as a time-limited course (e.g., eight sessions), with in-session mindfulness exercises, home practice, and e-coaching [22]. In one study, the exercises included body scan, breathing exercises, sitting meditation, lunch walking, and mindful grocery shopping. Training was presented in a group, but participants were asked to form pairs to discuss home practice and provide mutual support [23]. In another study, yoga practices were included along with body scan and breathing meditation [21]. When evaluated, worksite mindfulness programs have shown decreases in perceived stress, anxiety, depression, and fatigue among employees [24].

Do Workplace Wellness Programs Work?

Assessing the overall effectiveness of these programs has been a challenge. Programs vary greatly in content and quality. Some are better designed than others. Some provide little more than health screenings, while others provide multifaceted and comprehensive interventions. Participation rates are often low, and skewed toward younger and healthier employees, thus injecting a selection bias into the analysis. The studies evaluating these programs can also range in quality [25].

Still, there is an established peer-reviewed literature evaluating such programs. These studies evaluate whether the programs have achieved the health promotion outcomes that the programs were designed to achieve, and whether the businesses providing the programs to their employees are achieving positive results for the organizations, like overall savings in healthcare costs. The results in both cases are mixed [14].

Evaluations of single wellness programs at large companies like Prudential Insurance have shown positive improvements for employees in general fitness and physical activity [9]. One multisite study that evaluated wellness programs designed to reduce obesity and smoking at 32 worksites showed an average loss of 4.8 lb among participants and a 43 percent rate of smokers who quit [26]. Other studies of single wellness programs have shown positive results in some measures (e.g., lower blood pressure, more exercise, more consumption of fruits and vegetables), but not in others (e.g., no change in cholesterol, blood glucose, or body mass index) [27].

Large systematic reviews or meta-analyses that pool studies together have found some improvements in employees' health outcomes, but the effect sizes of such interventions have often been modest. One systematic review of 29 studies found modest improvements in weight-related outcomes, but no overall improvements in activity. Programs where employees had more contacts with counselors and employers made environmental modifications to promote wellness tended to have better results [15]. A meta-analysis of programs targeting physical activity showed positive but modest improvements in physical activity, fitness, lipids, work attendance, and stress [28]. In a review of 18 studies, improvements in health outcomes were significant but small, with more changes among younger employees and those who had more regular contact with the program [16].

Have businesses benefited from workplace wellness programs and gotten a return on their investment? Here again, the results are mixed. The RAND Corporation conducted a survey of employers in which they expressed confidence that their programs would reduce costs, absenteeism, and lost productivity due to employee health problems. But only about half of the employers surveyed actually conducted a formal evaluation of their programs to determine whether they met their goals. Of the ones that did conduct formal evaluations, only about 2 percent reported actual savings [8].

Some studies have demonstrated reductions in absenteeism and improvements in productivity. In one meta-analysis, absenteeism costs fell on average about $2.73 for every dollar spent on wellness programs [25]. Another meta-analysis found a small effect size in the reduction of absenteeism and lost productivity as a result of wellness programs [16].

When it comes to healthcare cost savings from wellness programs, some of the older studies have shown evidence of cost savings. A 2010 meta-analysis found that medical costs fell about $3.27 for every dollar spent on wellness programs [25]. But in an influential 2015 analysis by RAND of many workplace wellness programs, no cost savings from such programs were found [2]. This result caused many to rethink the cost-effectiveness of workplace wellness programs.

Conclusion

Providing wellness interventions to employees in the workplace is a rational response to the widespread health risks that pervade modern societies. The workplace makes for a natural setting in which to conduct health risk assessments so that workers can be apprised of potential or actual threats to their health. The workplace is a logical forum for employees to receive health-promotion education and, where needed, more intensive wellness interventions. It makes sense for employers to want a healthier workforce and to explore ways of containing rising healthcare costs.

There is empirical evidence suggesting that these programs can make a difference in improving the health of employees. But the realities of such programs do not always match up with their aspirations. Employee participation remains a challenge. The quality of programs is inconsistent and uneven, ranging from comprehensive to minimal. There is vigorous debate as to whether employers are actually getting a return on their investment in terms of cost savings. We need to do a better job of identifying the active ingredients that make such interventions effective and conducting rigorous and continuous program evaluation of them. It is hoped that model programs can be developed, evaluated, disseminated, and replicated in the future so that the true promise of workplace wellness interventions can be fulfilled.

References

1. RZ Goetzel, RJ Ozminkowski. The health and cost benefits of work site health-promotion programs. *Annu Rev Public Health* 2008; **29**: 303–323.

2. S Mattke, KA Kapinos, JP Caloveras, et al. Workplace wellness programs: services offered, participation, and incentives. *RAND Health Q* 2015; **5**(2): 7.

3. Centers for Medicare & Medicaid Services. The Affordable Care Act and wellness programs. 2012. www.cms.gov/CCIIO/Resou rces/Fact-Sheets-and-FAQs/wellness1120 2012a.html (accessed April 21, 2020).

4. B Ramazzini. *Diseases of Workers*. Classics of Medicine Library; Special ed., 1983.

5. S Mukherjee. *The Emperor of All Maladies: A Biography of Cancer*. New York, Scribner; 2010.

6. RN Stearns. *The Industrial Revolution in World History* (4th ed.). New York, Routledge; 2018.

7. TD Schneid. *Safety Law: Legal Aspects in Occupational Safety and Health*. Boca Raton, FL, CRC Press; 2018.

8. S Mattke, H Liu, J Caloyeras, et al. Workplace wellness programs study: final report. *RAND Health Q* 2013; **3**(2): 7.

9. DL Gebhardt, CE Crump. Employee fitness and wellness programs in the workplace. *Am Psychologist* 1990; **45**: 262–272.

10. F Isaac, P Flynn. Johnson & Jonson LIVE FOR LIFE Program: now and then. *Am J Health Promot* 2001; **15**: 365–367.

11. CA Heaney. Worksite health interventions: targets for change and strategies for attaining them. In: JC Quick, LE Tetrick, eds., *Handbook of Occupational Health Psychology* (2nd ed.). Washington, DC, American Psychological Association; 2014; 319–336.

12. M Shain, DM Kramer. Health promotion in the workplace: framing the concept; reviewing the evidence. *Occup Environ Med* 2004; **61**: 643–648.

13. L Linnan, M Bowling, J Childress, et al. Results of the 2004 national worksite health promotion survey. *Am J Public Health* 2008; **98**(8): 1503–1509.

14. S Mattke, C Schnyer, KR Van Busum. A review of the U.S. workplace wellness market. *RAND Health Q* 2013; **2**(4): 7.

15. EC Aneni, LL Roberson, W Maziak, et al. A systematic review of internet-based worksite wellness approaches for cardiovascular disease risk management: outcomes, challenges, & opportunities. *PLoS One* 2014; **9**(1): 1–11.

16. A Rongen, SJW Robroek, FJ van Lenthe, A Burdorf. Workplace health promotion: a meta-analysis of effectiveness. *Am J Prev Med* 2013; **44**(4): 406–415.

17. LM Anderson, TA Quinn, K Glanz, et al. The effectiveness of worksite nutrition and physical activity interventions for controlling employee overweight and obesity. *Am J Prev Med* 2009; **37**(4): 340–357.

18. CL Cooper, PJ Dewe, MP O'Driscoll. Employee assistance programs: strengths, challenges, and future roles. In: JC Quick, LE Tetrick, eds., *Handbook of Occupational Health Psychology* (2nd ed.). Washington, DC, American Psychological Association; 2014; 337–356.

19. LR Murphy. Stress management in work settings: a critical review of the health effects. *Am J Health Promot* 1996; **11**(2): 112–135.

20. KM Richardson, HR Rothstein. Effects of occupational stress management intervention programs: a meta-analysis. *J Occup Health Psych* 2008; **13**(1): 69–93.

21. KA Aikens, J Astin, KR Pelletier, et al. Mindfulness goes to work: impact of an online workplace intervention. *J Occup Environ Med* 2014; **56**(7): 721–731.

22. D Allexandre, AM Bernstein, E Walker, et al. A web-based mindfulness stress management program in a corporate call center: a randomized clinical trial to evaluate the added benefit of onsite group support. *J Occup Environ Med* 2016; **58**(3): 254–264.

23. J van Berkel, CRL Boot, KI Proper, et al. Process evaluation of a workplace health promotion intervention aimed at improving work engagement and energy balance. *J Occup Environ Med* 2013; **55**(1): 19–26.

24. T Lomas, JC Medina, I Ivtzan, et al. Mindfulness-based interventions in the workplace: an inclusive systematic review and meta-analysis of their impact upon wellbeing. *J Pos Psych* 2018. DOI:10.1080/17439760.2018.1519588.

25. K Baicker, D Cutler, Z Song. Workplace wellness programs can generate savings. *Health Affairs* 2010; **29**(2): 1–8.

26. RW Jeffery, JL Forster, SA French, et al. The healthy worker project: a work-site intervention for weight control and smoking cessation. *Am J Public Health* 1993; **83**(3): 395–401.

27. RM Merrill, A Anderson, SM Thygerson. Effectiveness of a worksite wellness program on health behaviors and personal health. *J Occup Environ Med* 2011; **53**(9): 1008–1012.

28. VS Conn, AR Hafdahl, PS Cooper, et al. Meta-analysis of workplace physical activity interventions. *Am J Prev Med* 2009; **37**(4): 330–339.

Wellness Interventions for Physicians and Healthcare Professionals

Matthew Goldenberg and Itai Danovitch

Introduction

Delivering healthcare is both a deeply gratifying and a demanding occupation. Physicians and healthcare professionals (clinicians) are trained to have a knowledge base and skill set that are firmly rooted in evidence and hard science. However, they must also be facile with the soft skills, exhibiting flexibility and creativity when addressing unknown or unexpected challenges. In today's highly matrixed healthcare environment it often is not enough for a clinician to be a skilled practitioner with a compassionate bedside manner; they may have to serve as scholar, expert, administrator, and leader of teams, managing staff without the benefit of clear lines of accountability. When all goes well, the clinician is able to sustain high levels of productivity over a long career, taking good care of patients and supporting health system transformation while simultaneously being engaged members of their family and fulfilling roles within their communities.

Over the last two decades, this aspirational balance has become more difficult. The scales have tipped as clinicians have experienced significant new work demands and fundamental changes to the context within which healthcare must be delivered. Well-intentioned efforts to increase standardization, improve quality, and reduce heterogeneity have contributed to what some have wryly described as the "Toyotization" of medicine [1–2]. With widespread adoption of time-consuming electronic health platforms, many providers have lamented diverting attention from patients to digital devices. Escalations in healthcare operating costs and widespread consolidation have reduced the number of individual and small-group practices, previously a source of decentralization and autonomy across medicine [3]. And perpetual change in the market for healthcare insurance has led to a dynamic in which patients cycle in and out of practices, undermining the vital physician–patient relationship.

When external demands exceed internal resources, the consequence is stress. Sustained stress can contribute to occupational burnout, a syndrome characterized by emotional exhaustion, depersonalization, and a low sense of personal accomplishment. The consequences of burnout have been well characterized [4–5]. For clinicians, burnout is associated with family and marital problems, an array of somatic symptoms and health problems, anxiety, depression, substance-use disorders, and suicide. For patients, clinician burnout is associated with decreased satisfaction, safety, and quality of care. And for healthcare practices or systems, burnout is associated with low morale and high clinician turnover, with significant replacement costs.

Perhaps because of the highly visible individual effects of burnout, initial efforts to develop remedies focused on individuals: calls for education on relaxation techniques, coaching on stress management, or encouragement to strive for personal life balance. However, in the face of continued nationwide escalation in the prevalence of burnout and a growing outcry from clinicians that it simply is not possible to solve widespread systemic challenges solely through personal stress management, a series of systems-oriented wellness models began to emerge.

As an example, the National Academy of Medicine (NAM) established an Action Collaborative of 50 organizations committed to reversing trends in burnout and promoting clinician well-being [4, 6]. Goals for the Action Collaborative include: improving baseline understanding of challenges to clinician well-being; raising the visibility of clinician stress and burnout; and elevating evidence-based, multidisciplinary solutions that will improve patient care by caring for the caregiver. This initiative developed a conceptual model with seven domains contributing to wellness, five of which were outside of the direct control of the clinician (Figure 21.1). The NAM model depicts the factors associated with clinician well-being and resilience, applies these factors across all healthcare professions, specialties, settings, and career stages, and emphasizes the link between clinician well-being and outcomes for clinicians, patients, and the health system.

The Stanford WellMD Center developed a similar model, highlighting three overarching domains contributing to professional fulfillment: (1) a culture of wellness (shared values, behaviors, and leadership qualities that prioritize personal and professional growth, community, and compassion for self and others); (2) efficiency of practice (workplace systems, processes, and practices that promote safety, quality, effectiveness, positive patient and colleague interactions, and work–life balance); and (3) personal resilience (individual skills, behaviors, and attitudes that contribute to physical, emotional, and professional well-being).

In 2017 the Accreditation Council for Graduate Medical Education (ACGME), the governing body for US-based residency programs, changed their core requirements to promote both resident and attending physician health and to require time be provided to allow physicians to address mental health needs [7]. The new requirements emphasize "that psychological, emotional, and physical well-being are critical in the development of the competent, caring, and resilient physician" [8].

These models and initiatives converged with and were fueled by a series of peer-reviewed publications, white papers, and position statements highlighting that widespread burnout is a symptom of widespread problems. These problems are heterogeneous, they vary by geography, care setting, and clinician type. And burnout itself is not a diagnosis, it is a syndrome, a final common pathway. Thus, rather than singular solutions, it is necessary to have a range of options and customizable strategies. In order to cultivate and sustain a workforce of clinicians characterized by ingenuity, flexibility, and perseverance, it is necessary to establish an environment and infrastructure that supports the attributes that enable thriving: self-reliance, interpersonal communication skills, adaptability, resilience, and stamina. This chapter reviews the approaches and interventions that promote well-being and thriving among clinicians in healthcare settings.

Wellness Promotion Strategies

Strategies to promote wellness can be thought of along two organizing principles. There are spheres of control, beginning with the individual clinician, and rising to the practice setting, the organization, and finally the healthcare system (Figure 21.2). And within each sphere, a continuum of strategies exists that ranges from prevention to intervention. Of course, these are interdependent concepts, and typically both individual interventions and organizational

EXTERNAL FACTORS

SOCIETY & CULTURE

- Alignment of societal expectations and clinician's role
- Culture of safety and transparency
- Discrimination and overt and unconscious bias
- Media portrayal
- Patient behaviors and expectations
- Political and economic climates
- Social determinants of health
- Stigmatization of mental illness

RULES & REGULATIONS

- Accreditation, high-stakes assessments, and publicized quality ratings
- Documentation and reporting requirements
- HR policies and compensation issues
- Initial licensure and certification
- Insurance company policies
- Litigation risk
- Maintenance of licensure and certification
- National and state policies and practices
- Reimbursement structure
- Shifting systems of care and administrative requirements

ORGANIZATIONAL FACTORS

- Bureaucracy
- Congruent organizational mission and values
- Culture, leadership, and staff engagement
- Data collection requirements
- Diversity and Inclusion
- Harassment and discrimination
- Level of support for all healthcare team members
- Power dynamics
- Professional development opportunities
- Scope of practice
- Workload, performance, compensation, and value attributed to work elements

LEARNING/PRACTICE ENVIRONMENT

- Autonomy
- Collaborative vs. competitive environment
- Curriculum
- Health IT interoperability and Usability/Electronic health records
- Learning and practice setting
- Mentorship program
- Physical learning and practice conditions
- Professional relationships
- Student affairs policies
- Student-centered and patient-centered focus
- Team structures and functionality
- Workplace safety and violence

HEALTH CARE RESPONSIBILITIES

- Administrative responsibilities
- Alignment of responsibility and authority
- Clinical responsibilities
- Learning/career stage
- Patient population
- Specialty related issues
- Student/trainee responsibilities
- Teaching and research responsibilities

INDIVIDUAL FACTORS

PERSONAL FACTORS

- Access to a personal mentor
- Inclusion and connectivity
- Family dynamics
- Financial stressors/economic vitality
- Flexibility and ability to respond to change
- Level of engagement/connection to meaning and purpose in work
- Personality traits
- Personal values, ethics and morals
- Physical, mental, and spiritual well-being
- Relationships and social support
- Sense of meaning
- Work-life integration

SKILLS & ABILITIES

- Clinical Competency level/experience
- Communication skills
- Coping skills
- Delegation
- Empathy
- Management and leadership
- Mastering new technologies or proficient use of technology
- Optimizing work flow
- Organizational skills
- Resilience skills/practices
- Teamwork skills

Figure 21.1 Factors affecting clinician well-being and resilience. Reprinted with permission from the National Academy of Sciences, Courtesy of the National Academies Press, Washington, DC (https://nam.edu/clinicianwellbeing/wp-content/uploads/2018/10/Factors-Affecting-Clinician-Well-Being-and-Resilience.pdf).

FACTORS AFFECTING CLINICIAN WELL-BEING AND RESILIENCE

This conceptual model depicts the factors associated with clinician well-being and resilience; applies these factors across all health care professions, specialties, settings, and career stages; and emphasizes the link between clinician well-being and outcomes for clinicians, patients, and the health system. The model should be used to understand well-being, rather than as a diagnostic or assessment tool. In electronic form, the external and individual factors of the conceptual model are hyperlinked to corresponding landing pages on the Clinician Well-Being Knowledge Hub. The Clinician Well-Being Knowledge Hub provides additional information and resources. The conceptual model will be revised as the field develops and more information becomes available.

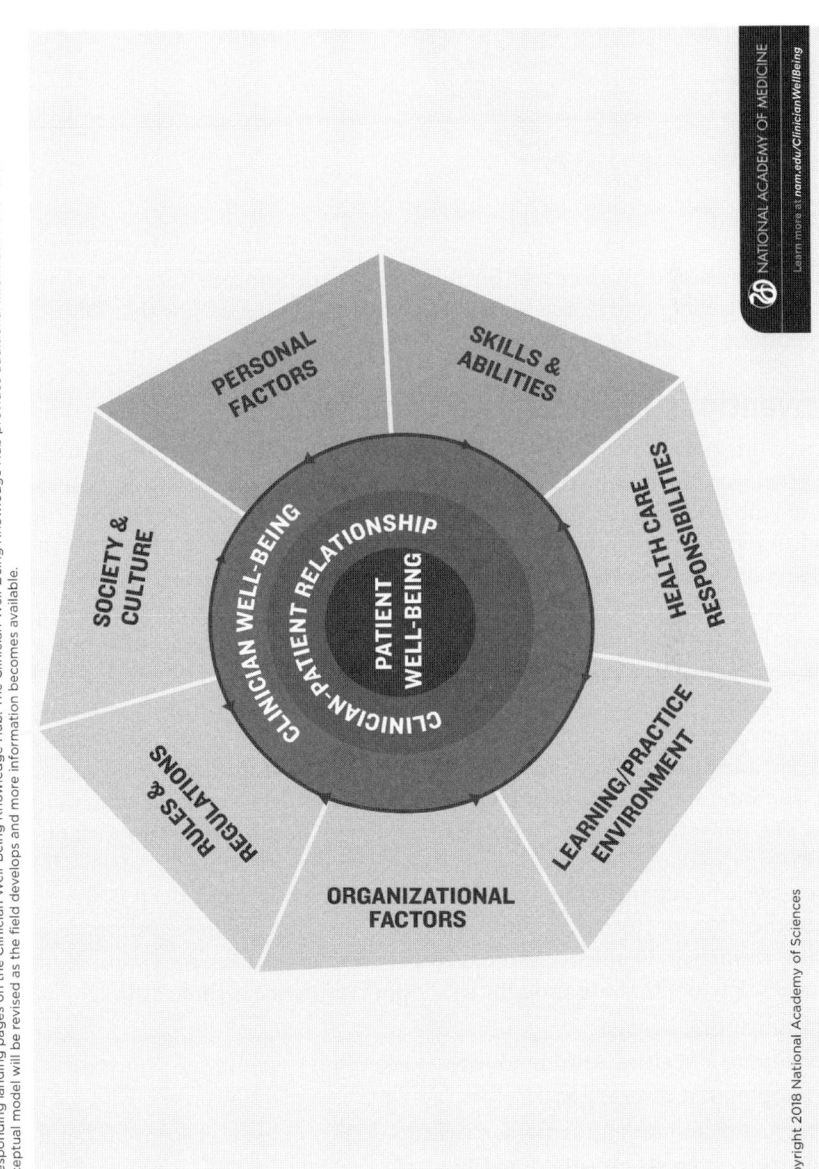

Copyright 2018 National Academy of Sciences

Figure 21.1 (cont.)

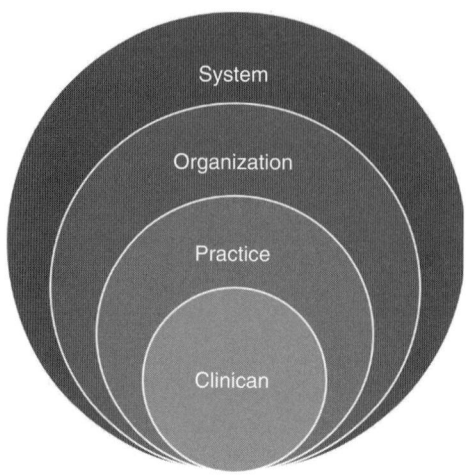

Figure 21.2 Levels of interventions for wellness promotion.

changes are needed to decrease burnout rates and improve the mental wellness of the healthcare provider workforce [9–10]. Nevertheless, in the review that follows, we organize interventions according to this rubric.

Interventions for Individual Clinicians

Effective integration of work and life activities is crucial to fostering a sustainable career [11]. However, for many clinicians, the practical challenge of setting boundaries, making personal life a priority, or simply taking time for self-care, feels like swimming upstream. A straightforward intervention addressing this issue is supporting utilization of regular vacations and off-work periods and managing work intrusions during off times by establishing coverage, or where coverage is not possible, clear parameters on communication. Physicians commonly have difficulty establishing distinct periods outside of work without work intrusions. One study found that physicians spend up to seven hours, after hours and on the weekends, per week utilizing electronic documentation and communication [12]. Encouraging clinicians to disconnect electronic devices during weekends and holidays, when an adequate coverage plan is in place, is an important component of fostering work–life integration and outside-of-work interests. Development of activities outside of work, whether it be interests, hobbies, or time with family, is also important. Additionally, prioritizing time outside of work may allow for some additional strategies for clinicians to improve well-being, including optimal nutrition, exercise, and sleep [13].

Another major priority for clinicians seeking to improve their wellness is to develop and enhance resilience. Resilience is vital to recovering after facing psychological stresses or challenges. Factors that are thought to support resilience include [14]:

- emotional intelligence;
- developing a healthy attitude toward work;
- developing self-awareness;
- recognizing and accepting personal limitations;
- nurturing interests outside of work;
- maintaining healthy personal and professional relationships.

While the above skills may seem somewhat abstract to a clinician who is experiencing symptoms of burnout and/or low mental wellness, with deliberate attention it is possible to cultivate them over time. For instance, emotional intelligence is the capacity to be aware of, control, and express one's emotions, and to handle interpersonal relationships judiciously and empathetically. By learning to identify their internal feelings and outward communication style, clinicians can become more empowered to regain control of what might be a chaotic and burnout-promoting working environment [15].

There is also ample evidence that mindfulness-based stress reduction and compassion cultivation increase resilience and decrease burnout [16–18]. Mindfulness is the state of being aware/being conscious of something. As a therapeutic process, mindfulness is a state achieved by focusing one's awareness on the present moment, acknowledging one's thoughts, feelings, and body sensations with compassion and without judgment. This is highly valuable for clinicians, particularly given the reality that medical training, while explicitly encouraging compassion, can at times inadvertently reinforce coping strategies that rely on suppressing emotions to manage expedience.

These interventions can be employed by clinicians at any stage of their career. However, there are specific interventions for medical students and residents, who are also susceptible to burnout. Autonomy, building of competence, and strong social relatedness have been found to be most associated with resident well-being. While working hour restrictions have come under critique for undermining training quality [19], there are also indications that increased sleep and time away from work are associated with greater resident well-being. Decreasing burnout and increasing well-being and resilience in residence has been found to be associated with increased empathy [20]. A new culture and standard are best set early in a clinician's training and medical schools and residency programs are well positioned to promote this cultural shift.

Another intervention for trainees is to find a well-being and wellness mentor. This would not be a clinical mentor, but instead one to help foster and promote development of behaviors that will lead to a sustainable career and enhanced mental well-being. Mentoring programs that pair trainees and early-career clinicians with more seasoned professionals can help fill in gaps in training about the day-to-day realities of the practice of medicine. Having support, someone to communicate with and model behavior after, and someone who can observe for signs of burnout can be a mutually beneficial relationship.

We encourage all clinicians to be proactive, to promote their own mental wellness and not wait until their mental health is suffering to seek help and assistance. However, when impairment is suspected, it is essential to have an evaluation by a professional who is experienced at evaluating healthcare professionals with suspected impairment. The evaluation should be customized to specifically answer the questions that need to be addressed, including current fitness for duty. California Public Protection and Physician Health (CPPPH), a non-profit organization based in California, has created guidelines on how to properly evaluate a healthcare provider with suspected impairment [21].

Practice-Level Interventions

Efficient working environments have optimized systems, process, and practices that help clinicians and their teams provide compassionate evidence-based care for their patients. Physicians who work in systems that restrict or impair their ability to provide optimal care for their patients experience decreased efficiency and increased risk of burnout. Factors commonly associated with inefficient practices include excessive time pressures and chaotic work environments. While it is important that the previously discussed individual interventions are available to clinicians, several meta-analyses have shown that both individual and organizationally led strategies are needed to effectively decrease rates of burnout. In fact, when directly compared, organization-directed approaches may have greater overall effects [9–10].

Electronic medical records (EMRs) are a major point of contention and focus. Those of us who were in practice around 2007–2012, when many institutions rolled out their EMRs, can recall clinicians who literally retired from the practice of medicine in response. For those who continued to practice, there needed to be a compromise between the way they were trained (and had been practicing) and what was now possible after the integration of EMRs into their practice. Many clinicians significantly increased their work hours in order to absorb new administrative requirements while maintaining practice volumes. Commonly, they adapted by increasing the work they brought home, completing notes during off-work hours, checking electronic inboxes on nights and weekends.

Two interventions that can have significant benefits for improving well-being are increasing teamwork and re-engineering practice workflows. Increased teamwork can be achieved by training staff and thoughtfully laying out the physical work areas of staff to enhance face-to-face verbal communication and decrease reliance on electronic messaging. Co-locating workstations enables clinicians to sit amid their colleagues and support staff (nurses, medical assistants, etc.), which facilitates both camaraderie and efficient flow of relevant information. Practices can also make changes to the workflow for clinicians and all staff to promote interaction with patients and decrease reliance on electronic messaging between visits. Pre-visit planning can be enhanced to include ordering of lab tests prior to the visit, so that lab results can be discussed in person. Utilizing a medical assistant or nurse to conduct a medication review, set agendas, complete forms, and close gaps in administrative care coordination can promote additional clinician time with patients.

Practices can also develop systems to filter electronic and paper information that would normally pass to clinicians by increasing verbal updates between staff. For example, normal laboratory results, prescription renewals, and other requests can be handled by delegates or well-trained assistants who brief the clinician with scheduled meetings throughout the day. The focus should be developing a team to support the indirect patient care tasks that typically burden the clinician, or bottleneck the team and make the practice less efficient. Having stable, well-trained teams that work together every day and meet regularly makes medical practices less chaotic, saves time, meets patients' needs more quickly, and increases sustainability for members of the care team.

One final example of a tool to improve the efficiency of the practice of medicine is the utilization of clerical documentation assistants, or "scribes." Along with the clinician, they can capture medical notes for the patient record, enter orders, prepare the after-visit summaries, and reinforce the care plan with the patient. In one study, utilizing pre-med students and others as scribes saved internists 75 minutes, and geriatricians 152 minutes, in a four-hour session. Scribes have been shown to save physicians more than three hours of work each day in some practices [22]. The AMA has created modules and online resources through www.stepsforward.org, where more specifics on interventions and implementation strategies can be reviewed for each goal.

Organizational Interventions

Organizations must also change and adapt to support the well-being of their clinicians and practices. Accordingly, senior leadership must be engaged in developing and evaluating interventions that support the physical and psychological health of the workforce. Ultimately, the case for clinician well-being is a case for a productive, sustainable, thriving organization with an engaged workforce delivering efficient practices, high-quality care, and satisfied patients [14].

A culture of wellness includes a set of normative values, attitudes, and behaviors that promote self-care, personal and professional growth, and compassion for colleagues, patients, and self [23]. Often lost in modern-day discussions about clinician well-being and the burnout epidemic is that caring and healing can be joyful activities. According to the Institute for Health Care Improvement, approaching solutions from an assets-based orientation (i.e., not just intervening where there are deficits) enables more innovative solutions and serves to promote primary prevention [24]. It is important for leadership to address fairness and equity as they are major contributors to bringing joy to the workplace. By taking an approach that gets full buy-in and engagement of all staff members in the mission, joy can be experienced by an entire team. The IHI developed a four-step model that encourages leaders to implement a wellness performance improvement pathway characterized by the following iterative steps [24] (Figure 21.3):

1. Ask staff, "What matters to you?"
2. Identify unique impediments to joy in work in the local context.

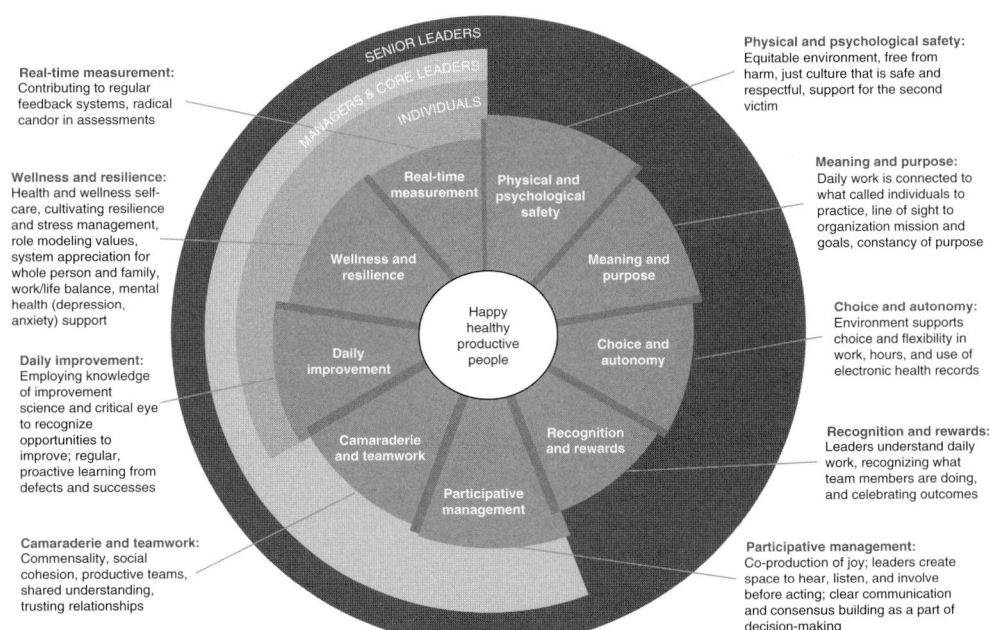

Figure 21.3 Institute for Healthcare Improvement framework for ensuring a joyful, engaging workforce.

3. Commit to a systems approach to making joy in work a shared responsibility at all levels of the organization.
4. Use improvement science to test approaches to improving joy in work in your organization.

Leaders can use their positions to raise awareness and make the case that improved clinician well-being improves patient outcomes and has meaningful financial implications. A key component of organizational wellness is committing to the collection of data and measures that are linked to staff engagement, well-being, and burnout. Such measures can be used to drive improvement initiatives, development of policies, assignment of resources, and to signal the seriousness with which the institution takes wellness.

If organizational leaders set a goal to improve and sustain a thriving workforce, a series of strategies can be employed to implement change. Given the significance of the clinical burden associated with the EMR, assigning appropriate resources to optimize workflows involving the EMR is a priority. Volume-based productivity goals may have their role in assessing clinician productivity, but they can lead to unintended consequences and are not an adequate mechanism to incentivize clinician behavior. Measuring and setting incentives around quality, value, and well-being may liberate teams and clinicians to develop local innovations that both improve efficiency and well-being.

Another important area of policy intervention involves work hours and access to wellness-promoting nutrition and activities while on-site. For example, organizations may be able to promote resilience of their workforce by limiting work hours and providing access to healthy food options, on-site exercise facilities, and places to practice relaxation, meditation, or to get rest during on-call, overnight, or long shifts [14].

While some clinicians may seek opportunities to take extra shifts to enhance their income, there are situations where lack of having a backup or having a fully staffed department prevent clinicians from taking desired time off. Even voluntary overtime has been linked to decreased health, and it is vital for healthcare organizations to minimize staffing arrangements that consistently rely on overtime [25]. Leadership should consider policies that impact the workforce even when they are off-site. For example, clinicians should not be discouraged from taking necessary leaves of absence to rehabilitate their health and wellness. If the institutional environment is supportive, it allows the individual clinician to take acceptance and accountability for their own work–life balance.

Another focus of leadership should be to increase job stability and fully staff required positions. Understaffing is a major source of need for overtime. Nurse absenteeism has been found to be related to violence at work. Decreased physical and mental health in nurses was found where violence was present in the workplace [26]. Healthcare systems therefore must establish a zero-tolerance environment in which violence will not be condoned, and safety is a priority.

Finally, hospital leadership, medical staff, and well-being committees should provide education about the signs of burnout. These include: isolation, withdrawing, irritability, falling behind on workload or taking more time to complete usual tasks, and increased substance-use or depression. An open, blame-free culture allows identifying workplace burnout and hazards, and the reporting of "near misses" and workplace incidents.

Systems Interventions

The practice of medicine by any clinician is embedded within the context of their practice, their organization, and the health system or health policy environment within which they practice. Over the last decade a series of reports by national organizations including, but not limited to, the AMA, the NAM, the Institute of Healthcare Innovation, and the Accreditation Council for Graduate Medical Education (ACGME) have made it clear that reducing burnout and promoting well-being are fundamental goals for our national healthcare system. These organizations have helped to bring attention to the importance of these issues and have mapped out a series of strategies at all levels of healthcare, from practice to policy. While many of their proposed strategies have been covered in the prior sections, there are several areas that exist within but also beyond the sphere of control of individual organizations.

Studies have shown that early-career physicians do not feel prepared for the stresses of medicine in their training [27]. Medical schools and residency programs can address this by incorporating specific attention to the stress and operational realities of medicine within their curricula. In 2017, the ACGME [7] revised the Common Program requirements for residency programs. They have mandated that residency programs must "make efforts to enhance the meaning that each resident finds in the experience of being a physician, including protecting time with patients, minimizing non-physician obligations, providing administrative support, promoting progressive autonomy and flexibility, and enhancing professional relationships." Their mandates also include the attending faculty, as well as the resident physicians. They have encouraged residency programs to develop policies and programs that "encourage optimal resident and faculty member well-being." Physician health and resilience competencies were adopted by the Royal College of Physicians and Surgeons of Canada and the College of Family Physicians of Canada [28].

Stigma continues to be a major barrier to prevention and early intervention among clinicians. Licensing boards commonly request information about historical psychological history unrelated to current functional status. Focusing on a distant history of psychiatric symptoms is potentially prejudicial and exacerbates secrecy and shame. It also increases fear of seeking help. A more enlightened approach would emphasize current functional status over lifetime impairment, and would be paired with accessible clinician wellness or diversion programs that offer support to potentially vulnerable clinicians rather than unjustified restrictive actions. Currently there is enormous state-to-state variability in clinician wellness programs.

There is a pressing need for research on the factors that contribute to well-being, as well as the interventions that are effective in preventing burnout and promoting well-being. Burnout is a syndrome, not a diagnosis, and there is a need to refine the reliability and validity of the construct, as well as its associations with other conditions and relevant outcomes. As specific interventions are rolled out or piloted, it is vital to use qualitative or quantitative methods to assess the impact of these interventions, and to determine what organizational or systems factors are necessary to facilitate widespread dissemination and implementation.

Conclusion

Providing outstanding, high-value patient care requires a workforce that is highly competent, agile, and innovative. In the current healthcare climate, symptoms of burnout among clinicians are highly prevalent, and there are not adequate resources, supports, and interventions to support the healthcare workforce. While every clinician has a responsibility to personally take care of themselves, it is imperative that we cultivate a context and environment that supports clinicians. We have provided a summary of the individual, practice-level, organizational, and system-wide strategies that can improve clinician wellness. We also encourage further efforts to destigmatize clinician mental health, to decrease the fear surrounding reaching out for help and the appropriate evaluation and treatment when needed.

References

1. J Moraros, M Lemstra, C Nwankwo. Lean interventions in healthcare: do they actually work? A systematic literature review. *Int J Qual Health Care* 2016; **28**(2): 150–165.

2. ST Teich, FF Faddoul. Lean management: the journey from Toyota to healthcare. *Rambam Maimonides Med J* 2013; **4**(2): e0007.

3. LR Burns, JC Goldsmith, A Sen. Horizontal and vertical integration of physicians: a tale of two tails. In: *Annual Review of Health Care Management: Revisiting the Evolution of Health Systems Organization*. Bingley: *Emerald Group Publishing*; 2014; 39–117.

4. T Brigham, C Barden, AL Dopp, et al. A journey to construct an all-encompassing conceptual model of factors affecting clinician well-being and resilience. NAM Perspectives Discussion Paper. National Academy of Medicine, Washington, DC; 2018. https://nam.edu/journey-construct-encompassing-conceptual-model-factors-affecting-clinician-well-resilience (accessed April 21, 2020).

5. LN Dyrbye, TD Shanafelt, CA Sinsky, et al. Burnout among health care professionals: a call to explore and address this underrecognized threat to safe, high-quality care. NAM Perspectives Discussion Paper. National Academy of Medicine, Washington, DC; 2017. https://nam.edu/burnout-among-health-care-professionals-a-call-to-explore-and-address-this-underrecognized-threat-to-safe-high-quality-care (accessed April 21, 2020).

6. VJ Dzau, DG Kirch, TJ Nasca. To care is human: collectively confronting the clinician-burnout crisis. *N Engl J Med* 2018; **378**(4): 312–314.

7. ACGME (Accreditation Council for Graduate Medical Education). Improving physician well-being, restoring meaning in medicine. www.acgme.org/What-We-Do/Initiatives/Physician-Well-Being (accessed April 21, 2020).

8. ACGME (Accreditation Council for Graduate Medical Education). ACGME common program requirements. www.acgme.org/What-We-Do/Accreditation/Common-Program-Requirements (accessed April 21, 2020).

9. M Panagioti, E Panagopoulou, P Bower, et al. Controlled interventions to reduce burnout in physicians: a systematic review and meta-analysis. *JAMA Intern Med* 2017; **177**(2): 195–205.

10. CP West, LN Dyrbe, PJ Erwin, TD Shanafelt. Interventions to prevent and reduce physician burnout: a systematic review and meta-analysis. *Lancet* 2016; **388** (10057): 2272–2281.

11. TD Shanafelt, CM Balch, GJ Bechamps, et al. Burnout and career satisfaction among American surgeons. *Ann Surg* 2009; **250**(3): 463–471.

12. BG Arndt, JW Beasley, MD Watkinson, et al. Tethered to the EHR: primary care physician workload assessment using EHR event log data and time-motion observations. *Ann Fam Med* 2017; **15**(5): 419–426.

13. MS Hamidi, MK Boggild, AM Cheung. Running on empty: a review of nutrition and physicians' well-being. *Postgrad Med J* 2016; **92**(1090): 478–481.

14. B Bohman, L Dyrbye, CA Sinksy, et al. Physician well-being: the reciprocity of practice efficiency, culture of wellness, and personal resilience. *NEJM Catalyst* 2017.

15. A Omid, F Haghani, P Adibi. Emotional intelligence: an old issue and a new look in clinical teaching. *Adv Bio Res* 2018; **7**(32). DOI:10.4103/2277-9175.225926.

16. T Singer, OM Klimecki. Empathy and compassion. *Curr Biol* 2014; **24**(18): R875–R878.

17. CP West, LN Dyrbye, JT Rabatin, et al. Intervention to promote physician well-being, job satisfaction, and professionalism: a randomized clinical trial. *JAMA Intern Med* 2014; **174**(4): 527–533.

18. MS Krasner, RM Epstein, H Beckman, et al. Association of an educational program in mindful communication with burnout, empathy, and attitudes among primary care physicians. *JAMA Intern Med* 2009; **302**(12): 1284–1293.

19. N Ahmed, K Devitt, I Keshet, et al. A systematic review of the effects of resident duty hour restrictions in surgery: impact on resident wellness, training, and patient outcomes. *Ann Surg* 2014; **259**(6): 1041–1053.

20. KS Raj. Well-being in residency: a systematic review. *J Grad Med Educ* 2016; **8**(5): 674–684.

21. CPPPH. Guidelines. www.cppph.org/cppph-guidelines (accessed April 21, 2020).

22. DB Reuben, J Knudsen, W Senelick, E Glazier, BK Kortez. The effect of a physician partner program on physician efficiency and patient satisfaction. *JAMA Intern Med* 2014; **174**(7): 1190–1193.

23. C Sinksy, T Shanafelt, ML Murphy, et al. Creating the organizational foundation for joy in medicine. 2017. https://edhub.ama-assn.org/steps-forward/module/2702510 (accessed April 21, 2020).

24. J Perlo, B Balik, S Swensen, et al. IHI framework for improving joy in work. IHI White Paper, Institute for Healthcare Improvement, Cambridge, MA; 2017.

25. DGJ Beckers, D van der Linden, PGW Smulders, et al. Voluntary or involuntary? Control over overtime and rewards for overtime in relation to fatigue and work satisfaction. *Work Stress* 2008; **22**(1): 33–50.

26. M Itzhaki, I Bluvstein, A Peles Bortz, et al. Mental health nurse's exposure to workplace violence leads to job stress, which leads to reduced professional quality of life. *Front Psychiatry* 2018; **9**(59): 10.3389/fpsyt.2018.00059.

27. RS Patel, R Bachu, A Adikey, M Malik, M Shah. Factors related to physician burnout and its consequences: a review. *Behav Sci (Basel)*. 2018; **8**(11): 98.

28. D Puddester, L Flynn, J Cohen. *CanMEDS Physician Health Guide: A Practical Handbook for Physician Health and Well-Being*. Ottawa, The Royal College of Physicians and Surgeons of Canada; 2009.

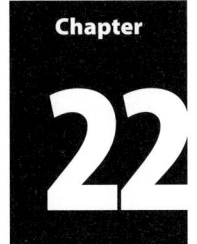

Chapter

Nutrition

James Lundy

Introduction

The field of wellness has a challenge. This challenge involves connecting wellness with the topic of nutrition. Logic would intuitively connect how a patient eats with how much wellness and vitality they exude. But this challenge is much more complex. Not only is how the field of nutrition is analyzed, measured, and quantified a tremendous confusion, but one must also carefully consider the individual biases of the researchers and any bureaucratic/institutional influence on those researchers.

From these multifactorial issues, many publications have arisen within the study of nutrition for each type of diet (or food consumption style) for humans. Each diet is "touted" as the best or most appropriate for some or all patients. Or certain foods are first banished as unhealthful, only to return to the limelight at a later date as now healthful. Obviously, these statements lead to significant and often contradictory messages to clinicians and patients alike. Therefore, this chapter will shed light on this vast topic and allow the reader to gain a better grasp of the topic for both personal and clinical use.

Diets, Wellness, and Health

Nutrition and diets have been traditionally studied from the context of health and not from a place of wellness. Any rational person would surmise that a "healthy" diet must result in a state of wellness. The difficulty is that wellness as a variable has been minimally measured in the context of nutrition or diets. A few studies have looked at happiness or subjective well-being in association with certain food types. However, the vast majority of diet/nutrition research has focused on health or biometric measures such as glycemic control, body weight, waist circumference, lipid factors, blood pressure, and other endocrine markers. These variables are then compared between two or three diets, trying to find significant support for the preferred "model" diet. But wellness, as a standalone variable, is usually not measured or even mentioned.

The minimal focus on nutrition and wellness in the research has focused on the brain and brain health. Some research suggests that nutrition can have some effect on the brain by way of gene expression [1]. Diet quality can also affect wellness measures of sleep duration and quality [2]. Other research has focused on brain health by studying diet's interaction with mental disorders. Depression is one disorder that has been linked and sought to treat through diet modification [3]. However, often food intake and diet quality is interconnected but not separated from other significant lifestyle modifications, such as exercise and smoking [4, 5]. As such, nutritional wellness with regard to brain health is not effectively elucidated.

Some very recent research has focused on the wellness topics of subjective well-being (happiness), general life satisfaction, and mental well-being with consumption of fruits and vegetables. In large, prospective, longitudinal panels in Australia and the United Kingdom, researchers note that increased consumption is positively and significantly associated with increased happiness and well-being [6, 7]. These results have often been dose-dependent, in that increased consumption per day or increased days per week consumed will result in higher levels of life satisfaction and improved mood. However, no other specific foods nor food categories have been directly compared to subjective well-being, either in clinical trials or epidemiological studies.

As such, wellness does not receive proper attention and focus. The physiology of the human body is easier to measure and report. Therefore, we will study human wellness in nutrition by proxy. Wellness will be implied by health, with a focus on more physiological factors and anthropometrics which are reported and measured within the research. It is reasonable to assume that when these factors improve by diet quality and choice, health improves as well as wellness.

In Search of the Perfect Diet

The ideal or perfect diet may be difficult to determine from the research. Some difficulty is inherent in how food and nutrition is studied, as previously noted. Another issue is how efficient and adaptive the human body can be in the many various locales, temperaments, and available foodstuffs. This ease of adaption means researchers may have more difficulty elucidating one style of eating over another.

With regard to adaption to foods and locations, humans can exist on diets ranging from 95 percent fat (as noted with the Inuits, who subsist on whale and seal with no vegetables) to 5 percent fat (as noted with the Ornish diet). The human physiology adapts to effectively metabolize any level of macronutrient consumed. And this adaptive nature allows humans to consume entirely meat-based diets, entirely plant-based diets, or combinations of the two. Ultimately this flexibility has allowed humankind to flourish no matter the location or whatever foods could be found, grown, or hunted. This adaptability should be considered remarkable and wonderful, and also demands significant respect. It may have been the one physiological component that allowed the human race to continue to subsist for thousands of years.

An additional challenge when seeking the perfect diet is studying deficiency diseases/chronic diseases and the incubation period. Compared to infectious diseases, which can develop with short incubation periods (hours to days) or drug clinical trials in which medication effects can be investigated very quickly, food consumption (healthy or unhealthy) takes long periods of time to develop disease conditions. The human system can exist for a reasonably long period of time before developing a disease of deficiency (e.g., scurvy requires vitamin C deficiency of 1–3 months to develop). Humans can consume inappropriate amounts of some substances for a long period of time before developing chronic diseases such as type 2 diabetes mellitus, hypertension, cardiovascular diseases, non-alcoholic liver disorder, and obesity. Since the nature of the human system is to remain vibrant and alive, metabolism has the flexibility to exist with both over- and underconsumption of healthy and unhealthy nutrients before diseases develop.

Thus, determining the perfect diet would require long periods of time-consuming study of various macronutrients, vitamins, minerals, etc. *while also in absence of any deficiency or chronic diseases*. This becomes challenging and expensive in research, which leads to the final challenge in nutrition research.

Aside from reductionist research to determine minimum amounts of each vitamin, mineral, etc., often research uses epidemiological studies to surmise the appropriate or perfect diet. The main challenge that exists as a huge challenge to epidemiology is causation versus correlation. Often, large population-based nutrition research using epidemiology makes correlations regarding nutrients and disease prevalence. But as all clinicians remember, correlation is not causation. These research findings cannot impart causation of disease from an individual food stuff because a third variable may be interacting or causing the disease. However, lay and professional publications commonly use associations/correlations as grounds for publishing and disseminating information. Some critics of nutritional epidemiology note that these study designs consistently present false and unreproducible conclusions which become the basis of public policy [8]. This research is often utilized or reported as a proxy of healthy/unhealthy consumption in the absence of large clinical trials. Therefore, the clinician must remain open-minded, as well as skeptical, whenever dealing with epidemiological nutritional research.

Investigating Various Diets

In this chapter, we will discuss the more common diets in the literature. These include the Mediterranean diet, Paleolithic diet, ketogenic diet, Dietary Approach to Stop Hypertension (DASH) diet, plant-based/vegetarian diet, FODMAP diet, modified Atkins diet, MIND diet, Ornish diet/lifestyle, and weight loss diets.

The word *diet* is used in this chapter as an easy manner to describe an eating style, paradigm, or system. There is no suggestion or indication that the word *diet* is meant for losing body fat or body weight, as what is commonly connoted with the word "diet." As you will see, each of the diets/food paradigms have supporting literature for their specific effectiveness in a variety of health concerns or diagnoses. Please keep an open mind as you read about each dietary style. We will compose a list of similarities at the end of this chapter.

Mediterranean Diet

The Mediterranean diet was first introduced by Ancel Keys in 1975 with his book *How to Eat Well and Stay Well the Mediterranean Way*, and had developed out of his Seven Countries Study that started in the late 1950s. The diet and food paradigm were further developed by an Italian research director named Anna Ferro-Luzzi and a Greek medical school professor named Antoina Tricholpoulou in the late 1980s. It gained popularity and was the subject of significant research after the landmark paper by Ferro-Luzzi in 1989 in which a workable definition of the diet was described and labeled [9].

The Mediterranean diet is not a specific form of eating but constitutes a general eating style that is modified and individualized by many countries surrounding the Mediterranean Sea. Thus, it has general properties but is not specific or dogmatic. It is hallmarked by the copious use of fruits, vegetables, whole grains, legumes, nuts, olive oil, and fish. Additionally, it recommends limited amounts of chicken, lamb, small amounts of dairy and red meat, as well as a moderate amount of wine consumed. The general percentage of macronutrients in research tends to be roughly 30 percent protein, 30 percent fat, and 40 percent carbohydrates.

The benefits of the Mediterranean diet are numerous:

1. reduced frailty in older persons [10, 11];
2. associated with lower rates of breast cancer [12–14], gastric cancer [15], nasopharyngeal cancer [16], endometrial cancer [17], pancreatic cancer [18], colorectal cancer [19], and prostate cancer [20];
3. decreased inflammation and insulin resistance with metabolic syndrome [21];
4. decreased BMI, waist circumference, inflammation, and insulin resistance [22];
5. reduced body weight [23] and waist circumference [24];
6. decreased diastolic blood pressure [25];
7. reduced cardiovascular disease/cardiovascular mortality [26];
8. reduced diabetes risk [27] and improved diabetes control [28, 29];
9. lower systemic inflammation and oxidative stress [30];
10. associated with reduced risk of depression [31];
11. better cognitive function [32] and lowered dementia rates [33], slower cognitive decline [34, 35], lowered Alzheimer's disease risk [36, 37], and delayed mortality from Alzheimer's disease [38];
12. decreased all-cause mortality [39].

Paleolithic Diet

The Paleolithic or "Paleo diet" is a food plan that is proposed as what was eaten prior to an agricultural era [40–42]. The proponents state that it mimics what our hunter-gatherer ancestors would have eaten by either foraging or hunting. Research on this diet has been extrapolated from modern and recent-past hunter-gatherer groups, as well as the stomach contents from unearthed ancient human remains.

Since the Paleo diet focuses on pre-agricultural foods, it limits or eliminates most agricultural products such as grains, corn, refined carbohydrates, and legumes (beans). Additionally, it limits other substances such as dairy, sugar, and all oils and salt (all of which would not have been present prior to agricultural development). The main components focus on lean meats, fruits, vegetables, nuts, and any substance grown wildly, which could include mushrooms, tubers, or other plants. One of the benefits extolled by this diet is the fiber content, estimated from historical data, which is significantly higher than typical modern diets.

The benefits of the Paleolithic diet are:

1. improved cardiovascular measures such as decreased blood pressure, reductions in total cholesterol, LDL cholesterol, and triglycerides [43];
2. improved glycemic control [44] and more satiating [45], improved glucose tolerance in type-2 diabetics [46];
3. significantly greater weight loss [47], and fat loss and weight loss in normal subjects [48, 49];
4. significantly satiating in normal subjects [50];
5. decreased fasting plasma leptin levels [51];
6. lowered systemic inflammation and oxidative stress [52];
7. lower risk of colorectal cancer [53];
8. decreased all-cause mortality [54].

Ketogenic Diet

The ketogenic diet or "keto diet" was first established in 1921 as a viable treatment for epilepsy [55]. It has since been extensively researched and consistently supported for this treatment. The discovery in 1967 that brain metabolism can use ketones as a viable energy source for brain function (instead of glucose/carbohydrates) altered how ketosis was viewed and respected [56].

Remember not to confuse ketosis with diabetic ketoacidosis. In ketosis, the ketone bodies circulating in the body are a very small magnitude (7/8 mmol/L of ketone bodies) and there is no change in pH of the blood. Conversely, *diabetic* ketoacidosis has substantially higher levels of circulating ketone bodies (>25 mmol/L) and acidic changes to blood pH [57]. Diabetic ketoacidosis is a very serious medical condition, whereas mild dietary ketosis is safe for months to years without any adverse concerns.

When the body is in a state of ketosis, it is utilizing free fatty acids either by diet or stored adipose tissue for metabolism and function. Glucose is still circulating throughout the bloodstream; however, ketones are utilized by cells in order to produce movement and activity. Traditionally, glucose has been considered the main energy source for the human body. But the ketone bodies are equally effective for brain and body energy. As such, consider ketosis and ketone bodies as a unique, different, and separate energy source for use by the human body. The benefit of multiple energy systems and this superb adaptability allows the human system to exist in different environments where different foods are available (summer, winter, mountain, desert, tropical, etc.)

The ketogenic diets has many benefits:

1. as an adjunct treatment with human cancer [58–60] and animal cancer studies [61, 62];
2. treatment for epileptic seizures [63–65];
3. weight loss [66–68] and body fat loss [69–71] while maintaining normal metabolic rate [72];
4. better hunger control [73];
5. improved serum cardiovascular biomarkers in normal subjects [74];
6. improved glucose control in diabetic animals [75], as well as weight loss in diabetic humans [76];
7. improved insulin control as well as weight loss [77].

Dietary Approaches to Stop Hypertension (DASH) Diet

The DASH diet was introduced in 1997 to examine healthy eating style in order to reduce or lower hypertension [78]. Additionally, it has focused on reducing mortality from these cardiovascular events, as well as strokes [79, 80]. The original research focused on ample fruits, vegetables, and low-fat dairy, as well as reduced saturated fat, total fat, and cholesterol.

Subsequently, a food questionnaire was developed that elucidated and stipulated components of the diet: (1) high intake of fruits, vegetables, whole grains, legumes and seeds, and low-fat dairy; and (2) low intake of red and processed meat, sugar-sweetened beverages, and sodium [80]. Reducing saturated fat was suggested by de-emphasizing red and processed meat. The DASH diet does not indicate specific macronutrient levels as a general rule.

The DASH diet has many benefits, including:

1. reduced systolic blood pressure [81, 82] and diastolic blood pressure [83];
2. improved cognitive function [84];
3. improved blood pressure in metabolic-syndrome and non-metabolic-syndrome subjects [85];
4. lower blood pressure within two weeks of starting the diet [86];
5. improved lipid components such as LDL and HDL cholesterol [87];
6. improves glycemic and oxidative stress in gestational diabetes [88] and obese patients [89];
7. decreased inflammation [90];
8. associated with lower risk of kidney disease [91];
9. decreased mortality in heart failure patients [92].

In contrast to the blood pressure changes, research from the Framingham study indicated that, in middle-aged adults, over a long period of time the DASH diet was not associated with decreased blood pressure or decreased hypertension [93]. As always, epidemiological research must be reviewed critically.

Plant-Based or Vegetarian Diet

The plant-based or vegetarian diet consists of a variety of grains, fruits, and vegetables, as well as the absence of animal protein in the form of beef, chicken, fish, pork, or eggs. Dairy is included in some and avoided in other vegetarian diets. Some vegetarians may eat eggs (ovo-vegetarian), dairy (lacto-vegetarian), or fish (pesce-vegetarian), or some combination of all three, in order to supplement their diets.

Vegans, in contrast, are the most restrictive, with the absence of all animal products of any kind. All nutrients for vegans come from plant-based products only. Plant or grain protein is the main source of protein for most vegetarians and for all vegan eaters.

The plant-based/vegetarian/vegan diet has many benefits:

1. decreased body fat [94, 95] and reduced body weight [96, 97];
2. improved insulin resistance and decreased diabetes risk [98, 99];
3. improved lipid biomarker profiles in addition to weight loss [100];
4. decreased blood pressure as well as improved lipid biomarkers [101, 102];
5. decreased total cholesterol, LDL cholesterol, and HDL cholesterol [103];
6. decreased cardiovascular risk [104], 105];
7. associated with lower colorectal cancer incidence, with pesco-vegetarians having the lowest incidence [106];
8. reduced all-cause [107] and cardiovascular/cancer mortality [108–110]; however, this is not consistent in all studies [111].

FODMAP Diet

The FODMAP diet (fermentable oligosaccharide, disaccharide, monosaccharide, and polyol) is a diet that restricts fermentable short-chain carbohydrates. It was originally developed from a diet based on fructose malabsorption in some patients [112]. It evolved to include other foods that can irritate patients with irritable bowel syndrome (IBS).

The mechanism of action suggests that these non-digested/fermented food fibers will create distension in the gut by both bacterial gas production and water retention affecting osmotic concentrations. This distension of the gut can cause the usual symptoms of bloating, flatulence, abdominal pain, and other symptoms.

The research for the use of the FODMAP diet has treatment and gastrointestinal (GI) ramifications:

1. reduced irritable bowel syndrome (IBS) symptoms in adults [113, 114] as well as children [115];
2. reduced exercise-induced GI distress in runners [116];
3. reduced symptoms with functional GI disorders with fructose/lactose intolerance [117];
4. improved GI symptoms such as bloating, gas, and constipation associated with IBS and inflammatory bowel disease [118, 119];
5. improved pain and GI symptoms with fibromyalgia [120];
6. altering microbiota in the colon of Crohn's disease patients [121].

Modified Atkins Diet

The modified Atkins diet is an extrapolation of the diet introduced by Robert Atkins, MD in 1992 in his book *Dr. Atkins' New Diet Revolution*. Dr. Atkins' food recommendations are based upon high protein, high fat, and low carbohydrates. It is similar to the ketogenic diet, with the same focus on higher fat and higher protein. However, the modified Atkins diet has a higher percentage of carbohydrate whereas the ketogenic diet is extremely low in carbohydrates (less than 30–50 g total per day).

The modified Atkins diet has many benefits:

1. reduced rate of epileptic seizures in children [122, 123], equal to the ketogenic diet [124];
2. weight loss [125] as well as improved risk factors for cardiovascular disease [126];
3. increased weight loss, decreased systolic blood pressure, improved glycemic control [127];
4. improved LDL/HDL cholesterol ratio [128];
5. reduced circulating glucose and improved glycohemoglobin levels (Hb1Ac) [129];
6. less hunger and negative affect accompanied with weight loss [130];
7. fewer food cravings for high carbohydrate/high sugar in addition to decreased appetite [131];
8. higher protein content does not affect kidney function compared to high carbohydrate diet in type-2 diabetics [132];
9. comparable to more restrictive ketogenic diet in the treatment of glucose transporter type-1 deficiency syndrome [133].

MIND Diet

The MIND Diet (Mediterranean-DASH Intervention for Neurodegenerative Delay) is a combination of the Mediterranean diet and the DASH diet. It is currently being investigated regarding brain health and mild weight loss. It includes 10 foods considered to be brain-healthy: whole grains, vegetables, berries, fish, poultry, beans, nuts, wine, and olive oil. Additionally, it limits five unhealthy foods such as: dairy, red meat, processed meat, sweets, and fast/fried foods. It is a relatively newer dietary intervention with the main focus on brain-related outcomes.

The MIND diet has been shown to:

1. reduce the incidence of Alzheimer's disease in those who strongly and moderately adhere to the diet [134];
2. reduce cognitive decline [135];
3. improve cognitive function [136];
4. improve verbal memory [137].

Ornish Diet/Lifestyle

The Ornish diet/lifestyle is a very low-fat (less than 10 percent of total energy) vegetarian diet with severe restrictions which focuses on the population with cardiovascular disease. The diet was initially studied along with exercise, behavior modification, stress reduction, and group support meetings in addition to the diet. As such, often the diet is associated with all-round positive changes, but as a diet it is a component of a multimodal treatment plan. A structured program is needed to maintain compliance, otherwise diet compliance drops notably [138];

The benefits of the Ornish Diet/Lifestyle include:

1. improved body weight, cardiac biomarkers, exercise capacity, and quality of life in patients with heart failure [139] and other cardiac patients [140, 141];
2. short-term improvement in cardiovascular status in 23 patients with ischemic heart disease [142];
3. reduced angina and delayed revascularization with cardiac patients [143];
4. regression of coronary atherosclerosis at one year [144] ;
5. regression of coronary atherosclerosis and fewer cardiac events at five years [145];
6. reduced BMI, body weight, and number of patients with angina; however, no change in atherosclerosis process in the carotid artery [146].

Weight Loss Diets

Several commercial and written diets have a focus on weight loss. These include: Weight Watchers Points Plus, Curves Complete 90-day Challenge, Jenny Craig at Home, and Nutrisystem Advance Select. These diets have been shown to reduce body weight equally well and better than controls [147]. In another study, four commercial diet systems (Slim Fast Plan, Weight Watchers Pure Points, Dr. Atkins' New Diet Revolution, and Rosemary Conley's "Eat Yourself Slim" Diet & Exercise Plan) resulted in loss of body weight and body fat at two and six months, but none significantly more than the others [148, 149]. Two other studies compared several diet plans (Atkins, Zone, Ornish, and Weight Watchers in 2005; Atkins, Zone, Ornish, and LEARN in 2007), with those on all diets losing similar amounts of weight, but usually the most weight was lost by subjects using the Atkins diet [125, 150]. Finally, in a recent meta-analysis of diets, the researchers suggested that all diets are equally effective at weight loss, and patients should be recommended a diet they will consistently follow [151].

Common Ideas Among All Diets

Diets are varied and diverse. Some use similar energy systems but with different macro-nutrient levels, such as the ketogenic and the modified Atkins diets. Some are used for individual-focused goals or have specific purposes, such as the FODMAP, Ornish, DASH diet, or MIND diets. Many diets exist to help people lose weight, and we have only touched upon several for which research exists. Some diets are meant for the general human population, such as the Mediterranean and Paleolithic diets.

With all of this diversity, here are some suggestions about all of them to consider when investigating your personal or patient's education:

1. All diets have research supporting their health- or disease-improving benefits. (Please read the research for yourself with a critical and skeptical nature – look for biases by the authors . . . there is usually one!)
2. No diet is superior in all aspects when compared to the other diets listed. (No diet works for all people [152].)
3. All diets consume whole foods and not ultra-processed foods, food substitutes, or imitation foods.
4. All diets are based upon different ratios of macronutrients (protein, fat, and carbohydrates).
5. All diets minimize or limit sugar (and often refined carbohydrate) intake.
6. Individuals are encouraged to avoid food allergens as necessary (common food allergies = dairy, gluten, nuts, shellfish, etc.).
7. Most diets do not emphasize dietary supplements such as vitamins or minerals (the only exception is B12 for vegans, who do not obtain this vitamin from plants and must take it as a supplement).
8. Most diets acknowledge the benefits of fiber, but vary in the amount or type of fiber (ketogenic having the least fiber volume and FODMAP having the most restriction on type of fiber).

This information gives a brief overview and the benefits of each type of diet. Please use this as a starting point with your patients in order to improve their health behaviors and lifestyles.

Discussion

In this chapter, we have investigated and presented characteristics of each diet and the respective research pertaining to these diets. The diets each impact multiple diseases and influence many biometric changes. However, for brevity's sake, only select and pertinent research has been presented; obviously more research is available for each diet paradigm. Additionally, other diets do exist in lay publications but do not have any scientific research or clinical trials to support their use. Therefore, only the most studied and validated diets were included here.

As would be expected, the research between diets can be conflicting, and overall research dearth is noted between wellness and diets. As such, we will focus exclusively on comparisons of different diet paradigms.

The two most common biometrics for comparing/validating diets in the literature are body weight loss or macronutrient compositions. Diet comparison trials, primarily focusing on weight and weight loss, often report other biometric benefits (glycemic control, lipids, blood pressure, etc.) as secondary gains. These trials usually use a specific disease population (such as obesity, diabetes, metabolic syndrome, hypertension) and normal controls in an effort to validate the diet of interest.

Other diet comparison studies attempt to elucidate which ratio of macronutrients is most beneficial for human consumption. These comparisons again use disease populations and apply differing amounts of protein, carbohydrate, and lipids (fat) in order to ascertain the most healthful ratios. These studies again use primarily biomarkers, including metabolic energy production, to support the diet of interest. However, these two components (weight and macronutrient types) will not give any indication as to improving human wellness. Instead, these studies aim to demonstrate which diet will support human physiology better. As we will find out, often many diets cannot claim superiority for all people.

In a recent meta-analysis, investigators sought to compare clinical trials for 20 of the most popular diets. These diets focused on weight loss without calorie restriction within each diet [153]. Unfortunately, the clinical research is limited, with only 16 total clinical articles for the 20 diets. The preponderance of the evidence suggests clinically meaningful weight loss with the Atkins diet in the short term (6 months) as well as long term (12 months). However, the other diets may be effective at weight loss but have limited clinical testing. In fact, many diets, although popular in the press, have no clinical testing to their credit.

In another recent meta-analysis, 11 randomized controlled trials focused on comparison of low-fat diets with low-carbohydrate diets. In this analysis, low-carbohydrate diets demonstrated significantly improved lipid changes (lowered triglycerides, increased HDL-C, increased LDL-C), as well as a greater reduction in bodyweight compared to the low-fat diets [154].

Another large-scale prospective randomized controlled trial involved comparing healthy low-fat (29 percent of calories) versus healthy low-carbohydrate (30 percent of calories) diets, but without calorie counting or restriction [155]. Both groups were instructed to increase consumption of vegetables, eat whole unprocessed foods, and minimize refined flours/sugars. Each study macronutrient (grams of fat or carbohydrate) was reduced significantly, then gradually added back into the participants' diets until they reached a level deemed sustainable for perpetuity. Thus, subjects had a healthy-eating focus, with an ideal ratio for maintenance. The results indicated that both diets were generally healthy and had improved lipid factors along with the weight loss. But weight loss was not significantly different between the groups, and no prognostic measure could help with allocating future patients to each of these two diets.

Finally, when comparing the Mediterranean, low-carbohydrate, and low-fat diets, all three result in weight loss, with most weight loss from the Mediterranean and low-carbohydrate diets. The lower-carbohydrate diets had greater reductions in total cholesterol to HDL-C ratio, and the Mediterranean diet improved diabetics' fasting plasma glucose and insulin levels relative to low-fat diets [156]. Another good study compared various levels of each macronutrient and found that with a reduction of 750 kilocalories per day, all subjects demonstrated improved lipid-related risk factors and insulin levels, regardless of percentages of each macronutrient [157].

In the context of research in nutrition, many lay publications and much clinical research focuses on body weight and weight loss. Obviously for obesity and general overweight patients, weight loss is important for many health reasons. As a general rule, weight loss occurs when fewer calories are consumed than metabolism and volitional activity require (i.e., hypocalorie). This is the calories in/calories out (CICO) model of thermodynamics to explain weight loss or weight gain. It stipulates that weight gain results from abundance of calories, whereas weight loss develops from a restriction of calories. A posit of this model is that calories of fat, carbohydrate, and protein are all equal; a calorie of sugar has an equal effect on the human body as a calorie of protein. Although this sounds simple and concise, it does not take into consideration physiology, and indicates that all weight loss or gain will always be linear. This is not the case: As more weight is lost, often fewer calories for metabolism are needed and often metabolism will decrease tremendously in periods of severe calorie restriction (i.e., fasting). Thus, weight loss in the CICO model will occur with any hypocalorie situation, regardless of diet style, as long as the hypocalorie situation remains constant.

In contrast, the endocrine model of metabolism suggests that body weight is affected more by endocrine factors than calories consumed. This model of weight gain suggests that inappropriate levels of endocrine factors (namely insulin = hyperinsulinemia) result from food choices. Various food choices affect endocrine hormone release and ultimately affect how calories are used during metabolism or stored. For example, a calorie of carbohydrate will release more insulin than a calorie of lipids/fat. Also, different carbohydrates, often based upon many structural factors, will release differing levels of insulin. Thus, hormonal control, as indicated by the endocrine model, has a larger impact on body weight than simple calorie intake.

From both a pragmatic and logical perspective, weight management is a complex interplay of both models, along with other unaccounted for contributors (e.g., the microbiome of the intestines). As such, both components should be addressed in any weight loss/gain program. Separation of these two models is short-sighted, naïve, and incomplete, and is often the result of the territorial nature of some researchers.

Practical Guidelines for General Nutrition

From the above information, it would appear that human nutrition is complex and must be relegated to someone with extensive training and daily practice with patients. However, for the general population, three rules of nutrition work for most people and most of the above diets. These rules do not address any food intolerances or allergies, which should naturally be avoided. As you become more familiar with these principles, you will feel more comfortable espousing this information to your patients.

1. Eat whole foods. As simple as this sounds, the goal is to eat minimally processed foods, especially avoiding ultra-processed foods. Ideally these should be as close to as found in nature, whether it be plant or animal. This rule does not state that one type of macronutrient is better than another, just that each macronutrient should be minimally processed. And as items are processed less, fewer additional ingredients (preservatives, coloring, additives, etc.) are added. Examples are: whole intact apples, which are better than apple sauce; whole corn, which is better than a corn tortilla; or natural protein (good-quality fish, chicken, steak, or beans) instead of manufactured protein (protein powder, bars, etc.). Whether you choose to eat animal proteins exclusively, plant matter exclusively, or a combination of both, seek to get as close to the whole, intact food, as close to nature as possible.

2. Focus on natural fiber. Foods with fiber, especially whole, intact cell walls, have a large number of proposed health benefits: glucose/cholesterol control, satiation, microbiome feeding, bile/cancerous trapping, increasing bioactive/phytonutrient consumption, lowered inflammatory markers, reduction in cancers/chronic diseases, and finally reduced mortality [158]. Fiber is not uniform, in that fiber is predominantly found in plant matter (fruits and vegetables) and animal proteins do not have any fiber. Certain patients have issues with some types of fiber (e.g., a low FODMAP diet may possibly help

some GI issues such as irritable bowel disease). Some diets downplay the role of fiber in the human diet, but they completely acknowledge that fibrous foods may contain some micronutrient/phytonutrient/other unknown food component that may be healthful to humans. The dietary reference intakes as stipulated by the Institute of Medicine recommend intake of 25 g/day fiber for adult females and 38 g/day for adult males. Most Western diets do not meet this minimum requirement. Therefore, always seek to eat some foods that contain fiber. If you follow the above rule about eating whole foods, the additional benefit of whole foods is the presence of fiber. So, another reason to eat whole foods!

3. Minimize sugar or high glycemic index/glycemic load foods. Foods that contain large amounts of sugar, usually added but also naturally occurring, will result in excessive glucose in the bloodstream and a corresponding hyperinsulemic situation will result. (Glycemic index rates the increase in blood glucose a food contains relative to the reference white bread; glycemic load uses glycemic index and accounts for overall portion size of the food, and more accurately describes the blood glucose rise of a food.) Additionally, high glycemic index or glycemic load foods will have the same effect on the glucose level of the body, as well as stimulating the reward centers of the brain. As indicated by the endocrine model, these rapid infusions of glucose and subsequent high insulin secretions cause many deleterious effects (hunger, mood issues, cravings, hypoglycemic events, increased subsequent meal volumes), which may set the stage for some of our chronic diseases (e.g., diabetes, obesity, metabolic syndrome, cardiovascular disease). Medium and low glycemic index/load foods will also cause a slower rise in blood glucose and often contain more fiber. The negative components of high glycemic index/load foods are often significantly blunted in more medium foods. Therefore, minimizing or eliminating sugar or high glycemic index/load foods is strongly recommended.

Conclusion

In this chapter, you have been presented with general knowledge of the various diets present in the literature. General diets have some influence on wellness and health biomarkers. Unfortunately, wellness is not often studied as a variable in nutrition research. However, additional research is ongoing and should be constantly monitored. Studies that connect nutrition to wellness should be continually encouraged.

The main point of this chapter revolves around the superior complexity of the human physiology to allow adaptability in any environment. Since it is complex, no definitive, all-encompassing, or ideal diet has been elucidated by the research. However, different diet paradigms work well for different populations, and this is what the research has consistently supported.

Each patient and practitioner must use this information to guide their dietary choices. Culture, ethics, and physiology may influence dietary choices and should be considered when giving nutrition advice. Also, individual motivations and basic nutrition knowledge can affect the guidance given to patients. As many research studies have demonstrated, diet education is not a one-time, prescriptive piece of advice; patients may often need ongoing support and encouragement to maintain appropriate diet adherence. Therefore, your involvement is key and integral to improving the wellness of patients, as well as yourself, through healthful nutrition.

References

1. MJ Dauncey. Recent advances in nutrition, genes and brain health. *Proc Nutr Soc* 2012; **71**(4): 581–591.

2. TC Mondin, AL Stuart, LJ Williams, et al. Diet quality, dietary patterns and short sleep duration: a cross-sectional population-based study. *Eur J Nutr* 2018; **58**: 641–651.

3. FN Jacka, A O'Neil, R Opie, et al. A randomised controlled trial of dietary improvement for adults with major depression (the "SMILES" trial). *BMC Med* 2017; **15**(1): 23.

4. J Hayward, FN Jacka, H Skouteris, et al. Lifestyle factors and adolescent depressive symptomatology: associations and effect sizes of diet, physical activity and sedentary behaviour. *Aust N Z J Psychiatry* 2016; **50** (11): 1064–1073.

5. FN Jacka, A Mykletun, M Berk. Moving towards a population health approach to the primary prevention of common mental disorders. *BMC Med* 2012; **27** (10): 149.

6. R Mujcic, J Oswald. Evolution of well-being and happiness after increases in consumption of fruit and vegetables. *Am J Public Health* 2016; **106**(8): 1504–1510.

7. N Ocean, P Howley, J Ensor. Lettuce be happy: a longitudinal UK study on the relationship between fruit and vegetable consumption and well-being. *Soc Sci Med* 2019; **222**: 335–345.

8. JPA Ioannidis. The challenge of reforming nutritional epidemiologic research. *JAMA* 2018; **320**(10): 969–970.

9. N Teicholz, *The Big Fat Surprise.* New York, Simon and Schuster; 2014.

10. Y Wang, Q Hao, L Su, et al. Adherence to the Mediterranean diet and the risk of frailty in old people: a systematic review and meta-analysis. *J Nutr Health Aging* 2018; **22**(5): 613–618.

11. G Kojima, C Avgerinou, S Iliffe, K Walters. Adherence to Mediterranean diet reduces incident frailty risk: systematic review and meta-analysis. *J Am Geriatr Soc* 2018; **66** (4): 783–788.

12. A Castelló, E Boldo, B Pérez-Gómez, et al. Adherence to the Western, Prudent and Mediterranean dietary patterns and breast cancer risk: MCC-Spain study. *Maturitas* 2017; **103**: 8–15.

13. PA van den Brandt, M Schulpen. Mediterranean diet adherence and risk of postmenopausal breast cancer: results of a cohort study and meta-analysis. *Int J Cancer* 2017; **140**(10): 2220–2231.

14. B Krusinska, I Hawrysz, L Wadolowska, et al. Associations of Mediterranean diet and a posteriori derived dietary patterns with breast and lung cancer risk: a case-control study. *Nutrients* 2018; **11**(10): 4.

15. D Praud, P Bertuccio, C Bosetti, et al. Adherence to the Mediterranean diet and gastric cancer risk in Italy. *Int J Cancer* 2014; **134**(12): 2935–2941.

16. F Turati, F Bravi, J Polesel, et al. Adherence to the Mediterranean diet and nasopharyngeal cancer risk in Italy. *Cancer Causes Control* 2017; **28**(2): 89–95.

17. M Filomeno, C Bosetti, E Bidoli, et al. Mediterranean diet and risk of endometrial cancer: a pooled analysis of three Italian case-control studies. *Br J Cancer* 2015; **112** (11): 1816–1821.

18. C Bosetti, F Turati, A Dal Pont, et al. The role of Mediterranean diet on the risk of pancreatic cancer. *Br J Cancer* 2013; **109**(5): 1360–1366.

19. A Castelló, P Amiano, N Fernández de Larrea, et al. Low adherence to the western and high adherence to the Mediterranean dietary patterns could prevent colorectal cancer. *Eur J Nutr* 2018; **58**: 1495–1505.

20. A Castelló, E Boldo, P Amiano, et al. Mediterranean Dietary pattern is associated with low risk of aggressive prostate cancer: MCC-Spain study. *J Urol* 2018; **199**(2): 430–437.

21. K Esposito, R Marfella, M Ciotola, et al. Effect of a Mediterranean-style diet on endothelial dysfunction and markers of vascular inflammation in the metabolic syndrome: a randomized trial. *JAMA* 2004; **292**(12): 1440–1446.

22. J Mattei, M Sotos-Prieto, SJ Bigornia, SE Noel, KL Tucker. The Mediterranean diet score is more strongly associated with favorable cardiometabolic risk factors over 2 years than other diet quality indexes in Puerto Rican adults. *J Nutr* 2017; **147**(4): 661–669.

23. A Lasa, J Miranda, M Bulló, et al. Comparative effect of two Mediterranean diets versus a low-fat diet on glycaemic control in individuals with type 2 diabetes. *Eur J Clin Nutr* 2014; **68**(7): 767–772.

24. J Álvarez-Pérez, A Sánchez-Villegas, EM Díaz-Benítez, et al. Influence of a Mediterranean dietary pattern on body fat distribution: results of the PREDIMED-Canarias intervention randomized trial. *J Am Coll Nutr* 2016; **35** (6): 568–580.

25. LS Rallidis, J Lekakis, A Kolomvotsou, et al. Close adherence to a Mediterranean diet improves endothelial function in subjects with abdominal obesity. *Am J Clin Nutr* 2009; **90**(2): 263–268.

26. R Estruch, E Ros, J Salas-Salvadó, et al. Primary prevention of cardiovascular disease with a Mediterranean diet supplemented with extra-virgin olive oil or nuts. *N Engl J Med* 2018; **378**: e34,

27. J Salas-Salvadó, M Bulló, R Estruch, et al. Prevention of diabetes with Mediterranean diets: a subgroup analysis of a randomized trial. *Ann Intern Med* 2014; **160**(1): 1–10.

28. K Esposito, MI Maiorino, G Bellastella, et al. A journey into a Mediterranean diet and type 2 diabetes: a systematic review with meta-analyses. *BMJ Open* 2015; **5**(8). DOI:10.1136/bmjopen-2015-008222.

29. O Ajala, P English, J Pinkney. Systematic review and meta-analysis of different dietary approaches to the management of type 2 diabetes. *Am J Clin Nutr* 2013; **97**(3): 505–516.

30. KA Whalen, ML McCullough, WD Flanders, et al. Paleolithic and Mediterranean diet pattern scores are inversely associated with biomarkers of inflammation and oxidative balance in adults. *J Nutr* 2016; **146**(6): 1217–1226.

31. U Fresán, M Bes-Rastrollo, G Segovia-Siapco, et al. Does the MIND diet decrease depression risk? A comparison with Mediterranean diet in the SUN cohort. *Eur J Nutr* 2018; **58**: 1271–1282.

32. EH Martínez-Lapiscina, P Clavero, E Toledo, et al. Mediterranean diet improves cognition: the PREDIMED-NAVARRA randomised trial. *J Neurol Neurosurg Psychiatry* 2013; **84**(12): 1318–1325.

33. CA Anastasiou, M Yannakoulia, MH Kosmidis, et al. Mediterranean diet and cognitive health: initial results from the Hellenic Longitudinal Investigation of Ageing and Diet. *PLoS One* 2017; **12**(8): e0182048.

34. C Féart, C Samieri, V Rondeau, et al. Adherence to a Mediterranean diet, cognitive decline, and risk of dementia. *JAMA* 2009; **302**(6): 638–648.

35. A Koyama, DK Houston, EM Simonsick, et al. Association between the Mediterranean diet and cognitive decline in a biracial population. *J Gerontol A Biol Sci Med Sci* 2015; **70**(3): 354–359.

36. V Berti, M Walters, J Sterling, et al. Mediterranean diet and 3-year Alzheimer brain biomarker changes in middle-aged adults. *Neurology* 2018; **90**(20): e1789–e1798.

37. B Singh, AK Parsaik, MM Mielke, et al. Association of Mediterranean diet with mild cognitive impairment and Alzheimer's disease: a systematic review and meta-analysis. *J Alzheimers Dis* 2014; **39**(2): 271–282.

38. N Scarmeas, JA Luchsinger, R Mayeux, Y Stern. Mediterranean diet and Alzheimer disease mortality. *Neurology* 2007; **69**(11): 1084–1093.

39. I Alvarez-Alvarez, I Zazpe, J Pérez de Rojas, et al. Mediterranean diet, physical activity and their combined effect on all-cause mortality: the Seguimiento Universidad de Navarra (SUN) cohort. *Prev Med* 2018; **106**: 45–52.

40. RS Kuipers, MF Luxwolda, DA Dijck-Brouwer, et al. Estimated macronutrient and fatty acid intakes from an East African Paleolithic diet. *Br J Nutr* 2010; **104**(11): 1666–1687.

41. M Konner, SB Eaton. Paleolithic nutrition: twenty-five years later. *Nutr Clin Pract* 2010; **25**(6): 594–602.

42. L Cordain, JB Miller, SB Eaton, et al. Plant–animal subsistence ratios and macronutrient energy estimations in worldwide hunter-gatherer diets. *Am J Clin Nutr* 2000; **71**(3): 682–692.

43. LA Frassetto, M Schloetter, M Mietus-Synder, RC Morris Jr, A Sebastian. Metabolic and physiologic improvements from consuming a paleolithic, hunter-gatherer type diet. *Eur J Clin Nutr.* 2009; **63**(8): 947–955. Erratum in: *Eur J Clin Nutr* 2015; **69**(12): 1376.

44. J Otten, A Stomby, M Waling, et al. Benefits of a Paleolithic diet with and without supervised exercise on fat mass, insulin sensitivity, and glycemic control: a randomized controlled trial in individuals with type 2 diabetes. *Diabetes Metab Res Rev.* 2017; **33**(1). DOI:10.1002/dmrr.2828.

45. T Jönsson, Y Granfeldt, S Lindeberg, AC Hallberg. Subjective satiety and other experiences of a Paleolithic diet compared to a diabetes diet in patients with type 2 diabetes. *Nutr J* 2013; **29**(12): 105.

46. S Lindeberg, T Jönsson, Y Granfeldt, et al. A Palaeolithic diet improves glucose tolerance more than a Mediterranean-like diet in individuals with ischaemic heart disease. *Diabetologia* 2007; **50**(9): 1795–1807.

47. A Genoni, P Lyons-Wall, J Lo, A Devine. Cardiovascular metabolic effects and dietary composition of ad-libitum Paleolithic vs. Australian guide to healthy eating diets: a 4-week randomised trial. *Nutrients* 2016; **8**(5). DOI:10.3390/nu8050314.

48. C Mellberg, S Sandberg, M Ryberg, et al. Long-term effects of a Palaeolithic-type diet in obese postmenopausal women: a 2-year randomized trial. *Eur J Clin Nutr* 2014; **68**(3): 350–357.

49. M Osterdahl, T Kocturk, A Koochek, PE Wändell. Effects of a short-term intervention with a Paleolithic diet in healthy volunteers. *Eur J Clin Nutr* 2008; **62** (5): 682–685.

50. HF Bligh, IF Godsland, G Frost, et al. Plant-rich mixed meals based on Palaeolithic diet principles have a dramatic impact on incretin, peptide YY and satiety response, but show little effect on glucose and insulin homeostasis: an acute-effects randomised study. *Br J Nutr* 2015; **113**(4): 574–584.

51. M Fontes-Villalba, S Lindeberg, Y Granfeldt, et al. Palaeolithic diet decreases fasting plasma leptin concentrations more than a diabetes diet in patients with type 2 diabetes: a randomised cross-over trial. *Cardiovasc Diabetol* 2016; **15**: 80.

52. KA Whalen, ML McCullough, WD Flanders, et al. Paleolithic and Mediterranean diet pattern scores are inversely associated with biomarkers of inflammation and oxidative balance in adults. *J Nutr* 2016; **146**(6): 1217–1226.

53. KA Whalen, M McCullough, WD Flanders, et al. Paleolithic and Mediterranean diet pattern scores and risk of incident, sporadic colorectal adenomas. *Am J Epidemiol* 2014; **180**(11): 1088–1097.

54. KA Whalen, S Judd, ML McCullough, et al. Paleolithic and Mediterranean diet pattern scores are inversely associated with all-cause and cause-specific mortality in adults. *J Nutr* 2017; **147**(4): 612–620.

55. A Paoli, A Rubini, JS Volek, KA Grimaldi. Beyond weight loss: a review of the therapeutic uses of very-low-carbohydrate (ketogenic) diets. *Eur J Clin Nutr* 2013; **67** (8): 789–796.

56. OE Owen, AP Morgan, HG Kemp, et al. Brain metabolism during fasting. *J Clin Invest* 1967; **46**(10): 1589–1595.

57. A Paoli, K Grimaldi, L Toniolo, et al. Nutrition and acne: therapeutic potential of ketogenic diets. *Skin Pharmacol Physiol* 2012; **25**(3): 111–117.

58. F Cavaleri, E Bashar. Potential synergies of β-Hydroxybutyrate and butyrate on the modulation of metabolism, inflammation, cognition, and general health. *J Nutr Metab* 2018; **2018**: 7195760.

59. KJ Martin-McGill, AG Marson, C Tudur Smith, MD Jenkinson. The modified Ketogenic diet in adults with glioblastoma: an evaluation of feasibility and

deliverability within the National Health Service. *Nutr Cancer* 2018; **70**(4): 643–649.

60. J Zhang, PP Jia, QL Liu, et al. Low ketolytic enzyme levels in tumors predict ketogenic diet responses in cancer cell lines in vitro and in vivo. *J Lipid Res* 2018; **59**(4): 625–634.

61. S Aminzadeh-Gohari, RG Feichtinger, S Vidali, et al. A ketogenic diet supplemented with medium-chain triglycerides enhances the anti-tumor and anti-angiogenic efficacy of chemotherapy on neuroblastoma xenografts in a CD1-nu mouse model. *Oncotarget* 2017; **8**(39): 64728–64744.

62. RJ Morscher, S Aminzadeh-Gohari, RG Feichtinger, et al. Inhibition of neuroblastoma tumor growth by ketogenic diet and/or calorie restriction in a CD1-Nu mouse model. *PLoS One* 2015; **10**(6). DOI:10.1371/journal.pone.0129802.

63. KJ Martin-McGill, MD Jenkinson, C Tudur Smith, AG Marson. The modified ketogenic diet for adults with refractory epilepsy: an evaluation of a set up service. *Seizure* 2017; **52**: 1–6.

64. EG Neal, H Chaffe, RH Schwartz, et al. The ketogenic diet for the treatment of childhood epilepsy: a randomised controlled trial. *Lancet Neurol* 2008; **7**(6): 500–506.

65. M Nei, L Ngo, JI Sirven, MR Sperling. Ketogenic diet in adolescents and adults with epilepsy. *Seizure* 2014; **23**(6): 439–442.

66. NB Bueno, IS de Melo, SL de Oliveira, T da Rocha Ataide. Very-low-carbohydrate ketogenic diet v. low-fat diet for long-term weight loss: a meta-analysis of randomised controlled trials. *Br J Nutr* 2013; **110**(7): 1178–1187.

67. B Moreno, D Bellido, I Sajoux, et al. Comparison of a very low-calorie-ketogenic diet with a standard low-calorie diet in the treatment of obesity. *Endocrine* 2014; **47**(3): 793–805.

68. AF Cicero, M Benelli, M Brancaleoni, et al. Middle and long-term impact of a very low-carbohydrate ketogenic diet on cardiometabolic factors: a multi-center, cross-sectional, clinical study. *High Blood Press Cardiovasc Prev* 2015; **22**(4): 389–394.

69. A Paoli, A Bianco, KA Grimaldi, A Lodi, G Bosco. Long term successful weight loss with a combination biphasic ketogenic Mediterranean diet and Mediterranean diet maintenance protocol. *Nutrients* 2013; **5**(12): 5205–5217.

70. D Gomez-Arbelaez, D Bellido, AI Castro, et al. Body composition changes after very-low-calorie ketogenic diet in obesity evaluated by 3 standardized methods. *J Clin Endocrinol Metab* 2017; **102**(2): 488–498.

71. B Moreno, AB Crujeiras, D Bellido, I Sajoux, FF Casanueva. Obesity treatment by very low-calorie-ketogenic diet at two years: reduction in visceral fat and on the burden of disease. *Endocrine* 2016; **54**(3): 681–690.

72. D Gomez-Arbelaez, AB Crujeiras, AI Castro, et al. Resting metabolic rate of obese patients under very low calorie ketogenic diet. *Nutr Metab (Lond)* 2018; **15**: 18.

73. AM Johnstone, GW Horgan, SD Murison, DM Bremner, GE Lobley. Effects of a high-protein ketogenic diet on hunger, appetite, and weight loss in obese men feeding ad libitum. *Am J Clin Nutr* 2008; **87** (1): 44–55.

74. MJ Sharman, WJ Kraemer, DM Love, et al. A ketogenic diet favorably affects serum biomarkers for cardiovascular disease in normal-weight men. *J Nutr* 2002; **132**(7): 1879–1885.

75. MK Badman, AR Kennedy, AC Adams, P Pissios, E Maratos-Flier. A very low carbohydrate ketogenic diet improves glucose tolerance in ob/ob mice independently of weight loss. *Am J Physiol Endocrinol Metab* 2009; **297**(5): E1197–E1204.

76. LR Saslow, AE Mason, S Kim, et al. An online intervention comparing a very low-carbohydrate ketogenic diet and lifestyle recommendations versus a plate method diet in overweight individuals with type 2 diabetes: a randomized controlled trial. *J Med Internet Res* 2017; **19**(2): e36.

77. J Tay, ND Luscombe-Marsh, CH Thompson, et al. A very low-carbohydrate, low-saturated fat diet

for type 2 diabetes management: a randomized trial. *Diabetes Care* 2014; **37**(11): 2909–2918.

78. LJ Appel, TJ Moore, E Obarzanek, et al. A clinical trial of the effects of dietary patterns on blood pressure. *N Engl J Med* 1997; **336**(16): 1117–1124.

79. A Salehi-Abargouei, Z Maghsoudi, F Shirani, L Azadbakht. Effects of Dietary Approaches to Stop Hypertension (DASH)-style diet on fatal or nonfatal cardiovascular diseases – incidence: a systematic review and meta-analysis on observational prospective studies. *Nutrition* 2013; **29**(4): 611–618.

80. TT Fung, SE Chiuve, ML McCullough, et al. Adherence to a DASH-style diet and risk of coronary heart disease and stroke in women. *Arch Intern Med* 2008; **168**(7): 713–720.

81. FM Sacks, LP Svetkey, WM Vollmer, et al. Effects on blood pressure of reduced dietary sodium and the Dietary Approaches to Stop Hypertension (DASH) diet. *N Engl J Med* 2001; **344**(1): 3–10.

82. M Siervo, J Lara, S Chowdhury, et al. Effects of the Dietary Approach to Stop Hypertension (DASH) diet on cardiovascular risk factors: a systematic review and meta-analysis. *Br J Nutr* 2015; **113**(1): 1–15.

83. P Saneei, A Salehi-Abargouei, A Esmaillzadeh, L Azadbakht. Influence of Dietary Approaches to Stop Hypertension (DASH) diet on blood pressure: a systematic review and meta-analysis on randomized controlled trials. *Nutr Metab Cardiovasc Dis* 2014; **24**(12): 1253–1261.

84. AAM Berendsen, JH Kang, O van de Rest, et al. The Dietary Approaches to Stop Hypertension Diet, cognitive function, and cognitive decline in American older women. *J Am Med Dir Assoc* 2017; **18**(5): 427–432.

85. F Hikmat, LJ Appel. Effects of the DASH diet on blood pressure in patients with and without metabolic syndrome: results from the DASH trial. *J Hum Hypertens* 2014; **28**(3): 170–175.

86. PR Conlin, D Chow, ER Miller 3rd, et al. The effect of dietary patterns on blood pressure control in hypertensive patients: results from the Dietary Approaches to Stop Hypertension (DASH) trial. *Am J Hypertens* 2000; **13**(9): 949–955.

87. S Chiu, N Bergeron, PT Williams, et al. Comparison of the DASH (Dietary Approaches to Stop Hypertension) diet and a higher-fat DASH diet on blood pressure and lipids and lipoproteins: a randomized controlled trial. *Am J Clin Nutr* 2016; **103**(2): 341–347.

88. Z Asemi, Z Tabassi, M Samimi, T Fahiminejad, A Esmaillzadeh. Favourable effects of the Dietary Approaches to Stop Hypertension diet on glucose tolerance and lipid profiles in gestational diabetes: a randomised clinical trial. *Br J Nutr* 2013; **109**(11): 2024–2030.

89. M Razavi Zade, MH Telkabadi, F Bahmani, et al. The effects of DASH diet on weight loss and metabolic status in adults with non-alcoholic fatty liver disease: a randomized clinical trial. *Liver Int* 2016; **36**(4): 563–571.

90. P Saneei, M Hashemipour, R Kelishadi, A Esmaillzadeh. The Dietary Approaches to Stop Hypertension (DASH) diet affects inflammation in childhood metabolic syndrome: a randomized cross-over clinical trial. *Ann Nutr Metab* 2014; **64**(1): 20–27.

91. CM Rebholz, DC Crews, ME Grams, et al. DASH (Dietary Approaches to Stop Hypertension) diet and risk of subsequent kidney disease. *Am J Kidney Dis* 2016; **68**(6): 853–861.

92. EB Levitan, CE Lewis, LF Tinker, et al. Mediterranean and DASH diet scores and mortality in women with heart failure: the Women's Health Initiative. *Circ Heart Fail* 2013; **6**(6): 1116–1123.

93. J Jiang, M Liu, LM Troy, et al. Concordance with DASH diet and blood pressure change: results from the Framingham Offspring Study (1991–2008). *J Hypertens* 2015; **33**(11): 2223–2230.

94. B Jakše, S Pinter, B Jakše, M Bučar Pajek, J Pajek. Effects of an ad libitum consumed low-fat plant-based diet supplemented with plant-based meal replacements on

body composition indices. *Biomed Res Int* 2017; **2017**: 9626390.

95. N Wright, L Wilson, M Smith, B Duncan, P McHugh. The BROAD study: a randomized controlled trial using a whole food plant-based diet in the community for obesity, ischaemic heart disease or diabetes. *Nutr Diabetes* 2017; 7 (3): e256.

96. F Sofi, M Dinu, G Pagliai, et al. Low-calorie vegetarian versus Mediterranean diets for reducing body weight and improving cardiovascular risk profile: CARDIVEG study (cardiovascular prevention with vegetarian diet). *Circulation* 2018; **137**(11): 1103–1113.

97. GM Turner-McGrievy, CR Davidson, EE Wingard, S Wilcox, EA Frongillo. Comparative effectiveness of plant-based diets for weight loss: a randomized controlled trial of five different diets. *Nutrition* 2015; **31**(2): 350–358.

98. Z Chen, MG Zuurmond, N van der Schaft, et al. Plant versus animal based diets and insulin resistance, prediabetes and type 2 diabetes: the Rotterdam Study. *Eur J Epidemiol* 2018. DOI:10.1007/s10654-018-0414-8.

99. A Satija, SN Bhupathiraju, EB Rimm, et al. Plant-based dietary patterns and incidence of type 2 diabetes in US men and women: results from three prospective cohort studies. *PLoS Med* 2016; **13**(6). DOI:0.1371/journal.pmed.1002039.

100. S Mishra, J Xu, U Agarwal, et al. A multicenter randomized controlled trial of a plant-based nutrition program to reduce body weight and cardiovascular risk in the corporate setting: the GEICO study. *Eur J Clin Nutr* 2013; **67**(7): 718–724.

101. YF Chiu, CC Hsu, TH Chiu, et al. Cross-sectional and longitudinal comparisons of metabolic profiles between vegetarian and non-vegetarian subjects: a matched cohort study. *Br J Nutr* 2015; **114**(8): 1313–1320.

102. Y Yokoyama, K Nishimura, ND Barnard, et al. Vegetarian diets and blood pressure: a meta-analysis. *JAMA Intern Med* 2014; **174**(4): 577–587.

103. Y Yokoyama, SM Levin, ND Barnard. Association between plant-based diets and plasma lipids: a systematic review and meta-analysis. *Nutr Rev* 2017; **75**(9): 683–698.

104. H Kahleova, S Levin, N Barnard. Cardio-metabolic benefits of plant-based diets. *Nutrients* 2017; **9**(8). pii: E848.

105. A Satija, SN Bhupathiraju, D Spiegelman, et al. Healthful and unhealthful plant-based diets and the risk of coronary heart disease in U.S. adults. *J Am Coll Cardiol* 2017; **70**(4): 411–422.

106. MJ Orlich, PN Singh, J Sabaté, et al. Vegetarian dietary patterns and the risk of colorectal cancers. *JAMA Intern Med* 2015; **175**(5): 767–776.

107. D Aune, E Giovannucci, P Boffetta, et al. Fruit and vegetable intake and the risk of cardiovascular disease, total cancer and all-cause mortality: a systematic review and dose–response meta-analysis of prospective studies. *Int J Epidemiol* 2017; **46**(3): 1029–1056.

108. T Huang, B Yang, J Zheng, et al. Cardiovascular disease mortality and cancer incidence in vegetarians: a meta-analysis and systematic review. *Ann Nutr Metab* 2012; **60**(4): 233–240.

109. PN Appleby, FL Crowe, KE Bradbury, RC Travis, TJ Key. Mortality in vegetarians and comparable nonvegetarians in the United Kingdom. *Am J Clin Nutr* 2016; **103**(1): 218–230.

110. TJ Key, GE Fraser, M Thorogood, et al. Mortality in vegetarians and non-vegetarians: a collaborative analysis of 8300 deaths among 76,000 men and women in five prospective studies. *Public Health Nutr* 1998; **1**(1): 33–41.

111. TJ Key, PN Appleby, EA Spencer, et al. Mortality in British vegetarians: results from the European Prospective Investigation into Cancer and Nutrition (EPIC-Oxford). *Am J Clin Nutr* 2009; **89** (5): 1613S–1619S.

112. JG Muir, PR Gibson. The Low FODMAP diet for treatment of irritable bowel syndrome and other gastrointestinal disorders. *Gastroenterol Hepatol (NY)* 2013; **9**(7): 450–452.

113. SS Rao, S Yu, A Fedewa. Systematic review: dietary fibre and FODMAP-restricted diet in the management of constipation and irritable bowel syndrome. *Aliment Pharmacol Ther* 2015; **41**(12): 1256–1270.

114. P Varjú, N Farkas, P Hegyi, et al. Low fermentable oligosaccharides, disaccharides, monosaccharides and polyols (FODMAP) diet improves symptoms in adults suffering from irritable bowel syndrome (IBS) compared to standard IBS diet: a meta-analysis of clinical studies. *PLoS One* 2017; **12**(8): e0182942.

115. BP Chumpitazi, JL Cope, EB Hollister, et al. Randomised clinical trial: gut microbiome biomarkers are associated with clinical response to a low FODMAP diet in children with the irritable bowel syndrome. *Aliment Pharmacol Ther* 2015; **42**(4): 418–627.

116. DM Lis, T Stellingwerff, CM Kitic, et al. Low FODMAP: a preliminary strategy to reduce gastrointestinal distress in athletes. *Med Sci Sports Exerc* 2018; **50**(1): 116–123.

117. CH Wilder-Smith, SS Olesen, A Materna, AM Drewes. Predictors of response to a low-FODMAP diet in patients with functional gastrointestinal disorders and lactose or fructose intolerance. *Aliment Pharmacol Ther* 2017; **45**(8): 1094–1106.

118. A Marsh, EM Eslick, GD Eslick. Does a diet low in FODMAPs reduce symptoms associated with functional gastrointestinal disorders? A comprehensive systematic review and meta-analysis. *Eur J Nutr* 2016; **55**(3): 897–906.

119. H Pourmand, A Esmaillzadeh. Consumption of a low fermentable oligo-, di-, mono-saccharides, and polyols diet and irritable bowel syndrome: a systematic review. *Int J Prev Med* 2017; **13**(8); 104.

120. AP Marum, C Moreira, F Saraiva, P Tomas-Carus, C Sousa-Guerreiro. A low fermentable oligo-di-mono saccharides and polyols (FODMAP) diet reduced pain and improved daily life in fibromyalgia patients. *Scand J Pain* 2016; **13**: 166–172.

121. EP Halmos, CT Christophersen, AR Bird, et al. Consistent prebiotic effect on gut microbiota with altered FODMAP intake in patients with Crohn's disease: a randomised, controlled cross-over trial of well-defined diets. *Clin Transl Gastroenterol* 2016; **14**(7); e164.

122. S Sharma, N Sankhyan, S Gulati, A Agarwala. Use of the modified Atkins diet for treatment of refractory childhood epilepsy: a randomized controlled trial. *Epilepsia* 2013; **54**(3): 481–486.

123. S Sharma, S Goel, P Jain, A Agarwala, S Aneja. Evaluation of a simplified modified Atkins diet for use by parents with low levels of literacy in children with refractory epilepsy: a randomized controlled trial. *Epilepsy Res* 2016; **127**: 152–159.

124. N Porta, L Vallée, E Boutry, et al. Comparison of seizure reduction and serum fatty acid levels after receiving the ketogenic and modified Atkins diet. *Seizure* 2009; **18**(5): 359–364.

125. CD Gardner, A Kiazand, S Alhassan, et al. Comparison of the Atkins, Zone, Ornish, and LEARN diets for change in weight and related risk factors among overweight premenopausal women: the A TO Z Weight Loss Study: a randomized trial. *JAMA* 2007; **297**(9): 969–977.

126. J Tay, GD Brinkworth, M Noakes, J Keogh, PM Clifton. Metabolic effects of weight loss on a very-low-carbohydrate diet compared with an isocaloric high-carbohydrate diet in abdominally obese subjects. *J Am Coll Cardiol* 2008; **51** (1): 59–67.

127. DA de Luis, O Izaola, R Aller, et al. Effects of a high-protein/low carbohydrate versus a standard hypocaloric diet on adipocytokine levels and insulin resistance in obese patients along 9

months. *J Diabetes Complications* 2015; **29** (7): 950–954.

128. ML Dansinger, JA Gleason, JL Griffith, HP Selker, EJ Schaefer. Comparison of the Atkins, Ornish, Weight Watchers, and Zone diets for weight loss and heart disease risk reduction: a randomized trial. *JAMA* 2005; **293**(1): 43–53.

129. MC Gannon, FQ Nuttall. Effect of a high-protein, low-carbohydrate diet on blood glucose control in people with type 2 diabetes. *Diabetes* 2004; **53**(9): 2375–2382.

130. FJ McClernon, WS Yancy Jr, JA Eberstein, RC Atkins, EC Westman. The effects of a low-carbohydrate ketogenic diet and a low-fat diet on mood, hunger, and other self-reported symptoms. *Obesity (Silver Spring)* 2007; **15**(1): 182–187.

131. CK Martin, D Rosenbaum, H Han, et al. Change in food cravings, food preferences, and appetite during a low-carbohydrate and low-fat diet. *Obesity (Silver Spring)* 2011; **19**(10): 1963–1970.

132. J Tay, CH Thompson, ND Luscombe-Marsh, et al. Long-term effects of a very low carbohydrate compared with a high carbohydrate diet on renal function in individuals with type 2 diabetes: a randomized trial. *Medicine (Baltimore)* 2015; **94**(47): e2181.

133. Y Ito, H Oguni, S Ito, M Oguni, M Osawa. A modified Atkins diet is promising as a treatment for glucose transporter type 1 deficiency syndrome. *Dev Med Child Neurol* 2011; **53**(7): 658–663.

134. MC Morris, CC Tangney, Y Wang, et al. MIND diet associated with reduced incidence of Alzheimer's disease. *Alzheimers Dement* 2015; **11**(9): 1007–1014.

135. MC Morris, CC Tangney, Y Wang, et al. MIND diet slows cognitive decline with aging. *Alzheimers Dement* 2015; **11**(9): 1015–1022.

136. CT McEvoy, H Guyer, KM Langa, K Yaffe. Neuroprotective diets are associated with better cognitive function: the Health and Retirement Study. *J Am Geriatr Soc* 2017; **65**(8): 1857–1862.

137. AM Berendsen, JH Kang, EJM Feskens, et al. Association of long-term adherence to the MIND diet with cognitive function and cognitive decline in American women. *J Nutr Health Aging* 2018; **22**(2): 222–229.

138. TL Franklin, KM Kolasa, K Griffin, C Mayo, DT Badenhop. Adherence to very-low-fat diet by a group of cardiac rehabilitation patients in the rural southeastern United States. *Arch Fam Med* 1995; **4**(6): 551–554.

139. CR Pischke, G Weidner, M Elliott-Eller, D Ornish. Lifestyle changes and clinical profile in coronary heart disease patients with an ejection fraction of <or=40% or >40% in the Multicenter Lifestyle Demonstration Project. *Eur J Heart Fail* 2007; **9**(9): 928–934.

140. SG Aldana, WR Whitmer, R Greenlaw, et al. Cardiovascular risk reductions associated with aggressive lifestyle modification and cardiac rehabilitation. *Heart Lung* 2003; **32**(6): 374–382.

141. N Chainani-Wu, G Weidner, DM Purnell, et al. Changes in emerging cardiac biomarkers after an intensive lifestyle intervention. *Am J Cardiol* 2011; **108**(4): 498–507.

142. D Ornish, LW Scherwitz, RS Doody, et al. Effects of stress management training and dietary changes in treating ischemic heart disease. *JAMA* 1983; **249**(1): 54–59.

143. D Ornish. Avoiding revascularization with lifestyle changes: the Multicenter Lifestyle Demonstration Project. *Am J Cardiol* 1998; **82**(10B): 72T–76T.

144. D Ornish, SE Brown, LW Scherwitz, et al. Can lifestyle changes reverse coronary heart disease? The Lifestyle Heart Trial. *Lancet* 1990; **336**(8708): 129–133.

145. D Ornish, LW Scherwitz, JH Billings, et al. Intensive lifestyle changes for reversal of coronary heart disease. *JAMA* 1998; **280** (23): 2001–2007.

146. SG Aldana, R Greenlaw, A Salberg, et al. The effects of an intensive lifestyle modification

program on carotid artery intima-media thickness: a randomized trial. *Am J Health Promot* 2007; **21**(6): 510–516.

147. C Baetge, CP Earnest, B Lockard, et al. Efficacy of a randomized trial examining commercial weight loss programs and exercise on metabolic syndrome in overweight and obese women. *Appl Physiol Nutr Metab* 2017; **42**(2): 216–227.

148. LM Morgan, BA Griffin, DJ Millward, et al. Comparison of the effects of four commercially available weight-loss programmes on lipid-based cardiovascular risk factors. *Public Health Nutr* 2009; **12**(6): 799–807.

149. H Truby, S Baic, A deLooy, et al. Randomised controlled trial of four commercial weight loss programmes in the UK: initial findings from the BBC "diet trials." *BMJ* 2006; **332**(7553): 1309–1314.

150. ML Dansinger, JA Gleason, JL Griffith, HP Selker, EJ Schaefer. Comparison of the Atkins, Ornish, Weight Watchers, and Zone diets for weight loss and heart disease risk reduction: a randomized trial. *JAMA* 2005; **293**(1): 43–53.

151. BC Johnston, S Kanters, K Bandayrel, et al. Comparison of weight loss among named diet programs in overweight and obese adults: a meta-analysis. *JAMA* 2014; **312**(9): 923–933.

152. MF Hjorth, C Ritz, EE Blaak, et al. Pretreatment fasting plasma glucose and insulin modify dietary weight loss success: results from 3 randomized clinical trials. *Am J Clin Nutr* 2017; **106**(2): 499–505.

153. SD Anton, A Hida, K Heekin et al. Effects of popular diets without specific calorie targets on weight loss outcomes: systematic review of findings from clinical trials. *Nutrients* 2017; **9**(8). DOI:10.3390/nu9080822.

154. N Mansoor, KJ Vinknes, MB Veierød, K Retterstøl. Effects of low-carbohydrate diets v. low-fat diets on body weight and cardiovascular risk factors: a meta-analysis of randomised controlled trials. *Br J Nutr* 2016; **115** (3): 466–479.

155. CD Gardner, JF Trepanowski, LC Del Gobbo, et al. Effect of low-fat vs low-carbohydrate diet on 12-month weight loss in overweight adults and the association with genotype pattern or insulin secretion: The DIETFITS randomized clinical trial. *JAMA* 2018; **319** (7): 667–679.

156. I Shai, D Schwarzfuchs, Y Henkin, et al. Dietary Intervention Randomized Controlled Trial (DIRECT) Group: weight loss with a low-carbohydrate, Mediterranean, or low-fat diet. *N Engl J Med* 2008; **359**(3): 229–241.

157. FM Sacks, GA Bray, VJ Carey, et al. Comparison of weight-loss diets with different compositions of fat, protein, and carbohydrates. *N Engl J Med* 2009; **360**(9): 859–873.

158. N Veronese, M Solmi, MG Caruso, et al. Dietary fiber and health outcomes: an umbrella review of systematic reviews and meta-analyses. *Am J Clin Nutr* 2018; **107** (3): 436–444.

Nutraceuticals and Wellness

Dax Volle and Katrina DeBonis

Introduction

According to the *Merriam-Webster English Dictionary,* a nutraceutical is defined as "a foodstuff (such as a fortified food or dietary supplement) that provides health benefits in addition to its basic nutritional value." Nutraceuticals may consist of a single food or plant ingredient or a combination of components that have multiple active ingredients.

Many nutraceutical products have demonstrated, either *in vitro* or *in vivo,* antioxidant, anti-inflammatory, and adaptogenic properties that may improve general health and well-being and may prevent or even treat certain diseases. Likewise, some nutraceuticals have been extensively studied and have a clearly delineated mechanism of action and established efficacy and safety data. However, unlike foodstuffs, which are regulated in the USA by the Food and Drug Administration (FDA) and by similar governmental agencies in many countries, nutraceuticals are subject to no such regulation and can be sold without proof of effectiveness or safety. Furthermore, some nutraceuticals have potential toxic or adverse effects and many interact with pharmaceutical agents through myriad biochemical pathways that may affect the safety and efficacy of those agents.

It is estimated that, in the year 2015, 60–70 percent of Americans consumed either a single or multiple dietary supplements each day, and that number is likely rising with growing awareness of nutraceuticals and their potential benefits [1]. However, clinicians are often not informed of nutraceutical use by patients and, even when informed, they largely have little guidance with regard to how to assist their patients in safely utilizing nutraceuticals to promote wellness and health or to treat disease. In keeping with the objective of this text, this chapter will examine the role of nutraceuticals in facilitating wellness and health, as well as the potential risks associated with various nutraceuticals and their possible interactions with pharmaceutical agents.

Given the large numbers of studies examining nutraceuticals but noting an unfortunate dearth of high-quality evidence for direct benefit in humans, this chapter will summarize only the results of high-quality *in vitro* studies with positive results, or *in vivo* studies with clear demonstration of benefit in humans. If an effect is not discussed in a section then there is not clear evidence for benefit in humans or only theoretical or preliminary evidence of benefit *in vitro*. A lack of evidence does not necessarily determine lack of possible benefit, but given the need for applicability to clinical use, theoretical or preliminary effects will largely be omitted from this chapter. This is to ensure that the focus can remain on established benefits, potential risks, and known interactions with pharmaceuticals.

According to Kalia, nutraceuticals can be categorized into seven distinct categories that will be reviewed systemically with regard to their established benefits, potential safety issues, and relation to pharmaceutical agents [2].

Dietary Fiber

Dietary fiber is food or plant material that is not broken down by gut enzymes but instead is digested by microflora throughout the digestive tract. Soluble components of fiber promote bulking of gut contents, which results in delayed gastric emptying and an increase in the uptake of nutrients, which stimulates satiety. Adequate intake of soluble fiber (25–30 g daily) has been shown to reduce LDL cholesterol and to reduce the risk of cardiovascular disease, stroke, hypertension, diabetes, obesity, and diverticulitis [3].

The main risk of excessive fiber consumption is diarrhea, though fiber may potentially interact with pharmaceuticals via altering pharmacokinetic properties of drug metabolism such as rate of absorption from the gastrointestinal tract. Specifically, one review found that fiber consumption lowered the plasma concentration of lithium, tricyclic antidepressants, and ethinylestradiol, and elevated the plasma concentration of levodopa. Interactions between dietary fiber and statins, hypoglycemic agents, carbamazepine, levothyroxine, and digoxin were varied, with studies often showing contradictory results and unable to draw firm conclusions with regard to these medications [4].

Probiotics and Prebiotics

A probiotic is defined as a live microbial supplement that, when consumed in an adequate amount, results in improved balance of the gut microbial flora. Probiotics generally include lactobacilli (e.g., *Lactobacillus acidophilus*, *L. casei*, *L. brevis*, etc.), gram-positive cocci (e.g., *Lactococcus lactis*, *Streptococcus salivarius*, *Enterococcus faecium*, etc.), and bifidobacteria (e.g., *Bifidobacterium bifidum*, *B. adolescentis*, *B. infantis*, etc.).

Prebiotics are dietary components that alter the composition or metabolism of the gut microbiota and mainly include short-chain polysaccharides found in foods such as chicory root, banana, tomato, alliums, beans, and peas. Prebiotics generally promote the growth of lactobacilli and bifidobacteria in the gut [3].

Both pro- and prebiotics have been shown to have beneficial effects, thought to be mediated through influence on the immune system, such as reduced severity of upper respiratory infections and reduced incidence of allergies [5]. Adverse effects are generally limited to gastrointestinal distress after overconsumption of prebiotics, and neither are thought to interact significantly with medications. Rare reports of systemic infections in immunocompromised individuals with bacteria found in probiotic cultures have been published, and caution should be used in this population [6].

Polyunsaturated Fatty Acids

Polyunsaturated fatty acids (PUFAs) are widely available in foods including fatty fishes (mackerel, salmon, herring, trout, blue fin tuna), flaxseed, soybeans, canola, walnuts, and red/black currants, as well as in supplements. Polyunsaturated fatty acids are divided into omega-3 fatty acids and omega-6 fatty acids. The primary omega-3 fatty acids are α-linolenic acid (ALA), eicosapentanoic acid (EPA), and docosahexanoic acid (DHA); the primary omega-6 fatty acids are linoleic acid (LA), γ-linolenic acid (GLA), and arachidonic acid (ARA).

Beneficial effects of PUFAs include reduced plasma lipid concentrations, reduced atherosclerosis, reduced risk of childhood asthma, improved symptoms of depression when used as an adjunctive treatment, improvement in illness course of bipolar disorder when added to the usual treatment, alleviation of premenstrual stress and anxiety, and they may reduce the risk of age-related cognitive dysfunction and development of neurodegenerative disorders [7–10].

Safety concerns with PUFAs are minimal and are generally related to tolerability issues and gastrointestinal distress. Review of the available literature found no consistent reports of harmful interactions between PUFA supplements and pharmaceutical agents.

Vitamins

Vitamins are organic molecules that serve as essential micronutrients in the human body to ensure proper functioning of human metabolism. They are not synthesized in the body and must be obtained from outside sources, generally either through diet or supplements. The 13 vitamins essential for healthy human metabolism are: vitamins A (all-trans-retinol, all-trans-retinyl-esters, as well as all-trans-beta-carotene and other provitamin A carotenoids), B1 (thiamine), B2 (riboflavin), B3 (niacin), B5 (pantothenic acid), B6 (pyridoxine), B7 (biotin), B9 (folic acid or folate), B12 (cobalamins), C (ascorbic acid), D (calciferols), E (tocopherols and tocotrienols), and K (quinones).

Vitamins have a diverse range of health benefits (Table 23.1) and supplementation either aims to utilize these health-promoting benefits or to correct vitamin deficiencies that may arise as a result of poor diet, malnutrition, or disease. Vitamins largely exert their benefits by

Table 23.1 Vitamins and their benefits [8, 9, 11]

Vitamin	Health benefit
A	Antioxidant, promotes vision health, treatment of certain skin conditions
D	Slightly reduces risk of acquiring respiratory tract infections, slightly reduces incidence of asthma exacerbations, adjunctive treatment of depression
E	Antioxidant
K	Essential for the proper functioning of coagulation
C	Antioxidant, promotes wound healing and bone health, may shorten duration of colds, high-dose sustained release formulations may reduce anxiety and stress
B1	Essential component of glucose metabolism, used to treat severe malnutrition
B2	May prevent migraines in adults
B3	Mixed results regarding prevention of cardiovascular disease; B3 supplementation increases HDL cholesterol but also increases risk for the development of diabetes
B6	Treatment of sideroblastic anemia, treatment of morning sickness, alleviation of premenstrual stress and anxiety
B7	May promote hair and nail health
B12	Supplementation may prevent deficiency in people taking H2-receptor antagonists, proton pump inhibitors, and/or metformin
Folic acid	Reduces incidence of neural tube defects when taken before and during pregnancy, promotes male sexual health and fertility, reduced risk of stroke, adjunctive treatment of depression

Table 23.2 Vitamin toxicity [12, 13]

Vitamin	Toxic dose	Toxic effect
A	>10,000 IU daily	Teratogen during first eight weeks of pregnancy, carotenemia
B1	No established toxic dose	None known
B2	No established toxic dose	None known
B3	>1500 mg daily	Hepatotoxicity, especially if dose not titrated slowly or in the presence of extant liver disease
B6	>300–500 mg daily	May be neurotoxic over time, especially if reduced renal function
B12	No established toxic dose	None known
C	Unknown	Rare, cases of hemolytic anemia in individuals with G6PD deficiency
D	>50,000 IU daily	Hypercalcemia
E	>1600–3200 IU daily	Increased risk of bleeding (only with alpha-tocopherol formulation)
K	No established toxic dose	None known
Folic acid	No established toxic dose	None known, doses >5000 µg daily may mask pernicious anemia

restoring normal biochemical functioning or by free-radical scavenging mechanisms and reduction of oxidative stress, which is theorized to promote health and reduce the incidence of disease and inflammatory disorders.

Vitamins are essential nutrients, but care must be taken when taking supplements, given the potential for significant toxicity or adverse events with supra-physiologic dosing (see Table 23.2).

Vitamins are generally safe with regard to nutrient–drug interactions, but there are several examples that must be kept in mind when counseling patients on the use of these substances with pharmaceuticals to avoid potential interactions (Table 23.3).

Polyphenols

Polyphenols form a large group of phytochemicals, which are compounds produced by plants as a byproduct of their metabolism. There are approximately 8000 different varieties of polyphenols, with the most salient to human health being the curcuminoids, flavonoids, and stilbenoids [3]. Polyphenols are of current interest mainly due to *in vitro* evidence that they demonstrate anti-carcinogenic, anti-atherogenic, antioxidant, anti-inflammatory, anti-microbial, anti-hyperglycemia, and cardioprotective effects, and that they may have a role in the prevention of neurodegenerative diseases via mitigation of age-related cellular damage [10, 15, 16]. However, the overwhelming majority of these compounds currently lack evidence for a direct causal relationship between isolated dietary polyphenols and prevention or treatment of any disease in humans, and more research is needed to clarify their therapeutic potential. The best evidence available to promote wellness and to reduce the risk

Table 23.3 Interactions between vitamins and pharmaceuticals [14]

Vitamin	Pharmaceutical	Interaction	Management of interaction
A	Retinoids	Toxicity including nausea, vomiting, dizziness, blurred vision, and poor coordination	Avoid concomitant use
B6	Levodopa Phenytoin	Decreased efficacy Risk of seizure	Carbidopa/levodopa combination Discontinue B6 use or increase dose of phenytoin
E	Warfarin	Increased risk of bleeding	Avoid doses >800 IU/day of vitamin E
K	Warfarin	Decreased efficacy, risk of thromboembolism	Maintain consistent intake of vitamin K
Niacin	Statins	Increased risk of myopathies	Avoid concomitant use
Calcium	Fluoroquinolones and tetracyclines	Decreased efficacy, risk of antibiotic failure	Avoid concomitant use
	Levothyroxine and bisphosphonates	Decreased efficacy, risk of hypothyroidism	Separate doses by at least four hours

of disease is the consumption of a well-balanced diet, rich in fruits and vegetables, and presumably polyphenols [3].

Polyphenols may interact with pharmaceuticals and impact their plasma concentration through effects on certain liver enzymes involved in drug metabolism (Table 23.4). These interactions are important to consider when counseling patients on diet and the use of supplements.

Spices

Spices have been used by humans for thousands of years to enhance the sensory quality of foods via the conference of characteristic flavors, smells, colors, or textures. The majority of spice ingredients are terpenes of phenolic compounds such as flavonoids, which were discussed previously.

Preliminary research demonstrates that dietary spices, even in small quantities, have a wide variety of antioxidant, anti-mutagenic, anti-inflammatory, and immune modulatory effects on cells and a wide range of potentially beneficial effects on human health via their action on the gastrointestinal, cardiovascular, respiratory, metabolic, reproductive, and nervous systems [3]. Despite this promising early research, well-constructed and controlled clinical trials evaluating individual ingredients of spice compounds are required to better characterize the preventive and therapeutic potential for the majority of spices.

Spices are generally harmless when used as food, but may exhibit toxicity when used at higher doses. At present, only high-dose garlic has demonstrated toxicity in humans [3].

Table 23.4 Known human interactions between plant polyphenols and pharmaceuticals [17]

Plant	Polyphenol	Molecular target	Interaction
Grapefruit	Flavonoids	Inhibits: CYP3A4, CYP1A2, MRP2, OATP-B, and P-glycoprotein	Calcium channel blockers, statins, immunosuppressants, antiviral agents, phosphodiesterase-5 inhibitors, antihistamines, antiarrhythmics, antibiotics
Orange	Flavonoids	Inhibits: CYP3A4, P-glycoprotein, OATP-A, OATP-B	Atenolol, ciprofloxacin, cyclosporine, celiprolol, levofloxacin, and pravastatin
Grapes	Stilbenes and flavonoids	Inhibits: CYP3A4 and CYP2E1	Cyclosporine
Cranberry	Flavonoids	Inhibits: CYP3A and CYP2C9	Warfarin

Adaptogens

Adaptogens are substances that theoretically enhance nonspecific stress resistance, which is a physiological response to general stressors that is likely mediated by the neuro–endocrine–immune axis. Animal and isolated cellular studies have demonstrated that adaptogens have a wide range of neuroprotective, anti-stress, antidepressive, anxiolytic, and nootropic effects, with some promising early results with specific adaptogens in humans for improving attention and mental endurance, reducing mental and physical fatigue, and for the treatment of depression and anxiety [18].

Adaptogens come from a wide variety of plant sources, including *Rhodiola rosea*, *Schisandra chinensis*, and *Eleutherococcus senticosus*, and these three have been the subject of most investigation. Adaptogen compounds typically contain complex phenolic acids or triterpenoids and are largely structurally similar to catecholamines or corticosteroids; this similarity may explain their interaction with the neuro–endocrine–immune axis. In fact, *in vitro* experiments have found adaptogens to be regulators of the mediators of the stress response, such as molecular chaperons (e.g., Hsp70), stress-activated c-Jun N-terminal protein kinase (JNK1), Forkhead box O (FoxO) transcription factor, cortisol, and nitric oxide (NO). In addition, the terpenoid glucoside rosiridin, an isolate from *Rhodiola rosea*, has been found to inhibit monoamine oxidases A and B *in vitro*, which may underlie its demonstrated benefit in depression [18].

Given their wide range of effects, adaptogens may not only have a role in the prevention and treatment of stress-induced and stress-related illness, but may serve as adjuvants to the standard treatment for many chronic illnesses with an inflammatory component, including cardiovascular and neurodegenerative diseases. However, clinical trials thus far have had significant methodological limitations, so further research is required before definitive conclusions can be made regarding where adaptogens fit into wellness and medicine.

Adaptogens are generally very well tolerated and are considered safe to use, with no serious side effects observed in clinical trials. Some people taking adaptogen compounds have reported dizziness and dry mouth, but causality was not determined. *In vitro* studies have shown that certain adaptogens interact with the cytochrome P450 system, specifically the 1A2, 2C9, 3A4, and 3A5 enzyme subtypes, which may cause the plasma level of drugs that are substrates of these specific enzymes to increase or decrease, though this effect has not been confirmed in human studies.

Specific Nutraceuticals with Toxic Potential

Many nutraceuticals are safe, though as we have shown, others have a toxic potential. For a large number of nutraceuticals, no toxicity or safety data exists due to a lack of pharmacological or toxicological studies. Furthermore, the safety of nutraceuticals may be jeopardized as a result of contamination or adulteration with pesticides, fertilizers, toxic plants, heavy metals, mycotoxins, and a wide range of other possible contaminants. This section will outline known toxicity issues with specific nutraceutical compounds that have not already been described previously in this chapter so that clinicians will be equipped with a well-rounded understanding of the benefits, as well as the potential risks of using nutraceuticals as part of an approach to wellness and health (Table 23.5).

Table 23.5 Specific nutraceuticals with toxic potential in humans [19]

Nutraceutical	Compound	Toxicity
Ackee (*Blighia sapida*)	Hypoglycin A, hypoglycin B	GI and CNS toxicity
Aconite	Aconite/aconitine	Ventricular tachycardia
Aristolochia	Aristolochic acid	GU tract toxicity, GU tract carcinomas
Artemisia spp. and *Salvia* spp.	Monoterpene ketones (α-thujone and β-thujone)	Neurotoxicity
Ayahuasca	B-carbolines and DMT	Hallucinations, tachycardia, hypertension, mydriasis, and vomiting
Bitter melon	Momordicins	Hypoglycemia, miscarriage
Black kohosh	Cimigenol, formononetin	Hepatotoxicity, vertigo, seizures
Blue-green algae	Microcystins	Hepatotoxicity
Chinese cinnamon	Cinnamaldehyde	Hepatotoxicity
Coffee	Caffeine	Anxiety, tremor, tachycardia, rarely death
Comfrey	Pyrrolizidine alkaloids	Hepatotoxicity
Ephedra	Ephedrine alkaloids	Cardiotoxicity, nephrotoxicity
Garcinia cambogia (found in some weight loss supplements)	(−)-hydroxycitric acid	Cardiotoxicity, hepatotoxicity, nephrotoxicity, rhabdomyolysis

Table 23.5 (cont.)

Nutraceutical	Compound	Toxicity
Ginkgo biloba	Ginkgotoxins	Spontaneous hemorrhage, seizures, interactions with the CYP450 system
Goldenseal	Berberine, hydrastine, canadine, canalidine	Tachycardia, seizures, metabolic disturbance, rarely death
Grapefruit	Furocoumarins	Multiple interactions with the CYP450 system
Camellia sinensis (green tea extract)	(−)-epigallocatechin-3-gallate	Hepatotoxicity
Kava	Kavalactones, flavokawain B, pipermethysticin, schaftoside	Hepatotoxicity
Kratom	Mitragynine, 7-hydroxymitragynine	Neurotoxicity, possible addiction
Lychee/litchi	Hypoglycin A, methylenecyclopropyl-glycine (MCPG)	Encephalopathy, hypoglycemia
Pennyroyal oil	Pulegone, menthofuran	Hepatotoxicity, GI bleeding, renal failure, coma, rarely death
St. John's wort	Hypericin, hyperforin, naphthodianthrones, pseudohypericin, sesquiterpenes	Seizures, bone marrow suppression
Valerian	Valerinic acid	Hepatotoxicity, CNS depression

Safety evaluation of nutraceuticals is complicated by several factors, including multiple chemical compounds potentially present in a single plant or extract, variability in chemical compounds due to climate, soil characteristics, cultivation practices, and geography, utilization of fertilizers and pesticides, plant stressors, lack of standard extraction procedures, and lack of defined quality control standards. These factors all determine the identity, purity, quality, quantity, composition, and strength of active nutraceutical ingredients and may result in large variability in effectiveness and safety from one manufacturer to another [19].

Case Example

J.M. is an adult female who has been diagnosed with breast cancer and is undergoing treatment at an integrative oncology center at a large academic medical center that, in addition to medical, surgical, and radiation oncology, offers psychotherapy, support groups, spiritual care, and nutritional counseling.

J.M. is currently taking tamoxifen, a chemotherapy medication used to treat some types of breast cancer and to prevent breast cancer recurrence in those who have already undergone treatment. Importantly, tamoxifen is partially metabolized by the CYP450 3A4 enzyme, as well as other P450 subtypes.

Additionally, J.M. began taking many supplements after her cancer diagnosis, including green tea extract, shark liver oil, vitamin A (5000 IU daily), vitamin D3 (5000 IU daily), vitamin K2 (500 μg daily), Ji Xue Teng, zinc picolinate (20 mg daily), a probiotic supplement, magnesium (400 mg daily), curcumin (200 mg daily), gingko biloba (120 mg daily), and a multivitamin. She also consumes 8 fluid ounces of grapefruit juice daily.

In addition to the side effects of chemotherapy, she is struggling with the stress of a cancer diagnosis, a leave from work, mild anxiety and depression, and a sense of demoralization about "being in the patient role," which she identified taking numerous supplements as a contributor to.

She meets with a nutritionist on staff to determine the utility of her current supplement regimen. The nutritionist advised her to follow a Mediterranean-type diet and exercise as tolerated. Shark liver oil, green tea extract, multivitamin, and the probiotic were continued. All other supplements were stopped, with special attention given to the discontinuation of gingko biloba and grapefruit juice, noting their potential interactions with CYP450 3A4 that could lead to reduced effectiveness of tamoxifen and potential progression or recurrence of her cancer. Fish oil and *rhodiola* extract were started to help manage her mild depression, anxiety, and stress related to her cancer diagnosis.

This patient reported overall improvement in her quality of life, stress level, anxiety, and depression, and continued to receive treatment for her cancer.

Practice Pearls

- Nutraceuticals have a broad range of demonstrated and theoretical benefits that may be harnessed to promote health and wellness and to prevent and treat certain diseases.
- Many nutraceuticals lack clear evidence for efficacy, but this is not lack of potential benefit given that many nutraceutical compounds are poorly understood and have not yet been adequately studied.
- Some nutraceuticals have specific side effects, toxicities, and potentially deleterious interactions with pharmaceutical agents that must be considered when prescribing these agents or counseling patients on using them.
- At present, nutraceuticals are not regulated by most government safety agencies, including the FDA, so they do not have to demonstrate efficacy or safety before being sold commercially, and their health claims are largely unmonitored.
- Before prescribing vitamins or minerals, it is prudent to check nutritional laboratory studies including: vitamin B12 level, folate level, 25-hydroxyvitamin D level, serum iron, ferritin level, red blood cell (RBC) magnesium level, and RBC zinc level, to determine whether there are any nutritional deficiencies that should be corrected.
- Always ask patients or clients about their use of supplements to ensure that potential risks or interactions with pharmaceuticals are not overlooked and that appropriate counseling is done.

References

1. CRN. Consumer survey on dietary supplements. 2015. www.crnusa.org/CRN-consumersurvey-archives/2015 (accessed April 21, 2020).

2. A Kalia. *Textbook of Industrial Pharmacognosy*. New Delhi, CBS Publishers & Distributors Pvt; 2011.

3. L Das, E Bhaumik, U Raychaudhuri, R Chakraborty. Role of nutraceuticals in human health. *J Food Sci Technol* 2011;**49** (2): 173–183.

4. A Canga, N Martínez, A Prieto, et al. Dietary fiber and its interaction with drugs. *Nutrición Hospitalaria* 2010; **25**(4): 535–539.

5. I Lenoir-Wijnkoop, M Sanders, M Cabana, et al. Probiotic and prebiotic influence beyond the intestinal tract. *Nutr Rev* 2007; **65**(11): 469–489.

6. S Doron, D Snydman. Risk and safety of probiotics. *Clin Infect Dis* 2015; **60**(suppl. 2): S129–S134.

7. J Liu. The effects and mechanisms of mitochondrial nutrient α-lipoic acid on improving age-associated mitochondrial and cognitive dysfunction: an overview. *Neurochem Res* 2007; **33**(1): 194–203.

8. J Sarris, J Murphy, D Mischoulon, et al. Adjunctive nutraceuticals for depression: a systematic review and meta-analyses. *Am J Psychiatr* 2016; **173**(6): 575–587.

9. D McCabe, M Colbeck. The effectiveness of essential fatty acid, B vitamin, vitamin C, magnesium and zinc supplementation for managing stress in women: a systematic review protocol. *JBI Database Syst Rev Implement Rep* 2015; **13**(7): 104–118.

10. G Duthie, P Gardner, J Kyle. Plant polyphenols: are they the new magic bullet? *Proc Nutr Soc* 2003; **62**(03): 599–603.

11. L Allen, T Covington, R Berardi, L Young *Handbook of Nonprescription Drugs*. Washington, DC, American Pharmaceutical Association; 1996.

12. M Rosenblum Vitamin toxicity. 2017. https://emedicine.medscape.com/article/819426-overview (accessed April 21, 2020).

13. D Rees, H Kelsey, J Richards. Acute haemolysis induced by high dose ascorbic acid in glucose-6-phosphate dehydrogenase deficiency. *BMJ* 1993; **306** (6881): 841–842.

14. M Sulli, D Ezzo. Drug interactions with vitamins and minerals. 2007. www.uspharmacist.com/article/drug-interactions-with-vitamins-and-minerals (accessed April 21, 2020).

15. A Scalbert, I Johnson, M Saltmarsh. Polyphenols: antioxidants and beyond. *Am J Clin Nutr* 2005; **81**(1): 215S–217S.

16. S Chen, D Volle, J Jalil, P Wu, G Small. Health-promoting strategies for the aging brain. *Am J Geriatr Psychiatr* 2019; **27**(3): 213–236.

17. L Rodríguez-Fragoso, J Martínez-Arismendi, D Orozco-Bustos, et al. Potential risks resulting from fruit/vegetable–drug interactions: effects on drug-metabolizing enzymes and drug transporters. *J Food Sci* 2011; **76**(4): 112–124.

18. A Panossian, G Wikman. Effects of adaptogens on the central nervous system and the molecular mechanisms associated with their stress-protective activity. *Pharmaceuticals* 2010; **3**(1): 188–224.

19. R Gupta, A Srivastava, R Lall. Toxicity potential of nutraceuticals. In: O Nicolotti, ed., *Computational Toxicology*. New York, Humana Press; 2018; 367–394.

Pharmaceuticals and Alternatives for Wellness

Thomas Parisi, Blaire Heath, Raymond Wen, and Waguih
William IsHak

Introduction

The relationship between mind, body, and spirit has inspired philosophers, artists, physicians, and scientists for centuries. Daring to reach for our dreams yet fearing to lose that which we have fought so hard to attain, the tools developed to navigate the human condition have pushed the limits of technological advancement. Although the landscape and its demands will continue to evolve, a common thread throughout time is humanity's desire to reach its potential, to function at peak capacity. This guiding light has led to the development of medicine, which has been utilized as a means by which to save the fragile yet resilient corporeal form, as well as an instrument to transcend its bounds. Medicine as an art involves the use of wide-ranging modalities, including pharmaceuticals. Experiencing health in all meanings of the word involves the absence of illness, as well as the optimization of health. Personalized medicine, or functional medicine, encompasses the ideal functioning of all organ systems and typically involves alternative or holistic medicine. As the standard tirelessly advances, wellness as a concept continues to encapsulate the mental, physical, emotional, and spiritual aspects of health.

Defining wellness can be highly involved, in light of the various organ systems, each patient's preferences, baseline health, and personal goals. Facets, such as attention and memory, emotional health, strength and stamina, living without or sustainably managing pain, cardiovascular fitness and metabolism are the underpinnings to the overall experience of wellness. Vitality, vibrancy, gusto, and drive encompass the intangibles of wellness, while the subtlety of the power to endure, the capacity to develop, quality of life, and the ability to maintain mental vigor provide the foundation. Table 24.1 includes wellness categories that can be utilized to explore patient objectives. Attention entails attaining and maintaining optimal focus. Memory has a variety of layers and discrete time frames, involving storage and manipulation. Emotional health regards a patient's experience of self and the ability to

Table 24.1 General wellness

Category	Description
Attention and memory	Focusing, storing, and manipulating information
Emotional health	Experience of self and engagement with environment
Strength and stamina	Application and performance over time
Experience of pain	Subjective level of physical comfort and ease
Cardiovascular fitness	Interconnectivity of respiratory, hepatic, and metabolic systems

engage the environment. Strength can be measured by application and stamina by performance over time. Pain denotes the subjective level of physical comfort and ease. Cardiovascular fitness is interconnected with respiratory, hepatic, and metabolic systems, dictating health outcomes across a broad spectrum. Factors that comprise metabolic health directly and indirectly affect weight, impacting a patient's subjective physical experience.

The World Health Organization defines health as a state of "complete physical, mental and social well-being and not merely the absence of disease or infirmity" [1]. There are a wide number of interventions from which healthcare providers can select, as they endeavor to help manage the various conditions faced by their patients. The point of departure from the treatment of diseases and their complications is to integrate wellness, with personalized medicine as the platform. Considering the interconnectedness of mental, physical, emotional, and spiritual well-being, pharmaceutical interventions will be highlighted, in the context of personalized medicine, with the aim being the overall optimization of human wellness.

Pharmaceutical Use to Target Wellness

Pharmaceuticals play a significant role in the healthcare regimens of a vast majority of the US population. The pharmaceutical industry in the USA accounts for 10 percent of overall health spending, or $328 billion annually (up to $450 billion when list prices and all transactions are included) [2]. Additionally, the number of prescriptions filled for American adults increased in 2016 to 4.5 billion, up from 2.4 billion in 1997, an 85 percent increase compared to the population increase during the same time span of 21 percent. It is important to note that nutraceuticals or dietary supplements in 2016 contributed $121.6 billion to the US economy. More than two-thirds of American adults take dietary supplements every year [3]. While pharmaceuticals and nutraceuticals play such a large role in patient's lives, the process leading to the availability of pharmaceuticals alone is exceptionally rigorous. The Food and Drug Administration (FDA) has a lengthy and detailed process for new drug approvals, with Stage I (Discovery and Development), Stage II (Preclinical Research), Stage III (Clinical Research), Stage IV (FDA Drug Review), and Stage V (FDA Post-Marketing Drug Safety Monitoring). The drug development stages, including early chemical development, dosing in healthy volunteers, and large-scale trials for indication in large scale double-blind randomized placebo-controlled trials, traditionally have strict guidelines for the manufacture and the continued monitoring of the respective safety profiles of the investigated agents. Conversely, the 1994 Dietary Supplement Health and Education Act (DSHEA) loosened the potential regulations of products intended to supplement the diet, with supplements including one or more dietary components. Ingredients already used prior to passage of the DSHEA were deemed safe based on previous use and new dietary ingredients reviewed, but not approved, by the FDA.

The aim of personalized medicine's focus on the gestalt of patient wellness involves improvement of quality of life, inclusive of feeling more vibrant, living longer, and minimizing polypharmacy and adverse side effects. Therefore, the pharmaceutical agents presented in this chapter may serve as part of the solution for goals such as mental health, neurocognitive wellness, vitality, and gastrointestinal (GI) health, which may have broad repercussions across a number of organ systems, cardiac health, metabolism, and pain reduction. Agents will be suggested as tools by which to navigate certain health goals, while mechanisms of action, common adverse reactions with black box warning (BBW), and dosing suggestions will likewise be presented.

Depression

Depression is a common mental disorder lasting at least two weeks, with characteristic symptoms of altered sleep or appetite, loss of interest in activities once enjoyed, guilt, loss of energy and concentration, psychomotor agitation or retardation, and sometimes suicidal ideation. Depression affects more than 300 million people of all ages worldwide [4]. It is the leading cause of disability and the major contributor to overall global burden of disease, affecting more women than men. Close to 800,000 people die annually by suicide. Despite effective pharmacological and therapy-based treatments, less than 50 percent of those affected in the world (in many countries less than 10 percent) receive treatment. Beyond the use of pharmaceuticals to manage the illness, optimizing patient functioning can lead to improvement in overall wellness. The use of antidepressants for lifestyle enhancement is controversial, yet deficiencies in functioning, not unrelated to basic processes such as sleeping or eating, as well as the facets of functioning that might go overlooked, such as the ability to awaken in the morning and start the day feeling motivated and focused, to meaningfully interact with loved ones and coworkers, or to vigorously engage professional responsibilities, merit clinical attention. Functional improvement, as well as increased quality of life, is seen in efficacious management of depression and has a direct bearing on overall patient wellness [5].

Example Pharmaceutical for Depression: Sertraline

Sertraline is a pharmaceutical that, based on comparing 21 active treatments and placebo, has been found best among the antidepressant classes as far as efficacy, tolerability, and cost in managing major depressive disorder (MDD) [6]. It is known to have both calming and mildly activating properties, making it a good choice for anxious depression, as well as for anxiety disorders, the latter for which higher doses can be reserved.

Mechanism of action: selective serotonin (5-HT) reuptake inhibition; dopamine (DA) transporter inhibition; sigma-1 receptor binding may contribute to the calming effect.

Adverse reactions: diarrhea, nausea, vomiting, abdominal pain, somnolence, decreased libido, hyponatremia, increased risk of bleeding; BBW associated with antidepressants includes increased suicidality in those less than 24 years of age.

Dosing: 25–200 mg by mouth daily or at bedtime with food.

Alternatives to Pharmaceuticals for Depression

St. John's Wort (SJW) has been shown to be more effective as monotherapy than placebo in the management of mild to moderate depression, though its lack of efficacy in MDD has made it less popular [7]. It is started at 300 mg by mouth three times daily then increased to 1500 mg daily within the first six weeks. It has likewise been shown to improve mental quality of life, though not subjective physical quality of life. Mental quality of life references self-perception overall, in terms of well-being, a sense of belonging, autonomy, and one's relationship to the experience of hope, whereas physical quality of life denotes functioning, activity level, and instrumental activities of daily living. Studies have shown that SJW has been associated with significantly more treatment responders than placebo, with depression symptoms significantly improved with SJW relative to placebo. The quality of the studies comparing SJW to pharmaceutical antidepressants, however, has not been of high enough caliber to offer a definitive conclusion. For low- to moderate- grade depression, it may be a viable option for patients who are concerned with the side-effect profile associated with pharmaceutical antidepressants. Patients who trialed SJW were also overall less likely to experience adverse reactions, compared to pharmaceutical antidepressants, and in fact experienced equivalent amounts of adverse reactions to placebo, though studies substantiating the first claim were not deemed high quality. There have also been concerns about persistence of effect and variations in agent preparation.

S-adenosyl-L-methionine (SAMe) is an endogenous molecule synthesized from L-methionine and adenosine triphosphate that is commercially available in the USA as a dietary supplement. Due to its abundance in the brain, it is proposed that SAMe increases monoamine synthesis through a variety of reactions as a methyl donor, thereby being intimately involved with the regulation of 5-HT, DA, and norepinephrine (NE), similar to existing antidepressants. Research has highlighted comparable efficacy between SAMe and escitalopram in patients with MDD, as well as similar adverse reactions primarily concerned with the intestines, the stomach, and mental acuity. However, the results did not indicate whether SAMe has an advantage over placebo or current therapeutics [8]. Despite the data being relatively positive, it is noted that the methodologies in these trials vary, which can hinder the clinical significance of administering SAMe for MDD. SAMe has not been tested to the same standards as its prescription counterparts by the FDA, which should be taken into consideration when recommended to patients for its relative efficacy. However, the risk and adverse reactions profile of SAMe weigh favorably compared to other prescription antidepressants, most notably the lack of sexual dysfunction and weight gain, which are the most common side effects patients report upon discontinuation. Note that serotonin syndrome can be a potential risk for patients taking both SSRIs and SAMe, which may result in complications in patients with treatment-resistant depression [9]. In addition, there are limited studies that suggest the efficacy of SAMe in patients with MDD who are not responding to first-line antidepressants, and it is still uncertain whether SAMe can serve as a monotherapy in patients with MDD, but rather potentially as a supplementary pharmacotherapy [10]. Additional clinical trials are warranted to explore its mechanism, pharmacokinetics, and long-term adverse reactions in order to strengthen SAMe as a viable antidepressant alternative and adjunction.

Dihydroepiandrosterone (DHEA) is a principle precursor for androsterone (ADT), testosterone, and estradiol that is co-released with cortisol secretion from the adrenal cortex in men and women [11]. While historically it has often been marketed commercially as a hormone and as an athletic supplement, it is also known to induce antidepressant and anxiolytic effects. The mechanisms by which DHEA leads to therapeutic effects are unclear, but downstream metabolites of DHEA are dominant modulators for the GABA-a receptor, which suggests one physiological pathway for its ability to mitigate stress and anxiety [12]. The literature suggests that patients who had a significantly elevated DHEA-to-cortisol ratio in plasma showed fewer dissociative symptoms, which can be interpreted as a resilience factor toward adrenocorticotropic hormone and stress [13]. Overall, while DHEA has been shown to improve mood through an elevation in plasma ADT levels, studies with larger sample sizes are necessary before determining its therapeutic efficacy.

5-hydroxtryptophan (5-HTP) is one of the major precursors for 5-HT in the brain, which is believed to be a principle neurotransmitter deficient in MDD. Currently, first-line antidepressants primarily act by inhibiting the reuptake of 5-HT, which elevates extracellular 5-HT (5-HT_{Ext}) and mediates their antidepressant effect [14]. While 5-HTP has been shown to increase 5-HT$_{Ext}$ levels in the brain, its poor pharmacokinetic properties make it difficult to sustain such levels. This poses a limitation because a constant, sustained elevation of 5-HT$_{Ext}$ is required to achieve therapeutic effect. At the moment, 5-HTP is not a therapeutic alternative or adjunct treatment for MDD, despite small trials that showed significant improvements when used in adjunct therapy [15]. Past studies suggest that 5-HTP monotherapy and adjunct therapy with SSRIs and SNRIs are not associated with serious adverse effects in patients with treatment-resistant depression [16]. While oral 5-HTP formulations have been shown to increase 5-HT$_{Ext}$ levels in the brain, its poor pharmacokinetic properties make it difficult to sustain such levels. Nonetheless, for 5-HTP to be a clinically viable antidepressant or part of augmentation therapy, a slow-release 5-HTP could be ideal, as it would deliver sustained 5-HT$_{Ext}$ levels, higher adherence among outpatients, and less adverse reactions; these qualities would draw parallel to current first-line antidepressants and make 5-HTP a daily or twice-daily therapeutic.

Botulinum toxin A (Botox) is the most frequent cosmetic treatment in the USA, with millions of applications annually. For some recipients, the effects of Botox go beyond physical benefits, with many patients reporting an increase in well-being, mood, and happiness [17]. Studies have shown that one injection of Botox in the glabellar region reduced the symptoms in patients with chronic and treatment-resistant MDD [18]. The mechanism by which botulinum toxin treats depression is unclear. It is speculated that the reduction in proprioceptive feedback from facial muscles plays a role in improving mood, as well as in increasing emotional perception. Interestingly, remission is not contingent on a positive preference to the cosmetic transition [19]. Botulinum toxin has several advantages over other conventional antidepressants. The long-lasting pharmacokinetics of botulinum toxin and its singular administration can aid patients in cases of poor therapy adherence. The therapy is also well tolerated, with bruising and irritation immediately after initial injection as the primary risks. However, one drawback to its use would be the long onset of action, as certain vulnerable patients with MDD cannot wait weeks before depressive symptoms alleviate.

Anxiety

Anxiety is characterized by worry, restlessness, easy fatigability, difficulty concentrating, irritability, muscle tension, sleep disturbances, and sometimes GI upset. With varying severity, it can engender a sense of negativity or avoidance, steering patients away from robustly engaging life. Anxiety disorders are the most common mental illness in the USA [20], with 40 million adults affected. Though manageable, less than 40 percent of people with anxiety get treatment. Patients with anxiety disorders are six times more likely to be hospitalized for psychiatric conditions than patients without anxiety. Though benzodiazepines can be employed for acute care, they are not suggested as ongoing treatment, as depression is frequently comorbid with anxiety and they can cause habituation; they can also show decreased efficacy over time.

Example Pharmaceutical for Anxiety: Fluoxetine

Fluoxetine has shown high response and remission among the antidepressant classes in the treatment of anxiety [21]. Referenced studies compared fluoxetine to duloxetine, escitalopram, lorazepam, paroxetine, pregabalin, sertraline, tiagabine, and venlafaxine. Fluoxetine has a long half-life (4–6 days), while its active metabolite has around a nine-day half-life.

The twofold benefit of this long half-life is that it reduces withdrawal reactions characteristic of sudden discontinuation of some medications and provides longer coverage in cases in which regimen adherence is questionable.

Mechanism of action: 5-HT2C antagonism; disinhibition of release of NE and DA.

Adverse reactions: nausea, anorexia, insomnia, headache, hyponatremia, decreased libido, increased risk of bleeding, insomnia; BBW associated with antidepressants includes increased suicidality in those under 24 years of age.

Dosing: 10–80 mg by mouth daily.

Alternatives to Pharmaceuticals for Anxiety

Kava is a natural herb that is known for its anxiolytic properties across many cultures when ingested as a supplement or drink. Anecdotal reports have touted kava kava as a major contributor to wellness in the native population of Fiji. Because it demonstrates anxiolytic effects without sedation or cognitive impairment, kava kava has been viewed as an attractive alternative to benzodiazepines and other anxiolytic prescriptions with notable side effects. Various kava extracts have been shown to exhibit efficacy similar to that of buspirone and opipramol in patients with general anxiety disorder (GAD) [22], and female patients have reported an increase in sex drive concurrent with reduced anxiety [23]. While kava is generally safe to consume for adults, hepatotoxicity has been reported, which has primarily been attributed to poor quality standards during kava extraction [24]. Although long-term uses have been associated with jaundice and scaly skin, which can limit patients who are taking kava for chronic GAD, kava remains a suitable and safe alternative for patients who want to utilize natural remedies for their anxiety disorders. Kava has been shown to be superior to placebo in the treatment of anxiety in three out of seven trials, according to a 2018 systematic review [25].

Cannabidiol (CBD) is a novel therapy initially designed to ameliorate epilepsy syndromes in children. Since then, clinical evidence has emerged that demonstrates the potential of CBD to be a therapeutic against a number of neuropsychiatric disorders. It has been used to treat various anxiety disorders, such as posttraumatic stress disorder, GAD, panic disorder, social anxiety disorder, and obsessive-compulsive disorder. Based on existing studies, CBD is speculated to work on 5-HT1ARs in the brain via the serotonergic system, which in turn demonstrates anxiolytic effects, minimal to no sedative effects, and almost no residual side effects [26]. While it is suggested that the activity of CBD at the 5-HT1A receptor also leads to its antidepressive effects, the mechanism and potential are still unclear and warrant further investigation [27]. Despite a lack of well-powered trials, existing results present CBD as a novel anxiolytic agent for several reasons. It is not psychoactive and does not have a detrimental effect on cognition. It has a moderate safety profile, fast onset, and ease of administration that makes it tolerable for patients of various health and age groups. Overall, current research demonstrates the reliable efficacy of CBD in reducing anxiety seen in various psychiatric disorders. More research is required to establish its anxiolytic mechanism in the brain, as well as the effects of chronic CBD administration in vulnerable patient populations.

Valerian root and its extracts have been used medicinally dating back to the early Renaissance. Today, valerian is widely used as a natural therapeutic for patients with anxiety and sleep disorders. The mechanism of valerian is similar to that of benzodiazepines, notable for binding to the GABA-a subunit and inducing an inhibitory effect, leading to its anxiolytic and sedative properties. Further, valerian exhibits partial 5-HT5a agonism, which suggests alternative pathways for its anxiolytic properties [28]. Studies have been conducted to test whether valerian has an indication for insomnia due to its sedating properties, with limited and inconclusive results [29]. While valerian is generally safe to use by adults for short periods of time, there is a lack of well-powered studies to accurately elucidate its therapeutic effects in patients with anxiety and MDD. A small study showed that valerian and diazepam showed similar efficacy in patients [30]. However, more studies with larger sample sizes are required before determining whether valerian root has clinical efficacy in treating anxiety and insomnia.

Essential oils have been a staple home remedy for mood alleviation and relaxation for decades due to their effects on the central nervous system, but recent studies have supported their indication in treating patients with a range of clinical psychiatric disorders, including GAD, subthreshold anxiety, and MDD [31, 32]. Specifically, the lavender oil derivative silexan has not only been shown to be as efficacious as paroxetine in treating patients with GAD, but has also demonstrated improved health-related quality of life [31]. Silexan also exhibited efficacy in patients who suffer from subthreshold anxiety, a type of anxiety that is often undertreated due to its inconspicuous symptoms [32]. Other essential oil therapies, such as aromatherapy massage, have only been effective in temporarily alleviating comorbid anxiety and depression in cancer patients, suggesting that essential oil-based therapy could be used for short-term management, or as an adjunct therapy for vulnerable patient populations with comorbid anxiety and depression [33]. Overall, essential oil therapies are generally safe and well tolerated in patients with anxiety disorders, and can be used as an alternative for patients looking for natural remedies.

Cognition

Cognition encompasses the mental processes of acquiring, storing, manipulating, and retrieving information. The ability to appreciate context, substance, purpose, and nuance is facilitated by healthy cognition, helping patients achieve goals, navigate complexity, and feel a sense of mastery in their lives. Age-related declines in working memory and in processing speeds impact wellness and quality of life, including personal interactions and meaningful engagement with professional endeavors, and can contribute to depression. While cholinesterase inhibitors or stimulants are the cornerstone in the respective treatments of dementia or attention disorders, cognition is herein explored as a facet directly related to overall wellness, with a nutraceutical suggested as an option for healthy patients.

Example Pharmaceutical for Cognition: Methylphenidate

Methylphenidate is approved for the treatment of attention-deficit/hyperactivity disorder. However, off-label uses of methylphenidate include the treatment of depression, fatigue, low motivation, and faltering scholastic performance, facets of cognition all linked to self-rated well-being.

Mechanism of action: stimulates central nervous system activity; blocks reuptake and increases release of NE and DA in extraneuronal space.

Adverse reactions: nervousness, insomnia, tachycardia, headache, anorexia, weight loss, dependence, psychosis, mania, myocardial infarct, stroke.

Dosing: 10–60 mg by mouth daily.

Alternatives to Pharmaceuticals for Cognition

Gingko biloba has shown modest, significant increased accuracy, non-significant reduction in reaction time, a modest increase in working memory accuracy, and trends toward faster reaction times for working memory in healthy individuals, and has also been found in healthy individuals to produce a dose-dependent improvement in speed of attention [34]. Gingko biloba dose is 120–600 mg by mouth twice daily. Side effects can include diarrhea, nausea, vomiting, headache, and tearing. More robust studies that reveal the effect of gingko biloba on memory in healthy individuals are needed.

Sleep

Sleep is a natural, cyclical, physiological process, the lack of which has been shown to have wide-ranging adverse short- and long-term effects [35]. Short-term consequences of lack of sleep include pain, mood changes, cognition deficits, heightened startle response, and impaired productivity. Long-term consequences of lack of sleep include hypertension, dyslipidemia, cardiovascular disease, type-2 diabetes, metabolic syndrome, and overall reduced quality of life. A focus on healthy sleep habits is paramount in efforts toward overall wellness. Primary sleep disorders regard at least one month of difficulty initiating or maintaining sleep, unrelated to medical conditions, psychiatric conditions, or the effects of substances, thereby leading to impaired daytime functioning. Delayed sleep phase causes around a 3–6-hour interruption between usual sleep and wake times and can be seen in depression. While a wide variety of sleep aids might aid in the short- or long-term management of insomnia, many have habituating properties, with effects that wane over time, so will be excluded.

Example Pharmaceutical for Sleep: Trazodone

Trazodone was originally introduced as an antidepressant at doses of 150–300 mg daily. Evidence emerged for its use in primary and secondary insomnia at doses ranging from 25 mg to 100 mg at bedtime, and it has been shown to improve quality of life and overall ratings of well-being. Side effects are dose-dependent.

Mechanism of action: antagonizes 5-HT2A/c and alpha-1 adrenergic receptors; inhibits 5-HT reuptake.

Adverse reactions: somnolence, headache, dizziness, fatigue, confusion, ataxia, tremor, malaise.

Dosing: 25–100 mg by mouth at bedtime for sleep.

Alternatives to Pharmaceuticals for Sleep

Melatonin has shown the most convincing evidence for reducing sleep onset latency in primary insomnia and in delayed sleep phase syndrome [36]. The pineal gland secretes endogenous melatonin, low levels of which are associated with aging. The optimal dose is 2 mg by mouth four hours before sleep. Exogenous melatonin is not known to cause tolerance, dependence, or morning somnolence. It can induce phase shifts in the circadian timing system, lower core body temperature, and decrease alertness, all characteristics that lead to successful sleep.

Pain

Pain management involves considerations for acute management of disease-specific pain. Over 23 million adults in the USA alone experience significant levels of pain [37]. Adults with more severe pain have been shown to have worse health, utilize more healthcare, and suffer from more disability than those with less severe pain. While the field of pain management has delivered much-needed pain control to a wide range of pain patients suffering with varying types and degrees of pain, the addictive properties of a number of analgesics have proven problematic. Patients who struggle with pain can face daily challenges in functioning, interpersonal relationships, and the overall experience of wellness. When pain is not effectively treated or relieved, it can have highly unfavorable effects on quality of life [38]. Musculoskeletal disorders specifically affect mortality, morbidity, and quality of life [39]. While pain management typically focuses on tertiary prevention, there are efforts that can be made to prevent the development of conditions that cause pain and facets of pain that can be chronically managed or acutely treated. The focus herein will be on bone pain, joint pain, inflammation, and general pain. Approximately 10 million Americans have osteoporosis and another 44 million have low bone density [40]. Aside from the structural changes caused by osteoporosis, which can lead to fractures – some of which can turn out to be fatal – the associated pain is commonly experienced as cramps, bone pain, and muscle aches, all of which limit daily activities and decrease overall wellness and quality of life, thus hindering vitality [41]. Hip fractures secondary to osteoporosis cause the greatest morbidity and mortality, and risk exponentially increases with age. Osteoarthritis, on the other hand, is a degenerative joint disease, usually of the articular cartilage. Joint pain is chiefly associated with aging, with the most frequently affected joints being knees, hips, fingers, and lower spine. It is one of the 10 most disabling diseases of the developed world [42]. An estimated 10 percent of men and almost 20 percent of women over the age of 60 have symptomatic arthritis, with 25 percent of said population being so limited as to be unable to perform usual daily activities. Inflammation due to symptoms of arthritis, including osteoarthritis or rheumatoid arthritis, is commonly accompanied by pain, stiffness, swelling, and decreased range of movement. Though much pain is disease-specific, it can also be quite generalized, with compromised bone health and joint health, as well as inflammation, likewise contributing to an insidious decline in overall wellness. As such, the following suggestions might be considered modest components of the complex picture of optimizing health, also in the context of averting specific health conditions.

Example Pharmaceutical for Pain: Diclofenac

Diclofenac is the most effective NSAID in terms of improving osteoporotic (and rheumatic) pain and function [43]. It has been found at 150 mg daily to be more effective in alleviating pain than celoxocib 200 mg daily, naproxen 1000 mg daily, ibuprofen 2400 mg daily, or etoricoxib 60 mg daily. A 100 mg daily dose of diclofenac has been found to be comparable to the aforementioned agents, while at 100 mg daily or at 150 mg daily diclofenac has also been found to improve physical function in a manner comparable to said agents. Patient global assessment of disease severity at 100 mg or 150 mg was found to be superior to or comparable to that of the other agents. Platelet effect and major cardiovascular events were similar across all agents. Upper GI events with diclofenac were lower compared to naproxen or ibuprofen, yet comparable to celecoxib. Withdrawal risk with diclofenac was lower compared to ibuprofen, similar to celecoxib or naproxen, yet higher than etoricoxib.

Mechanism of action: inhibits cyclooxygenase, reducing prostaglandin and thromboxane synthesis.

Adverse reactions: dyspepsia, nausea, vomiting, abdominal pain, increased bleeding; BBW of increased risk of serious and potentially fatal cardiovascular thrombotic events, such as myocardial infarction and stroke; increased bleeding and ulcers.

Dosing: 50–150 mg by mouth daily.

Alternatives to Pharmaceuticals for Pain

Curcumin is the extracted, active compound in the turmeric plant. Pain, stiffness, and function have all been shown to improve with curcumin when dosed at 1 g by mouth daily [44]. Evidence shows that curcumin is supported in the treatment of arthritic inflammation, yet larger studies of higher quality are merited to confirm the therapeutic efficacy.

Conclusion

Personalized medicine translates to optimal care for each patient, best accomplished through accountability and continuity of care within the healthcare system. Checkpoints – from prescriber, to dispensing, to administration, inclusive of healthcare education – facilitate patient ownership of treatment regimens. Table 24.2 offers suggestions for providers and patients that might assist in the implementation of tailored treatment plans. Patients are encouraged to have a single primary care provider and a single pharmacy or pharmacy chain, permitting ideal monitoring in the hopes of minimizing agent interactions and duplications, as well as promoting regimen adherence. Minimizing the number of agents prescribed, as well as the complexity of their administration, lends to improved adherence. The use of combination pills or long-acting formulations can simplify drug administration, as well as minimize adverse reactions. An added benefit of long-acting formulations is that often there is a more consistent drug release rather than an abrupt peak after administration. Encouraging patients to access their pharmacist can also help reinforce concerns related to polypharmacy, pharmaceuticals and natural alternatives, agent–agent interactions, or adverse reactions. A list containing the active pharmaceutical and alternative agents can serve as a crucial communication tool, facilitating simplicity, as well as potentially guiding interventions in the cases of emergency.

As pharmaceutical developments advance, the gap between prevention and health optimization may narrow. Lifestyle medication could garner a deserved spot on the top shelf among the repertoire of clinical interventions. Even after scaling to this zenith, patients and physicians will yet strive to seize the much-prized goal of wellness. Though understanding will evolve, the relationship between body, mind, and spirit may never be fully grasped, while efforts will continue such that it might mystify less over time. Whether it be conveyed by vitality, wellness, *joie de vivre*, longevity, or vigor, the thrust of medical care is toward a condition greater than that of merely being free of disease. Pharmaceuticals, natural alternatives, and nutraceuticals serve as critical vehicles on the road toward whole-person wellness.

Table 24.2 Overview of implementation of treatment regimens

Encourage a single primary care provider
Suggest patient have one pharmacy or pharmacy chain
Minimize number of agents, drug interactions, and duplications
Reduce administration complexity
Create a list of health conditions and treatment agents

References

1. World Health Organization. WHOQOL: measuring quality of life. 2019. www.who.int/healthinfo/survey/whoqol-qualityoflife/en (accessed April 7, 2019).

2. Health Affairs. Spending on prescription drugs in the US: where does all the money go? 2018. www.healthaffairs.org/do/10.1377/hblog20180726.670593/full (accessed April 7, 2019).

3. Council for Responsible Nutrition Foundation. Economic impact of the dietary supplement industry. 2016. www.crnusa.org/resources/economic-impact-dietary-supplement-industry (accessed April 7, 2019).

4. World Health Organization. Depression. 2018. www.who.int/news-room/factsheets/detail/depression (accessed April 8, 2019).

5. WW IsHak, W Bonifay, K Collison, et al. The recovery index: a novel approach to measuring recovery and predicting remission in major depressive disorder. *J Affect Disord* 2017; **208**: 369–374.

6. A Cipriani, T Furukawa, G Salanti, et al. Comparative efficacy and acceptability of 21 antidepressant drugs for the acute treatment of adults with major depressive disorder: a systematic review and network meta-analysis. *Lancet* 2018; **391**: 1357–1366.

7. EA Apaydin, AR Maher, R Shanman, et al. A systematic review of St. John's wort for major depressive disorder. *Syst Rev* 2016; **5**: 148.

8. GI Papakostas, D Mischoulon, I Shyu, JE Alpert, M Fava. S-adenosyl methionine (SAMe) augmentation of serotonin reuptake inhibitors (SRIs) for SRI- non-responders with major depressive disorder: a double-blind, randomized clinical trial. *Am J Psychiatr* 2010; **167**: 942–948.

9. D Mischoulon, LH Price, LL Carpenter, et al. A double-blind, randomized, placebo-controlled clinical trial of S-adenosyl-L-methionine (SAMe) versus escitalopram in major depressive disorder. *J Clin Psychiatry* 2014; **75**: 370–376.

10. J Sarris, GI Papakostas, O Vitolo, D Mischoulon. S-adenosyl methionine (SAMe) versus escitalopram and placebo in major depression RCT: efficacy and effects of histamine and carnitine as moderators of response. *J Clin Psychiatr* 2014; **75**: 855–863.

11. M Bradley, M McElhiney, J Rabkin. DHEA and cognition in HIV-positive patients with non-major depression. *Psychosomatics* 2012; **53**: 244–249.

12. R Ben Dor, CE Marx, LJ Shampine, DR Rubinow, PJ Schmidt. DHEA metabolism to the neurosteroid androsterone: a possible mechanism of DHEA's antidepressant action. *Psychopharmacology (Berl)* 2015; **232**: 3375–3383.

13. SJ Russo, JW Murrough, MH Han, DS Charney, EJ Nestler. Neurobiology of resilience. *Nat Neurosci* 2012; **15**: 1475–1484.

14. JP Jacobsen, AD Krystal, KR Krishnan, MG Caron. Adjunctive 5-hydroxytryptophan slow-release for treatment-resistant depression: clinical and preclinical rationale. *Trends Pharmacol Sci* 2016; **37**: 933–944.

15. LJ Van Hiele. L-5-Hydroxytryptophan in depression: the first substitution therapy in psychiatry? The treatment of 99 out-patients with "therapy-resistant" depressions. *Neuropsychobiology* 1980; **6**: 230–240.

16. EH Turner, JM Loftis, AD Blackwell. Serotonin a la carte: supplementation with the serotonin precursor 5-hydroxtryptophan. *Pharmacol Ther* 2006; **109**: 325–328.

17. JI Davis, A Senghas, F Brandt, KN Ochsner. The effects of BOTOX injections on emotional experience. *Emotion* 2010; **10**: 433–440.

18. E Finzi, NE Rosenthal. Treatment of depression with obotulinumtoxinA: a randomized, double-blinded, placebo controlled trial. *J Psychiatr* 2014; **52**: 1–6.

19. MA Woller, C de Boer, N Kalak, et al. Facing depression with botulinum toxin: a randomized controlled trial. *J Psychiatr* 2012; **45**: 574–581.

20. National Institute of Mental Health. Anxiety disorders. 2018. www .nimh.nih.gov/health/topics/anxiety-disorders/index.shtml (accessed April 25, 2019).

21. D Baldwin, R Woods, R Lawson, et al. Efficacy of drug treatments for generalised anxiety disorder: systematic review and meta-analysis. *BMJ* 2011; **342**: d1199.

22. RJ Boerner, H Sommer, W Berger, et al. Kava-kava extract LI 150 is as effective as opipramol and buspirone in generalised anxiety disorder: an 8-week randomized, double-blind multi-centre clinical trial in 129 outpatients. *Phytomedicine* 2003; **10**: 38–49.

23. J Sarris, C Stough, R Teschke, et al. Kava for the treatment of generalized anxiety disorder RCT: analysis of adverse reactions, liver function, addiction, and sexual effects. *Phytother Res* 2013; **27**: 1723–1728.

24. A Rowe, LY Zhang, I Ramzan. Toxicokinetics of kava. *Adv Pharmacol Sci* 2011; **2011**: 326724.

25. K Smith, C Leiras. The effectiveness and safety of Kava Kava for treating anxiety symptoms: a systematic review and analysis of randomized clinical trials. *Complement Ther Clin Pract* 2018; **33**:107–117.

26. EM Blessing, MM Steenkamp, J Manzanares, CR Marmar. Cannabidiol as a potential treatment for anxiety disorders. *Neurotherapeutics* 2015; **12**: 825–836.

27. S Shannon, N Lewis, H Lee, S Hughes. Cannabidiol in anxiety and sleep: a large case series. *Perm J* 2019; **23**: 18-041.

28. S Jerome, P Alexander, S Isaac, S Con, S Andrew. Herbal medicine for depression, anxiety and insomnia: a review of psychopharmacology and clinical evidence. *J Eur Coll Neuropsychol* 2011; **21**: 841–860.

29. S Bent, A Padula, D Moore, M Patterson, W Mehling. Valerian for sleep: a systematic review and meta-analysis. *Am J Med* 2006; **119**: 1005–1012.

30. LS Miyasaka, ÁN Natallah, B Soares. Valerian for anxiety disorders. *Cochrane Database Syst Rev* 2006; **4**: CD004515.

31. K Siegfried, G Markus, EM Walter, V Hans-Peter, et al. Lavender oil preparation silexan is effective in generalized anxiety disorder: a randomized, double-blind comparison to placebo and paroxetine. *Int J Neuropsychopharmacol* 2014; **17**: 859–869.

32. K Siegfried, EM Walter, V Hans-Peter, et al. Silexan in anxiety disorders: clinical data and pharmacological background. *World J Biol Psychiatry* 2018; **19**: 412–420.

33. SM Wilkinson, SB Love, AM Westcombe, et al. Effectiveness of aromatherapy massage in the management of anxiety and depression in patients with cancer: a multicenter randomized controlled trial. *J Clin Oncol* 2007; **25**: 532–539.

34. DO Kennedy, AB Scholey, KA Wesnes. The dose-dependent cognitive effects of acute administration of *Ginkgo biloba* to healthy young volunteers. *Psychopharmacology (Berl)* 2000; **4**: 416–423.

35. WW IsHak, K Bagot, S Thomas, et al. Quality of life in patients suffering from insomnia. *Innov Clin Neurosci* 2012; **9**: 13–26.

36. F Auld, EL Maschauer, I Morrison, et al. Evidence for the efficacy of melatonin in the treatment of primary adult sleep disorders. *Sleep Med Rev* 2017; **34**: 10–22.

37. National Center for Complementary and Integrative Health. NIH analysis shows Americans are in pain. 2015. https://nccih .nih.gov/news/press/08112015 (accessed April 1, 2019).

38. N Katz. The impact of pain management on quality of life. *J Pain Symptom Manage* 2002; **1**(Suppl.): S38–S47.

39. C Beaudart, E Biver, O Bruyére, et al. Quality of life assessment in musculo-skeletal health. *Aging Clin Exp Res* 2018; **5**: 413–418.

40. World Health Organization. Scientific Group on the Assessment of Osteoporosis at Primary Health Care Level: summary meeting report Brussels, Belgium. 2004. www.who.int/chp/topics/Osteoporosis.pdf (accessed April 2, 2019).

41. RW Moskowitz. The burden of osteoarthritis: clinical and quality-of-life

issues. *Am J Manage Care* 2009; 8(Suppl.): S223–S229.

42. T Neogi. The epidemiology and impact of pain in osteoarthritis. *Osteoarthr Cartil* 2013; 9: 1145–1153.

43. A van Walsem, S Pandhi, RM Nixon, et al. Relative benefit–risk comparing diclofenac to other traditional non-steroidal anti-inflammatory drugs and cyclooxygenase-2 inhibitors in patients with osteoarthritis or rheumatoid arthritis: a network meta-analysis. *Arthritis Res Ther* 2015; 17: 66.

44. JW Daily, M Yang, S Park. Efficacy of turmeric extracts and curcumin for alleviating the symptoms of joint arthritis: a systematic review and meta-analysis of randomized controlled clinical trials. *J Med Food* 2016; 8: 717–729.

Chapter

25

Exercise, Dance, Tai Chi, Pilates, and Alexander Technique

Ziya Altug

Introduction

Movement is essential for life. Our ability to move not only enhances our function in daily activities, but also keeps our minds and bodies tuned for whatever challenges the world brings our way. Perhaps our ancient ancestors did not focus on exercise since their daily activities frequently involved walking, carrying, lifting, bending, climbing, and reaching. Modern society is dominated by tasks such as sitting for work (e.g., driving to work, office jobs) and leisure-time activities (e.g., sitting at home and at the movies to watch the screen, or at concerts or sporting events). For this reason, the current society needs to exercise either in the home, at a gym, or outdoors to offset our sedentary work and leisure activities. This chapter will briefly touch upon areas where individuals can engage in various forms of movement.

Exercise

According to the 23rd edition of *Taber's Cyclopedic Medical Dictionary*, exercise is a form of physical or mental activity to restore, maintain, and increase normal capacity to improve fitness or manage a particular medical condition. The physical aspects of exercise include the maintenance or development of strength, flexibility, endurance, balance, and agility. Mental exercise, on the other hand, involves tasks and activities to improve concentration, problem-solving, and memory. Exercise in general is needed to prevent conditions such as heart disease, falls, osteoporosis, depression, and sarcopenia, and also to maintain normal blood pressure and sugar levels. Finally, physical activity and exercise are needed to promote a sense of well-being and maintain independence with activities of daily living. Box 25.1 outlines the basic benefits of exercise, and Box 25.2 highlights some elements a clinician needs to consider when prescribing therapeutic exercise.

According to the American College of Sports Medicine global health initiative on Exercise is Medicine, healthcare providers should include physical activity as a part of treatment plans. The American Physical Therapy Association's Guide to Physical Therapist Practice defines therapeutic exercise as a "systematic performance or execution of planned physical movements, postures, or activities intended to enable the patient/client to 1) remediate or prevent impairments, 2) enhance function, 3) reduce risk, 4) optimize overall health, and 5) enhance fitness and well-being." Additionally, therapeutic exercise may be used to foster recovery after injury or surgery and to prevent complications after illness or injury. Finally, the factors determining the exercise prescription include the patient's/client's medical history, medical evaluation, history of injury, goals, preferences, response (in other words, how they tolerate movement and activity), fitness level (beginner, intermediate, or advanced), equipment availability, other clinician programs (i.e., what was done before), and the best available research.

Box 25.1 Benefits of Exercise

- Increases endurance (stamina) and strength
- Reduces stress, anxiety, and depression
- Decreases blood pressure
- Lowers low-density lipoprotein (LDL) cholesterol
- Raises high-density lipoprotein (HDL) cholesterol
- Improves sleep
- Improves control of blood sugar levels
- Improves flexibility, balance, coordination, agility, and reaction time
- Improves mood, self-confidence, cognitive processing speed, and attention span
- Improves posture and daily function (such as the ability to get out of a chair with ease)
- Improves pelvic floor strengthening before and after pregnancy
- Improvement in musculoskeletal issues (for example, less knee or shoulder pain)
- Improves function after orthopedic surgery, such as after a total knee or hip replacement surgery, rotator cuff surgery, or back and neck surgery
- Serves as an adjunct to improving and controlling medical conditions, such as asthma, diabetes, facial palsy, stroke, peripheral neuropathy, and back and neck pain
- Slows age-related decline in bone mineral density and improves bone density
- Slows age-related decline in muscle mass and strength, as well as improving muscle mass and strength
- Reduces risk of falling by improving strength, flexibility, and balance
- Reduces body fat and excess weight in cases of obesity and overweight

Box 25.2 Elements of Therapeutic Exercise

The following are some elements a clinician needs to consider when prescribing therapeutic exercise:

- Indication – why you are doing the exercise?
- Contraindications – what are key areas you should avoid?
- Precautions – what are key areas you should be cautious of?
- Type – what type of exercise is needed? For example, does the person need flexibility, strength, aerobic, anaerobic, balance, coordination, speed, or agility training?
- Frequency – how many days per week should the exercise be performed?
- Intensity – how hard should the exercise be performed?
- Time – for how long should the exercise be performed?
- Volume – how much total time should be spent doing the exercise?
- Pattern – how much rest is needed between sets, exercises, and training days?
- Progression – how should the person progress their exercise?
- Maintenance – what is the minimum amount of training needed to maintain gains?

What Does Selected Research Say about Exercise?

- A high-intensity resistance and impact training program enhances indices of bone strength and functional performance in healthy postmenopausal women with low to very low bone mass [1].

- Resistance training improved global cognitive function in adults with mild cognitive impairment [2].
- A 12-month resistance training program benefited the executive cognitive function among senior women aged 65–75 years [3].
- A landmark study in the *New England Journal of Medicine* showed that high-intensity resistance exercise training is effective in counteracting muscle weakness and physical frailty in individuals aged 72–98 years [4].
- A landmark study in *JAMA* concluded that high-resistance weight training led to significant gains in muscle strength and functional mobility among frail residents of nursing homes up to 96 years of age [5].

Case Vignette: Exercise

Bob, a 54-year-old male, works indoors as an accountant for a large company. He is overweight and stopped exercising when his knees and lower back started to hurt about 10 years ago. In addition to his sedentary lifestyle, he has been diagnosed with hypertension and moderate osteoarthritis of his knees. Upon his physician's suggestion, he scheduled an appointment with a physical therapist. After a complete evaluation, the physical therapist not only created a clinical treatment strategy for Bob, but the therapist also prescribed a simple short-duration and intermittent exercise program. Bob now performs 10 minutes of walking before work after he parks his car, 10 minutes at lunch, and 10 minutes after work for a total of 30 minutes per day. After three months, Bob notices that he has significantly less knee and back pain, and he lost about 15 pounds. His physician informs him that his blood pressure has dropped and if he continues he may be able to further reduce his blood pressure. Overall, Bob enjoys his outdoor walks in the fresh air and sunshine. His mood has improved and he no longer feels like he does not have time for exercise since he includes activity in his work schedule.

For additional information, refer to:

- Academic Consortium for Integrative Medicine & Health (www.imconsortium.org)
- American College of Sports Medicine (www.acsm.org)
- American Physical Therapy Association (www.apta.org)
- Exercise is Medicine (www.exerciseismedicine.org)
- National Center for Complementary and Integrative Health (https://nccih.nih.gov)
- National Strength and Conditioning Association (www.nsca.com)
- SHAPE America (www.shapeamerica.org)

Dance

Dance is perhaps one of the oldest forms of activity and exercise. Dance can be a fun way to engage in weight-bearing exercise. Plato, an ancient Greek philosopher, said "Life must be lived as play." Maybe dance combined with the therapeutic benefits of music and art may regain the top spot as an ideal form of fitness and therapeutic activity. In recent years, dance therapy has been used to help treat conditions such as autism, Alzheimer's disease, balance disorders, cancer, cerebral palsy, cognitive impairment, depression, heart disease, Parkinson's disease, post-stroke, schizophrenia, socialization and well-being, and stress reduction. See Table 25.1 for the different types of dance.

Table 25.1 Types of dance

• Argentine tango	• Mambo
• Ballet	• Merengue
• Belly dancing	• Modern dance
• Bolero	• Paso doble
• Cha cha cha	• Quickstep
• Charleston	• Rumba
• Country two step	• Salsa
• Flamenco	• Samba
• Foxtrot	• Square dancing
• Freestyle	• Tap dancing
• Hustle	• Waltz
• Jitterbug	• Viennese waltz
• Jive	• West coast swing
• Lambada	• Zumba
• Lindy hop	

What Does Selected Research Say about Dance?

• Dance can improve motor parameters of Parkinson's disease and functional mobility [6].
• Ballroom dancing serves as a non-pharmacological intervention that may benefit cognitive functions [7].
• A dance-based exercise program improved cardiorespiratory capacity, and decreased postexercise heart rate and fatigue in obese postmenopausal women [8].
• Dance therapy may improve health-related quality of life and exercise capacity in patients with chronic heart failure [9].
• Tango dance and mindfulness meditation could be used as complementary adjuncts for the treatment of depression and/or included in stress management programs [10].

Case Vignette: Dance

Mary is a 41-year-old stay-at-home mother of two children under the age of 10. She gives private piano lessons from her home. Mary has gained about 30 pounds of weight after having her children and has been diagnosed with anxiety and osteopenia. Her doctor has advised her to exercise, but she has never found an exercise program she enjoys. In high school and college, Mary was never interested in athletics but focused on playing music and became a music teacher. Once her kids are in high school she plans to teach music at a local school. Mary has tried many forms of exercise, including joining a gym, yoga, Pilates, and walking outdoors, but none are forms of activity she can stay with for any length of time. For her birthday, Mary's friend gives her a gift card to attend a dance studio with her husband. After they complete six sessions of dance classes they are both hooked. Mary and her husband decide to take regular dance classes twice per week and go dancing at a club another two times per week while her parents watch the children. After six months, both Mary and her husband lose weight, and Mary feels good about doing her fun weight-bearing exercise to help improve her bone density.

For additional information, refer to:

- American Dance Therapy Association (https://adta.org)
- American Music Therapy Association (www.musictherapy.org)

Tai Chi

Tai chi (also known as T'ai Chi Ch'uan or Tai Qi) is a form of traditional Chinese martial art or exercise in which a series of slow, controlled, multidirectional movements helps to improve balance, flexibility, strength, and agility, and also helps to improve mental concentration and promote relaxation. Tai chi is sometimes considered as a mind in action or meditation in motion. The exact origin of tai chi is unknown, but it is said that this martial art developed many centuries ago, when animal movements were imitated to recover physical and mental health.

There are several styles of tai chi, such as the Yang (a very popular form), Chen, Wu, Hao, and Sun styles, with some forms having around 108 postures and movements (considered the long form), and other forms around 24 movements (considered the short form). The benefits of the short form include that is it easier to learn and consumes less time. The long form, on the other hand, benefits a person more since it is physically and mentally more challenging.

In practical terms, tai chi may be used with patients and clients who need to improve their endurance, mobility, posture, balance, and cognitive function, and their ability to manage stress and pain, prevent falls, and socialize, using a low-cost and low-tech form of activity.

What Does Selected Research Say about Tai Chi?

- May be considered a therapeutic option in the multidisciplinary management of fibromyalgia [11].
- Shows demonstrable effects on body composition when compared to inactive controls [12].
- Can improve exercise capacity in individuals with chronic obstructive pulmonary disease [13].
- Can reduce pain intensity and self-reported disability in individuals experiencing long-term low back pain symptoms [14].
- Effective in decreasing the number of falls, the risk for falling, and the fear of falling, and improves functional balance and physical performance in individuals aged 70 years or older [15].

Case Vignette: Tai Chi

Jane, an 82-year-old retired math teacher, noticed that she and her husband of 52 years no longer had stamina when they went shopping, and their balance was getting worse when doing daily activities. They both do gardening and periodically go to a community center for fundraising events. They both feel somewhat isolated since their kids live in other states. Upon the suggestion of a neighbor, they attended a new tai chi class at a nearby park. To their surprise, there were about 25 individuals from their community in attendance. After performing tai chi twice weekly for six weeks, Jane and her husband have noticed that they have more stamina and improved balance. They now have a new social group and the participants meet regularly every week to attend shows and events in their community.

For additional information, refer to:

- American Tai Chi and Qigong Association (www.americantaichi.org)
- International Medical Tai Chi and Qigong Association (www.imtqa.org)

Pilates

The Pilates system is a form of body work that uses controlled movements and poses to improve strength, flexibility, balance, and mental concentration. German-born Joseph H. Pilates (1880–1967) is the creator of this system. Throughout his career, he developed many original exercise machines (the Reformer, Cadillac, Wunda Chair, and Ladder Barrel), created a mat exercise series, wrote two books, and formulated his own exercise theories.

The original mat and apparatus based exercises can be modified to accommodate those with pain and/or injury, and to challenge the elite athlete. In practical terms, Pilates may be used with patients and clients who need to work on core stability and strength, and also work on posture, balance, and mobility.

What Does Selected Research Say about Pilates?

- Effective in patients with chronic nonspecific low back pain in the management of disability, pain, and kinesiophobia [16].
- Resulted in improvement of pain, function, quality of life, and reduction of the use of analgesics in individuals treated for chronic mechanical neck pain [17].
- Provided better outcomes in pain and disability than advice alone for patients with nonspecific chronic low back pain [18].
- Equipment-based Pilates was superior to mat Pilates for the outcomes of disability and kinesiophobia in individuals with chronic nonspecific low back pain [19].
- A clinical Pilates program produced similar benefits on self-reported disability, pain, function, and health-related quality of life as a general exercise program in individuals with chronic low back pain [20].

Case Vignette: Pilates

Jessica, a 27-year-old engineer, competed in gymnastics until she graduated from college. In her last year of competition, her team physician diagnosed her with spondylolisthesis (forward-slipping of one vertebra on the one below it) in her lower back. After completing an eight-week course of physical therapy, her physical therapist recommended she try going to a Pilates studio for additional core stabilization exercise as a supplement to her current home program. Being a former completive athlete, Jessica found that she enjoyed challenging herself not only with the Pilates mat exercises, but also by using Pilates apparatus such as the Reformer and Cadillac. She found that she could perform the controlled movements without back pain while getting a great workout.

For additional information, refer to:

- Pilates Method Alliance (www.pilatesmethodalliance.org)
- Polestar Pilates Education (www.polestarpilates.com)

Alexander Technique

Frederick M. Alexander (1869–1955) created the Alexander technique, which is a form of body work that promotes postural health. His system helps to reeducate the whole body in proper movement patterns and postural habits.

In practical terms, the Alexander technique may be used by musicians, performers, and individuals who want to improve performance and posture, reduce pain and tension, and want to move more easily in common daily activities, such as going from a sit to a stand position. The technique can also help individuals breathe and walk better, and also help improve balance.

What Does Selected Research Say about the Alexander Technique?

- Lessons promote self-efficacy and self-care, and reductions in chronic neck pain [21].
- Lessons may improve performance anxiety in musicians [22].
- Alexander technique lessons and acupuncture sessions both led to significant reductions in neck pain and associated disability compared with usual care [23].
- It is a cost-effective approach to treatment of back pain in primary care [24].
- Lessons are likely to lead to sustained benefit for people with Parkinson's disease on the Beck Depression Inventory and the Attitudes to Self Scale [25].

Case Vignette: Alexander Technique

John, a 47-year-old dentist at a university medical clinical practice, noticed that he was starting to have neck pain during patient care. Since John was also a professor at the dental school, he had many hours of computer use every week to complete his administrative duties. Prolonged computer use exacerbated his neck symptoms. He knew about the university ergonomics program and scheduled a consultation to determine what type of new chair and other equipment might be needed for his symptoms. The ergonomic specialist was also trained as an Alexander technique practitioner. After completing his ergonomic assessment and getting some new office equipment and lots of useful ergonomic tips, John decided to work privately with the Alexander technique teacher. He wanted to work on his posture and also learn more efficient ways to perform his work as a dentist without creating neck pain. After six sessions with the Alexander technique teacher, John found new ways to use his dental instruments without pain. John also used his new knowledge to improve his posture during his daily walking program.

For additional information, refer to:

- Alexander Technique International (www.alexandertechniqueinternational.com)
- American Society for the Alexander Technique (www.amsatonline.org)
- The Complete Guide to the Alexander Technique (www.alexandertechnique.com)

Conclusion

The best form of sustainable exercise and activity is the one the patient/client considers enjoyable and will actually engage in on a consistent basis. It is the responsibility of the clinician to introduce patients/clients to a variety of exercises and activities based on their needs, goals, and preferences. Not every type of exercise or activity covers the full spectrum of fitness and therapeutic needs for a patient. For this reason, a person may need to engage in a multimodal approach, such as performing tai chi several days per week and perhaps walking, dancing, and engaging in Pilates or the Alexander technique on the alternate days.

References

1. SL Watson, BK Weeks, LJ Weis, et al. High-intensity resistance and impact training improves bone mineral density and physical function in postmenopausal women with osteopenia and osteoporosis: the LIFTMOR randomized controlled trial. *J Bone Miner Res* 2018; 33: 211–220.

2. MA Fiatarone Singh, N Gates, N Saigal, et al. The study of mental and resistance training (SMART) study-resistance training and/or cognitive training in mild cognitive impairment: a randomized, double-blind, double-sham controlled trial. *J Am Med Dir Assoc* 2014; 15: 873–880.

3. T Liu-Ambrose, LS Nagamatsu, P Graf, et al. Resistance training and executive functions: a 12-month randomized controlled trial. *Arch Intern Med* 2010: 170: 170–178.

4. MA Fiatarone, EF O'Neill, ND Ryan, et al. Exercise training and nutritional supplementation for physical frailty in very elderly people. *N Engl J Med* 1994; 330: 1769–1775.

5. MA Fiatarone, EC Marks, ND Ryan, et al. High-intensity strength training in nonagenarians: effects on skeletal muscle. *JAMA* 1990; 263: 3029–3034.

6. M Dos Santos Delabary, IG Komeroski, EP Monteiro, et al. Effects of dance practice on functional mobility, motor symptoms and quality of life in people with Parkinson's disease: a systematic review with meta-analysis. *Aging Clin Exp Res* 2018; 30: 727–735.

7. I Lazarou, T Parastatidis. A Tsolaki, et al. International ballroom dancing against neurodegeneration: a randomized controlled trial in Greek community-dwelling elders with mild cognitive impairment. *Am J Alzheimers Dis Other Demen* 2017; 32: 489–499.

8. J Casilda-Lopez, MC Valenza, I Cabrera-Martos, et al. Effects of a dance-based aquatic exercise program in obese postmenopausal women with knee osteoarthritis: a randomized controlled trial. *Menopause* 2017; 24: 768–773.

9. M Gomes Neto, MA Menezes, V Oliveira Carvalho. Dance therapy in patients with chronic heart failure: a systematic review and a meta-analysis. *Clin Rehabil* 2014: 28: 1172–1179.

10. R Pinniger, RF Brown, EB Thorsteinsson, et al. Argentine tango dance compared to mindfulness meditation and a waiting-list control: a randomised trial for treating depression. *Complement Ther Med* 2012; 20: 377–384.

11. C Wang, CH Schmid, RA Fielding, et al. Effect of tai chi versus aerobic exercise for fibromyalgia: comparative effectiveness randomized controlled trial. *BMJ* 2018; 360: k851.

12. LK Larkey, D James, M Belyea, et al. Body composition outcomes of tai chi and qigong practice: a systematic review and meta-analysis of randomized controlled trials. *Int J Behav Med* 2018; 25: 487–501.

13. AW Chan, A Lee, DT Lee, et al. The sustaining effects of tai chi qigong on physiological health for COPD patients: a randomized controlled trial. *Complement Ther Med* 2013; 21: 585–594.

14. M Hall, CG Maher, P Lam, et al. Tai chi exercise for treatment of pain and disability in people with persistent low back pain: a randomized controlled trial. *Arthritis Care Res (Hoboken)* 2011; 63: 1576–1583.

15. F Li, P Harmer, KJ Fisher, et al. Tai chi and fall reductions in older adults: a randomized controlled trial. *J Gerontol A Biol Sci Med Sci* 2005; 60: 187–194.

16. D Cruz-Diaz, M Romeu, C Velasco-Gonzalez, et al. The effectiveness of 12 weeks of Pilates intervention on disability, pain and kinesiophobia in patients with chronic low back pain: a randomized controlled trial. *Clin Rehabil* 2018; 32: 1249–1257.

17. L de Araujo Cazotti, A Jones, D Roger-Silva, et al. Effectiveness of the Pilates method in the treatment of chronic mechanical neck pain: a randomized controlled trial. *Arch Phys Med Rehabil* 2018; **99**: 1740–1746.

18. GC Miyamoto, KFM Franco, JM van Dongen, et al. Different doses of Pilates-based exercise therapy for chronic low back pain: a randomised controlled trial with economic evaluation. *Br J Sports Med* 2018; **52**: 859–868.

19. MA da Luz, LO Costa, FF Fuhro, et al. Effectiveness of mat Pilates or equipment based Pilates exercises in patients with chronic nonspecific low back pain: a randomized controlled trial. *Phys Ther* 2014; **94**: 623–631.

20. H Wajswelner, B Metcalf, K Bennell. Clinical Pilates versus general exercise for chronic low back pain: randomized trial. *Med Sci Sports Exerc* 2012; **44**: 1197–1205.

21. J Woodman, K Ballard, C Hewitt, et al. Self-efficacy and self-care-related outcomes following Alexander technique lessons for people with chronic neck pain in the ATLAS randomised, controlled trial. *Eur J Integr Med* 2018; **17**: 64–71.

22. SD Klein, C Bayard, U Wolf. The Alexander technique and musicians: a systematic review of controlled trials. *BMC Complement Altern Med* 2014; **14**: 414.

23. H MacPherson, H Tilbrook, S Richmond, et al. Alexander technique lessons or acupuncture sessions for persons with chronic neck pain: a randomized trial. *Ann Intern Med* 2015; **163**: 653–662.

24. S Hollinghurst, D Sharp, K Ballard, et al. Randomised controlled trial of Alexander technique lessons, exercise, and massage (ATEAM) for chronic and recurrent back pain: economic evaluation. *BMJ* 2008; **337**: a2656.

25. C Stallibrass, P Sissons, C Chalmers. Randomized controlled trial of the Alexander technique for idiopathic Parkinson's disease. *Clin Rehabil* 2002; **16**: 695–708.

Sleep, Rest, and Relaxation in Improving Wellness

Ashley Ngor and Waguih William IsHak

Introduction

Sleep, rest, and relaxation are often undervalued factors that contribute to the maintenance and improvement of wellness. Sleep cycles and their given durations have been clinically proven to influence essential aspects of human life: cardiovascular health, metabolic health, mental health, immunologic health, human performance, and mortality, to name a few [1]. Inadequate sleep has known associations with increased risks of mortality, cardiovascular disease, cerebrovascular disease, obesity, diabetes, cancer, and depression. Rest, in the context of this chapter, is not necessarily synonymous with sleep – for instance, sleep can still occur without rest and its improvements on overall functioning [2]. Relaxation often corresponds to feelings of peace, comfort, body laxity, mental laxity, and positive emotions. Relaxation as a wellness tool can take a variety of forms, such as abdominal breathing and progressive muscle relaxation techniques [3]. While each of these components has its own effects on health, they should all be considered and practiced in one's journey to attaining better health and optimizing wellness.

Sleep

Optimal Sleep

The crucial role of sleep in improving wellness is a universally accepted construct and has been proven time and time again in a multitude of studies and reports. In a 2018 prospective cohort study with a total of 13,423 adult participants, Loprinzi et al. found that better health-related quality of life (HRQOL) and a reduction in all-cause mortality both result from optimal levels of sleep [4]. Even after the consideration of factors such as age, gender, race/ethnicity, body mass index, education, smoking, white blood cell level, iron level, red blood cell distribution width, mean platelet volume, blood pressure, diabetes, coronary artery disease, physical activity, and depression, there was a 19 percent reduced risk of premature all-cause mortality for those sleeping 7–9 hours every night.

Good sleep also has a positive effect on mental health, athletic performance, and academic performance. After three years of follow-up, 969 Japanese workers in a longitudinal study were found to exhibit greater mental well-being due to feelings of being well rested after sleep [5]. In another cohort of older adults, good sleep was associated with greater eudaimonic well-being – greater feelings of purpose in life, greater environmental mastery, and greater positive relationships [6]. Proper sleep has also proven influential on athletic performance, with collegiate athletes sleeping less than eight hours per night being 1.7 times more likely to have a musculoskeletal injury than athletes sleeping over eight hours per night; furthermore, athletes who slept more than eight hours during weekdays had a 61% lower likelihood of musculoske-letal injury than their unrested counterparts [7]. Higher grade point averages (GPA) have also been correlated with students with more than seven hours of nighttime sleep, more consistent sleep schedules, lower levels of daytime sleepiness, and less weekend "catch up" sleep.

Long-Term and Short-Term Sleep

The importance of sleep in improving wellness is especially evident in its lack or abun-dance – both extremes can significantly and detrimentally affect the wellness of the human body. Kim et al. found a U-shaped relationship between sleep time and quality of life (QOL) using a 2015 nationwide cross-sectional survey of 28,178 subjects from the Korea National Health and Nutrition Examination Survey (KNHANES) IV–V [8]. Korean men and women sleeping ≤4 hours per day or ≥10 hours per day had significantly worse QOL, independent of perceived health status and depressive disorder, than their counterparts who slept for seven hours per day. A US study of adults came to the same conclusion, finding positive, linear relationships between both (1) shorter sleep periods and poor perceived health and (2) longer sleep periods and poor perceived health.

Excess sleep has especially strong associations with cardiovascular disease, diabetes mellitus, cognitive impairment, depression, and limitations in physical function, and may even be a possible predictor of mortality [9]. The European Prospective Investigation into Cancer – Norfolk found an increased risk of stroke with long-term sleeping, based on a cohort study of 9692 adults aged 42–81 that lasted for 9.5 years [5]. A cohort study of 3820 older adults in Spain found that long sleep duration was associated with seven-year mortality, even in those with optimal perceived health, good cognitive function, quality of life greater than the cohort median, no depressive symptoms, and no disabilities [9]. National Health and Nutrition Examination Surveys carried out from 2005 to 2008 support this finding, discovering an association between all-cause mortality and long-term sleep.

Sleep deprivation leads to a variety of cognitive, emotional, and physical function declines, as depicted in Figure 26.1: reduced work performance and social participation, feelings of isolation, and a number of health problems. However, treatment for the sleep disorder has been proven to improve QOL [5].

Acute and chronic sleep deprivation have similar effects on affected persons, such as a reduction in executive functioning, memory, reaction time, attention/concentration, and emotional regulation [10], as shown in Table 26.1. In fact, the decline in cognitive psychomotor performance experienced by individuals who are awake for 14–26 hours is comparable to that experienced by individuals who have a 0.04 percent increase in blood alcohol concentration.

A great example to demonstrate the possible daily effects of sleep deprivation would be resident physicians. In a systematic review, Mansukhani et al. accumulated a few of the many effects of sleep loss on the wellness and performance of resident physicians [10]. Some effects include a 20 percent increase in errors, 14 percent more time required to complete tasks, a lack of empathy and concern for patients, problems with relationships and parent-ing, and an increase in the consumption of alcohol and drugs. While the dangers of sleep loss are harmful alone, awareness of sleepiness diminishes over time and may result in an individual eventually becoming oblivious to impairments; for a resident physician, this could threaten the safety and quality of life of both their patients and themselves. The realities of sleep deprivation can be seen in the case of an 18-year-old patient, Libby Zion, who died as a direct result of a resident physician's lack of sleep. Since then, actions have

Table 26.1 Effects of sleep loss on cognitive functioning

Cognitive function	Effects of sleep loss
Executive functions	Difficulty with shifting tasks, errors during task performance, deterioration of performance as complexity increases.
Memory	Impairment of visuospatial memory and digit recall.
Reaction time	Slow response time and accuracy.
Attention and concentration	Decreased psychomotor vigilance.
Emotional regulation	Decreased self-esteem, empathy, impulse control, and positive thinking.

Adapted from: MP Mansukhani, BP Kolla, S Surani, J Varon, K Ramar. Sleep deprivation in resident physicians, work hour limitations, and related outcomes: a systematic review of the literature. *Postgrad Med* 2012; **124**(4): 241–249.

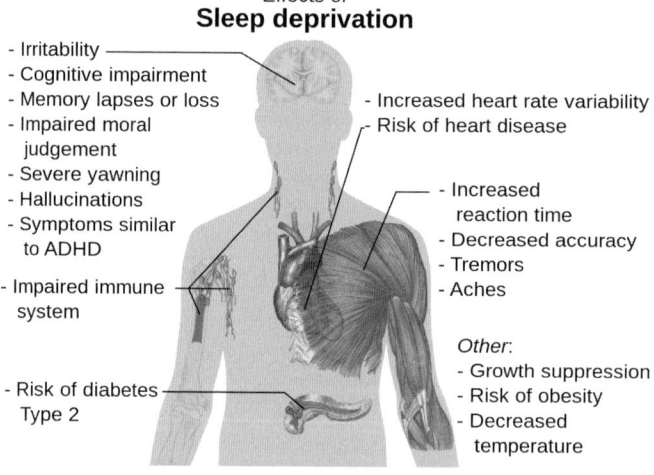

Figure 26.1 The effects of sleep deprivation (reprinted from: https://commons.wikimedia.org/wiki/File:Effects_of_sleep_deprivation.svg, Creative Commons).

been taken to limit resident work hours, first seen in 1989 when New York State limited it to 80 hours per week. It should be noted, however, that short-term sleep characteristics may have less of a negative impact on well-being than long-term sleep characteristics. In one meta-analysis, short-term sleep problems were found to have a smaller increase in vascular risk than long-term sleep problems [5].

Sleep may also have an effect on neurodegenerative diseases. It has been found that Alzheimer's disease, Parkinson's disease, and Huntington's chorea are similar in having circadian rhythm alterations as an early symptom, which suggests that the molecular mechanisms of the circadian system may play either a cause or effect role in neurological disease progression [5]. In older workers and those with neurodegenerative diseases or mild cognitive impairment, these sleep disorders may also be correlated with the onset of dementia.

Furthermore, sleep disorders have influence on metabolic conditions such as obesity, which is affected by genetic, environmental, and lifestyle factors. From the observation of 119,859 European adults, one study indicated a change in phenotypic expression of obesity by varying sleep characteristics such as sleep duration, chronotype, sleeping habits, and shift work. This study was able to conclude that insufficient sleep magnifies the genetic risk of obesity and phenotypic measures such as BMI and abdominal circumference. In obese adults specifically, reduced sleep duration has been found to affect body composition, dietary intake, and QOL. Absolute fat mass, relative fat mass, and truncal fat mass were all higher in obese subjects sleeping ≤300 minutes per day when compared to their counterparts sleeping >300 minutes per day. Subjects sleeping ≤300 minutes per day also had a higher carbohydrate consumption per day than their counterparts [11]. A lack of sleep may lead to obesity, and from there an even greater propensity for more severe obesity and poor QOL.

Susceptibility to accidents also corresponds to sleep deprivation. A meta-analysis of 27 observational studies came to the conclusion that 13 percent of work injuries could be attributed to sleep problems [5]. One survey encompassing emergency medicine residents from 78 participating programs discovered that nearly three-quarters of motor vehicle accidents and near-miss accidents occurred after a night shift, overall illustrating a positive linear relationship between the number of night shifts worked per month and motor vehicle accidents [10]. Obstructive sleep apnea (OSA), a common sleep disorder, has been correlated to a 100 percent increased risk of accidents and increased risk of occupational non-driving injury by 15-fold [5]. In 2014, it was estimated that simply early OSA diagnosis and treatment could prevent up to one million work accidents, 1000 deaths, and 20,000 cases of permanent disability every year in Italy.

Rest

The effects of rest on overall well-being are related and comparable to those resulting from sleep. Helvig et al. define rest as being the pathway to inner tranquility and mental health, while acting as a base of support for physical health [2]. One study that encompasses the importance of rest found that workers with fewer rest days in between work days reported greater muscular pain and worse mental health.

Rest as a Pathway to Mental Health

The positive influence of rest is evident in its beneficial effects on mental health. Rest can result in modest improvements in anxiety, depression, and dementia that are not seen in individuals who do not rest or cannot rest because of altered circadian rhythms. Rest may prove especially beneficial in workplace environments involving a substantial amount of sedentary behavior, which has been known to be correlated with premature mortality, cardiovascular disease, diabetes, some cancers, and other chronic diseases [12]. In a 2017 eight-week study of 49 sedentary female employees, short, frequent breaks were found to improve arousal, fatigue, and mood levels better than longer, planned breaks. This suggests that short-interval rests may be useful in increasing the energy and overall well-being of individuals in a workplace environment.

In a 2016 10-week study of 59 white-collar workers, a 10-minute daily active rest program was enacted, in support of the idea that moderate exercise may allow quicker fatigue recovery than passive rest [13, 14]. This intervention resulted in improvement of friendliness, interpersonal stress, and support from superiors, colleagues, family, and friends. In turn, rest allowed for an overall advancement of relationships and mental health in the workplace [13]. The same authors conducted a similar study to determine the effect of the active rest program with 130 workers over the course of eight weeks [14]. They discovered that "vigor" and work engagement increased with the program, implying validity for active rest in the workplace as a means of improving mental stamina and individual health-related work productivity loss.

Patterson et al. investigated the effect of inter-shift recovery (recuperative rest between shifts) on emergency medical services clinicians, and found an association between longer recovery between shifts with longer shift lengths and greater feelings of cheerfulness, calmness, and alertness, and thus greater emotional content and mental stamina [15]. A rest recovery interval of 11 hours or less between work days was revealed by another systematic review to have unfavorable influence on sleep, sleepiness, and fatigue – and problems with sleep may have an adverse effect on well-being and correspond to anxiety, depression, and shift-work disorder [16]. Interestingly, rest can also take the form of light activity – one study found a reduction in fatigue due to three minutes of light activity every 30 minutes, as compared to sitting without interruption [12].

Rest as a Base of Support

Rest also plays a significant role as a base of support for physical health. The most widespread use of rest is in the field of rehabilitation; its efficacy was seen in one study in which time to rest allowed cardiac surgery patients to recuperate at a better and faster rate [2]. A quasi-experimental study of 135 individuals conducted by Cáceres-Muñoz et al. investigated the effect of a rest pause program and information leaflets on musculoskeletal pain, and found a 20 percent reduction in neck pain and a 17 percent reduction in lumbar spine pain over seven days, and an overall reduction in pain in all body regions [17]. The control group, in contrast, only had musculoskeletal pain reduction in the lumbar spine that was less than the reduction experienced by the intervention group. Similarly, Henning et al. found that short, frequent breaks from computer work alongside stretching exercises can result in improvements of productivity and eye, leg, and foot comfort, thereby contributing to and improving the health and safety of workers [18]. More specifically, results from another study showed that short, frequent 10-minute breaks can reduce leg discomfort, while infrequent long breaks can reduce lower back discomfort [19].

Ikeda et al. found, from their one-month observational study involving 54 daytime employees, that workers with a shorter daily rest period (DRP) generally had a higher diastolic blood pressure. A higher diastolic blood pressure was found among workers with a DRP <14 hours than among workers with a DRP >14 hours [16]. Due to diastolic blood pressure having associations to hemorrhagic stroke, stroke, and coronary heart disease, it can be concluded that a DRP >14 hours may reduce cardiovascular health risks in workers. A DRP >14 hours was also proven to ensure an optimal amount of sleep, thereby demonstrating the relationship between rest and sleep on influencing wellness.

Similar to sleep, rest also has an impact on the likelihood of accidents occurring. A 2010 study evaluating 407 observations from a national truckload carrier determined that fatigue-related crash risk can be reduced by increasing total rest-break duration [20]. Key findings from this study are that 30-minute rest breaks are effective as a whole, early rest breaks do not increase effectiveness, and three or more rest breaks do not increase effectiveness. Rest breaks may be a crucial tool in preventing fatalities due to commercial truck accidents.

Relaxation

In addition to sleep and rest, a majority of evidence supports how relaxation can be used as a tool in improving wellness. In order to combat the detrimental effects of stressors on immune function (such as the secretion of glucocorticoids), relaxation techniques enhance body immunity by releasing β-endorphins that increase the number of NK cells [21]. An increase in QOL was found after relaxation techniques were used in an elderly population undergoing open heart surgery [22]. Forbes et al. investigated the health and well-being of 3472 patients with diabetes, chronic obstructive pulmonary disease, and irritable bowel syndrome over the course of one year and found that relaxation had a greater positive effect on self-perceived feelings of happiness than did exercise [23]. In a majority of the studies systematically reviewed by Klainin-Yobas et al., older adults who received relaxation interventions were also shown to have more significant depression and anxiety reductions than their respective controls [3]. Surprisingly, some of the relaxation interventions had effects lasting 14–24 weeks after the interventions. Greater social support, well-being, life satisfaction, self-awareness, and connections with others or with a higher power are generally seen with many relaxation and calming approaches [21].

Psychological Relaxation

A majority of psychological relaxation techniques are geared to improve mental well-being. Reig-Ferrer et al. found a decrease in psychological distress and an improvement in QOL at the three-month follow-up mark after use of a relaxation technique aimed at increasing psychological well-being [21]. Relaxing training (RT) in the form of breath control and meditation has resulted in better QOL and significantly lower arterial blood pressure due to slow breathing increasing baroreflex sensitivity, decreasing muscle sympathetic nerve activity, and decreasing chemoreflex activation [24]. Relaxing training has also proved beneficial in autonomic balance, respiratory control, and reducing blood pressure in those with hypertension. Another program using mindfulness-based stress reduction in healthy older adults led not only to a decrease in loneliness, but also to downregulation of proinflammatory NF-κB-related gene expression over the course of eight weeks [21].

Physiological Relaxation

Physiological relaxation techniques are those primarily involving muscular relaxation. The Jacobson-type muscle relaxation technique, which involves tensing and relaxing of muscle groups, has been reported to improve cellular immune response in elderly adults [21]. A popular form of physiological relaxation, termed progressive muscular relaxation (PMR), has resulted in improvements in chronic disease symptoms (in disorders such as rheumatoid arthritis, irritable bowel syndrome, chronic pain, and pulmonary hypertension), psychological tension, anxiety, depression, pain, salivary cortisol levels, blood pressure, headaches, efforts against immunoglobulin, heart rate, cardiac rehabilitation management, QOL, and emotional balance [22, 24]. A study by Hassanpour-Dehkordi and Jalali supports the use of PMR, with its finding that PMR can promote improvements in fatigue, physical function, individual independence, and overall QOL for elderly patients suffering from multiple sclerosis, prostate cancer, irritable bowel syndrome, and posttraumatic stress disorder [22]. Parás-Bravo et al. came to a similar conclusion, finding improvements in the perceived QOL of cancer patients after PMR intervention [25]. A study involving 272 cancer patients showed how PMR can significantly improve emotional, functional, and physical well-being in addition to social and familial relationships. Several articles also attribute to PMR decreasing pain and distress specifically in breast cancer patients [22]. A two-month PMR intervention on unemployed people in Greece led to better management of depression, anxiety, and stress symptoms, in addition to MSC (sense of coherence) and MCS (mental component summary) [24].

Conclusion

In conclusion, an overwhelming amount of evidence suggests that the three factors of sleep, rest, and relaxation can all have extensive influence on the betterment of one's overall health and well-being. The most important consequence of proper sleep is a decreased risk of mortality, and its true importance is mostly seen in the repercussions of improper sleep – both a lack of sleep and an abundance of sleep are correlated with decreased health, QOL, and well-being. The use of rest periods has been determined to positively affect both mental health and physical health, notably in high-stress workplace environments and in the field of rehabilitation. Relaxation in the sense of this chapter takes the form of psychological relaxation, such as meditation, and physiological relaxation, such as muscular relaxation, which both lead to greater mental and bodily function and thus greater wellness.

The low-risk, low-cost attributes of resting techniques and relaxation techniques may one day have widespread applications in the field of medicine. As more and more promising evidence in regards to sleep, rest, and relaxation comes to light, these elements are increasingly becoming more accepted as effective interventions for optimizing wellness.

References

1. Consensus Conference Panel, NF Watson, MS Badr, et al. Joint consensus statement of the American Academy of Sleep Medicine and Sleep Research Society on the recommended amount of sleep for a healthy adult: methodology and discussion. *Sleep* 2015; **38**(8): 1161–1183.

2. A Helvig, S Wade, L Hunter-Eades. Rest and the associated benefits in restorative sleep: a concept analysis. *J Adv Nurs* 2016; **72**(1): 62–72.

3. P Klainin-Yobas, WN Oo, PY Suzanne Yew, Y Lau. Effects of relaxation interventions on depression and anxiety among older adults: a systematic review. *Aging Mental Health* 2015; **19**(12): 1043–1055.

4. PD Loprinzi, C Joyner. Meeting sleep guidelines is associated with better health-related quality of life and reduced premature all-cause mortality risk. *Am J Health Promot* 2018; **32**(1): 68–71.

5. N Magnavita, S Garbarino. Sleep, health and wellness at work: a scoping review. *Int J Environ Res Public Health* 2017; **14**(11): 1347.

6. A Steptoe, K O'Donnell, M Marmot, J Wardle. Positive affect, psychological well-being, and good sleep. *J Psychosom Res* 2008; **64**: 409–415.

7. E Kroshus, J Wagner, D Wyrick, et al. Wake up call for collegiate athlete sleep: narrative review and consensus recommendations from the NCAA Interassociation Task Force on Sleep and Wellness. *Br J Sports Med* 2019; **53**: 731–736.

8. JH Kim, EC Park, KB Yoo, S Park. The association between short or long sleep times and quality of life (QOL): results of the Korea National Health and Nutrition Examination Survey (KNHANES IV-V). *J Clin Sleep Med* 2015; **11**(6): 625–634.

9. AE Mesas, E López-García, LM León-Muñoz, P Guallar-Castillón, F Rodríguez-Artalejo. Sleep duration and mortality according to health status in older adults. *J Am Geriatr Soc* 2010; **58**: 1870–1877.

10. MP Mansukhani, BP Kolla, S Surani, J Varon, K Ramar. Sleep deprivation in resident physicians, work hour limitations, and related outcomes: a systematic review of the literature. *Postgrad Med* 2012; **124**(4): 241–249.

11. EL Poggiogalle, C Lubrano, L Gnessi, et al. Reduced sleep duration affects body composition, dietary intake and quality of life in obese subjects. *Eat Weight Disord* 2016; **21**: 501–505.

12. EL Mailey, SK Rosenkranz, E Ablah, A Swank, K Casey. Effects of an intervention to reduce sitting at work on arousal, fatigue, and mood among sedentary female employees: a parallel-group randomized trial. *J Occup Environ Med* 2017; **59**(12): 1166–1171.

13. R Michishita, Y Jiang, D Ariyoshi, et al. The practice of active rest by workplace units improves personal relationships, mental health, and physical activity among workers. *J Occup Health* 2017; **59**(2): 122–130.

14. R Michishita, Y Jiang, D Ariyoshi, et al. The introduction of an active rest program by workplace units improved the workplace vigor and presenteeism among workers: a randomized controlled trial. *J Occup Environ Med* 2017; **59**: 1140–1147.

15. PD Patterson, DJ Buysse, MD Weaver, CW Callaway, DM Yealy. Recovery between work shifts among emergency medical services clinicians. *Prehosp Emerg Care* 2015; **19**(3): 365–375.

16. H Ikeda, T Kubo, S Izawa, et al. Impact of daily rest period on resting blood pressure and fatigue: a one-month observational study of daytime employees. *J Occup Environ Med* 2017; **59**(4): 397–401.

17. VS Cáceres-Muñoz, A Magallanes-Meneses, D Torres-Coronel, et al. Efecto de un programa de pausa activa más folletos informativos en la disminución de molestias musculoesqueléticas en trabajadores administrativos. *Rev Peru Med Exp Salud Publica* 2017; **34**(4): 611–618.

18. RA Henning, P Jacques, GV Kissel, AB Sullivan, SM Alteras-Webb. Frequent short rest breaks from computer work: effects on productivity and well-being at two field sites. *Ergonomics* 1997; **40**(1): 78–91.

19. IA Rahman, N Mohamad, JM Rohani, RM Zein. The impact of work rest scheduling for prolonged standing activity. *Ind Health* 2018; **56**(6): 492–499.

20. C Chen, Y Xie. The impacts of multiple rest-break periods on commercial truck driver's crash risk. *J Saf Res* 2014; **48**: 87–93.

21. A Reig-Ferrer, R Ferrer-Cascales, A Santos-Ruiz, et al. A relaxation technique enhances psychological well-being and immune parameters in elderly people from a nursing home: a randomized controlled study. *BMC Complement Altern Med* 2014; **14**: 311.

22. A Hassanpour-Dehkordi, A Jalali. Effect of progressive muscle relaxation on the fatigue and quality of life among Iranian aging persons. *Acta Med Iran* 2016; **54**(7): 430–436.

23. H Forbes, E Fichera, A Rogers, M Sutton. The effects of exercise and relaxation on health and wellbeing. *Health Econ* 2017; **26**(12): e67–e80.

24. K Merakou, K Tsoukas, G Stavrinos, et al. The effect of progressive muscle relaxation on emotional competence: depression–anxiety–stress–sense of coherence – health related quality of life and well being of unemployed people in Greece: an intervention study. *Explore (NY)* 2019; **15**(1): 38–46.

25. P Parás-Bravo, P Salvadores-Fuentes, C Alonso-Blanco, et al. The impact of muscle relaxation techniques on the quality of life of cancer patients, as measured by the FACT-G questionnaire. *PLoS One* 2017; **12**(10): e0184147.

Chapter 27

Sex, Intimacy, and Well-Being

Kailee Marin, Gabriel Tobia, Atef Bakhoum, Lancer Naghdechi, Samuel Korouri, and Waguih William IsHak

Introduction

Sex is on the mind of many people, whether they admit it or not. What makes "good sex" elusive is the relatively subjective nature of what that means and the varying opinions on how to attain it. Moreover, theories exist on the differences in the biological and psychological sexual response and expectations regarding sex between males and females. In this chapter, we define several key elements, suggest factors important to achieving sexual well-being, and suggest practical "real-world" techniques that may be helpful to the clinician advising patients on sex or intimacy, along with methods to optimize this area of life.

What Is Sex?

To understand sexual wellness, it is important to understand sex. So, what is sex and how do we define it? Sex can mean different things to different people. Does thinking about sex count as sex? To some, the idea of sex is enough. Is thought a form of sexual activity? For some, watching or listening is preferred, whereas for others physical contact is essential. Colored by the lens of life, sex may be seen differently depending on many factors, including life experience, culture, sexual orientation, gender, age, socioeconomic status, even geography. Sex keeps the heart and immune system strong, enhances sleep, relieves pain, and has added health benefits, briefly described in Table 27.1. More than just for reproductive purposes, sex is a pleasurable activity that is part and parcel of overall well-being because of its relationship to all the biopsychosocial aspects of life. In addition to being important toward the act of intercourse or masturbation, sexual wellness is related to overall wellness.

Is Arousal Enough?

Arousal is biologically defined as different physiological processes in the body. The stages of arousal vary between men and women. As seen in Figure 27.1, the stages of arousal include sexual excitement, sexual plateau, orgasm/ejaculation, and resolution. Men have a more predictable sexual response, while the level of arousal is more variable for women and may fluctuate between stages. Men experience a refractory period, during which subsequent orgasms cannot be achieved. Women do not necessarily experience a refractory period. This means that women might have multiple consecutive orgasms. Alternatively, women may reach and maintain the plateau phase without reaching orgasm at all [3].

Table 27.1 Health benefits of sex

Benefit	Mechanism
Heart health	• Sex can be a decent cardio workout (one 30-minute session can burn 70 calories) [1]. • People who had sex an average of 12 times per month were shown to have greater heart rate variability [1]. • May lower the risk of developing heart disease, the leading cause of death for women [1].
Immune strength	• College students who reported "frequent" (one to two times per week) sexual encounters had significantly higher levels of salivary IgA than students reporting zero, infrequent (less than once a week), and very frequent (three or more times per week) encounters [2].
Sleep better	• Relaxing effects of the post-coital oxytocin surge help some reduce stress and fall asleep more quickly.
Feel better	• Oxytocin and other endorphins released help relieve physical pain.

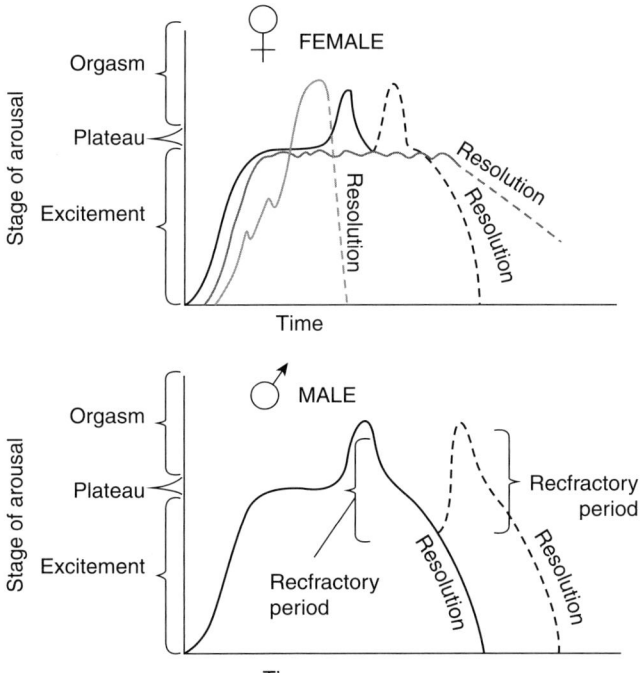

Figure 27.1 Sexual response, differences between the sexes.

In Figure 27.1, arousal peaks in the orgasm phase. According to this model, orgasm is the summit, and some may say it's the goal. Colloquially, orgasm signals the end of the encounter, so with that end are daily orgasms enough in and of itself? Most would agree that simply having orgasms would not lead to the same fulfillment compared to a close emotional and physical connection with another person, i.e., an intimate sexual relationship with a partner.

What Is Intimacy?

Intimacy is developed with repetitive encounters or exchanges that may be either verbal or non-verbal. It has long been considered a primary psychological need [4]. Intimacy is closeness between people. The intimate exchange occurs when trust and sensitivity are present while one party shares something personal or private with another. Attentive listening and conveyance of understanding are concepts that have been included in the description of intimacy [5]. Intimacy depends not only on what is said or done, but the setting in which the exchange occurs.

Intimacy is important because it has been shown to increase one's sense of well-being [6, 7]. A longitudinal study of 182 individuals showed intimacy as key to well-being. In the study, the cohort was assessed on four occasions throughout a 40-year period of their adult lives. These assessments showed positive correlations between increased intimacy and well-being [7].

Is Intimacy Enough?

Consider someone who is in the "friend zone" to be your sexual partner for life. They satisfy certain needs (such as being a supportive shoulder to cry on), but elicit no sexual attraction in the first place. You may have an intimate relationship with this individual, but would you be able to sustain a sexually fulfilling relationship with him/her? There are other examples that might also suggest that intimacy is not enough. For example, maybe the physical attraction disappears through various means – psychological or physical. When one partner lets him/herself go but the relationship remains emotionally close, can it be sustained? It is difficult to maintain sexual wellness once the attraction dissipates. Sometimes people grow apart and intimacy alone is not enough to sustain well-being in the sexual relationship. To this end, the remainder of the chapter will focus on ways to increase intimacy, as well as other factors that may enhance overall sexual well-being.

Enhancing Intimacy for Wellness

Sexual wellness is unequivocally linked to stress. Everyone experiences stress in their lives, and chronic stress can make it difficult to achieve sexual well-being. Chronic stress triggers release of hormones such as cortisol, which shifts hormone production in men and women so that our bodies can deal with a stressor at the expense of our sexual well-being [8]. Intimacy in relationships has consistently been shown to have a strong positive impact on well-being [9]. Enhancing intimacy can be a good way to reduce the effects of chronic stress. In one study, 51 couples reported time spent engaging in intimate interactions and provided saliva samples for the purpose of cortisol assessment every three hours over a one-week time frame. The study showed a significant association between intimacy and reduced salivary cortisol levels, suggesting that intimacy can mitigate the stress response [10]. The decrease in cortisol brought about by increasing intimacy can reverse the hormonal effects of the stress response, thereby also leading to increases in sexual wellness. Thus, it is important to enhance intimacy in a relationship in order to boost sexual well-being, and consequently overall well-being.

One way of enhancing intimacy between partners is through developing habits of honesty that will allow them to become more honest as the relationship persists. It is noted, however, that the opposite often occurs. One example of this is the "white lie" that occurs when one partner tells the other what they think they want to hear, with the justification (conscious or not) that they are being sensitive to the feelings of their partner. Even this superficially harmless dishonesty creates distance in the intimate relationship. By developing habits of dishonesty, the partners end up becoming more closed, and more distant. The importance of honesty has been asserted with the argument against common cases of justified dishonesty, i.e., scenarios in which it is widely thought permissible to lie. Expanding on the depths of honesty, the concept of "meta-honesty" is explained as honesty about one's own efforts at communication, including one's efforts to be honest. This is an important component of the intimate relationship [11].

One study exploring the effectiveness of solution-focused brief couples therapy found the approach facilitated changes that helped couples become hopeful about the future of their relationship. These changes are attributed to the increase in the use of mutual constructive communication patterns and the decrease in the use of mutual avoidant and demand/withdrawal communication patterns. Participants succeeded in replacing hostile and negative feelings toward their partner, which helped to create a more intimate feel in the relationship. Intimacy between a couple increases when the relationship is constructive, and as the study concludes, solution-focused couples therapy has been shown to promote the constructive relationship [12].

Building intimacy isn't always butterflies and rainbows. Having the desire to create intimacy is not enough if there is no direction in which to begin. Sometimes it's hard to be vulnerable, and sometimes the truth is ugly. See Table 27.2 for practical advice to increase intimacy in your relationship [6]. The table is arranged in a logical order, starting with a tool to assess willingness to engage in your desired level of closeness. This is important to understand early in the relationship, as many relationships are doomed from the beginning due to a mismatch in core values around the desire and need for intimacy. Important in developing a strong sense of self is understanding that some core values might not necessarily be desirable to everyone. Some core values are negative, or bring forth traits that most would want to avoid. Those who meet the criteria for personality disorders may have a sense of self that is based on such things as devaluing others (narcissistic), inflicting pain on others (sadistic), committing crimes (antisocial), or partaking in other socially unacceptable behaviors. With regard to the dynamic nature of intimacy, it is notable that everyone will have a level of desire and capacity for intimacy that will ebb and flow with mood or circumstance. Some situations aren't appropriate for deep levels of intimacy that are at times desired. For example, talking to your partner on the phone while you're at work could be much different from the conversation you would have over a candlelit dinner. This is healthy and to be expected. A comfortable balance of closeness and independence will help to keep the relationship from becoming stagnant. There is some ability to set expectations in both directions when you set the environment to match the level of desired intimacy.

Pharmacological Sexual Enhancement

Pharmacological interventions may be appropriate for patients who are continually dissatisfied with their sexual experiences. It is important to always weigh the risks and benefits

Table 27.2 Creating intimacy

Goal	How to get there	Examples
Does their desire for closeness match yours?	Open up to the depth you desire; ask them to do the same and gauge their reaction.	• "I feel really sad that my mom's not here." • "My dream is to write children's books."
Vulnerability	Share openly about yourself.	• What makes you cry? • When did you last cry? • When have you felt weakest? Strongest? • What do you hide from people? Are you hiding anything from someone right now? • What embarrasses you? When were you last embarrassed?
Strong sense of self	Know your core values.	• Trust • Loyalty • Honesty • Sense of humor • Money
Intimacy is dynamic	Be flexible with yourself and your partner. Understand that needs change over time, and you have to allow for this.	• Remember that this is healthy and can be helpful. • Respond appropriately to the situation and circumstances.
Set the mood	Control the environment.	• Privacy • Engage the senses – visual (view), tactile (leather vs lace), taste (wine, chocolate), smell (scented candle, perfume), auditory (music).

of these interventions. If the provider is able to work with the patient to find a pharmacologic intervention that enhances the sexual experience, with little or no adverse reactions, there could be a significant increase in the patient's overall quality of life [13]. The advent of oral phosphodiesterase-5 (PDE-5) inhibitors, starting with sildenafil, has revolutionized the pharmacological treatment of sexual disorder, in particular erectile dysfunction. Differences to consider when selecting a specific PDE-5 inhibitor include onset and duration of action, as well as dosing modifications. See Table 27.3 for a summary of PDE-5 inhibitors [14].

Pharmacologic interventions outside of the PDE inhibitor class are summarized in Table 27.4 [14]. These medications work under various mechanisms, and include alprostadil, apomorphine, bupropion, flibanserin, and testosterone. Although the treatment of female sexual disorder was long overlooked, flibanserin may signal the arrival of a new generation of drugs going in that direction.

Table 27.3 Summary of PDE-5 inhibitors

Medication	Mechanism	Common side effects	Serious side effects	Contraindications

• Avanafil
• Sildenafil
• Tadalafil
• Vardenafil
	Block the degradation of cyclic-GMP by cGMP-specific PDE-5 in the smooth muscle cells lining the blood vessels supplying the corpus cavernosum	Headache, flushing, nasal congestion, diarrhea, dizziness, photosensitivity, dyspepsia, myalgia	Priapism, hypersensitivity reaction, sudden hearing loss, vision loss, myocardial infarction, arrhythmias, stroke, seizures, cerebrovascular hemorrhage, dyspnea, hypotension, Stevens–Johnson syndrome	• Simultaneous use of:
				  – Nitrates
				  – Serotonin receptor antagonists

Table 27.4 Other pharmacologic interventions

Medication	Mechanism	Indication	Side effects	Notes
• Alprostadil	Synthetic PGE1, increased cAMP, decreased norepinephrine	• Erectile dysfunction	Penile pain, bleeding at injection site, priapism	• Intra-cavernosal injection Intraurethral suppository
• Apomorphine	Dopamine receptor agonist	• Male erectile disorder • Female hypoactive sexual desire disorder	Nausea, sweating, dizziness, drowsiness, dyskinesia, hallucinations, orthostatic hypotension, syncope, cardiac events, priapism, abuse potential	• Contraindications – Nitrates – Guanylate cyclase stimulators
• Buproprion	Norepinephrine and dopamine reuptake inhibitor	• Female hypoactive sexual desire disorder • Reverse SSRI-induced hypoactive sexual disorder	Nausea, dry mouth, constipation, headache, insomnia, arrhythmias, angle closure glaucoma, suicidal thoughts	• Contraindications – Seizures – Eating disorders
• Flibanserin	Serotonin agonist and antagonist	• Female hypoactive sexual desire disorder	Somnolence, fatigue, dizziness, hypotension, syncope, accidental injury, appendicitis, CNS depression	• Contraindications – EtOH – CYP3A4 inhibitors – Hepatic impairment
• Testosterone	Naturally occurring androgen hormone	• Increases sexual function in severely hypogonadal men • Increases libido in women with SSRI or SNRI-associated loss of sexual desire	Headache, depression, diarrhea, fatigue, confusion, application site reaction, rash, acne, back pain, prostate hypertrophy and prostatitis, venous thromboembolism, stroke, myocardial infarction, priapism, oligospermia, prostate cancer	• Effectiveness in men with normal testosterone level is limited • Transdermal testosterone used for women

Table 27.5 Dietary supplements

Supplement	Notes	Side effects
L-Arginine	Amino acid available over the counter. Studies on its effect on sexual desire and arousal in both premenopausal and postmenopausal women are encouraging [3]	Abdominal pain, diarrhea, gout, asthma exacerbation, hypotension
Dehydroepiandrosterone (DHEA)	Naturally occurring weak steroid hormone. Some studies have shown some positive effect of both oral and intravaginal DHEA on postmenopausal women with vaginal atrophy and dyspareunia. Research of the effect of the supplement on men is less conclusive [3]	Abdominal pain, acne, fatigue, hirsutism, alopecia, menstrual irregularities, voice changes, headache, hypertension, hypoglycemia, nasal congestion, psychosis

Dietary Supplements

Dietary supplements are inexpensive and typically convenient for the average patient to obtain. Like the abovementioned pharmacologic interventions, supplements have side effects that should be considered. With more evidence of effectiveness in women than in men, supplements enhancing the sexual experience may also enhance overall wellness [13]. Example dietary supplements are described in Table 27.5.

Food and Herbal Remedies

Since antiquity, some foods and herbal remedies have had a reputation of increasing libido and improving sexual function. Most traditional remedies have either never been studied closely or were not shown to be superior to placebo. However, some "naturally" have sexual enhancement effects supported by some scientific evidence, although the quality of the latter may be lacking. If food and herbal remedies can be utilized to enhance sexual experiences, they may become useful in promoting overall wellness. By enhancing the sexual experience, sexual well-being can be cultivated [13]. Table 27.6 provides an overview of some such remedies. Furthermore, some traditional food-based diets have been shown to increase sexual health, particularly in men [15]. If these diets can enhance the sexual experience, then it follows that they can also promote well-being [13]. Table 27.7 provides an overview of these diets.

Non-pharmacological Sexual Enhancement

The promotion of a close emotional and sexual relationship is an essential component of sexual wellness. Additionally, exercise, nutrition, sufficient sleep, and stress reduction have all been associated with improved sexual satisfaction, as has the use of erotic materials such as erotica,

Table 27.6 Non-traditional remedies

Remedy	Notes
MACA root	Grows exclusively in the Andes. Human studies have shown a potential positive effect on sexual desire in both men and women [16].
Ginseng	Native to Korea, possible positive effect on erectile function in men, improved sexual arousal in menopausal women, sexual frequency and satisfaction in perimenopausal women [16].
Yohimbine	Yohimbine is an indole alkaloid extracted from the bark of the *Pausinystalia* yohimbe tree, the *Rauwolfia* root, and the *Aspidosperma* quebracho tree. It is an alpha-2 adrenoceptor antagonist that has been used in traditional medicinal treatment for erectile dysfunction in West Africa for centuries. Studies have shown it to be effective in erectile function [17], as well as decreased sexual desire, particularly caused by antidepressant use [18]. Side effects include hyperglycemia, urinary retention, irritability, tremor, nausea, vomiting, headache, and nervousness. Serious side effects include hypertension and respiratory depression [16].

Table 27.7 Traditional food diets

Diet	Notes
Mediterranean	Based on available foods found in countries that border the Mediterranean Sea. Diet includes an abundance of plant foods (fruits, vegetables, whole grains, nuts, and legumes), olive oil, cheese and yogurt, fish and poultry, red meat, fresh fruit for dessert, and wine [19]. Studies have shown that erectile dysfunction lessens in men adhering to this diet, and deterioration of erectile function lessens over time [15].
Low-fat, low-calorie	Studies show that weight loss through the use of this diet alleviates erectile dysfunction in overweight and obese men [15]. Studies also suggest an improvement in testosterone levels in overweight and obese men losing weight via this diet [15].

sensual clothing, and toys [3]. Several additional nonpharmacological interventions are outlined below for those who have failed or are reluctant to try pharmacologic interventions.

Cognitive-Behavioral and Mindfulness-Based Therapies

Cognitive-behavioral therapy (CBT) is one of the most well-known and well-researched forms of treatment for sexual dysfunction. These interventions target thoughts and/or behaviors that may be contributing to the cause or maintenance of sexual dysfunction. Specific cognitive and behavioral factors targeted, as well as some of the tools utilized, in CBT are listed below [20]:

- Cognitive factors:
  - myths regarding sexual activity
  - negative sexual self-schemas

- distraction during sexual activity
- judgmental focus on one's sexual performance or body image
- Behavioral factors:
  - avoidance of sexual activity
  - difficulties engaging in sexual communication with partners
- Tools
  - psychoeducation
  - cognitive restructuring
  - communication training
  - directed masturbation
  - relaxation training
  - sensate focus

Mindfulness-based therapy (MBT) involves purposeful awareness of the individual's present experience – physical, mental, and cognitive. The awareness needs to be free of judgment, focusing on accepting current thoughts and emotions for what they are. This differs from CBT, which aims to restructure one's thinking [20]. Small changes in one's perspective can lead to significant enhancement of sexual and intimate experiences, and with this improvement of sexual well-being there should be a following improvement in overall life satisfaction or general well-being [13].

Stimulation of the Anterior Fornix Erogenous (AFE) Zone

The stimulation of the area in the inner half of the anterior fornix of the vagina has been shown to increase vaginal lubrication and facilitation of orgasm [21].

Sex Positions and the Coital Alignment Technique

The coital alignment technique (CAT) aims at facilitating contact between the male pubic bone and base of the penis with the female clitoris during penile–vaginal intercourse. It was shown to increase coital female orgasm frequency and simultaneous orgasms, in addition to improving sexual satisfaction [22].

Orgasm Synchronization and Other Techniques

Orgasm synchronization, or simultaneous orgasm, is associated with greater sexual satisfaction. *Start–stop,* and the *squeeze technique* both aim at delaying male ejaculation to prolong the duration of intercourse [3].

Sensate Focus

First described by Masters and Johnson, sensate focus is a sex therapy aimed at focusing the participants on their own sensory perceptions. Participants are invited to touch each other in turn in a mindful way and explore each other's sexual responses, at first without an involvement on breasts and genitals [23].

For more tips to facilitate sexual wellness, see Figure 27.2, adapted from Caitlin Cantor's "Tips for sexual wellness in 2018" [24].

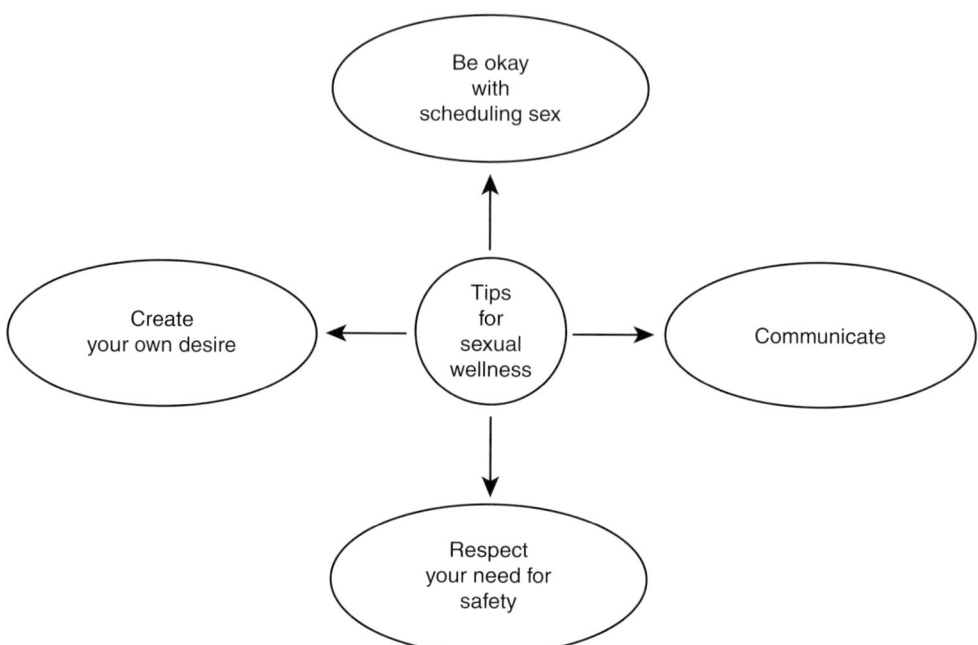

Figure 27.2 Tips for sexual wellness. www.psychologytoday.com/us/blog/modern-sex/201801/tips-sexual-wellness-in-2018. Data from Caitlin Cantor. Tips for sexual wellness in 2018. *Psychology Today,*

Conclusion

Sex is multidimensional and can mean different things to different people. Whether sex occurs through masturbation or sexual relations between people, there are countless iterations and no individualized answer for how to obtain optimal sexual well-being. It is suggested that arousal and intimacy are important, again to varying degrees, and depending on various factors. With it being likely that neither arousal nor intimacy in itself is enough, there is a necessity for a combination of the two. There is also the need to enhance intimacy through developing honesty and open communication with your partner, in order to increase wellness. Enclosed within the umbrella of wellness is sexual well-being, and the job of enhancing wellness mandates that we provide methods to improve sexual well-being. Sex, in addition to occupying a fundamental function of human beings, can be fun, feel great, and actually benefit your health. It's a way of not only expressing yourself, but has the potential to share expression with someone close to you. The solutions to some of the problems with achieving optimal sexual well-being are biopsychosocial in nature. As sex permeates countless aspects of human existence, we have covered potential pharmacologic, non-pharmacologic, and dietary interventions to enhance sexual well-being. As we go forward in life there are many things we strive for in career and relationships; rightfully so, sexual well-being is often one of those things. For some it is highly important, while for others it is less so. The variation in the value of sexual wellness between individuals raises the question: Why? Several possibilities exist, from physical dyspareunia to cultural/social taboos that surround the topic. This can make even the mere idea of sex uncomfortable. And there is always the possibility of denial – it's easier to say you don't want something that you don't have or have never experienced in the first place. However, one thing remains clear: Achieving sexual well-being, whether it be through enhancing intimacy or the actual sexual experience itself, can increase overall well-being and quality of life.

References

1. H Liu, LJ Waite, S Shen, DH Wang. Is sex good for your health? National study on partnered sexuality and cardiovascular risk among older men and women. *J Health Soc Behav* 2016; **57**(3): 276–296.

2. CJ Charnetski, FX Brennan. Sexual frequency and salivary immunoglobulin A (IgA). *Psychol Rep* 2004; **94**(3): 839–844.

3. WW IsHak. *The Textbook of Clinical Sexual Medicine*. Cham, Springer; 2017.

4. AH Maslow. *Toward a Psychology of Being*, vol. **2**. New York, Van Nostrand Reinhold; 1968.

5. K Prager. *The Psychology of Intimacy*. New York, Guilford Press; 1995.

6. SK Whitbourne. We all need some intimacy in our lives. *Psychology Today* 2012. www.psychologytoday.com/us/blog/fulfillment-any-age/201210/we-all-need-some-intimacy-in-our-lives (accessed August 31, 2019).

7. JR Sneed, S Whitbourne, SJ Schwartz, S Huang. The relationship between identity, intimacy, and midlife well-being: findings from the Rochester Adult Longitudinal Study. *Psychol Aging* 2012; **27**: 318–323.

8. A Goliszek. The stress–sex connection. *Psychology Today* 2014. https://www.psychologytoday.com/us/blog/how-the-mind-heals-the-body/201412/the-stress-sex-connection (accessed August 31, 2019).

9. K Tan, L Tay. Relationships and well-being. In R Biswas-Diener, E Diener, eds., *Psychology*. Champaign, IL, DEF publishers; 2019.

10. B Ditzen, C Hoppmann, P Klumb. Positive couple interactions and daily cortisol: on the stress-protecting role of intimacy. *Psychosom Med* 2008; **70**(8): 883–889.

11. H LaFollette, G Graham. Honesty and intimacy. *J Soc Pers Relatsh* 1986; **3**(1): 3–18.

12. E Abusaidi, K Zahrakar, F Mohsenzadeh. Effectiveness of solution-focused brief couple therapy in improvement of communication patterns and marital intimacy in women. *J Res Health* 2018; **6**: 555.

13. KR Stephenson, CM Meston. The conditional importance of sex: exploring the association between sexual well-being and life satisfaction. *J Sex Marital Ther* 2015; **41**: 25–38.

14. M Khera. Treatment of male sexual dysfunction. 2018. www.uptodate.com/contents/treatment-of-male-sexual-dysfunction (accessed August 1, 2019).

15. J La, NH Roberts, FA Yafi. Diet and men's sexual health. *Sexual Med Rev* 2018; **6**(1): 54–68.

16. J Melnyk, M Marcone. Aphrodisiacs from plant and animal sources: a review of current scientific literature. *Food Res Int* 2011; **44**: 840.

17. K Reid, DH Surridge, A Morales, et al. Double-blind trial of yohimbine in treatment of psychogenic impotence. *Lancet* 1987; **2**(8556): 421–423.

18. FM Jacobsen. Fluoxetine-induced sexual dysfunction and an open trial of yohimbine. *J Clin Psychiatry* 1992; **53**(4): 119–122.

19. J McManus, D Kaherine. A practical guide to the Mediterranean diet. Harvard Health Blog, March 21, 2019. www.health.harvard.edu/blog/a-practical-guide-to-the-mediterranean-diet-2019032116194 (accessed September 2, 2019).

20. KR Stephenson, J Kerth. Effects of mindfulness-based therapies for female sexual dysfunction: a meta-analytic review. *J Sex Res* 2017; **54**(7): 832–849.

21. CC Ann. A proposal for a radical new sex therapy technique for the management of vasocongestive and orgasmic dysfunction

in women: the AFE zone stimulation technique. *Sex Marital Ther* 1997; **12**(4): 357–370.

22. DF Hurlbert, C Apt. The coital alignment technique and directed masturbation: a comparative study on female orgasm. *J Sex Marital Ther* 1995; **21**(1): 21–29.

23. WH Masters, VE Johnson. *Human Sexual Inadequacy*. Boston, MA, Little, Brown; 1970.

24. CG Cantor, Tips for sexual wellness in 2018. *Psychology Today* 2018. www .psychologytoday.com/us/blog/modern-sex/201801/tips-sexual-wellness-in-2018 (accessed September 2, 2019).

Chapter

28

Mindfulness, Meditation, and Yoga

Kayse Budd

One step, the first step, is the most important one you can take.

Background: Why this Topic?

In my twenties I lived at Satchidananda yoga ashram in Buckingham, VA. I took an atypical three-year "sabbatical" between medical school and residency. During this time away from medicine, I lived at the ashram, became a yoga instructor, taught yoga professionally, created a mind–body skills course for adolescents, studied nutrition and herbalism, trained in energy medicine, explored astrology, made art, and studied with healers in Peru. Medical training was challenging for me. Yoga, meditation, nutrition, nature, art, energy medicine, astrology, and herbs were part of my healing. In time, they became part of the "medicine pouch" I can draw from to help others.

To make a long story short, I did eventually return to medicine. I was committed to becoming a new paradigm physician. Currently, I am working online as a holistic psychiatrist, writer, and educator. Up until December 2019 I was the "integrative psychiatrist" on staff at the Chopra Center in Carlsbad, California. It was an Ayurvedically inspired yoga and meditation center founded by Deepak Chopra and David Simon in 1996. At the Chopra Center we offered "panchakarma" (Ayurvedic cleanse) programs with vegetarian meals, meditation instruction, yoga classes, Ayurvedic bodywork, holistic medical evaluations, and lectures on nutrition, meditation, Ayurveda, and related topics. I miss working at the Center, but I continue to be inspired by the wisdom of yoga and Ayurveda every single day.

Mindfulness

For those new to meditation or Eastern spirituality, *mindfulness is acute awareness of the present moment*. Being mindful, we are able to more fully take in the sights, sounds, and smells that reach our senses. We can more carefully respond to the questions or comments that come our way. Mindfulness encourages *gratitude*, as well as compassion, and improves our ability to respond without reacting if something unexpected happens.

With practice, it's possible to use mindfulness to help us *surrender to the flow of Grace in each moment*. In doing this, we *trust* that the things that happen are exactly perfect – happening as they are for a reason. Most likely that reason is our own growth, learning, and spiritual development (and the growth and development of others involved, as well).

A Bit of Backstory

There are many wonderful teachers of mindfulness. One of my favorites is Thich Nhat Hanh. His books offer a beautiful, articulate explanation of the power and practice of mindfulness [1]. I had the fortune of studying directly with Thich Nhat Hanh during a retreat at his monastery in Escondido, California in 2009. The experience included lectures on mindfulness, seated meditation, mindful eating, mindful walking, mindful talking, and mindful listening. It was an incredible experience that affected my heart in a powerful way.

If able to put down judgments, the heart starts to purely experience, appreciate, and *delight* in life. This can happen in yoga and meditation, too! The experience of *pure presence in joy* has a blissful, heart-warming effect that makes it one of the most precious feelings in life.

Another excellent teacher of mindfulness is Jon Kabat-Zinn. He wrote a beautiful book called *Wherever You Go, There You Are* [2]. The book teaches that cultivating mindful loving acceptance allows us to walk with beauty wherever the journey of life takes us. Similarly, if distress, anger, and fear fill our minds, then no matter where we go or what we do, we are likely to recreate conditions that perpetuate those mind states.

Jon Kabat-Zinn developed a training program in mindfulness, yoga, and meditation called "mindfulness-based stress reduction" (MBSR). Inspired by the useful way this program presented information to patients, I did professional training in MBSR years ago with Dr. Kabat-Zinn himself. There have been quite a few studies on MBSR published in medical journals, so I will draw from that literature to present some data on mindfulness.

Research

A 2015 meta-analysis from the *Journal of Psychosomatic Research* looked at MBSR in "healthy" populations and found large effects on *stress* and moderate effects on *anxiety, depression, quality of life*, and *distress* [3]. An older 2004 meta-analysis reported statistically significant benefits for *stress, cancer adaptability, anxiety*, and *depression* [4]. A 2007 study published in *Arthritis and Rheumatism* found improvements in *depression* in patients with fibromyalgia who received MBSR [5].

It makes sense that mindfulness can improve both stress and mood because mindfulness *changes attitudes*. If we see ourselves as part of the whole, expanding our awareness outside of the sphere of our own realities, the stresses of everyday life become increasingly less significant. We begin to see challenges as tools to improve our tolerance, rather than catastrophes that could ruin our lives.

An interesting 2014 study found a statistically significant increase in *telomere length* in participants of an MBSR group for breast cancer [6]. Telomeres are the tips of chromosomes, and longer telomeres have been associated with *longevity*. Thus, mindfulness and meditation interventions may be very helpful in extending longevity, with implications for individuals with cancer as well as the general public.

A 2015 review paper in *Cancer Management and Research* found benefit of mindfulness therapies for *sleep* and *insomnia* problems [7]. The review also catalogued a few physiologic benefits of mindfulness-based interventions, such as decreased cytokine production, decreased cortisol, increased telomere length, increased NK cells, and more. A 2014 article in the journal *Psychology & Health* described a randomized controlled trial applying a mindfulness intervention to a pregnant population [8]. The control segment of the trial included a reading experience, while the active arm received mindfulness training. Participants in both groups improved, but those receiving the mindfulness training had more significant improvements in *pregnancy-related anxiety and worry*.

A similar study from Australia in 2014 looked at a mindfulness intervention in pregnant women and found statistically significant improvements in *depression and anxiety* [9]. Because mindfulness encourages us to be *aware* without reacting, it trains us to observe our fears rather than let them run wild. Mindfulness challenges the ruminative nature of depression, offering the patient another experience. Ruminative thoughts can be witnessed with compassion and then released. If we can catch negative thinking early and lovingly redirect the mind, we stand a good chance of having an episode of negative thinking rather than a full-blown depression.

How to Incorporate Mindfulness

I recommend using this chapter as inspiration to get started on your own personal journey with mindfulness (and meditation and yoga). Look into some of the teachers and references mentioned. And go beyond them, if truly interested. One thing leads to another in life, and this is no different. Healing is a spiral. The deeper you go, the more humble you become . . . as you realize there is always further to go.

Mindfulness paves the way for much higher, more advanced spiritual concepts and pursuits. It is step one for an awakened life. All you have to do to begin is *become aware of some part of yourself witnessing this moment*. In this moment you are reading. In another moment, you will be walking or talking or washing dishes. By becoming aware of yourself *be*-ing in those moments fully, you are practicing mindfulness. It's pretty easy when nothing challenging is happening! It's more difficult during emotionally intense moments, but that's also where it can be of greatest help (Box 28.1).

Box 28.1 Indications for Mindfulness

Consider mindfulness for these issues:
- stress*
- anxiety*
- depression*
- cancer diagnosis*
- fibromyalgia*
- ADHD*
- binge eating*
- addiction/smoking cessation*
- pregnancy (anxiety, depression, stress) *
- headaches*
- feeling disconnected/isolation
- identity confusion
- major life change
- easily triggered/frustrated
- relationship issues

*evidence-based

Meditation

Taking a step beyond mindfulness, which can be done in any moment, we move on to meditation. Meditation is like "applied mindfulness." It involves discrete "practice" periods of formal, mindful awareness. There are various different types of meditation – sitting, walking, chanting, movement, visual, and more. Really, almost anything can be a meditation, and in that way the boundary between mindfulness and meditation is quite subtle.

In the usual sense, however, meditation is more structured than mindfulness. It classically involves periods of sitting with eyes closed, awareness turned inward. Focus is on the breath (with or without a sacred sound or mantra) with gentle, open observation of both body and mind. Using the "vehicle" of the breath or sound, meditation has the potential to carry an individual to expanded states of consciousness.

That's really what meditation is, *a journey into consciousness*. It's a tool for travel ... through and beyond the mind into vast realms of space and pure awareness. It's possible to be purely aware with eyes open (mindful), but with eyes closed one can e x p a n d. Meditation gives us the opportunity to consciously merge our individual consciousness with the underlying consciousness permeating everything.

Role of Breathing in Meditation

Breath is a key factor in meditation and in controlling the mind state. There are many good breathing exercises (pranayama) that can help prepare one's mind for meditation. My favorite is "nadi suddhi"– alternate nostril breathing. This practice involves breathing in one nostril while covering the other, holding the breath for a few seconds, then breathing out the previously covered nostril while covering the one that was just open. You hold the breath again; then reverse the process. It is a soothing practice that calms and balances both mind and physiology.

Learning to favorably manipulate our brain waves and neurochemistry is an important part of self-care, in my opinion. I endeavor to teach all my patients natural techniques (combined with food and herbal medicines) they can use to create mind–body environments that feel amazing. If we are happy, calm, balanced, and inspired, it's likely our bodies and minds are healing in some way. Similarly, if we feel stressed, anxious, depressed, and confused, it's probable that our bodies and minds are hurt by these energies. Cytokines are generated, cortisol is rising, serotonin is dropping ... leading to depression, inflammation, immune dysfunction, and so on.

Mind or Gnat?

In the beginning, meditation is difficult. The mind is restless and flits about, like a gnat. It buzzes in your ear, making you think you have other things to do that are more important. But really, those things can wait. You are on the cushion to learn to master the mind, not get up and follow its every whim. Only in relative mastery will you be free of anxieties and worries – free of being pulled here and there by the mind. To achieve mastery at something, one has to practice. One has to develop discipline. To do this we must sit through the mind's buzzing. We must redirect it to stillness. Let thoughts go. Reorient to our breathing. In meditation, starting over is perpetual. It occurs with every out-breath.

A peaceful place is inside us all. Once we find it, we can be at home anytime! But, like any home, our "inner home" must be cultivated into a nourishing environment. Meditation helps us purify our body temple – making our inner landscape more inviting. With meditation, we cleanse our minds of negative, random thoughts by lovingly letting them go. Meditation cleanses the body, too. It calms the nervous system, which helps our body switch into detoxification mode.

An additional way that meditation cleanses the body and mind is via "prana," which is lifeforce "energy" in Sanskrit. Meditation increases prana, making us feel light and clear. It raises our vibration by bringing more energy into our system. Meditation refines our sensitivities, making us slowly more aware of subtle vibrations. We begin to notice that freshly prepared vegetables, fruits, and juices keep us feeling clear and light (enhance prana), whereas heavier, processed, fried or rich foods tend to slow us down (reduce prana). If we honor these observations, we will gradually make healthier choices with the food, as well as the images, sounds, and experiences we "consume."

Some Research on Meditation

There are many excellent studies, reviews, and meta-analyses about meditation. An NCBI search using key words "meta-analysis and meditation" revealed 130 listings. These studies reported positive benefits for *headaches, depression, insomnia, hypertension, cognitive performance, anxiety, stress, quality of life after cancer diagnosis, chronic pain, PTSD, asthma, bipolar disorder, smoking cessation, negative affect, prosocial behavior, insomnia,* and *telomere length.* I will discuss just a few of the interesting papers I found and encourage you to pursue any of the conditions that limited space caused me to omit.

A meta-analysis published in the journal *Depression and Anxiety* in 2012 reported statistically significant benefits of meditation interventions for *anxiety* [10]. A more comprehensive meta-analysis in 2018 analyzed 171 randomized controlled trials with 12,005 participants [11]. This review found consistent support for meditation in *depression, pain, addictive disorders,* and *smoking cessation.*

A 2018 meta-analysis from the *Chinese Medical Journal* examined 10 randomized controlled trials and one clinical trial (315 patients total) and found that meditation significantly improved intensity and frequency of *headaches* [12]. An older 2014 meta-analysis from *JAMA Internal Medicine* found moderate improvements in *anxiety, depression,* and *pain* with meditation, and lower but still statistically significant improvements in *stress/distress* and *quality of life* [13].

A meta-analysis from the *Annals of the New York Academy of Sciences* published in December 2018 looked at 18 trials (1684 participants) and found a significant benefit of meditation on *sleep quality* [14]. I personally teach all my insomnia patients to meditate, both sitting on a cushion and "in the bed" (lying on the back with hands over the heart). Strict meditation teachers may not appreciate this suggestion, but I find it really does help patients with insomnia. I encourage these patients to develop strong discipline with their thoughts and *not allow* themselves to think *at all* while in bed. If they wake up, they are encouraged to *diligently maintain emptiness* within their minds to calm themselves down.

A 2017 review from the journal *Psychological Trauma* found meditation to be effective for *PTSD* (and *depression*) when compared with a control [15]. *Quality of life* and *anxiety* were also improved, but to a lesser degree. One particularly helpful "type" of meditation intervention for trauma is the "Mind–Body Skills Group" (MBSG), designed by psychiatrist Jim Gordon, MD. I trained in this modality with Jim Gordon in 2002. I also helped organize a MBSG group for my medical school peers at the University of Michigan (with a UM faculty member trained by Dr. Gordon). Some might say medical training itself is traumatic (especially for sensitive people). The nurturing MBSG group helped my school experience be less stressful and more meaningful, for at least a little while. If the program could have continued for the duration of my education, it would have profoundly impacted my experience. I believe medical training needs to move in the direction of greater balance and nurturance *within the curriculum* if we want those qualities reflected in physicians at the end.

There are numerous studies on MBSGs, and one of the most informative is from Jim Gordon himself (plus his team) [16]. This study included 82 adolescents with PTSD in Kosovo. The groups, administered by trained high-school teachers, included meditation, journaling, drawing, movement, genograms, and biofeedback. There is extensive evidence that creative expression is healing. I am an artist, as well as a dancer, poet, and musician, so I love that this program incorporates all of that, plus meditation. Biofeedback offers participants proof that the meditation is indeed calming their physiology. Genograms allow students to examine their families for patterns, leading to enhanced objectivity, improved coping, and often a more spiritual interpretation of life.

The MBSR intervention in the study resulted in statistically significant improvement in PTSD scores. I personally facilitated MBSGs for both adolescents and adults in Telluride, Colorado between medical school and residency. I did not publish my results, but I did collect data. I found notable improvements in multiple areas of life – stress, self-esteem, anxiety, mood, sleep quality, family and social relationships, spirituality, and energy level. It was one of the most meaningful things I have done in my career.

Learning to Meditate

To illustrate the process of learning to meditate, I offer this poem:

MEDITATION
The mystery of NOW
Repeats itself.
Meanwhile . . .
Silence fishes
For fresh thoughts.

Kayse Budd, 2008

If you are serious about becoming skilled at meditation, you will need to practice every day (Box 28.2). Thirty minutes, twice a day, is an ideal investment for anyone desiring significant benefits relatively quickly. I usually tell my patients that if they absolutely cannot do 30 minutes, then do 15. If 15 is not possible, then do 5. If the end of the day arrives, and you still have not meditated, then sit on the edge of the bed and clear your mind for a minute or two.

A minute or two of meditation is not going to make someone a skilled meditator. Progress and brain changes are proportional to effort, but a little *is* better than nothing. Even clearing the mind for a minute makes a statement to yourself: *I am committed to this. I am willing and able to exist without thoughts.* It takes a certain amount of dedication to meditate even for a few minutes every day. This commitment and small display of discipline can lead to a greater investment in time.

Box 28.2 Meditation Instructions

- Choose a relatively quiet place (ideally).
- Sit comfortably, with your spine elongated and shoulders relaxed.
- Close your eyes.
- Become aware of the body resting.
- Gently bring your awareness to the heart.
- Become aware of your breathing.
- Take a few slow, deep breaths, or practice the nadi suddhi breathing technique.
- Become aware of the mind. Notice if any thoughts are present.
- If yes, meet them kindly, but choose not to engage them. Let them go and return to the breath.
- Center yourself in pure awareness.
- Stay there as long as possible.
- Consider placing the tip of the tongue on the bump behind the upper front two teeth. This creates a subtle, balancing energetic current (tip of tongue = female yin meridian; incisive papilla = yang masculine meridian).
- Consider focusing awareness on the heart or at a point, like a pearl, between the eyebrows in the center of the head.
- Experiment with different mudras (hand positions that channel energy and subtly change the feeling of the meditation). "Gyan mudra" is a classic – the tip of the first finger touching the thumb on the same hand.

Yoga

Yogas Citta Vritti Nirodhah

Yoga is the restraint of the modifications of the mind-stuff.

Pantajali Yoga Sutra 2

Yoga means union, specifically the union of mind, body, and spirit. The above sutra (verse) from the ancient text on yoga, *The Yoga Sutras of Patanjali*, defines the key goal of yoga. Yoga is a way to limit mind activity or "modifications" of the otherwise clear consciousness. The entire science of yoga is really based on this one ideal. Learning to control the mind – to stop it from worrying, wishing, and really thinking at all – is the goal and purpose of yoga.

The experience and wisdom gained while learning to control the mind . . .

That is yoga.

With yoga, we learn that the mind creates our suffering . . . and our liberation. If we want to have some control over life, which is ultimately a mystery, possibly the best we can do is learn to control our minds. If you can control your mind, nothing in this world can bind you.

For a yogi, *everything that happens is yoga*. All of life's events *and challenges* are perfectly designed and timed. They are "for us." All we have to do is *trust*. And maybe look for the lesson. Practicing this kind of faith, we learn surrender. We find freedom.

Yoga actually contains eight different parts or "limbs," and each of these parts helps us to develop a different aspect of ourselves. The eight together form a complete instruction manual or system for living. Yoga is thus not just about physical postures. That is only one limb of yoga. I highly encourage anyone interested in further exploration of the material introduced here to read the Yoga Sutras translated by Sri Swami Satchidananda [17]. It is an incredible interpretation of this still-relevant ancient text.

The Eight Limbs of Yoga

1. Yamas – ethical guidelines

    a. Ahimsa – nonviolence
    b. Satya – truthfulness
    c. Asteya – non-stealing
    d. Bramacharya – respect for sexual activity
    e. Aparigraha – non-coveting

2. Niyamas – practices that inform worldview

    a. Saucha – purity
    b. Santosha – contentment
    c. Tapas – discipline
    d. Svadhyaya – study of sacred texts, scriptures, and ultimately, the Self
    e. Ishvara Pranidhana – surrender to God, faith

3. Asanas – physical postures
4. Pranayama – breathing techniques
5. Pratyahara – sense-withdrawal
6. Dharana – concentration
7. Dhyana – awareness
8. Samadhi – transcendence

Many Meanings of Yoga

When I was living at the yoga ashram, I learned that one of the intentions of yoga is to *prepare the body for meditation*. Anyone desiring to reach the highest states of meditation will most likely want to learn yoga to support the mind–body system in that pursuit. At the ashram, we often had meditation sessions following asana class.

This was one *physical* way we practiced the idea that yoga prepares the body for meditation. I truly did reach deeper states of meditation in those sittings. To just meditate straight-away is difficult. Asana practice, by engaging the body harmoniously, effectively stills the mind.

When the mind is clear, we can see our true selves. Our true nature is peace, clarity, and love. Emptying the mind, we return to our natural state. Meditation is *unifying* because when people strip away the stories and thoughts of their individual minds, they are all left with the *same pure awareness*. The same consciousness enlivens every person. And, really, it enlivens everything else, too.

Behind All Changing Phenomena Is a Completely Stable Oneness

Through yoga we come to rest more and more in this Oneness – in the never-changing awareness that lies underneath all fluctuations of mind and matter.

Yoga, for the true seeker, never ends. It is a lifelong, constant pursuit. It requires patience, earnestness, and conviction. Yoga is about being willing to go on the *journey of Mastery*. Every single step, every little thing that occurs is part of the practice of yoga. All difficulties are part of a yogi's process of unique refinement.

Asana Yoga

Most of the yoga that Westerners know is asana yoga, the physical yoga of postures. "Hatha" yoga is a general category of asana practice that includes many styles. Even among the different styles there can be huge variations, depending on the teacher, as each brings his or her wisdom and experiences to the classroom.

Yoga asanas improve blood flow to the parts of the body activated by the session. This brings oxygen and healing chemicals to places where they may be needed, and it takes away products of metabolism and inflammation where they exist. This "nutrient exchange" is very important in the constant detoxification necessary for physical health. Ayurveda and yoga place more emphasis on detoxification and "cleansing" than Western medicine. I personally believe there is incredible wisdom in this ancient approach, which is why I have chosen to study Ayurveda as well as allopathic medicine. It is possible to detoxify the body with herbs, fasting, and even some astringent/bitter foods (e.g., beets, dandelion greens, parsley, cilantro, seaweed). Even more gentle is yoga, which detoxifies the body through movement and flow of energy, breath, blood, and lymph.

Flexibility is essential in life, according to yoga. Flexibility in the body can help support flexibility in the mind (and vice versa), as all things are connected. Some body types are naturally more flexible, but all can improve with practice, dedication, and intention.

Yoga Is Devotion

Yoga is a sacred practice. It is devotional – a "moving prayer." It is a conversation between body, mind, soul, and God. Yoga can connect us to nature (sun/moon salutations, tree pose, fish pose, etc.) and help us feel more integrated with all of life. This is especially useful for depressed people, who may feel disconnected from the earth and their purpose here.

The "grounding" aspects of yoga – the subtle ways it helps us connect to our bodies and the earth – can be helpful for anxiety and insomnia. Yoga is soothing to the nervous system, too. Many of the poses activate the parasympathetic nervous system (through stretching of the spinal column and nerve roots), calming us down. This is helpful for everyone, but perhaps especially useful for those with worry, ADHD, or stress.

Research on Yoga

Most, if not all, of the research on yoga is on Hatha-style asana yoga. I found positive studies on Pubmed for many things, but most notably *depression, type-2 diabetes, lower back pain, PTSD, quality of life after breast cancer diagnosis, stress, anxiety, smoking cessation, prenatal depression, fibromyalgia, arthritis, sleep, ADHD,* and *hypertension.* I reviewed quite a bit of data and found the strongest/most convincing evidence for *depression, PTSD, type-2 diabetes,* and *fibromyalgia and other functional pain syndromes.*

A 2013 meta-analysis looked at 12 randomized controlled trials with 619 participants. Moderate evidence of improvement was found for patients with diagnosable *depressive disorders* [18]. This meta-analysis also revealed improvement in *anxiety disorders.* A 2012 review by Balasubramaniam et al. looked at the impact of yoga on various neuropsychiatric conditions [19]. This research team found benefit for *depression,* as an adjunct to pharmacotherapy in *schizophrenia,* and in children with *ADHD.* This review also found evidence for the impact of yoga on *sleep.*

One of the more interesting evidence-supported indications for yoga is *type-2 diabetes.* A 2016 review found that yoga practices could significantly improve several parameters relevant to type-2 diabetes, including body composition, glycemic control, and lipid levels [20]. They also found modest evidence that yoga could *lower blood pressure, reduce oxidative stress, enhance pulmonary function,* improve mood, *extend sleep,* and increase quality of life. A 2017 study out of India found adherence to a weekly yoga program resulted in a significantly *lower hemoglobin A1C* after three months [21].

One of the most useful indications for yoga, in my opinion, is *fibromyalgia.* A 2010 randomized controlled trial looked at yoga for fibromyalgia and found improvements in fatigue, pain, mood, acceptance, negative thinking, and coping [22]. Yoga may actually benefit many different "functional pain syndromes." A review published in 2016 found "modest efficacy" for yoga in *chronic fatigue, headaches, irritable bowel, pelvic pain, back pain, neck pain,* and *somatoform pain* [23].

I personally have held a theory for years that *emotional stress causes oxidation* in the body, which results in increased free radicals/cytokines/inflammation. This then results in pain (and mental health issues). It is wonderful that scientists are finally talking about this [24]! If the process continues unabated, a pain syndrome or mental illness is often created. Consuming plants with high antioxidant value (as food and/or supplements) improves functional pain syndromes (and mental illness), presumably by buffering this process. Sleep, the universal healer, also improves pain syndromes (melatonin is an antioxidant). And finally, *yoga increases glutathione,* which is one of the body's strongest endogenous antioxidants [25]. Yoga is thus a true and legitimate treatment for stress, and all the conditions that come with it! Box 28.3 presents some guidelines on how to incorporate yoga into your practice.

Box 28.3 How to Incorporate Yoga into Your Practice

- Try it yourself. Observe the benefits in your life.
- Learn what is available in your community.
- Look for lower-cost classes at community centers and libraries.
- Educate clients about "exercise style" vs. restorative and other styles. Help them choose a style that fits their needs.
- Consider online videos or downloadable yoga classes. (This way you or your patients can learn enough to craft a 10–30 minute home practice.)
- Commit to 10 minutes of yoga per day for a week and see if improves your life. Expand from there.

Tying It All Together

Mindfulness, meditation, and yoga are, simply put, *tools for evolution*. They make us better humans. And yes, they are also evidence-based for a number of "problems" (problems are *teachers* in yoga). Ultimately, the proof is in the doing. You can feel your brain calming when you meditate. You can perceive your patience growing when you choose to be mindful. You can feel your mood and energy rising during yoga asana practice. Reading yogic parables inspires us to make more selfless, kind choices . . . the type of choices that advance the soul.

Mindfulness, meditation, and yoga all have one important thing in common: *presence*. They are each about *pure presence in the moment – without thoughts* in our minds. Cultivating time in pure presence, we learn to be less attached and more receptive. We reduce suffering by learning to *trust* the universe. After trust comes *acceptance*. Joys and sorrows are both viewed more neutrally. We eventually realize that we alone are responsible for our minds, moods, and contentment. If we use mindfulness to face things directly, then we can more *efficiently* take responsibility for all that we can do right now to be happy, develop our hearts, and move forward on the spiritual path.

The Bhavagad Gita verse 12.12 says, "Knowledge is better than practice; meditation is better than knowledge; and best of all is surrender, which soon brings peace" [26].

Aided by mindfulness, yoga and meditation offer a kind of "heart development" that can facilitate an individual soul's constant *surrender to the grace of the mystery*. The *secret peace* we are all looking for has been inside us all along. Peace comes not only from surrender, but from making our own hearts *home*. Offering a key to the locked door at the gateway to the heart, yoga is one of the most profound technologies on our planet. I feel blessed by its guiding presence in my life and hope I have inspired you to know it, too.

The result of yoga is *LOVE*.

Namaste!

References

1. TN Hanh. *The Miracle of Mindfulness.* Boston, MA, Beacon Press; 1999.

2. J Kabat-Zinn. *Wherever You Go, There You Are.* New York, Hyperion; 1994.

3. B Khoury, M Sharma, SE Rush, et al. Mindfulness-based stress reduction for healthy individuals: a meta-analysis. *J Psychosom Res* 2015; **78**(6): 519–528.

4. P Grossmand, L Niemann, S Schmidt, et al. Mindfulness-based stress reduction and health benefits: a meta-analisis. *J Psychosom Res* 2004; **57**(1): 35–43.

5. SE Septon, P Salmon, I Weissbecker, et al. Mindfulness meditation alleviates depressive symptoms in women with fibromyalgia: results of a randomized clinical trial. *Arthritis Rheum* 2007; **57**(1): 77–85.

6. CA Lengacher, RR Reich, KE Kip, et al. Influence of mindfulness-based stress reduction on telomerase activity in women with breast cancer. *Biol Res Nurs* 2014; **16**(4): 438–447.

7. CR Rouleau, SN Garland, LE Carlson. The impact of mindfulness-based interventions on symptom burden, positive psychological outcomes, and biomarkers in cancer patients. *Cancer Manag Res* 2015; 7: 121–131.

8. CM Guardino, C DunkelSchetter, JE Bower, et al. Randomised controlled pilot

trial of minfulness training for stress reduction during pregnancy. *Psychol Health* 2014; **29**(3): 334–349.

9. H Woolhouse, K Mercuri, F Judd, et al. Antenatal mindfulness intervention to reduce depression, anxiety and stress: a randomized controlled trial of the mindbabybody program in an Australian tertiary maternity hospital. *BMC Pregnancy Childbirth* 2014; **14**: 369.

10. KW Chen, CC Berger, E Manheimer, et al. Meditative therapies for reducing anxiety: a systematic review and meta-analysis of randomized controlled trials. *Depress Anxiety* 2012; **29**(7): 545–562.

11. SB Goldberg, RP Tucker, PA Greene, et al. Mindfulness-based interventions for psychiatric disorders: a systematic review and meta-analysis. *Clin Psychol Rev* 2018; **59**: 52–60.

12. Q Gu, JC Hou, XM Fang. Mindfulness meditation for primary headache pain: a meta-analysis. *Chin Med J* 2018; **131**(7): 829–838.

13. M Goyal, S Singh, EM Sibinga, et al. Meditation programs for psychological stress and well-being: a systematic review and meta-analysis. *JAMA Intern Med* 2014; **174**(3): 357–368.

14. HL Rusch, M Rosario, A Olivera, et al. The effect of mindfulness meditation on sleep quality: a systematic review and meta-analysis of randomized controlled trials. *Ann N Y Acad Sci* 2018. www.ncbi.nlm.nih.gov/pubmed/30575050 (accessed April 8, 2019).

15. L Hilton, AR Maher, B Colaiaco, et al. Meditation for posttraumatic stress: systematic review and meta-analysis. *Psychol Trauma* 2017; **9**(4): 453–460.

16. JS Gordon, JK Staples, A Blyta, et al. Treatment of posttraumatic stress disorder in postwar Kosovar adolescents using mind–body skills groups: a randomized controlled trial. *J Clin Psychiatry* 2008; **69**(9): 1469–1476.

17. SS Satchidananda, transl., *The Yoga Sutras of Patanjali*. Yogaville, Integral Yoga Publications; 1987.

18. H Cramer, R Lauche, J Langhorst, et al. Yoga for depression: a systematic review and metaanalysis. *Depress Anxiety* 2013; **11**: 1068–1083.

19. M Balasubramaniam, S Telles, PM Doraiswamy. Yoga on our minds: a systematic review of yoga for neuropsychiatric disorders. *Front Psychiatry* 2012; **3**: 117.

20. KE Innes, TK Selfe. Yoga for adults with type 2 diabetes: a systematic review of controlled trials. *J Diabetes Res* 2016; **2016**: 697370.

21. P Angadi, A Jagannathan, A Thulasi, et al. Adherence to yoga and its resultant effects on blood glucose in type 2 diabetes: a community-based follow-up study. *Int J Yoga* 2017; **10**(1): 29–35.

22. JW Carson, KM Carson, KD Jones, et al. A pilot randomized controlled trial of the yoga of awareness program in the management of fibromyalgia. *Pain* 2010; **151**(2): 530–539.

23. R Sutar, S Yadav, G Deasi. Yoga intervention and functional pain syndromes: a selective review. *Int Rev Psychiatry* 2016; **3**: 316–322.

24. S Salim. Oxidative stress and psychological disorders. *Curr Neuropharmacol* 2014; **12**(2): 140–147.

25. SV Hedge, P Adhikari, VJ Pinto, et al. Effect of 3-month yoga on oxidative stress in type 2 diabetes with or without complications: a controlled clinical trial. *Diabetes Care* 2011; **34**(10): 2208–2210.

26. S Mitchell, transl., *Bhavavad Gita*. New York, Three Rivers Press; 2000.

Chapter 29

Forgiveness, Gratitude, and Spirituality

Sindhu A. Idicula, Natasha Thrower, and James Lomax

Introduction

Forgiveness, gratitude, and spirituality are all areas that have been studied in the literature as having an impact on an individual's well-being. While they are associated topics, they also stand on their own and independently have effects on individuals and their wellness. Forgiveness involves a period of growth for an individual following an interpersonal transgression, allowing them to process and let go of the negative affects they may feel due to the experience. Gratitude is related to an individual's tendency to tune into one's gifts or benefits, and to be thankful for them, and also shows powerful effects on their ability to promote wellness in their lives. Spirituality is often connected with religion, but also stands independently, and serves as a powerful factor in improving the outcomes of individuals. All three show tremendous potential and are explored in this chapter.

Forgiveness

Forgiveness has been discussed as a process that helps facilitate an individual's growth from interpersonal hurts or transgressions. Interpersonal hurts, whether minor or major, occur frequently, for an array of reasons and in a variety of different contexts. These contexts may range from war and sociopolitical disputes, to more ordinary and frequent ones, and may include issues such as bullying, child abuse, intimate partner violence, and elder abuse. They may also stem from unhealthy relationships, as well as occur in otherwise healthy relationships, such as when individuals feel unacknowledged or rejected. These may lead to a variety of emotions, such as anger and hostility, and may promote a cycle of violence in the seeking of revenge. Carrying feelings of anger and hostility may also contribute to physical and mental health problems [1].

While there has been controversy about the definition of forgiveness, a few concepts emerge to better define the term. There are three concepts that are core to forgiveness. The first includes recognizing an injury to self or others causing resentment, anger, or hatred. The second is being able to let go of negative emotions, perceptions of injury, or past events. The third is freedom from the desire for retaliation or punishment of the offender [2]. The concept of "pseudoforgiveness," or false forgiveness, is both confounding and distinct, defined as a tendency to utilize the opportunity to gain power over the other by reminding them of their failures or displaying moral superiority [2]. Forgiveness does not imply a state of amnesia in which the injury is forgotten or ignored; rather, forgiveness implies a deliberate and thoughtful remembering of past injuries [3].

The literature has pointed to a connection between the ability to forgive and the improvement in health and wellness. Several authors have examined the role of forgiveness and cardiovascular parameters – they found that forgiveness was associated with lower heart rate, lower blood pressure, fewer medications, less alcohol use, and fewer physical symptoms of anger and cardiovascular recovery from stress [3]. Researchers have postulated that disorders such as fibromyalgia and chronic fatigue syndrome are ripe for study for forgiveness interventions, given that interventions may work on the negative emotions, such as anger, resentment and stress, that often accompany these disorders [4].

Self-forgiveness robustly predicted psychological well-being when looking at aggregate measures of depression, anxiety, life satisfaction, and general mental health [5]. Forgiveness has been associated with improved psychological health in a variety of groups, including incest survivors, college students, older women, and men whose partners underwent abortion [2]. In all four groups, who all harbored ill-will over past harms, participants were assigned to a forgiveness therapy group versus a control group. After participating in forgiveness therapy, all four groups showed improvement in their measures. The incest survivors had improved self-esteem and hope, and lowered depression and anxiety scores. The college students had greater improvements on their willingness to forgive, their attitudes toward their parents, hope, and anxiety. The older women exhibited improvements in self-esteem, depression, and anxiety compared to controls. The men displayed greater improvements in forgiveness, anxiety, anger, and grief [2]. Meta-analyses also show similar results. Recine's 2009 meta-analysis showed improved mental and physical health [6].

Similarly, unforgiveness has been associated with poorer outcomes. Toussaint in 2012 showed that a failure to arrive at forgiveness was associated with a negative health impact [7]. Individuals who placed conditions on forgiveness also appeared to have poorer health outcomes, as well as greater mortality risk [7]. Unforgivingness is emotionally complex, and may involve multiple feelings such as residual anger, fearfulness, depression, bitterness, and resentment [8]. Unforgiving has been conceptualized as developing from rumination about the nature of the transgression, its consequences for the victim or the relationships, and the attribution about the motivation of the transgressor [8].

Mindfulness has also been hypothesized to play a role in mediating forgivingness. Mindfulness was found to help facilitate "letting go" of the painful experiences by paying mindful attention to them and moving toward forgiveness. It is suggested that mindfulness does this by its metacognitive monitoring of internal experiences with an open and accepting stance and allowing oneself to respond to the current moment experiences, a process known as decentering [9].

Interventions that help facilitate forgiveness in individuals may help clinicians be able to help patients who might be struggling with unforgiveness. The literature suggests that interventions may be effective in helping people move toward a place of forgiveness, and in association, help improve their well-being and overall health. In multiple meta-analyses looking at what contributed to effective forgiveness interventions, Recine noted that, in general, interventions are more effective when they are longer, individual rather than group, involved a process rather than a cognitive decision-making approach, and addressed mental and emotional health, not just improving morals [6].

Two models of forgiveness interventions have been used widely. The first, promoted by Enright and the Human Development Study Group, includes 20 units covering cognitive, affective, and behavioral elements. Structured around four phases, it includes the following elements: (1) an uncovering phase, meant to explore defenses, emotions over the offense, and acknowledging psychological harm; (2) a decision phase, exploring what it means to forgive and considering it as a possibility; (3) cognitive reframing, seeing the offender in a new light and developing compassion and empathy for them; and (4) a deepening phase, in which participants may look for meaning in their suffering and recognize their own past mistakes [2]. The second model, developed by Worthington, is the REACH program, an acronym for a five-step forgiveness approach. First, participants recall (R) the hurt, second develop empathy (E) for the offender, third consider forgiveness as an altruistic (A) gift, fourth commit (C) to forgive, and finally hold (H) on to forgiveness in times of difficulty [1, 4].

Gratitude

Gratitude has been described when individuals can attend to the benefits and gifts that are attributable to the kindness of others or a tendency to express thankfulness consistently across situations and over time [9, 10]. There is some disagreement about the construct of gratitude – if gratitude is the thankfulness for the kindness of others, it fails to encapsulate those aspects of life in which individuals may be grateful for aspects of life not attributable to a benefactor [11]. An example may be gratitude for such events as "waking up in the morning" [3]. This has expanded the concept of gratitude to include, at a dispositional level, that gratitude may be part of a wider life orientation toward noticing and appreciating the positive in the world [11].

Gratitude is robustly associated with well-being, with regards to lack of psychopathology, general emotional functioning, existential functioning, and humanistic conceptions [11]. Gratitude may be associated with specific personality traits in the individual. With the Big Five traits, grateful people are typically more extroverted, agreeable, open, conscientious, and less neurotic. Individuals displaying high degrees of gratitude typically have more positive emotional functioning, positive social relationships, and less dysfunction [11]. They often are less angry or hostile, less depressed or emotionally vulnerable, and expressed experiencing positive emotions much more frequently. Grateful people often were more emotionally warm, gregarious, activity-seeking, trusting, altruistic, and tender-minded. They tended to be more open to feelings and ideas and values, and felt greater competence, dutifulness, and achievement-striving [11].

Gratitude has been studied in relationship to various psychopathological conditions. Studies on depression find that higher gratitude is associated with a positive life orientation, one incompatible with the "negative triad" of beliefs about self, world, and future which may be associated with depression, predicted lower rates of major depression, generalized anxiety, phobia, bulimia nervosa, poor body image, alcohol dependence, nicotine dependence, and drug abuse or dependence. Notably, thankfulness was more robustly and more consistently predictive of psychopathology than other aspects of religiosity measured, albeit a broader measure than gratitude. Gratitude has been studied in those who have been traumatized as well, suggesting that gratitude is lower in individuals with PTSD, and those individuals with PTSD who have higher gratitude have better daily functioning, regardless of symptomatology. Gratitude has also been shown to help facilitate posttraumatic growth, aiding in the recovery from traumatic experience [11].

Gratitude has additionally been associated with subjective well-being, a finding that is consistent with survey data that indicate that over 90 percent of American teens and adults note that expressing gratitude made them "extremely happy" or "somewhat happy" [11]. It has also been linked to "eudemonic" or psychological well-being, with higher autonomy, environmental mastery, personal growth, purpose in life, and self-acceptance [11]. Gratitude also seems to be related to more humanistic constructs, including authentic living and a tendency to not experience self-alienation [12]. In relationships, gratitude appears to be related to willingness to forgive and seems to promote relationship formation and maintenance [11, 12].

Most studies have looked at the adult population, but some have extended into the adolescent population as well. Studies in the adolescent literature have pointed to positive associations between gratitude and positive affect, life satisfaction, optimism, social support, and prosocial behavior, mostly even when controlling for positive affect. These studies have been extended to cultures outside of Western culture, and one study showed that gratitude is uniquely associated with less suicidality in Chinese adolescents, which builds on theories of positive emotions, arguing that gratitude can broaden and build one's psychological and social resources and promote growth and development in life [10].

Given the significant amount of research correlating gratitude to well-being, several promising clinical interventions have been designed to help foster positive functioning and psychological strengths, thus potentially improving disorders. Gratitude interventions can be divided into those that cultivate appreciative feelings or those that strengthen relationships [13]. Two interventions in the first category include gratitude lists and gratitude contemplation [11]. Gratitude lists include writing lists of things one is grateful for on a regular basis. The most popular approach in the literature, it is easy to implement clinically, and participants often note it is enjoyable and self-reinforcing. An example might be to ask an individual to write down three things in a diary for which they are grateful, immediately before going to bed. This strategy also lends itself to online websites and downloaded workbooks, allowing them to be low-cost and to substantially increase access to services. Grateful contemplation is a more generalized activity – it asks for individuals to write or think about things for which one is grateful in a more global fashion. Grateful contemplation is also a brief exercise, one that may only last for five minutes or so, and may have implications in being able to help raise mood more immediately [11].

The second category includes interventions that strengthen relationships. This may include activities such as gratitude visits, where an individual may write a letter to a benefactor, visit them, and read it to them in person. As this is an interpersonal rather than solitary activity, it has the benefit of building and strengthening the relationship. Compared to a control group who wrote about childhood memories, the group participating in a gratitude visit reported more happiness and less depression immediately and one month later. Compared to the other interventions studied, the gratitude visit was the most short-lived but also yielded the highest effect size [11].

Studies looking at the efficacy of these interventions have shown similar usefulness and social acceptability of all interventions. Some studies point to gratitude journaling allowing participants to feel more efficacious, which increased self-initiation and completion of the intervention. Individual differences may account for the differences as well [13].

Specific individuals may be best targeted for gratitude interventions. Depressed people are the least likely to initiate a gratitude intervention and the most likely to benefit from interventions that specifically target positive emotions such as gratitude [14]. Curiosity plays a big role in predicting intentions and behaviors, and it is hypothesized that interventions that help instill curiosity may motivate individuals to initiate well-being interventions, perhaps like motivational interviewing [14].

Hypothesized mechanisms of action of gratitude include a variety of different constructs. In the schematic hypothesis, an explanation of gratitude includes that individuals who were more grateful had specific schematic biases toward viewing help as more beneficial [12]. In the coping hypothesis, gratitude was associated with three categories of coping: (1) grateful individuals were more likely to seek out and use both instrumental and emotional social support; (2) grateful people used more active coping, planning, and positive reinterpretation, and tried to look for the potential for growth; and (3) grateful people were less likely to disengage, deny the problem, or escape through maladaptive substance-use [11]. In the positive affect hypothesis, gratitude, which functions as a positive emotion, may change the balance of positive and negative emotions [15]. In the broaden-and-build hypothesis, positive emotions are seen as serving a unique evolutionary purpose. Here, positive emotions such as gratitude serve to broaden thought and encourage cognitive and behavioral activities that build resources that can be utilized during the next stressful period. These include such factors as creativity, curiosity, planning, or other enjoyable activities that build resources [16].

Spirituality

Spirituality and health have been linked within most cultures for centuries [17], with billions of people considering religious practices and spiritual beliefs to be vital components of medical treatment and well-being. Yet, over time a shifting emphasis on science in the practice of modern medicine has led many in the medical community to doubt or reject its potential therapeutic effects [18]. In the early 1990s, however, spirituality returned to the purview of modern medical science after several national and global health organizations, including the Association of American Medical Colleges, the American Medical Association, the American College of Physicians, and the Joint Commission, began calling attention to the role of spirituality in patient care [19]. Since then, there has been a surge of literature published across medical, social, and behavioral sciences that examines and debates the connection between spirituality and mental and physical wellness.

Spirituality is a multidimensional term without a widely accepted definition, although Ken Pargament offers a "non-reductionistic" definition that is a clinically useful construct for translating empirical research conducted by him and his colleague Annett Mahoney [20]. For Pargament and Mahoney, spirituality involves "seeking the sacred," which can be either a theistic or a nontheistic striving. Some consider spirituality to be separate from organized religion, while others do not. The terms spirituality and religion overlap in that they are generally thought to share a common belief in transcendence, or connectedness to something beyond the physical world. Robert Cloninger provides a succinct version of how to nurture transcendence in "Fostering spiritualty and well-being in clinical practice" [21], and more comprehensive research support in *Feeling Good: The Science of Well Being* [22]. Both versions are based on his extensively documented seven-factor model of temperament and character utilizing the temperament and character inventory (TCI) instrument [23]. Religion is typically thought to involve dogma and traditional practices centered around a god, while modern spirituality is a broad concept thought to encompass a person's journey toward and connection with a higher power and ultimately influences one's deepest values and the meanings by which they live.

According to a 2016 Gallup Poll of 1025 adults in the USA, 89 percent believe in God or a universal spirit, and 75 percent consider religion of considerable importance [24]. In the face of illness or medical crisis, many patients look to spirituality and religion for strength and solace. Spirituality allows humans to feel connected to a higher entity, or sources of power and peace. Finding harmony with the universe, with oneself, and with others is also considered to be an important component of spiritual wellness. Individuals seek spiritual wellness through engagement in a variety of activities consistent with their spiritual or religious values. The process of seeking spiritual wellness can involve practices such as exercising faith and optimism; practicing prayer, meditation, or self-reflection; and expressing compassion, gratitude, and forgiveness.

Many studies support the idea of spirituality as a distinctive resource that can be drawn on to facilitate health and well-being [25]. In 2001, Koenig et al. published the *Handbook of Religion and Health*, which reviewed over 1200 studies investigating the relationship between religion and various indicators of health [26]. This comprehensive review of research published between 1900 and 2000 noted that most studies had observed a positive association between religion and physical and mental health. In more recent years, data from a range of disciplines has demonstrated the benefit of spiritual beliefs in supporting health, providing psychological comfort and improving outcomes such as quality of life [27, 28]. Scientific literature from around the world consistently supports a positive link between spirituality/ religiosity and health outcomes, such as diminished mortality, ability to cope with illness, and quality of life [19, 29]. Additionally, religion and spirituality appear to have protective effects for mental health outcomes such as depression, anxiety, substance abuse, and suicide risk [30].

Studies indicated that patients tend to rely on their religion more heavily after receiving a serious diagnosis and while coping with major illness [31]. Relying on spirituality or religion may assist with assuaging fear and pain and help patients to overcome feelings of helplessness by instead focusing on hope and determination [26, 32]. In general, spirituality appears to be a useful resource for coping with stress and it may enhance positive cognitions and emotions, giving patients a sense of hope and meaning during difficult life circumstances, and promoting better self-care. However, some studies suggest that negative spiritual or religious beliefs can lead to distress and an increased burden of illness [33, 34].

The notion that spiritual or religious beliefs can have a positive impact on physical health and mortality is common, yet remains controversial. Research conducted on this topic has yielded mixed results, with several studies showing both positive and negative effects of spiritual beliefs on health outcomes [34]. Studies aimed at examining the link between spiritual beliefs and physical health have been criticized for weak study design, and most demonstrated only a weak association, or no association at all [35, 36].

The mechanisms underlying the effects of religiosity or spirituality are not well understood, although there is some evidence to suggest that religious attendance may contribute to well-being by promoting social integration/support and altruism, and discouraging certain unhealthy lifestyle practices [37, 38].

Multiple studies suggest that even though most patients desire spiritual care [17, 39], few receive it. Some potential barriers include physician attitudes regarding the acceptability and importance of engaging patients in spiritual discussion, religious and cultural differences between patients and their practitioners, and a lack of provider training on addressing patients' spiritual needs [40].

More explicit focus on spirituality could improve patient-centered approaches to well-being; thus physicians should inquire about patients' religious and spiritual beliefs and seek to understand what function they serve for a given patient. Taking a spiritual history can often be a powerful intervention in itself [41]. Several assessments tools exist to help physicians approach the topic of spirituality openly and address the spiritual needs of their patients [42].

Clinicians may also need to recognize when a patient's spiritual or religious beliefs are distorted, limiting, and contribute to pathology rather than alleviating it. Providers should understand and respect the role of spiritual leaders, clergy, and cultural healers, and be able to effectively communicate and collaborate with them. By avoiding reductionistic perspectives, clinicians can engage patients with an open perspective allowing a more collaborative, respectful, and productive relationship with diverse individuals and communities [30].

References

1. S Akhtar, J Barlow. Forgiveness therapy for the promotion of mental well-being: a systematic review and meta-analysis. *Trauma Violence Abuse* 2016; **19**: 107–122.

2. BL Brush, EM Mcgee, B Cavanagh, M Woodward. Forgiveness. *J Holistic Nurs* 2001; **19**: 27–41.

3. WC Stewart, KE Reynolds, LJ Jones, JA Stewart, LA Nelson. The source and impact of specific parameters that enhance well-being in daily life. 2015. https://inside .fammed.wisc.edu/files/webfm-uploads/doc uments/our-dept/whole-me/Stewart_forgive ness_gratitude_hope_empathy_2015.pdf (accessed May 22, 2019).

4. L Toussaint, M Overvold-Ronningen, A Vincent, et al. Implications of forgiveness enhancement in patients with fibromyalgia and chronic fatigue syndrome. *J Health Care Chaplain* 2009; **16**(3–4): 123–139.

5. DE Davis, MY Ho, BJ Griffin, et al. Forgiving the self and physical and mental health correlates: a meta-analytic review. *J Couns Psychol* 2015; **62**: 329–335.

6. AC Recine. Designing forgiveness interventions: guidance from five meta-analyses. *J Holistic Nurs* 2014; **33**: 161–167.

7. AG Recine, L Recine, T Paldon. How people forgive: a systematic review of nurse-authored qualitative research. *J Holistic Nurs* 2019. DOI:10.1177/ 0898010119828080.

8. JW Berry, EL Worthington, LE O'Connor, L Parrott, NG Wade. Forgivingness, vengeful rumination, and affective traits. *J Pers* 2005; **73**: 183–225.

9. JC Karremans, HT van Schie, I van Dongen, et al. Is mindfulness associated with interpersonal forgiveness? *Emotion* 2019. DOI:10.1037/emo0000552.

10. D Li, W Zhang, X Li, N Li, B Ye. Gratitude and suicidal ideation and suicide attempts among Chinese adolescents: direct, mediated, and moderated effects. *J Adolesc* 2011; **35**: 55–66.

11. AM Wood, JJ Froh, AWA Geraghty. Gratitude and well-being: a review and theoretical integration. *Clin Psychol Rev* 2010; **7**: 890–905.

12. AM Wood, J Maltby, N Stewart, PA Linley, S Joseph. A social-cognitive model of trait and state levels of gratitude. *Emotion* 2008; **8**: 281–290.

13. American Psychological Association. PsycNET [database]. https://psycnet .apa.org/record/2014-57426-007 (accessed May 23, 2019).

14. LD Kaczmarek, TB Kashdan, D Drążkowski, et al. Why do people prefer gratitude journaling over gratitude letters? The influence of individual differences in motivation and personality on web-based interventions. *Pers Individ Differ* 2015; **75**: 1–6.

15. WR Miller, S Rollnick. *Motivational Interviewing: Preparing People for Change* (2nd ed.). New York, Guilford Press; 2002.

16. D Watson, K Naragon-Gainey. On the specificity of positive emotional dysfunction in psychopathology: evidence from the mood and anxiety disorders and schizophrenia/schizotypy. *Clin Psychol Rev* 2010; **7**: 839–848.

17. TB Kashdan, J Rottenberg. Psychological flexibility as a fundamental aspect of health. *Clin Psychol Rev* 2010; **30**: 865–878.

18. H Koenig, D King, V Carson. *Handbook of Religion and Health* (2nd ed.). New York, Oxford University Press; 2012.

19. C Puchalski, R Vitillo, S Hull, N Reller. Improving the spiritual dimension of

whole person care: reaching national and international consensus. *J Palliat Med* 2014; **17**(6): 642–656.

20. KI Pargament. *APA Handbook of Psychology, Religion, and Spirituality, Content, Theory, and Research.* Washington, DC, American Psychological Association; 2013.

21. CR Cloninger. Fostering spirituality and well-being in clinical practice. *Psychiatr Ann* 2006; **36**(3). DOI:10.3928/00485713-20060301-07.

22. CR Cloninger. *Feeling Good: The Science of Well-Being.* Oxford, Oxford University Press; 2004.

23. CR Cloninger, KM Cloninger. Person-centered therapeutics. *Int J Pers Cent Med* 2011; **1**: 43–52.

24. Gallup. Religion. 2019. www.gallup.com/poll/1690/religion.aspx (accessed June 26, 2019).

25. KI Pargament, A Mahoney, EP Shafranske. *APA Handbook of Psychology, Religion, and Spirituality*, vol. 2. Washington, DC, American Psychological Association; 2013.

26. HG Koenig, ME McCullough, DB Larson. *Handbook of Religion and Health.* New York, Oxford University Press; 2001.

27. T Gall, C Charbonneau, N Clarke, et al. Understanding the nature and role of spirituality in relation to coping and health: a conceptual framework. *Can Psychol* 2005; **46**: 88–104.

28. R Panzini, B Mosqueiro, R Zimpel, et al. Quality-of-life and spirituality. *Int Rev Psychiatr* 2017;**29**: 263–282.

29. V Counted, A Possamai, T Meade. Relational spirituality and quality of life 2007 to 2017: an integrative research review. *Health Qual Life Outcomes* 2018; **16**: 75.

30. H Koenig. Research on religion, spirituality, and mental health: a review. *Can J Psychiatr* 2009; **54**: 283–291.

31. G Ironson, R Stuetzle, MA Fletcher. An increase in religiousness/spirituality occurs after HIV diagnosis and predicts slower disease progression over 4 years in people with HIV. *J Gen Intern Med* 2006; **21** (Suppl. 5): S62–S68.

32. HG Koenig, DB Larson, SS Larson. Religion and coping with serious medical illness. *Ann Pharmacother* 2001; **35**: 352–359.

33. KI Pargament, HG Koenig, N Tarakeshwar, J Hahn. Religious coping methods as predictors of psychological, physical and spiritual outcomes among medically ill elderly patients: a two-year longitudinal study. *J Health Psychol* 2004; **9**: 713–730.

34. KI Pargament, BW Smith, HG Koenig, L Perez. Patterns of positive and negative religious coping with major life stressors. *J Sci Study Relig* 1998; **37**: 710.

35. F Kier, D Davenport. Unaddressed problems in the study of spirituality and health. *Am Psychologist* 2004; **59**(1): 53–54.

36. RP Sloan, E Bagiella, T Powell. Religion, spirituality, and medicine. *Lancet* 1999; **9153**: 664–667.

37. ME Mccullough, WT Hoyt, DB Larson, HG Koenig, C Thoresen. Religious involvement and mortality: a meta-analytic review. *Health Psychol* 2000; **19**(3): 211–222.

38. S Li, M Stampfer, D Williams, T VanderWeele. Association of religious service attendance with mortality among women. *JAMA Int Med* 2016; **176**: 777.

39. M Balboni, A Sullivan, A Amobi, et al. Why is spiritual care infrequent at the end of life? Spiritual care perceptions among patients, nurses, and physicians and the role of training. *J Clin Oncol* 2013; **31**: 461–467.

40. F Curlin, M Chin, S Sellergren, C Roach, J Lantos. The association of physicians' religious characteristics with their attitudes and self-reported behaviors regarding religion and spirituality in the clinical encounter. *Med Care* 2006; **44**: 446–453.

41. P Kinnersley, N Stott, TJ Peters, I Harvey. The patient-centeredness of consultations and outcome in primary care. *Br J Gen Pract* 1999; **49**: 711–716.

42. DD Kincheloe, LMS Welden, A White. A spiritual care toolkit: an evidence-based solution to meet spiritual needs. *J Clin Nurs* 2018; **27**: 1612–1620.

Positive Neuropsychology, Cognitive Rehabilitation, and Neuroenhancement

Patricia A. Pimental, John B. O'Hara, Jennifer M. Christopher, and Anna M. Ciampanelli

Introduction

The mind and body are connected in a myriad of ways that we as healthcare providers still do not fully comprehend. Recent research has demonstrated that there are biological, neurocognitive, psychological, spiritual, and social features of diseases and disorders, and there has been movement within the healthcare field toward the integrative biopsychosocial approach in the provision of healthcare services. Addressing these aspects allows the healthcare provider to tailor treatment to a patient's unique needs. This chapter covers interventions in the areas of positive neuropsychology/cognitive health, cognitive rehabilitation, and neuroenhancement.

Positive Neuropsychology and Cognitive Health

Pimental [1] discussed trending and future directions involving the integration of positive psychology, or psychology focused on positive behaviors such as gratitude, authenticity, and hopefulness, with neuropsychology and cognitive health. Positive neuropsychology, described by Randolph [2] as "A practice and academic orientation focused on the study and promotion of cognitive health," has been a popular topic within neuropsychological research in recent years. Pimental et al. [3] discussed some advantages of embracing positive neuropsychology, including "decentralizing the historical focus on deficits, disorders, and diagnoses, and optimizing peak performance, anti-aging, and longevity-based practices throughout the lifespan." In acknowledgment of this, Pimental et al. [3] described a paradigm shift in brain-based treatments and rehabilitation programs which could impact the world economy and refocus global attention on cognitive health throughout the life span. Pimental et al. [3] proposed a novel cognitive wellness and cognitive health service delivery model entitled BRAIN SMART^{SM} (see Figure 30.1).

Brain-Stimulating Activities

Promotion of cognitively stimulating activities, such as doing crossword puzzles and listening to music, has been associated with improved brain health and prevention of neurocognitive disorders such as dementia [4, 5]. Neurofeedback, such as audiovisual entrainment (AVE), has also demonstrated utility as an intervention that improves cognitive health through promotion of dendritic growth, altered cerebral blood flow, and normalized EEG activity [6]. Elderly adults between the ages of 53 and 87 who received

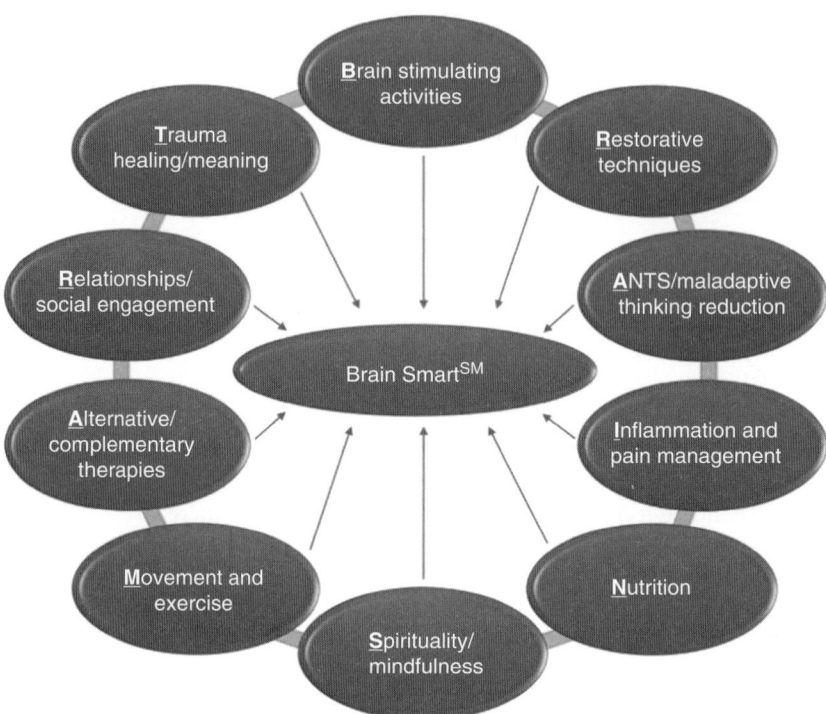

Figure 30.1 Brain Smart^{SM} infographic. ANTS, automatic negative thoughts.

three-weekly AVE sessions over four months demonstrated improvement on tests of neurocognitive ability and memory [7].

Restorative Techniques

There are several psychotherapeutic techniques that can promote optimal physiological functioning. Insufficient sleep or poor sleep quality has been associated with executive dysfunction, including attentional disturbance and deficits in processing speed [8]. Cognitive-behavioral therapy for insomnia (CBT-i) is a psychotherapeutic intervention geared toward restructuring of dysfunctional thoughts and beliefs pertaining to sleep. This intervention has demonstrated effectiveness in reduction of insomnia symptomatology and can be used in conjunction with pharmacologic treatments [9].

Lowered heart rate variability (HRV), which refers to varying beat-to-beat intervals against breathing rhythm, is correlated with autonomous nervous system dysfunction, physical disorders (e.g., diabetes, sleep disturbance), and emotional disturbances, and serves as a biomarker for generalized stress [10]. Physical activity, mindfulness exercises, and HRV biofeedback have all demonstrated utility in reducing stress and depressive symptoms, while improving sleep quality [11].

Automatic Negative Thoughts and Maladaptive Thinking Reduction

Maladaptive behaviors can negatively impact health status [12]. Cognitive-behavioral therapy (CBT) demonstrates effectiveness in promoting behavioral change through identification and change of maladaptive thinking patterns. Specific techniques include development of problem-solving skills, coping skills psychoeducation and practice, cognitive restructuring, stress-inoculation, and positive imagery [13].

Inflammation and Pain Management

Chronic inflammation has been identified as a contributor to several physiological maladies, with some researchers claiming that this generates free radicals and lipid peroxidation products, and can affect neurons, glial cells, the blood–brain barrier, and blood vessels supplying both nutrients and oxygen [14]. Some researchers have gone so far as to claim that inflammation may contribute to certain neurodegenerative disorders such as Alzheimer's disease, Parkinson's disease, Huntington disease, amyotrophic lateral sclerosis (ALS), and centrally sensitized pain.

Transcutaneous electrical nerve stimulation (TENS) consists of a device that is a noninvasive, non-pharmacological method of pain management and segmental pain control based on neuromodulation techniques that were proposed by Melzac and Wall in their gate control theory of pain [15, 16]. The TENS unit delivers low-voltage electrical pulses across the skin and along nerve pathways, delivering direct electrical stimulation to the area of pain, resulting in an analgesic effect. High-frequency stimulation is delivered to the skin via electrodes, which then activate afferent fibers within the spinal cord. This stimulation intercepts and inhibits nociceptive neurons located within the dorsal horn of the spinal cord [17].

In a study that addressed the effectiveness of transcutaneous electrical nerve stimulation as a non-pharmacological treatment for hyperalgesia and pain, DeSantana et al. [18] pointed out that both clinical trials and basic science research are continuing to support the use of TENS with sufficient intensity and duration for efficacious pain relief.

Nutrition and Diet

Recent research suggests that diet plays a central role in healthy cognitive aging. The Finnish Geriatric Intervention Study to Prevent Cognitive Impairment and Disability (FINGER) was a comprehensive whole-health program designed to determine how successful management of metabolic and vascular risk factors would improve cognitive abilities, specifically executive functions, in a geriatric patient population [19]. This program included dietary interventions, monitoring of cardiovascular risks, cognitive training, and social engagement. Participants adhered to a Mediterranean-style diet, received vitamin D supplementation, and restricted sugar, salt, and alcohol intake. Research suggests that the Mediterranean diet can be neuroprotective, reducing risk of neurodegenerative disorders [20]. The Mediterranean-DASH Intervention for Neurodegenerative Delay (MIND) diet [21] integrates the Mediterranean and DASH (Dietary Approaches to Stop Hypertension) diets. The MIND diet was developed around foods that could possibly inhibit beta amyloid, a widely researched Alzheimer's disease biomarker. Research suggests that the MIND diet may contribute to improvement on memory tasks and processing speed, as well as slowing of neurodegenerative disease processes.

Burgeoning interest in the human microbiome has led to a great deal of research in this domain in the past few years. Various neurocognitive and psychological disorders have been associated with dysfunctional immune regulation in humans [22]. Changes in human microbiota can have a direct impact on neurotransmitter (e.g., serotonin) production [23]. Probiotic supplements can also moderate cognitive and affective functions [24].

Spirituality and Mindfulness

Mindfulness exercises have been widely studied from many vantage points, including their utility in psychological interventions and their neurocognitive mechanisms of action. Mindfulness has been described as attending to the present moment in a purposeful, non-judgmental, and non-reactive manner [25]. Several studies have identified that mindfulness/meditation exercises can enhance neuroplasticity, an important neuro-modulation factor in several neural structures [26].

Movement and Exercise

The cognitive benefits of aerobic exercise have been well documented in the scientific research literature. Early research revealed that aerobic exercise could improve cerebrovascular network efficiency [27]. More recently, analysis of MRI data suggests exercise promotes angiogenesis and neurogenesis in the hippocampal formations [28]. Interestingly, improvements in executive functions can be seen in persons who engage in aerobic exercise, regardless of their level of physical fitness [29].

Alternative and Complementary Therapies

Biofeedback is a therapeutic intervention that is aimed at helping a patient develop a greater sense of control over physiological processes; this is accomplished via the manipulation of visually and aurally presented signals that serve to make an individual more cognizant of internal physiological processes previously thought to be outside of one's voluntary control [30]. Biofeedback can be easily integrated with many other psychological interventions, and demonstrates effectiveness with many different biopsychosocial disorders [31].

Relationships and Social Engagement

Early life experiences that are lacking in emotional support, accompanied by a preponderance of negative emotions, can have latent effects on biological aspects of aging, such as shortened telomere length [32]. A healthy social support network can be neuroprotective, so promotion of social engagement is an important recommendation to promote healthy cognitive aging [33]. For patients with more challenging family or social dynamics, psychotherapeutic interventions aimed at forgiveness, grieving/mourning, and relationship restoration can serve to enhance cognitive resilience [34].

Trauma Healing and Meaning

Exposure to repetitive, prolonged severe stressors can result in neurobiological change, notably dysregulation of circuitry connecting the prefrontal cortex and limbic system [35]. A summary by Pimental et al. [3] states that:

> Eye Movement Desensitization and Reprocessing (EMDR), is an evidence-based method that integrates components of the adaptive information processing model (AIP), affective neuroscience, attachment theory, interpersonal neurobiology, polyvagal theory, and structural dissociation theory [36, 37]. The primary objective of EMDR is to positively assimilate and integrate cognitive, affective, and somatic information. The subcortical areas of the brain contain inherent raw emotion circuits that are shaped by an individual's experiences.

Repeated arousal states such as terror and fear may become more readily activated to the point that they become characteristic traits of the individual [36]. It has been suggested by some researchers that the use of EMDR may influence the brain by promoting the stimulation and retraining of the ventral vagal branch of the ANS . . . [35, 36].

Gupta and Gupta [38] described other uses for EMDR, including dermatologic disorders influenced by stress, but more data is needed to substantiate these claims.

Cognitive Rehabilitation

According to Haskins et al., the main goal of cognitive rehabilitation is "to improve injury-related deficits in order to maximize safety, daily functioning, independence, and quality of life" [39]. Patients gradually improve as they strive toward a number of long-term goals, including problem orientation, awareness, goal-setting, compensation, internalization (i.e., automatizing practiced strategies), and generalization of skills.

Cognitive rehabilitation interventions are classified as restorative or compensatory [40]. Restorative treatments aim to strengthen patients' impaired functioning by means of intensively and continuously practicing a cognitive process. During this type of treatment, the level of difficulty increases as the patient demonstrates improved performance. If patients exhibit residual deficits that impact their ability to perform activities of daily living, compensatory treatments are utilized. "Bottom-up" interventions focus on restoring abilities through repetition of a basic skill; in contrast, "top-down" interventions focus on more complex tasks and require self-monitoring and self-regulating [41].

Interventions can also be classified as contextualized or decontextualized [40]. Decontextualized approaches often follow a standardized format targeting a specific cognitive process (e.g., a computer program targeted at treating attentional deficits that requires a patient to press a certain key when presented with a cue). Contextualized treatments focus on improving cognitive impairment during specific activities and skills (e.g., noticing attentional deficits while driving).

Additionally, treatment can be considered modular or comprehensive (Figures 30.2 and 30.3) [40]. Modular treatment focuses on treating impairment in one cognitive domain. For example, if a patient sustains a focal brain injury resulting in notable impairment in a specific cognitive domain (e.g., memory), a modular model of treatment (Figure 30.2) focused solely on improving that specific domain (e.g., memory) would be implemented. In contrast, a comprehensive approach (Figure 30.3) targets the impaired cognitive domain and other psychosocial deficits associated with brain injury.

Cicerone described three main approaches to cognitive rehabilitation: process-specific training, functional skills training, and metacognitive training [42]. Process-specific, or skill-specific, training includes specific interventions that home in on cognitive domains. This approach presumes that through repetitively engaging in a cognitive retraining exercise, reorganization of higher neurological and cognitive processes occurs. This model also assumes that training the specific cognitive domain will improve skills that can be generalized to everyday tasks. Functional skills training aims to address domain-specific, context-specific areas by focusing on the activities that the patient is unable to accomplish rather than the independent cognitive skill. This approach does not anticipate that skills will be generalized to situations. Metacognitive training focuses on the patient's subjective knowledge and awareness of deficits. This approach aims to train patients to

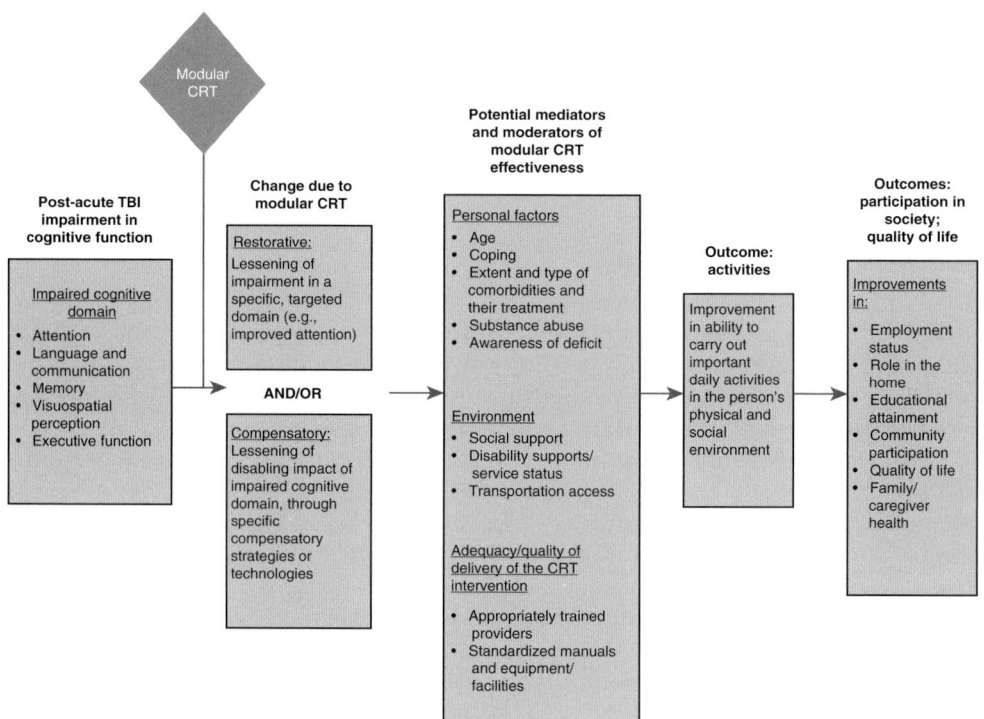

Figure 30.2 Model for modular CRT (reprinted with permission from Committee on Cognitive Rehabilitation Therapy for Traumatic Brain Injury. Defining cognitive rehabilitation therapy. In: R Koehler, EE Wilhelm, I Shoulson, eds., *Cognitive Rehabilitation Therapy for Traumatic Brain Injury: Evaluating the Evidence*. Washington, DC, National Academies Press; 2011).

identify deficits, self-monitor symptoms, and recognize when a compensatory strategy is warranted.

Remediation interventions may include cognitive and perceptual tabletop activities, parquetry blocks, specialized computer software programs, cancellation tasks, block designs, pegboard design copying, puzzles, sequencing cards, gesture imitation, picture matching, and design copying [43]. Compensatory interventions may include meal preparation, dressing, creating a shopping list, or balancing a checkbook. Other environmental adaptions may be made as well, such as placing all grooming items on one side of the bathroom for a person with a neglect, or setting an alarm as a medication reminder for individuals with memory impairment. External strategies might include the use of notebooks, planners, electronic devices, computerized systems, and auditory or visual cueing (e.g., calendars, cue cards). Internal strategies include the use of an image, word, or action sequence to help patients address their problem [39].

Research has elucidated the effectiveness of cognitive rehabilitation therapy in enhancing functioning and increasing independence in patients who have sustained cognitive impairments secondary to brain damage or disease [44]. Cicerone et al. conducted a systematic review of the literature examining a total of 370 cognitive rehabilitation interventions for patients who sustained traumatic brain injuries (TBIs) and cerebrovascular accidents (CVAs). The researchers established recommended *Practice Standards*,

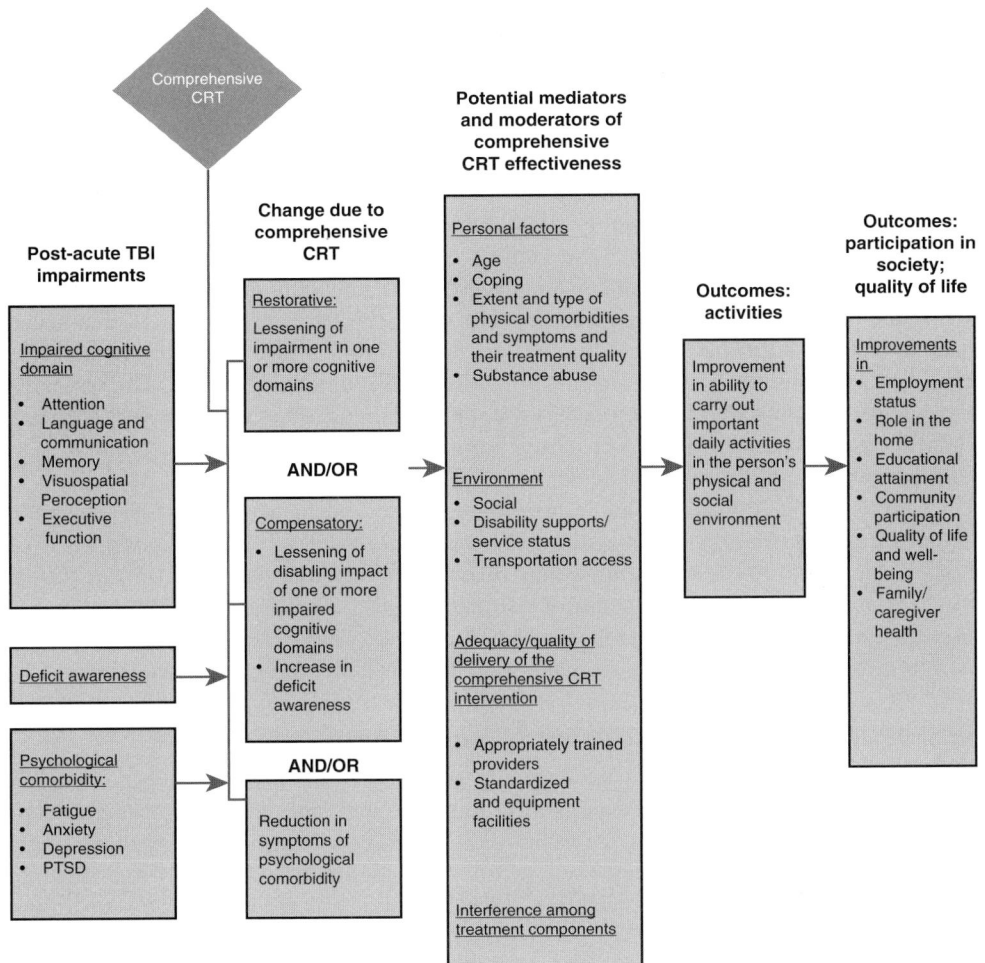

Figure 30.3 Model for multimodal/comprehensive CRT (reprinted with permission from Committee on Cognitive Rehabilitation Therapy for Traumatic Brain Injury. Defining cognitive rehabilitation therapy. In: R Koehler, EE Wilhelm, I Shoulson, eds., *Cognitive Rehabilitation Therapy for Traumatic Brain Injury: Evaluating the Evidence.* Washington, DC, National Academies Press; 2011)

Practice Guidelines, and *Practice Options* (classified based on the strength of the research) for each cognitive domain (i.e., attention, executive functioning, visuospatial functioning, language and communication, and memory).

Cicerone et al. emphasized the importance of direct attention training and metacognitive training to help patients learn compensatory strategies and to promote generalization in everyday tasks (*Practice Standard*) [44].

Cicerone et al. also recommended metacognitive strategy training as a *Practice Standard* to address executive functioning deficits [44]. A *Practice Guideline* indicated the benefits of learning formal problem-solving strategies to aid in functional activities and everyday situations.

Cicerone et al. recommended that visual scanning training be used as a treatment modality for left visual neglect following a right hemisphere CVA (*Practice Standard*) [44]. Another *Practice Standard* recommended the use of gestural or strategy training to address apraxia during acute rehabilitation secondary to a left hemisphere CVA. The researchers also provided a *Practice Guideline* that discouraged the use of microcomputer exercises aimed at improving a left neglect following a CVA, as this treatment method was found to be ineffective.

Cicerone et al. discussed two *Practice Standards* for remediation of language and communication challenges [44]. One standard recommended that cognitive-linguistic therapies be utilized as treatment for language deficits following a left hemisphere CVA during the acute and the post-acute stages. The other standard recommended that social communication skill deficits (including pragmatic communication) secondary to a TBI be addressed with specific interventions for functional communication deficits. The researchers indicated that cognitive interventions for specific language impairments (e.g., reading comprehension) be employed when a patient experiences a language deficit secondary to left hemisphere damage (*Practice Guideline*).

Cicerone et al. indicated that to remediate memory deficits in patients with mild memory impairments associated with a TBI, memory strategy training should be used (*Practice Standard*) [44]. This training may incorporate internalized strategies (e.g., visual imagery) and externalized compensatory strategies (e.g., memory journals). A *Practice Guideline* recommended for patients who have sustained severe memory deficits includes the use of external compensatory strategies that directly address functional activities.

Neuroenhancement/Cognitive Enhancement

Cognitive status can be enhanced through therapeutic interventions and emerging biomedical technology. Specifically, cognitive enhancement and neuroenhancement techniques can be used for all patients, regardless of health status. Cognitive enhancement refers to external tool-based technology used to improve cognition [45]. Tools may include pharmaceutical drugs and non-pharmacological cognitive enhancers (NPCEs), including nutrition, exercise, music, and yoga. Neuroenhancement uses neuroscience-based techniques to directly alter functional circuitry in the brain, which may contribute to improved performance on cognitive tasks.

Brain Stimulation

Neuroenhancement methods involve electromagnetic brain stimulation to relieve neurological and psychiatric symptoms [46]. Brain-stimulating technologies can be used to alleviate pain and improve cognitive processes while reducing drug toxicity and cost of treatment. Transcranial direct current stimulation (tDCS) is a noninvasive technique that targets brain areas and underlying mechanisms associated with perceptual, motor, and cognitive functioning [47]. This technique has been used in many clinical populations, including those with mild cognitive impairments, Alzheimer's disease, depression, and CVA. A hypothesized mechanism of action is that tDCS increases metabolic activity, which enhances learning, perception, and memory [46]. After receiving tDCS, participants engaged in learning through a visual search task, and there was an increase in performance accuracy and signal detection [48]. Overall, this technique contributed to improvements in sustained attention and allowed participants to maintain goal-directed behavior.

Transcranial magnetic stimulation (TMS) is another intervention that alters cortical excitability; when the pulse frequency is altered, there is an increase in excitability. Transcranial magnetic stimulation produces performance enhancement in perceptual discrimination, visual search tasks, motor learning, attention, memory, and language [49]. The mechanism is suggested to directly stimulate the cortical region or associated networks and influence specific cognitive functions. After a month of TMS, sequencing performance was significantly increased, displaying long-term or slow motor learning.

Comparisons between these methods suggest that tDCS influences a larger region of the cortex, involves fewer physiological effects (e.g., muscle twitches or auditory phenomena), and is easier to administer. However, research suggests that there may be additional benefits if both treatments are used in tandem [47].

An alternative neuroenhancement technique to tDCS is transcranial cerebellar direct current stimulation (tcDCS) [50]. This technique is commonly used for normal and pathological conditions with cerebellar dysfunction through the process of delivering direct current through surface electrodes over the cerebellum. This technique enhanced motor control, affect, learning, and working memory [46]. Also, tcDCS influenced cerebellar brain interactions induced by TMS, showing that therapies can be combined and result in reduced cerebellar dysfunction, improved psychiatric conditions, and enhanced neurorehabilitation [50].

Physical Exercise

Physical exercise, as a non-pharmacological neuroenhancement technique, is relatively safe, routine, and culturally accepted. Research suggests that after a week of physical exercise, improvements can be seen in mood and cognition [51]. Furthermore, aerobic exercise was associated with improvements in cognitively healthy adults in the domains of attention, memory, processing speed, and executive functioning. The intensity or duration of exercise did not appear to mediate the effects of neurocognitive improvements. With physical exercise, individuals with mild cognitive impairments displayed greater improvements in memory compared to cognitively healthy adults. For those diagnosed with probable Alzheimer's disease and/or Parkinson's disease, exercise can be used as a preventive measure and assist with improving gait, balance, mobility, and muscle power. Exercise also has long-term benefits and protective factors. Physical activity has been associated with neurobiological changes to the prefrontal and medial temporal areas of the brain, as well as increased hippocampal blood flow.

Individuals between the ages of 35 and 40 who engaged in exercise displayed faster response times and benefited in planning and execution of responses. There was also less hyperactivity in the prefrontal cortex, indicating that exercise could counteract overactivity [52].

Meditation and Yoga

Meditation has been associated with enhancements in attention and cognitive flexibility. Meditation is a non-physical activity that focuses on mental relaxation, attention to breathing, and one's own thoughts [53]. Several different meditation techniques have been associated with improvements in attention, processing speed, memory, and executive functioning in younger, middle-aged, and older adults. Research suggests that meditation can be used to offset age-related cognitive decline.

Meditation can reduce anxiety symptoms, similar to relaxation therapy and mindfulness interventions [54]. Neuroimaging data suggest that adults who regularly meditate display:

(1) thicker prefrontal cortices; (2) increased functional activity in the prefrontal cortices; (3) increased thickness of the right anterior insula; and (4) increased gray matter density in the left hippocampus, posterior cingulate cortex, and temporoparietal junction. An apparent benefit of meditation is increased cortical thickness in the sensory and spatial processing areas of the parietal lobe, which can lead to enhanced self-awareness [55].

Yoga is a combination of meditation, breathing techniques, and body postures, and has been associated with several health benefits. Older adults who practiced yoga demonstrated improved performance, relative to their non-yoga-practicing peers, on tasks measuring processing speed, sustained attention, and working memory [56]. In addition to the cognitive benefits, older adults who practiced yoga also demonstrated enhanced physical mobility [57] and a decrease in inflammatory processes [58].

Yoga has also been associated with reduction of various psychological symptoms. Older adults who practiced yoga in addition to treatment as usual reported a reduction of depressive symptoms [57]. Yoga may also be helpful in reducing symptoms of anxiety [59]. There are many hypotheses as to the mechanisms involved that may contribute to anxiety symptom reduction. One hypothesis stated that 60 minutes of yoga practice may contribute to an increase of GABA, an inhibitory neurotransmitter, that helps to decrease feelings of anxiety. Another hypothesis stated that brain-derived neurotrophic factor, which promotes development, survival, and plasticity of neurons in the nervous system, may contribute to a decrease in both depression and anxiety. However, more data is needed to substantiate these claims. Taken together, meditation and yoga practices are safe, effective, and inexpensive compared to other therapies [58].

Music

Music is an alternative method used to enhance cognition [45]. Music therapy is important for neuropsychological, cognitive, and social improvements in dementia. It is an ideal intervention due to the absence of side effects, convenience, and cost-effectiveness. The techniques can be modified to fit patients' needs, which can include listening to music, music-based intervention (i.e., music therapy), background music, multisensory stimulation, singing songs, and music with activities [60]. Music therapy can be divided into categories of receptive music, which includes listening to music in different formats, and active music, which consists of being actively involved in making music [45]. Receptive music has been associated with significant improvements in spatiotemporal tasks. Music therapy can help with reducing social isolation and may also improve one's emotional range [45]. Researchers hypothesize that music therapy may promote the release of endorphins, dopamine, nitric oxide, and endocannabinoids. The involvement of these neurotransmitters suggests that music may play a role in the reward, stress, arousal, and social affiliation systems [61].

Conclusion

In conclusion, advancements in positive neuropsychology and cognitive wellness have revealed several behavioral and health interventions that show great promise in helping to promote longevity and healthy cognitive aging. Several of these multimodal interventions are cost-effective and easily implemented in clinical settings, which may help to improve access to care in areas with greater healthcare disparity. Increased availability of these interventions may help to reduce systemic barriers to lifelong wellness and cognitive health.

References

1. PA Pimental. The brave new world of positive neuropsychology. *Appl Neuropsychol Adult* 2017; **24**(2): 99.

2. JJ Randolph. Positive neuropsychology: a framework for cognitive health. *NAN Bull* 2015; **29**(2): 25–26.

3. PA Pimental, JB O'Hara, J Jandak. Neuropsychologists as primary care providers of cognitive health: a novel comprehensive cognitive wellness service delivery model. *Appl Neuropsychol Adult* 2018; **25**(4): 318–326.

4. JA Pillai, CB Hall, DW Dickson, et al. Association of crossword puzzle participation with memory decline in persons who develop dementia. *J Int Neuropsychol Soc* 2011; **17**(6): 1006–1013.

5. GM Bidelman, C Alain. Musical training orchestrates coordinated neuroplasticity in auditory brainstem and cortex to counteract age-related declines in categorical vowel perception. *J Neurosci* 2015; **35**(3): 1240–1249.

6. D Siever. Audio-visual entrainment: History and physiological mechanisms. *Biofeedback* 2003; **31**(2): 21–27.

7. T Budzynski, HK Budzynski, HY Tang. Brain brightening: restoring the aging mind. In: JR Evans, ed., *Handbook of Neurofeedback: Dynamics and Clinical Applications.* New York, Haworth Medical Press; 2007.

8. F Waters, RS Bucks. Neuropsychological effects of sleep loss: implications for neuropsychologists. *J Int Neuropsychol Soc* 2011, **17**(4): 571–586.

9. MI Perlis, M Sharpe, MT Smith D Greenblatt, D Giles. Behavioral treatment of insomnia: treatment outcome and the relevance of medical and psychiatric morbidity. *J Behav Med* 2011; **24**(3): 281–296.

10. S Evans, LC Seidman, JC Tsao, et al. Heart rate variability as a biomarker for autonomic nervous system response differences between children with chronic pain and healthy control children. *J Pain Res* 2013; **6**: 449–457.

11. JE van de Zwan, W de Vente, AC Huizink, SM Bogels, E deBruin. Physical activity, mindfulness meditation, or heart rate variability biofeedback for stress reduction: a randomized control trial. *Appl Psychophysiol Biofeedback* 2015; **40**(4): 257–268.

12. M Ring. Integrative approaches to fibromyalgia. *Pain Practitioner* 2017; **27**(1): 13–15.

13. CD Belar, WW Deardorff. *Clinical Health Psychology in Medical Settings: A Practitioner's Guidebook* (2nd ed.). Washington, DC, American Psychological Association; 2009.

14. RL Blaylock. Food additive excitotoxins and degenerative brain disorders. *Med Sentinel* 1999; **4**(6): 212–215.

15. P Pimental. The psychology of pain: diagnosis, treatment and multidisciplinary management with a focus on musculoskeletal factors. In: C Schwab, ed., *Musculoskeletal Pain.* Philadelphia, PA, Hanley & Belfus; 1991.

16. R Veyilmuthu S Govindan, M Venugopalan, S Panicker. Effect of transcutaneous electrical nerve stimulation on labour pain relief among primigravida and multigravida mothers. *Int J Reprod Contracep Obstet Gynecol* 2017; **6**(3): 980–985.

17. AH Astokorki, AR Mauger. Transcutaneous electrical nerve stimulation reduces exercise induced perceived pain and improves endurance exercise performance. *Eur J Appl Psychol* 2016; **117**(3): 483–492.

18. JM DeSantana, DM Walsh, C Vance, BA Rakel, KA Sluka. Effectiveness of transcutaneous electrical nerve stimulation for treatment of hyperalgesia and pain. *Curr Rheumatol Rep* 2008; **10**(6): 492–499.

19. M Kivipelto, A Solomon, S Ahtiluoto, et al. The Finnish geriatric intervention study to prevent cognitive impairment and disability (FINGER): study design and progress. *Alzheimers Dementia* 2013; **9**(6): 657–665.

20. A Sánchez-Villegas, MA Martínez-González, R Estruch, et al. Mediterranean dietary pattern and depression: the PREDIMED randomized trial. *BMC Medicine* 2013; **11**: 1–11.

21. MC Morris, CC Tangney, Y Wang, et al. MIND diet associated with reduced incidence of Alzheimer's disease. *Alzheimers Dementia* 2015; **11**(9): 1007–1014.

22. CA Lowry, DG Smith, PH Siebler, et al. The microbiota, immunoregulation, and mental health: implications for public health. *Curr Environ Health Rep* 2016; **3**(3): 270–286.

23. JM Yano, K Yu, GP Donaldson, et al. Indigenous bacteria from the gut microbiota regulate host serotonin biosynthesis. *Cell* 2015; **161**(2): 264–276.

24. K Tillisch, J Labus, L Kilpatrick, et al. Consumption of fermented milk product with probiotic modulates brain activity. *Gastroenterology* 2013; **144**(7): 1394–1401.

25. NA Farb, ZV Siegel, H Mayberg, et al. Attending to the present: mindfulness meditation reveals distinct neural modes of self-reference. *Soc Cogn Affect Neurosci* 2017; **2**(4): 313–322.

26. KC Fox, ML Dixon, S Nijeboer, M Girn. Functional neuroanatomy of meditation: a review and meta-analysis of 78 functional neuroimaging investigations. *J Neurosci Biobehav Rev* 2016; **65**: 208–228.

27. HL Hawkins, AF Kramer, D Capaldi. Aging, exercise, and attention. *Psychol Aging* 1999; **7**(4): 643–653.

28. AC Pereira, DE Huddleston, AM Brickman, et al. An in vivo correlate of exercise-induced neurogenesis in the adult degenerate gyrus. *PNAS* 2007; **104**(13): 5638–5643.

29. AL Smiley-Oyen, KA Lowry, SJ Francois, ML Kohut, P Ekkekakis. Exercise, fitness, and neurocognitive function in older adults: the "selective improvement" and "cardiovascular fitness" hypothesis. *Ann Behav Med* 2008; **36**(3): 280–291.

30. J Basmajian. *Biofeedback: Principles and Practice for Clinicians.* Baltimore, MD, Williams & Wilkins; 1989.

31. DE Krebs, TL Fagerson. Biofeedback in neuromuscular reeducation and gait training. In: MS Schwartz, F Andrasik *Biofeedback: A Practitioner's Guide.* New York. Guilford Press; 2003.

32. GH Brody, T Yu, I Shalev. Risky family processes prospectively forecast shorter telomere length mediated through negative emotions. *Health Psychol* 2017; **36**(5): 438–444.

33. CM deFrias, RA Dixon. Lifestyle engagement affects cognitive status differences and trajectories on executive functions in older adults. *Arch Clin Neuropsychol* 2014; **29**(1): 16–25.

34. EL Worthington, M Scherer. Forgiveness is an emotion-focused coping strategy that can reduce health risks and promote health resilience: theory, review, and hypothesis. *Psychol Health* 2004; **19**(3): 385–405.

35. JD Bremner. Traumatic stress: effects on the brain. *Dialog Clin Neurosci* 2006; **8**(4): 445–461.

36. AM Gomez. *EMDR Therapy and Adjunct Approaches with Children: Complex Trauma, Attachment and Dissociation.* New York, Springer; 2013.

37. F Shapiro. *Eye Movement Desensitization and Reprocessing (EMDR) Therapy: Basic Principles, Protocols and Procedures* (3rd ed.). New York, Guilford; 2008.

38. MA Gupta, AK Gupta. Use of eye movement desensitization and reprocessing (EMDR) in the treatment of dermatologic disorders. *J Cutan Med Surg* 2002; **6**(5): 415–421.

39. EC Haskins, K Cicerone, K Dams-O'Connor, et al. *Cognitive Rehabilitation Manual: Translating Evidence-Based Recommendations into Practice.* Reston, VA, ACRM Publishing; 2012. https://acrm.org/wp-content/uploads/pdf/COG_Manual_020413_frontSection.pdf (accessed March 1, 2020).

40. Committee on Cognitive Rehabilitation Therapy for Traumatic Brain Injury. Defining cognitive rehabilitation therapy. In: R Koehler, EE Wilhelm, I Shoulson, eds., *Cognitive Rehabilitation Therapy for Traumatic Brain Injury: Evaluating the*

Evidence. Washington, DC, National Academies Press; 2011.

41. C Prince, ME Bruhns. Evaluation and treatment of mild traumatic brain injury: the role of neuropsychology. *Brain Sci* 2017; 7(8): 105.

42. KD Cicerone. Cognitive rehabilitation. In: ND Zasler, DI Katz, RD Zafonte, eds., *Brain Injury Medicine* (2nd ed.). New York, Demos Medical Publishing, LLC; 2013.

43. G Gillen. *Cognitive and Perceptual Rehabilitation: Optimizing Function*. St. Louis, MO, Mosby Elsevier; 2009.

44. KD Cicerone, DM Langenbahn, C Braden, et al. Evidence-based cognitive rehabilitation: updated review of the literature from 2003 through 2008. *Arch Phys Med Rehab* 2011; 92(4): 519–530.

45. A Sachdeva, K Kumar, KS Anand. Non-pharmacological cognitive enhancers: current perspectives. *J Clin Diagn Res* 2015; 9(7): 1–6.

46. VP Clark, R Parasuraman. Neuroenhancement: enhancing brain and mind in health and in disease. *NeuroImage* 2013; 85: 889–894.

47. HL Filmer, PE Dux, JB Mattingley. Applications of transcranial direct current stimulation for understanding brain function. *Trends Neurosci* 2014; 37(12): 742–753.

48. VP Clark, BA Coffman, MC Trumbo, C Gasparovic. Transcranial direct current stimulation (tDCS) produces localized and specific alterations in neurochemistry: a 1h magnetic resonance spectroscopy study. *Neurosci Lett* 2011; 500(1): 67–71.

49. B Luber, SH Lisanby. Enhancement of human cognitive performance using transcranial magnetic stimulation (TMS). *NeuroImage* 2014; 85: 963–972.

50. R Ferrucci, A Priori. Transcranial cerebellar direct current stimulation (tcDCS): motor control, cognition, learning and emotions. *NeuroImage* 2014; 85: 920–925.

51. PJ Smith, JA Blumenthal, BM Hoffman, et al. An aerobic exercise and neurocognitive performance: a meta-analytic review of randomized controlled trials. *Psychosom Med* 2010; 72(3): 239–252.

52. M Berchicci, G Lucci, F DiRusso. Benefits of physical exercise on the aging brain: the role of the prefrontal cortex. *J Gerontol A Biol Sci Med Sci* 2013; 68: 1337–41.

53. T Gard, BK Hölzel, SW Lazar. The potential effects of meditation on age-related cognitive decline: a systematic review. *Ann NY Acad Sci* 2014; 1307: 89–103.

54. T Krisanaprakornkit, W Sriraj, N Piyavhatkul, M Laopaiboon. Meditation therapy for anxiety disorders. *Cochrane Database Syst Rev* 2006; 1: 1–24.

55. L Miller, R Bansal, P Wickramaratne, et al. Neuroanatomical correlates of religiosity and spirituality: a study in adults at high and low familial risk for depression. *JAMA Psychiatr* 2014; 71(2): 128–135.

56. R Prakash, P Rastogi, I Dubey, et al. Long-term concentrative meditation and cognitive performance among older adults. *Neuropsychol Dev Cogn B Aging Neuropsychol Cogn* 2012; 19: 479–494.

57. N Cooper, P Suri, A Litman, DC Morgenroth. The effect of yoga on balance and mobility in populations with balance and mobility impairment: a systematic review with meta-analysis. *Curr Phys Med Rehabil Rep* 2018; 6(1): 1–14.

58. BR Cahn, MS Goodman, CT Peterson, R Maturi, PJ Millis. Yoga, meditation and mind–body health: increased BDNF cortisol awakening response, and altered inflammatory marker expression after 3-month yoga and meditation. *Front Hum Neurosci* 2017; 11: 1–13.

59. H Cramer, R Lauche, J Langhorst, G Dobos. Yoga for depression: a systematic review and meta-analysis. *Depress Anxiety* 2013; 20: 1068–83.

60. R Fang, S Ye, J Huangfu, DP Calimag. Music therapy is a potential intervention for cognition of Alzheimer's disease: a mini-review. *Translational Neurodegeneration* 2017; 6(2): 1–8.

61. ML Chanda, DJ Levitin. The neurochemistry of music. *Trends Cogn Sci* 2013; 17: 179–193.

Acupuncture, Herbs, and Ayurvedic Medicine

Lucy Postolov and Suzanne Gilberg-Lenz

Acupuncture and Chinese Herbs

Introduction

Traditional Chinese medicine (TCM) is a rich medical system dating back 2500 years [1]. The philosophical underpinnings and theoretical framework emphasize the ideology of holism within the human body, and extend to the close relationship between the human body and nature [2]. In the core theorem, balance is needed between the opposite influences on the body – Yin and Yang – to prevent disease and achieve good health [3]. Energy flow, called Qi, streams along 12 different meridians throughout the body, which keeps the Yin and Yang forces balanced. "Yin" represents the concept of cold, slow, and passive, and "Yang" represents energy that is hot, fast, and active [4]. Illness is caused by a disruption or blockage among the forces. Cultivating Yin/Yang harmony within the body and with nature is achieved through two main treatment modalities – herbal and manual treatment [2].

Acupuncture

Acupuncture (Figure 31.1), a commonly used manual TCM treatment modality, is the insertion of very fine needles to puncture the skin and tissue at specific acupoints along meridians to elicit specific therapeutic effects [2]. The discovery of acupuncture was first credited to the Chinese Emperor Huangdi in 2500 BCE [5]. The first document describing an organized system of diagnosis and treatment which was recognized as acupuncture is *The Yellow Emperor's Classic of Internal Medicine*, dating from about 100 BCE [6]. Acupuncture continued to develop over the centuries and gradually became one of the standard therapies used in China, alongside herbal medicine [6]. During the Ming Dynasty (1368–1644), *The Great Compendium of Acupuncture and Moxibustion* was published, which formed the basis of modern acupuncture. Acupuncture was introduced to the USA in the 1970s when a member of President Nixon's press corps received it during recovery from surgery. Over the next several decades, many states legalized the practice of acupuncture and by 1994 Americans made more than nine million visits for acupuncture treatments [5]. With the growth of public interest and utilization of acupuncture, Western scientists set out to mechanistically understand the application of acupuncture and test its effectiveness.

Mechanisms of Action: Traditional Chinese Medicine

The diagnostic process begins with the recognition of patterns based on history and physical examination. The information is organized into specific domains in the body, called "organ systems," with distinct physiologic attributes from Western organs [7]. Overarching

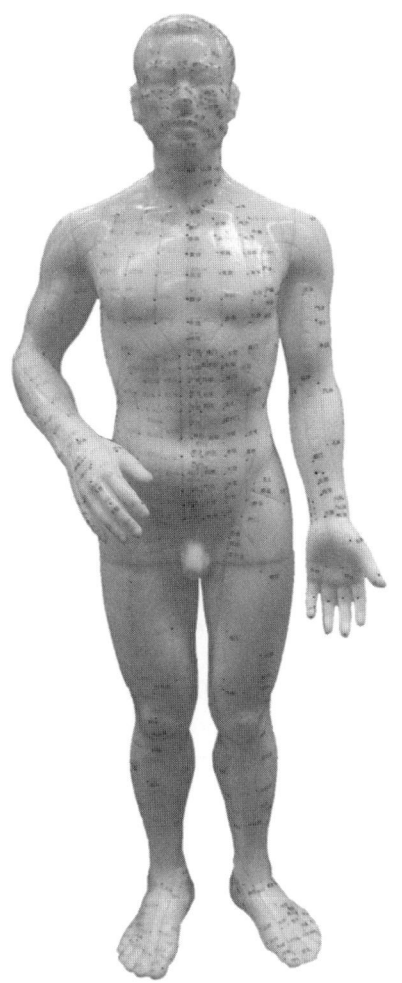

Figure 31.1 Acupuncture points and meridians.

"whole-body" characteristics including Yin/Yang and excess/deficiency are then also integrated in the formation of a standard diagnosis (e.g., deficient Yin of the kidney) caused by an obstruction or deficiency of Qi flow [7]. The insertion of fine needles (equivalent to a 36-gauge hypodermic needle) in acupuncture points located on meridians restores the flow of Qi and thereby health [5]. The depth of the needles and the location of the points depends on the nature of the problem.

Mechanism of Action: Allopathic Medicine

In allopathic medicine, diagnosis consists of signs, symptoms, and physical findings, supported with laboratory tests and diagnostic imaging [7]. The information is classified into physiologic systems and an overarching pathologic process is determined, then treated with lifestyle modification, pharmacologic treatment, or interventions as needed [7]. The anatomic and physiologic properties of acupuncture points and meridians are elusive to those trained in Western medicine [8]. From an anatomical perspective, meridians have been aligned with various neural and inter/intramuscular structures, while physiologically, some acupoint locations coincide with trigger points [8]. Others have postulated that needling results in deformation of connective tissues and alters fibroblasts; the resulting micro-injury causes release of ATP, whose byproducts act as antinociceptive agents to block pain [9]. Furthermore, functional magnetic resonance imaging (fMRI) of the brain has demonstrated specific changes in brain networks through acupoint stimulation, including modulation of the limbic network, an important intrinsic regulatory system of the human brain [10].

Application to Disease States

Chronic Low Back Pain

Chronic low back pain (LBP), defined as pain below the costal margin and above the gluteal folds for more than 12 weeks' duration, is one of the most frequently encountered musculoskeletal disorders [9]. Current treatment guidelines recommend starting with non-pharmacologic interventions, including acupuncture, given associated side effects and variable efficacy of pharmacologic therapy [11]. This recent recommendation was made after many acupuncture trials demonstrated efficacy. In 2002, the World Health Organization (WHO) confirmed the effectiveness of acupuncture for 28 diseases, one of which was LBP [12]. Later, a meta-analysis of 33 randomized controlled trials (RCTs) of acupuncture for LBP showed favorable results compared to controls (including sham) [13]. Likewise, the German Acupuncture Trials (GERAC) demonstrated efficacy in over 1000 patients, with a twofold improvement with acupuncture compared to conventional therapy at six months [14]. Mechanisms explaining its usefulness include local increases in circulation, improvement of myofascial dysfunction, and modulations of pain through antinociceptive effects of micro-injury and ATP/adenosine release [9]. fMRI studies have also shown effects of acupuncture stimulation in basal forebrain (and limbic) areas related to somatosensory and effector functions in relation to pain [10].

Multiple Sclerosis

Acupuncture has demonstrated effectiveness in multiple sclerosis (MS), an autoimmune neurological disease leading to debilitating weakness, pain, and fatigue, although studies are limited in both quantity and quality. In a systematic review of 12 studies, Karpatkin et al. found that acupuncture improved quality of life, energy and fatigue levels, urinary frequency, and pain [15]. In murine models, rats treated with electroacupuncture had lower pathogenic inflammatory cell levels as well as disease activity [15]. Although the number of large trials is low, there are many case reports of acupuncture treatment helping MS symptoms, validating the up to 21 percent usage rate in the MS population [15].

Essential Hypertension

Up to one billion people are affected by essential hypertension. Anti-hypertensive medication for essential hypertension can come with various side effects and safety concerns, such as drug resistance and non-compliance issues [16]. In a meta-analysis of 23 studies, Zhao et al. found that overall the addition of acupuncture to Western medicine yielded favorable results compared to medication alone [16]. In two trials of 170 patients, the combination of acupuncture and Western medicine more effectively decreased blood pressure compared to Western medicine alone, with a difference of 7.5 mmHg in systolic blood pressure and 4.2 mmHg in diastolic blood pressure [16].

Cancer

Acupuncture plays an important adjunctive role for symptom management during cancer treatment. During the 2017 National Cancer Institute's Conference on Acupuncture, it was reported that pain, fatigue, xerostomia, and nausea/vomiting improved with acupuncture treatment [17]. Patients with primary cancer-related pain experienced quicker and more sustained pain relief with acupuncture and pharmacotherapy compared to pharmacotherapy alone [17]. Several randomized acupuncture and electroacupuncture trials have demonstrated sustained pain relief for medication-related side effects, including aromatase inhibitor-associated arthralgias and chemotherapy-related neuropathic pain, in addition to improved functioning [17]. Xerostomia related to head and neck chemoradiation can be prevented and treated with acupuncture, resulting in significant improvement compared to standard of care methods [17]. Finally, patients suffering from fatigue and nausea/vomiting showed improved outcomes when acupuncture was used in combination with standard of care methods [17].

Chinese Herbal Medicine

Chinese herbal medicine uses herbs (including plants, minerals, and animal products) that are combined in a prescription according to Chinese medicine theories [2]. All parts of a plant can be used as each part is thought to have different therapeutic actions. There are approximately 4000 different Chinese herbs in the Chinese Materia Medica, with more than 11,000 prescriptions [2]. The understanding of use of Chinese herbs is extremely nuanced and beyond the scope of this chapter. As a general overview, herbs are categorized based on their actions on the body with flavor and temperature, among other descriptions correlating with Yin and Yang [2]. As in all TCM practices, Chinese herbal treatment is focused on balancing Yin and Yang in disease states. Herbs are thought to enter specific meridians and travel to particular organs where therapeutic action occurs.

Combination herbal therapy prescriptions, also known as formulas, are classified based on origins and are labeled classical, modified, or custom-made. Each formula is composed based on the principle of "chief," "deputy," "assistant," and "envoy." The "chief" herb of a formula is the essential ingredient, added in the largest quantity for the main therapeutic effect. The "deputy" herb has two functions: treat the main disease/symptom and treat the associated or coexisting disease/symptom. The "assistant" herb has three functions: reinforce the effect of the "chief" herb, counteract toxicity, and work with the chief herb to treat complex and serious disorders. The last component, "envoy," has two functions: act as a channel guiding the herb to the affected areas of the body, and harmonize the herbs within the formula. It is important to note that this component is usually applied in small doses.

There are many Chinese herbal formulas that are produced in the USA and Europe, and are tested for safety by an independent third-party laboratory (Figure 31.2).

While not regulated by the FDA, US and European Chinese herbal companies do not condone the use of endangered animals and plants, and advocate for clean products and manufacturing. It is advised that herbs be taken with caution and in moderation. Unfortunately, similar standards are not the norm in China, where some formulas are adulterated with pharmaceuticals that lead to extreme effects and side effects. Chinese

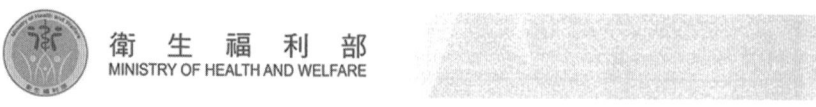

衛 生 福 利 部
MINISTRY OF HEALTH AND WELFARE

CERTIFICATE OF GOOD MANUFACTURING PRACTICE

Issue Date: August 5, 2016

Issued following an inspection in accordance with Article 57 of the Pharmaceutical Affairs Law and relevant Regulations of the Republic of China (Taiwan).

The competent authority of the Republic of China confirms the following:
The manufacturer: TTY Biopharm Company Limited Lioudu Factory
Site address: No.5, Gongjian W. Rd., Qidu District, Keelung, Taiwan, R.O.C.
Manufacturer's licence number: (AP) 0008055

is the manufacturer of medicinal products for human use that has been inspected with the following pharmaceutical dosage forms:
-Sterile products: Lyophilized powder for injection (aseptic preparation), injection (aseptic preparation and terminal sterilization)
-Non-Sterile products:
Solid dosage forms: film coated tablet (tablet), capsule

From the knowledge gained during inspection performed on November 3-4, 2015 and April 25-28, 2016, it is considered that the manufacturer complies with the Pharmaceutical Inspection Convention/Co-operation Scheme Guide to Good Manufacturing Practice (PIC/S GMP) for medicinal products.

This certificate is valid until February 6, 2019.
This certificate may be revoked at anytime as warranted.

Signed by

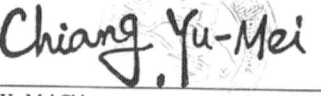

Yu-Mei Chiang
Director-General
Food and Drug Administration
(http://www.fda.gov.tw/TC/index.aspx)

Under the delegated authority of
Tzou-Yien Lin, M.D.
Minister
Ministry of Health and Welfare
Republic of China (Taiwan)

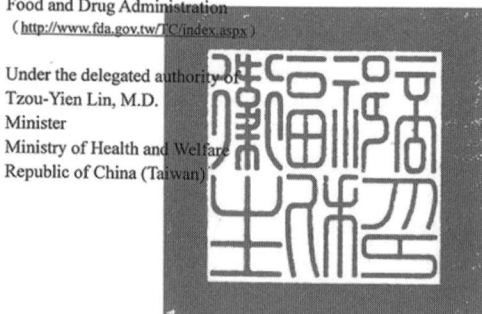

3179

Figure 31.2 Certificate of good manufacturing practice.

herbal therapy supplements are becoming more common, and are being taught at large academic institutions such as Cleveland Clinic, Duke University, University of California, San Francisco, and the Mayo Clinic. Formulae can be prepared as loose herbs, granules, or capsules. The most popular Chinese herbs include: turmeric (Yu Jin), goji berry (Gou Qi Zi), ginseng (Hong Shen), and licorice (Gan Cao).

Turmeric is a cousin root of ginger and is most commonly known for its bright orange color. It is sold in stores as a dried powder, which makes it easy to measure and cook with. It is also known for the beverage "Golden Milk," which acts as a reagent that regulates the liver and relieves patterns of stagnant Qi in relation to pain. In a 2016 systematic review and meta-analysis of RCTs, Daily et al. evaluated the efficacy of turmeric for alleviating symptoms of osteoarthritis [18]. Using two arthritis pain indices, they showed turmeric significantly reduced pain and increased function. When compared to pain medication, it was just as effective but with fewer side effects. They concluded that 1000 mg/day of curcumin was effective for the treatment of osteoarthritis.

The goji berry fruit is a festive red berry usually prepared in a dried form similar to a raisin. The goji berry is a traditional Chinese herb that has been used to prevent chronic diseases and has been found to improve visual, liver, and immune system function [19]. The effect is likely related to betaine, a metabolic product of choline thought to increase methylation, which generally wanes with age [19]. Goji berries also have high levels of antioxidants, including beta-carotene and phenolic compounds. One of the most popular uses of the goji berry is to make goji wine, in which the function of the wine is to be used against aging and aging-related diseases [19].

Licorice is the most prescribed herb in Chinese medicine, and can come in many forms. Licorice has been shown to soothe and relieve stomach pain and act as an anti-inflammatory and anti-arthritic remedy. The active components of licorice – glycyrrhizin and glycyrrhetinic acid – exert anti-inflammatory effects through suppression of COX-2 and its downstream product TxA2. Licorice is thought to both potentiate the therapeutic effects as well as decrease adverse effects of NSAIDS or DMARDs through the COX-2/TxA2 pathway [20].

Ginseng is another widely used herbal remedy in Chinese medicine that has been used for a variety of conditions, including improvement of physical performance, sexual function, diabetes, and hypertension [21]. Ginseng is a slow-growing root that can be classified as fresh, white, or red. In a systematic review of the Korean literature, Choi et al. found support for improved blood flow, improved exercise capacity, and reduced erectile dysfunction. Similarly, in an international systematic review, Lee et al. found benefits for glucose metabolism, psychomotor function, and pulmonary disease [22].

Chinese Herbs and Chemotherapy/Cancer

Chinese herbal medicines can be used to reduce the side effects caused by chemo- and radiotherapy. Both single herb and formula preparations have been found to be effective. Ginseng was found to synergize with standard cancer therapies, boost immune system function, and ameliorate chemo- and radiotherapy toxicity [23]. Likewise, astragalus root has been shown in clinical trials to reduce symptoms, improve quality of life, and delay progression of chemotherapy-induced peripheral neuropathy. A systematic review found that astragalus-containing formulas are effective at protecting against radiation pneumonitis when used during radiotherapy [23]. Many formulas are also effective adjuvants, including Shi-Quan-Da-Bu-Tang, a 10-herb combination used for many years for inflammatory conditions, which was recently found to modulate immune responses and reduce side effects of treatment, including in anorexia [23]. Bu-zhong-yi-qi-tang is a seven-herb formula, and is the top formula prescribed for lung cancer patients. It has been studied for its ability to reduce the incidence of chemotherapy resistance and mucositis, and to improve quality of life and fatigue levels in patients with cancer [23].

Diarrhea, nausea, and vomiting are the most common side effects among patients receiving chemo- or radiotherapy. Liu-jun-zi-tang, a six-herb combination formula used for appetite enhancement, protection against gastric mucosal injury, and improving the gastric accommodation reflex, reduced chemotherapy-associated anorexia and maintained food intake in an RCT evaluating chemotherapy-induced gastrointestinal side effects [23]. Fatigue is another side effect of both cancer and cancer treatment. A systematic review of RCTs including 10 trials and 751 participants found that Chinese herbal medicine plus chemotherapy or supportive care was superior to either alone in improving quality of life related to fatigue [23]. Finally, pain continues to be a difficult-to-treat symptom despite standard of care analgesia, with up to 50 percent of patients reporting undertreated pain. Wen Jing Zhi Tong Fang, a four-herb formula, when combined with the classic analgesic ladder treatment, was effective in relieving cancer-related pain and allowing reduced dosing of analgesic medications, fewer adverse reactions, and improved quality of life [23].

Conclusion

Traditional Chinese medicine, and in particular acupuncture and herbology, are increasing in popularity. Increasing patient use has resulted in trials evaluating efficacy and safety. Limitations of the available trials include sample size and methodology, but with the involvement of groups from major academic centers the shift toward improved quality is underway. While there remain differences in the knowledge of mechanism of action, fostering a common understanding is being motivated by patient interest. When administered by a licensed professional, acupuncture has very minimal risk. Similarly, when herbs are prescribed and monitored by a licensed professional, are known to be from a good source (preferably from the USA or Europe), and are safety tested, the downside is low. Given the low risk profile and the beneficial outcomes, the addition of acupuncture and/or herbs to standard of care methods for a variety of illnesses is worthwhile to the patient and cost-effective. Most Eastern and Western medical professionals will agree that by combining standard of care with TCM, the patient truly achieves an integrative care system with the potential for the best results.

Ayurvedic Medicine

Introduction

According to the *Merriam-Webster Dictionary*, Holism is "a theory that the determining factors, especially in living nature, are an irreducible whole" [24]. This acknowledges connections and interdependencies between preexisting systems of nature and humanity, in contradistinction to the more conventional Western reductionist view of a drive toward independence. This concept of holism leads to integration, or the "form[ation] of a whole" and "incorporation into a larger unit" namely, humans, families, communities, and environment [24]. By this definition, the body is inherently self-regulating, self-organizing, and self-healing. It is homeostatic or designed to restore its own natural state of balance. Holistic health and traditional, holistic health systems therefore focus on all levels of health, not merely the physical body, but also the mind (mental and emotional health) and spirit. Additionally, these systems employ diagnostic and therapeutic methodologies that demonstrate and support the concept of integration of the individual into the larger "whole" or the natural environment.

Ayurveda, the Science of Life

Ayurveda, loosely translated as "the science of life," is the traditional holistic health system of India. The term derives from Sanskrit – Ayus meaning life or longevity, and Veda meaning knowledge, learning, or science. Its origin can be found in the Indian subcontinent approximately 4000–5000 years ago (possibly in parallel with the development of TCM, with which it shares many concepts) and it is perhaps best known in the West as the sister science of yoga.

Ayurveda's mind–body–spirit approach is based in the Rig Veda, the ancient Hindu spiritual texts, and what is known as Sankhya philosophy [25]. The earliest overtly medical and surgical texts appeared around 1500 BC in the Carak Samhita and texts by the scholar Shushruta. In these early medical textbooks, we see specific recommendations on lifestyle, diet, and what is the foundation of Ayurveda and Dinacharya, or unique and individualized daily practices. The nomenclature of Ayurveda is revealed and enumerated via various states of balance and imbalance. Preventive practices and treatments including surgical techniques, body therapies, use of botanical medicine, and herbs are detailed. Ayurveda emphasizes the health of the individual within local, seasonal, communal, and natural, or environmental, contexts.

Ayurveda's philosophical underpinnings determine the pathophysiology of disease and its approach to diagnosis and management [26]. Misuse of the senses, failure of intellect, time, and motion are primary causes of dysfunction and disease. But the primordial cause of all disease is forgetting our true nature as spirit. In other words, health fails when individuals disconnect from their most essential self as spiritual. The building blocks of life, or the pancha maha bhutas, are the "five elements": ether, air, water, fire and earth. These elements are further characterized as hot or cold, dry or moist, heavy or light, and stable or mobile. These elements and their assigned characteristics are the core of the three doshas, or the mind–body constitutions according to which all humans can be described, understood, and ultimately healed. Vata is ether and air: primarily cold, dry, mobile, and light. Pitta is water and fire: hot, moist, light, and unstable. Kapha is water and earth: cold, moist, heavy, and stable. Doshic body types, characteristics of mind (thinking and feeling), and all manner of highly detailed expressions of health and personal habits, from sleep to digestion and elimination, sexual activity to social interaction, are determined and influenced by the individual's unique dosha. Humans are born with a specific doshic combination and these are set and influenced during fetal development.

Ayurveda's fascinating descriptions of physiology and pathophysiology precede any access to modern tissue dissection or laboratory science. The dhatus, or tissues, are detailed and include modern correlations to blood, lymph, immune system, central and peripheral nervous systems, musculoskeletal tissues, and digestive and reproductive tracts. The srotas are the channels via which biological energy and information travel: blood vessels, nerve tissue, and lymphatics. Samprapti are meticulously detailed charts of pathogenesis that have been developed to describe almost every conceivable medical or mental health issue from anxiety to kidney stones, heavy menses to hypertension, specific cancers to various types of diabetes. Pathology or illness develops as a consequence of a longstanding aggravation or imbalance in the individual's lifestyle that results in ama – toxin – production. If the root cause of this ama is not addressed, it accumulates then overflows and disturbs the overall balance of the individual's constitution, initially at the site of abnormality then ultimately spreading throughout and to remote body–mind locations. Left unattended, over time overt manifestations, or what we would call symptoms of disease, appear.

The individual's specific complaints are seen as imbalances, or vikruti, and movement away from the homeostatic set point of their innate prakruti, or actual doshic nature and health. Evaluation is performed via a complete health history with a specific focus on the minutiae of daily habits. Physical examination includes attention to the body type, height and weight, skin, facial features, tongue, and pulse. In the most traditional setting, bodily fluids are also examined. The goal of this examination is to understand the individual's constitution and imbalances so that they can be realigned via a treatment plan that addresses not only the individual and his or her daily practices of diet, sleep, exercise, and consumption of food, but also sensory experiences. The tools of Ayurvedic healing include lifestyle counseling and support, dietary recommendations, and herbal medicines – many of which are uniquely formulated for the individual based on his or her unique dosha or constitution. In some cases, application of aroma, sound/color therapy, body work such as specific types of oil massage and oil applications to the head or body, yoga, meditations, and purification or cleansing techniques are also employed.

Botanic, or herbal, medicine is used extensively in Ayurveda, but one of the most important approaches involves rasayana, or "that which enters rapidly into the essence of the physiology." These preparations are said to have the most rejuvenative properties because of their powerful ability to penetrate tissues and the subtlest realms of the mind–body–spirit [2]. In this way they promote and support the harmony and health of the individual from the cellular to the spiritual level. Some of these rasayanas include ashwagandha (*Withania somnifera*), shatavari (*Asparagus racemosus*), amalaki (*Emblic myrobalan*), bibhitaki (*Beleric myrobalan*), brahmi (*Centella asiatica*), guggulu (*Commiphora mukul*), pippali (*Piper longum*), and haritaki (*Chebulic myrobalan*). There are also classic combinations of these herbs prescribed for specific doshic or constitutional support and for particular imbalances and conditions. Prevention of disease via daily use of rasayana is also promoted.

Other key and unique concepts of Ayurveda are those of agni, ojas, and prana. Agni is the digestive fire or capacity to assimilate what we take in from our food, but also from our senses. The idea is that all that we consume is used to make the building blocks of our very beings – body, mind, and spirit. Ojas are the subtle nourishment that exists in each and every cell. Ojas exist at the boundary of body and mind, and could be considered most akin to the allopathic concept of immunity. It is what gives us strength and resilience on the deepest level. Prana, or breath, is much more than the oxygen that enters and carbon dioxide that exits our lungs. It is another essential element to our life force. To be specific, when agni is weak or the wrong foods and lifestyle are consumed, ama accumulates and disease progresses unless interventions and changes are made in accordance with the individual's specific constitutional needs. When agni is strong and the correct lifestyle is observed, ojas are produced and the individual experiences greater health and harmony.

Ayurvedic Practice

Although Ayurveda is not a licensed practice in the USA, it is regulated state by state as an alternative health practice. National organizations are working on setting criteria for education, competency, and future licensing. In India, the Bachelor of Ayurvedic Medicine and Surgery or Doctor of Ayurvedic Medicine and Surgery degree is offered and is considered somewhat equivalent to a BA/MA/MD in North America. More than 150 accredited schools exist in India. The training involves 4–6 years in an accredited postgraduate setting with opportunities for specialty and subspecialty training beyond that. Some opportunities for combination allopathic–Ayurvedic degrees exist in India. According to the National Institutes of Health National Center for Complementary and Integrative Health, there are approximately 240,000 users of Ayurveda in the USA [27]. This represents only 0.1 percent of all users of complementary and alternative medicine, but the wild growth in yoga and the use of some of the more spa-friendly treatments like shirodara, in which a stream of heated herb-infused oil is poured on the forehead, abhyangha, a coordinated two-person medicated herbed oil massage, and pancha karma, a series of purifying and rejuvenating practices performed over the course of 5–20 days, has introduced Ayurveda more widely to the West than can be easily measured. Some of Ayurveda's most prized and potent botanical medicines, ashwagandha and cooking spices like turmeric, have also captured the popular imagination for their unique healing properties.

Evidence for Efficacy

So how can we better understand this important medical system and evaluate its effectiveness? Complementary, alternative, and integrative medicines (CAIMs) are very difficult to assess. Mason et al. found that the wide spectrum of disciplines, practices, and philosophies that differ from conventional medicine were barriers [28]. Randomized controlled trials and conventional methodologies are reductionist by nature, while many CAIM practices embrace holism. The influence of individual practitioners is a component of CAIM treatments. This is partly attributed to an area of study called MAC – meaning and context. And what of the placebo effect? Healing touch? Bedside manner? What are appropriate outcome measures? How does science assess spiritual or personal growth as a health impact or predictor? Lastly, funding for this type of research is difficult to source.

Perhaps the field of psychoneuroimmunology (PNI) presents the Western paradigm that Ayurveda most closely resembles. This is the interdisciplinary study of the relationships between mind and body – or what allopathy refers to as mental and physical health – from neurologic and immune system physiology to disorders and dysfunction such as autoimmune disease, hypersensitivities, and immune deficiency. Psychoneuroimmunology explicitly studies the relationships between mind (psyche), brain (neuro), and immune systems, and has enjoyed more than three decades of recognition in the scientific and medical research communities. In the 1970s, we discovered that immune cells have receptors for neuropeptides involved in mood and brain function – i.e., the immune system and the nervous system appear to be designed to communicate with each other – but why? Walter Cannon, who taught at Harvard University between the 1910s and the 1930s, described homeostasis as the need for mental and physical balance throughout the organism, and the fight-or-flight reaction as a behavior observed in animals under duress.

Hans Selye described the "general adaptation syndrome," noting that animals under mental and physical stress were able to recover and heal, but that there were physical consequences to prolonged exposure to stress that were initiated and mediated by communication between the immune, hormonal, and nervous systems. Chiefly, his work noted that adaptation resulted from brief alarm, and resistance resulted from prolonged exposure, but the final result of unrelenting stress was terminal exhaustion and death. Reams of evidence for this have accumulated over the last century. In 1964, George Solomon demonstrated that actively psychotic patients underwent measurable immune alterations. When vaccinated, they developed a markedly less robust antibody response when compared with healthy controls.

The classic foundational study was performed in 1975 at the University of Rochester by Dr. Ader (a psychologist) and Dr. Cohen (an immunologist) [29]. While conducting a study of classic Pavlovian conditioning, they came upon some unexpected results that ended with the coining of the term PNI. Rats were conditioned with sweetened water laced with a chemotherapy agent in order to induce nausea and food aversion, in addition to suppressing the immune system. Surprisingly, after the rats were conditioned, merely feeding them the sweetened water without the chemotherapy agent was associated with immune suppression and even death. Further investigation proved that a signal via the nervous system (taste) was directly affecting immune function. This sounds much like the classic Ayurvedic concept of taste and consumption affecting doshic expression, strength of agni, and development of ama or ojas.

Many studies have repeatedly demonstrated that the brain and immune systems represent in many regards a single integrated system of defense, but in 1973 Candace Pert proved that this integration came in the form of neuropeptide-specific receptors present on cell walls in the brain and immune system [30]. These systems appear to have been designed to communicate directly and to function synergistically. This also demonstrates how emotions (neuropeptides), central nervous system, brain, and immunity all affect each other [31].

The body's primary means of managing acute and chronic stress is the hypothalamic–pituitary–adrenal (HPA) axis. Its intimate communications with the sympathetic and parasympathetic nervous systems are clear in this regard. Inflammatory cytokine release activates ACTH and cortisol release. Glucocorticoids suppress inflammatory cytokine production. Cytokines – while primarily considered part of the humoral immune response – are also produced in the brain, especially the hypothalamus, which we know is a seat of hormone system control. Proinflammatory cytokine processes take place during depression and manic and bipolar flares, and also influence autoimmune hypersensitivity and chronic infections. Chronic stress impairs our natural ability to repair and self-heal via inappropriate activation of our proinflammatory factors. We know at this point that many of the most commonly encountered disease states like cardiovascular disease, cancer, metabolic syndrome, and obesity-related illness are actually proinflammatory conditions, and this has led to the promotion of the prophylactic and therapeutic use of anti-inflammatories – vitamin D, omega-3 fatty acids, coq10, and other antioxidants. Chronic secretion of stress hormones (glucocorticoids and catecholamines) may reduce the effectiveness of neurotransmitters such as serotonin, norepinephrine, and dopamine, and their receptors in the brain. These differences can also produce functional changes in immune cells. In a 1984 study of medical students during finals, stress, attitude, and specific cellular immunity were found to be intimately related. Those with more stress demonstrated less immunity [32]. A meta-analysis by Herbert and Cohen in 1993 reviewed 38 studies of stressful events and immune function in healthy adults and showed consistent changes in specific cellular immunity [33]. Stress induced increases in total WBC count and decreases in helper T cells, suppressor cells, and NK cells, among others. In 2001, Zorrilla et al. replicated this meta-analysis and its findings with 75 studies [34].

We know that stress impairs immune function and the Ayurvedic model could be construed to correlate. But what about solutions to stress-induced illness? Critical areas of study include how behavior can induce alterations in immune function and immune alterations can induce behavior change; this could have major impacts in therapy and clinical application. This is where we can best demonstrate the benefits of Ayurvedic approaches such as yoga, meditation, lifestyle, and spiritual practices.

Nelson et al. at the University of California, Irvine, published a study in *Clinical Cancer Research* in 2008 [35]. The intervention in this study was psychological telephone counseling offered to cervical cancer survivors. Those in the experimental group showed a statistically significant improvement in quality of life (QOL), and those with an increased QOL showed a statistically significant improvement in immune function, measured by T cell helper function and various interleukins. Support increases survival by measurable biological markers. The authors concluded that "adaptive immunity supports integration of chronic stress response into biobehavioral models of cancer survivorship and suggests a novel mechanistic hypothesis by which interventions leading to enhanced QOL could result in improved clinical outcomes including survival." This conclusion demonstrates recognition of the mind–body connection and the potential power of PNI, thus providing further support for a foundation of biobehavioral paradigms like Ayurveda, and postulating potential mechanisms by which a psychosocial intervention might influence cancer survivorship.

The same 1984 medical student study mentioned above also looked at positive influences on immunity and found quite a few [32]. Satisfying personal relationships, social support, personal sharing, disclosure of traumatic experiences, humor and laughter, hypnosis and relaxation techniques, physical exertion and aerobic exercise, group intervention, and support all increased specific cellular and non-cellular immune function and response.

Evidence: Meditation

We know from observation that positive emotional experiences boost the immune system. Can we extrapolate that other intense and positive experiences, such as those found in spirituality, community, and ritual, do the same? Meditation is an activity of daily living with a spiritual- or ritual-oriented dimension that is regularly prescribed as part of the Ayurvedic lifestyle.

In 1972, Harvard University's Dr. Herbert Benson set out to study what was becoming a popular phenomenon introduced from India to America – meditation [36]. This groundbreaking study opened the conventional academic medical and research communities to non-conventional modalities. His work demonstrated the "relaxation response" and its beneficial physiological repercussions. It was hypothesized to serve as an antidote to "fight-or-flight." As meditation and mindfulness are detailed in previous chapters, we won't elaborate further other than to note that research specifically aimed at examining Ayurvedic-inspired mantra meditation, such as transcendental meditation (TM), have demonstrated mental and physical health benefits as well as longevity in diverse populations [37, 38].

Evidence: Botanic Medicine

Botanic medicine has been extensively reviewed and studied, and although nothing considered a "landmark" study exists, solid data does. Aggarwal et al. identify 175 Ayurvedic plants, their components, and their molecular targets, concluding that this reverse pharmacology approach is a viable means of developing Western pharmaceuticals for the prevention of cancer, cardiovascular disease, diabetes, and pulmonary, neurologic, and other chronic conditions [39]. Vayalil et al. proffer data on this class of Ayurvedic medicine's immunostimulatory capacity via quenching free radicals, enhancing cellular detoxification mechanisms, repairing damaged cells, inducing proliferation of cells, and inducing the self-renewal of damaged proliferating tissues in addition to replacing damaged or mutated cells with fresh cells [40]. In a truly comprehensive review of Ayurvedic botanic medicine, Khan and Balick review clinical, *in vivo* studies, with 43–63 percent of these studies conducted on humans and animals in a wide variety of clinical settings – dermatology, diabetes, renal, blood, and immune system, cardiovascular, anti-mutagen, nervous system, liver, antimicrobial, pain and inflammation, and gastrointestinal [41]. These authors, as well as many others, note that product consistency and purity are essential to evaluate, as purchase and use are not well regulated. Chainanu-Wu conducted a phase I, 25-subject human trial, and this was the sixth study of its kind to find no toxicity in three months of use of high-dose daily turmeric and its specific molecular anti-inflammatory impacts via enzymatic pathways [42]. Shatavari's traditional Ayurvedic indications for use have been validated in small, similar studies like that of Gautam et al. in the *Journal of Ethnopharmacology* [43]. Shatavari is said to give women the strength of "one hundred husbands" and reproductive as well as general resilience. Animals treated with *Asparagus racemosus* were found to have a beneficial CD3 and CD4 to CD8 ratio, which indicated T cell activation. They also demonstrated increased IL-2, IFNG, and IL-4, antibody titers, and lymphocytic proliferation.

Evidence: Lifestyle

An assessment set up as an RCT at Gujarat Ayurvedic University compared three interventions in the management of menopausal syndrome; all patients were treated for 45 days and followed up for 1 month [44]. Group A was treated with conjugated estrogens 0.625 mg once daily, Group B was treated with saraswatarishta (a traditional rasayana containing brahmi, haritaki, shatavari, ashwagandha, shankpushpi, calamus, vidari, and gotu kola) 20 ml mixed with water and taken before meals twice a day, and Group C was treated with shirodhara with bala taila, 30 min per sitting (alternating seven days of the shirodhara intervention with three days off). Compared to the other two groups, patients who received shirodhara had better relief. This treatment is a traditional practice of pouring medicated oil onto the forehead. Topical penetration of the forehead to the level of the muscularis has a local vasodilatory effect. It is postulated to impact hypothalamic function via antianxiety and antidepressant effects, endocrine balance, and inhibition of the autonomic nervous system ("fight-or-flight") [44]. The study included 48 women aged 40–50 with typical perimenopausal and menopausal complaints of hot flashes, insomnia, gastrointestinal problems, low libido, pain, weight gain, and fatigue, as well as mood issues like anxiety, depression, and irritability. The subjects underwent 45 days of treatment and were then assessed via Ayurvedic and Western rating scales.

All three groups experienced significant improvement in many symptoms. Both Ayurvedic experimental groups showed superior improvement compared to traditional hormone replacement therapy according to the Hamilton anxiety scale, and group C (shirodara) demonstrated the best effect on the menopause rating scale with respect to hot flashes, mood, and sleep. There were no reported untoward side effects in any group.

Conclusion

Ayurveda presents a wealth of opportunities to better understand the origins of today's emphasis on individualized wellness and lifestyle medicine. When we consider our recent developments in understanding the microbiome, the mind–gut connection and its impact on mood and immunity, epigenetics, and even stem cell regenerative medicine, Ayurveda seems prescient in its approach to the whole-person medicine we seek to deliver today.

References

1. PU Unschuld. *Traditional Chinese Medicine: Heritage and Adaptation.* New York, Columbia University Press; 2018.

2. P Leung. *A Comprehensive Guide to Chinese Medicine* (2nd ed.). Singapore, World Scientific; 2016.

3. JD Adams, EJ Lien. The traditional and scientific bases for traditional Chinese medicine: communications between traditional practitioners, physicians and scientists. In: J Adams, E Lien, eds., *Traditional Chinese Medicine: Scientific Basis for Its Use.* Cambridge, RSC Publishing; 2013; 1–10.

4. D Chiaramonte, C D'Adamo, B Morrison. Integrative approaches to pain management. In: H Benzon, J Rathmell, eds. *Practical Management of Pain* (5th ed.). Philidelphia, PA, Mosby Inc.; 2014; 658–668.

5. GG Hong. Acupuncture: the historical basis and its US practitioners. *Lab Med* 1998; **3:** 163–166.

6. A White, E Ernst. A brief history of acupuncture. *Rheumatology* 2004; **5:** 662–663.

7. HM Langevin, RN Schyner. Reconnecting the body in Eastern and Western medicine. *J Altern Complement Med* 2017; **4:** 238–241.

8. V Napadow, A Ahn, L Lao, et al. The status and future of acupuncture mechanism research. *J Altern Complement Med* 2008; **7:** 861–869.

9. T Lim, Y Ma, F Berger, G Litscher. Acupuncture and neural mechanism in the management of low back pain: an update. *Medicines* 2018; **3:** 63.

10. KS Hui, V Napadow, J Liu, et al. Monitoring acupuncture effects on human brain by fMRI. *J Vis Exp* 2010; **38:** 1190.

11. A Qaseem, TJ Wilt, RM McLean, MA Forciea. Noninvasive treatment acute, subacute, and chronic low back pain: a clinical practice guideline from the American Colleges of Physicians. *Ann Intern Med* 2017; **7:** 514–530.

12. X Zhang. *Acupuncture: Review and Analysis of Controlled Clinical Trials.* Geneva, World Health Organization; 2002.

13. E Manheimer, A White, B Berman, K Forys, E Ernst. Meta-analysis: acupuncture for low back pain. *Ann Intern Med* 2005; **142:** 651–663.

14. M Haake, HH Müller, C Schade-Brittinger, et al. German Acupuncture Trials (GERAC) for chronic low back pain: randomized, multicenter, blinded, parallel-group trial with 3 groups. *Arch Intern Med* 2007; **167:** 1892–1898.

15. HI Karpatkin, D Napolione, B Siminovich-Blok. Acupuncture and multiple sclerosis: a review of the evidence. *Evid Based Complement Alternat Med* 2014. DOI:10.1155/2014/972935.

16. X Zhao, H Hu, J Li, et al. Is acupuncture effective for hypertension? A systematic review and meta-analysis. *PLoS One* 2015; **10.** DOI:10.1371/journal.pone.0127019.

17. FZ Zia, O Olaku, T Bao, et al. The National Cancer Institute's Conference on acupuncture for symptoms management in oncology: state of the science, evidence and

research gaps. *JNCI Monogr* 2017; **52**; 68–73.

18. JW Daily, M Yang, S Park. Efficacy of tumeric extracts and curcumin for alleviating the symptoms of joint arthritis: a systematic review and meta-analysis of the randomized clinical trials. *PLoS One* 2013; **8**. DOI:10.1089/jmf.2016.3705.

19. Y Song, B Xu. Diffusion profiles of health beneficial components from goji berry (*Lyceum barbarum*) marinated in alcohol and their antioxidant capacities as affected by alcohol concentration and steeping time. *Foods* 2013; **3**: 32–42.

20. Q Huang, M Wang, X Chen, et al. Can active components of licorice, glycyrrhizin and glycyrrhetinic acid, lick rheumatoid arthritis? *Oncotarget* 2015, 7. DOI:10.18632/oncotarget.6200.

21. J Choi, T Choi, M Lee, T Kim. Ginseng for health care: a systematic review of randomised controlled trials in Korean literature. *BMJ Quality Safety*. 2013. DOI:10.1136/bmjqs-2013-002293.131.

22. N-H Lee, C-G Son. Systematic review of randomized controlled trials evaluating the efficacy and safety of ginseng. *J Acupunct Meridian Stud* 2011 **4**: 85–97.

23. Z Wang, F Qi, Y Cui, et al. An update on Chinese herbal medicines as adjuvant treatment of anticancer therapeutics. *BioScience Trends* 2018 **12**: 220–239.

24. Standard International Media. *Webster's Dictonary & Thesaurus: 2014 Edition*. Naples, FL, Standard Intl Media; 2017.

25. M Halpen, *Principles of Ayurvedic Medicine* (11th ed.). Independently published; 2018.

26. D Simon, D Chopra. *The Wisdom of Healing: A Natural Mind Body Program for Optimal Wellness*. New York, Harmony Books; 1997.

27. National Center for Complementary and Integrative Health. Ayurvedic medicine: in depth. http://nccih.nih.gov/health/ayurveda/introduction.htm (accessed January 14, 2019).

28. S Mason, P Tovey AF Long. Evaluating complementary medicine: methodological challenges of randomised controlled trials. *BMJ* 2002; **325**(7368): 832–834.

29. R Ader, N Cohen. Behaviorally conditioned immunosuppression. *Psychosomatic Medicine* 1975; **37**: 333–340.

30. CB Pert, SH Snyder. Opiate receptor: demonstration in nervous tissue. *Science* 1973; **179**: 1011–1014.

31. CB Pert, D Chopra. *Molecules of Emotion: Why You Feel the Way You Feel*. New York, Simon and Schuster; 1997.

32. R Glaser, JK Kiecolt-Glaser, JC Stout, et al. Stress-related impairments in cellular immunity. *Psychiatr Res* 1985; **16**(3): 233–239.

33. TB Herbert, S Cohen. Stress and immunity in humans: a meta-analytic review. *Psychosom Med* 1993; **55**: 364–379.

34. EP Zorrilla, L Luborsky, JR McKay, et al. The relationship of depression and stressors to immunological assays: a meta-analytic review. *Brain Behav Immun* 2001; **15**(3): 199–226.

35. EL Nelson, LB Wenzel, K Osann, et al. Stress, immunity, and cervical cancer: biobehavioral outcomes of a randomized clinical trial [corrected]. *Clin Cancer Res* 2008; **14**(7): 2111–2118.

36. JF Beary, H Benson. A simple psychophysiological technique which elicits the hypometabolic changes of the relaxation response. *Psychosom Med* 1974; **36**(2): 115–120.

37. JE Bormann, D Oman, JK Kemppainen, et al. Mantram repetition for stress management in veterans and employees: a critical incident study. *J Adv Nurs* 2006; **53**(5): 502–512.

38. TE Seeman, LF Dubin, M Seeman. Religiosity/spirituality and health: a critical review of the evidence for biological pathways. *Am Psychologist* 2003; **58**: 53–63.

39. BB Aggarwal, S Prasad, S Reuter, et al. Identification of novel anti-inflammatory agents from Ayurvedic medicine for prevention of chronic diseases: "reverse pharmacology" and "bedside to bench" approach. *Curr Drug Targets* 2011; **12**(11): 1595–1653.

40. PK Vayalil, G Kuttan, R Kuttan. Rasayanas: evidence for the concept of prevention of diseases. *Am J Chin Med* 2002; **30**: 155–171.

41. S Khan, MJ Balick. Therapeutic plants of Ayurveda: a review of selected clinical and other studies for 166 species. *J Altern Complement Med* 2001; 7(5): 405–515.

42. N Chainani-Wu. Safety and anti-inflammatory activity of curcumin: a component of turmeric (*Curcuma longa*). *J Altern Complement Med* 2003; **9**: 161–168.

43. M Gautam, S Saha, S Bani, et al. Immunomodulatory activity of *Asparagus racemosus* on systemic Th1/Th2 immunity: implications for immunoadjuvant potential. *J Ethnopharmacol* 2009; **121**: 241–247.

44. K Santwani, VD Shukla, MA Santwani, G Thaker. An assessment of Manasika Bhavas in menopausal syndrome and its management. *Ayu* 2010; **31**(3): 311–318.

Chapter

The Role of Aesthetics in Wellness

Asbasia A. Mikhail and Ashley Ngor

Introduction

While wellness is a concept that has no universally accepted definition [1], researchers have been able to determine eight dimensions crucial to wellness: physical, emotional, social, spiritual, intellectual, financial, occupational, and environmental [2]. The physical dimension includes physical health, self-image, body image, and appearance. The notion of "look good – feel good" has been gaining traction, and there is emerging scientific evidence supporting it [3, 4]. This chapter focuses on the popular aesthetic techniques of cosmetic procedures and styling, in addition to how such aesthetic techniques can improve overall wellness during and after recovery from surgical, medical, and psychiatric illness.

Cosmetic Procedures and Wellness

Cosmetic procedures, surgical as well as minimally invasive (Table 32.1), have continued to grow in popularity worldwide. The evidence for their role in improving overall wellness will be highlighted here.

In the USA alone, the American Society of Plastic Surgeons (ASPS) states that over 17.5 million surgical and minimally invasive cosmetic procedures were performed in 2017 – a 2 percent increase from the previous year [5]. While this may not seem significant, ASPS later compared the number of total cosmetic procedures performed in 2018 (17,721,671) to the number performed in 2000 (6,748,610) [5], determining that the total number of cosmetic procedures had increased by 163 percent. The reason for such a drastic increase is largely considered to be due to the increased prevalence of minimally invasive procedures, the number of which rose by 228 percent (15,909,931 procedures) between 2000 and 2018 [6]. More and more physicians of all specialties have given up their traditional medical practices solely to practice in the thriving industry of aesthetic medicine, due in part to the change in popular opinion. Hojjat et al. found that national and international media coverage from 2008 to 2017 on cosmetic procedures was overall positive, which contrasts heavily with the popular consensus just a few years before [7]. Although opinions regarding cosmetic procedures may vary, evidence supports the notion that how we perceive ourselves and how we are perceived on the outside positively affects how we feel on the inside. A 2013 systematic review by Bensoussan et al. of 28 studies looking at both surgical and minimally invasive cosmetic procedures found that they had positive effects on the quality of life of the patients receiving them [8]. In a research study evaluating 130 women and psychosocial changes in the five years following cosmetic surgery, analyses revealed improvement not only in satisfaction with their general appearance and the body part operated on, but also in self-esteem and well-being [9].

Table 32.1 Cosmetic procedures

Breast	Face and neck
Augmentation mammoplasty	Brow lift
Breast implant removal	Buccal fat removal
Breast implant replacement	Cheek augmentation
Breast lift (mastopexy)	Chin surgery (mentoplasty)
Reduction mammoplasty	Ear surgery (otoplasty)
Breast augmentation with fat grafting	Eyelid surgery (blepharoplasty)
Fat reduction	Facelift surgery (rhytidectomy)
Liposuction (lipoplasty)	Facial implants
Laser/ultrasound assisted liposuction	Neck lift (lower rhytidectomy)
Nonsurgical fat reduction	Nose surgery (rhinoplasty)
Body lifts	**Minimally invasive**
Arm lift (brachioplasty)	Botulinum toxin (Botox®, Dysport®, Xeomin®, Jeuveau®)
Body contouring	Chemical peel
Body lift	Dermabrasion
Gluteal augmentation and lift	Dermal fillers
Mommy makeover	Laser hair removal
Thigh lift	Laser skin resurfacing
Tummy tuck (abdominoplasty)	Microdermabrasion
Male-specific plastic surgery	Skin rejuvenation and resurfacing
Male breast reduction for gynecomastia	Spider vein treatment (sclerotherapy)
Hair transplant	Tattoo removal
Vaginal rejuvenation	

Source: adapted from www.plasticsurgery.org/cosmetic-procedures.

Minimally Invasive Cosmetic Procedures

Minimally invasive surgeries are gaining popularity in tandem with traditional surgeries.

The results of noninvasive facial rejuvenation [10] are sometimes comparable to surgical procedures, as shown in Figure 32.1.

Research studies have showed that compared to controls, individuals seeking botulinum toxin A (used in the minimally invasive procedure of Botox injection) and dermal filler injections had no signs of body dysmorphic disorder or personality disorders, and experienced higher health-related quality of life ratings [11]. Noninvasive procedures such as laser hair removal are being utilized far more frequently than ever before. Using the Dermatology Life Quality Index (DLQI), Roche et al. demonstrated that in 142 women laser hair removal greatly and sustainably increased quality of life for 12–30 months, in addition to significantly and less sustainably decreasing the magnitude of emotional burden caused by hirsutism [12].

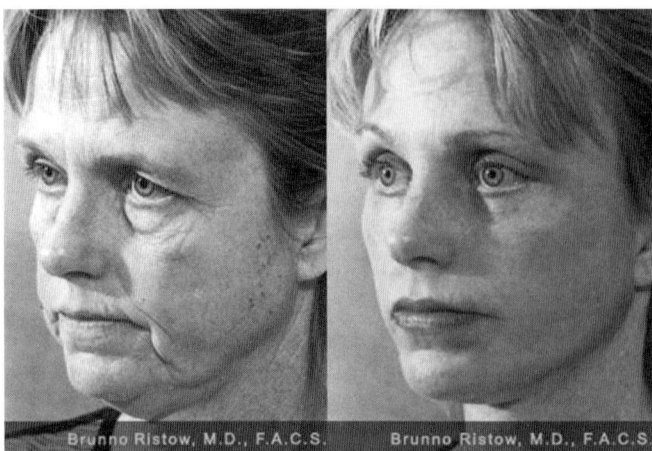

Figure 32.1 Facial rejuvenation included maintaining all the patient's natural fat (except under the chin), elevation of low eyebrows, eyelid operations and restoration of the natural fullness of the lips. Reprinted from: https://commons.wikimedia.org/wiki/File:Face_Lift_01_Dr._Ristow.jpg with permission from Creative Commons.

Surgical Cosmetic Procedures

Surgical cosmetic procedures (as highlighted in Table 32.1) include removing the signs of aging, such as facelifts (rhytidectomy or rhytidoplasty) [13], nose reshaping (rhinoplasty) [14], tummy tuck (abdominoplasty) [15], liposuction [16], and breast cosmetic surgeries [17]. One representative procedure is the *mommy makeover* depicted in Figure 32.2, showing pre-op and six-month post-op photos of a patient who underwent a breast lift, abdominoplasty, and liposuction of the flanks [18].

Surgical cosmetic procedures have been found to improve wellness [19]. A 2005 rhytidoplasty study revealed significant improvements in self-esteem and quality of life, leading to substantial advancements in health status and psychological functioning [20]. In multiple studies, facelifts have been proven to enhance the quality of life in one form or another by increases in well-being, comfort during social situations, self-confidence, quality of life, work situations, and new opportunities in the form of jobs, relationships, promotions, or raises [21]. In a 2014 study by Alderman et al., 611 female patients who had undergone breast augmentation were found to have substantially increased levels of breast satisfaction, psychosocial wellness, and sexual wellness at both six weeks and six months following the operation [22]. Similarly, breast-reduction surgery was found by Kececi et al. to increase self-esteem, satisfaction, and quality of life in 94 women for over four months after the procedure [23]. In a sample of 840 female patients, increased quality of life was detected after one-stage breast reconstruction with an acellular dermal matrix and anatomic implant muscle-sparing technique [24]. Men with gynecomastia that was corrected using cosmetic surgery with also saw improved well-being ratings [25].

The Importance of Aesthetics for Wellness during and after Recovery from Surgical, Medical, and Psychiatric Illness

While aesthetics may prove beneficial in the maintenance of wellness, it can also act as a form of rehabilitation for those recovering from surgical, medical, and psychiatric illness. Those with chronic illness or those recovering from serious illness undergo many changes to their physical appearance that may lower their overall feeling of wellness.

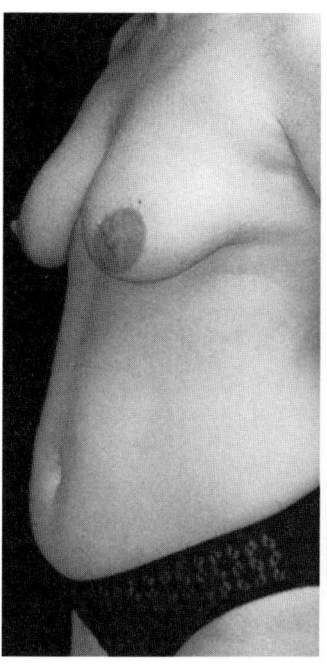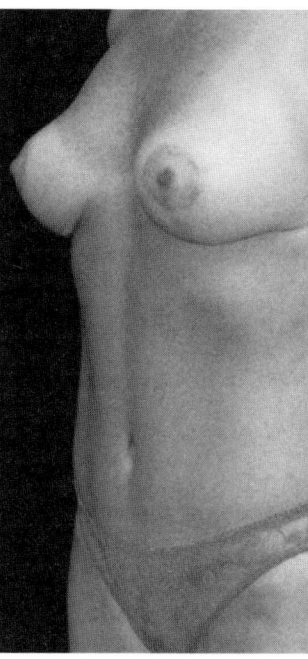

Figure 32.2 Mommy makeover pre-op (a) and six-month post-op (b) photos of a patient who underwent a breast lift, abdominoplasty, and liposuction of the flanks. Reprinted from:(a) https://commons.wikimedia.org/wiki/File:Mommy_Makeover_Patient_3_perioperative_photo.jpg, and (b) https://commons.wiki media.org/wiki/File:Mommy_Makeover_Patient_3_post-op_photo.jpg with permission from Creative Commons.

Cosmetic Procedures as a Form of Recovery

Cosmetic procedures have been implemented successfully as a recovery strategy for various illnesses. A 2018 systematic review found that the effects of cosmetic procedures and the effects of antidepressant treatments on health-related quality-of-life improvement are comparable [26]. While antidepressant treatment correlated with greater improvements, both had great impact on mental health and role emotional scales. Some individuals living with human immunodeficiency virus (HIV) suffer from facial lipoatrophy, with the loss of facial volume changing their appearance negatively because of antiviral medication use; as a result, many of these individuals avoid taking their necessary medications [27]. The use of minimally invasive facial dermal fillers to treat facial lipoatrophy has been shown to result in self-reported feelings of happiness and generally more compliant patients.

In the management of transient blepharoptosis after botulinum toxin injection, double eyelid cosmetic glue was used to induce a deeper eyelid crease and thus elevate the upper eyelid temporarily, as shown in Figure 32.3 [28]. Because all patients included in this study reported satisfactory improvement in the appearance of their transient blepharoptosis, double eyelid cosmetic glue and other cosmetic products may be viable recovery techniques for this condition. Botulinum toxin was also shown by Roche et al. in 2015 to be a safe and effective self-rehabilitation technique aimed to improve gait in chronic stroke patients and thus improve quality of life [29].

In mastectomy patients who underwent reconstructive surgery, research revealed that having surgery immediately after their mastectomies, as shown in Figure 32.4, protected patients from psychosocial stress, body image issues, diminished sexual well-being, fatigue, pain, and arm symptoms more so than for patients who underwent breast reconstruction at a later time [30–32].

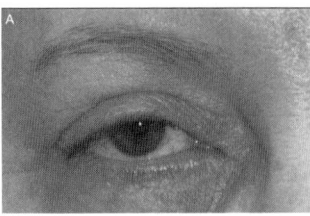
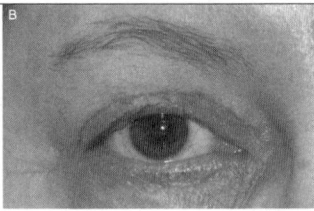

Figure 32.3 Eyelid make-up to manage transient blepharoptosis after botulinum toxin injection. This 58-year-old woman presented with (a) right upper eyelid ptosis, noted one week after botulinum toxin A injection. (b) Her right upper eyelid ptosis was temporarily treated with eyelid make-up and an improvement of 2 mm in her margin reflex distance 1 (MRD-1) could be observed immediately after application of the product. Reprinted from *Aesthetic Surgery Journal* with permission from Oxford University Press.

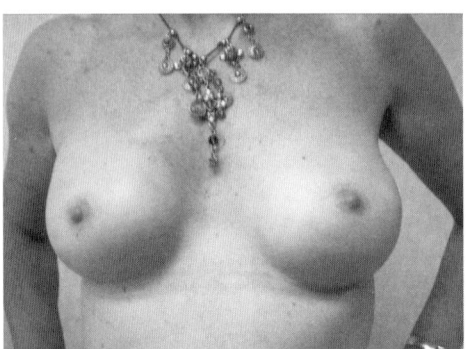

Figure 32.4 Bilateral nipple-sparing mastectomy and implant reconstruction for bilateral breast cancer in a 57-year-old woman. Reprinted from: https://commons.wiki media.org/wiki/Category:Breast_reconstruction#/medi a/File:Breast_reconstruction_15.jpg with permission from Creative Commons.

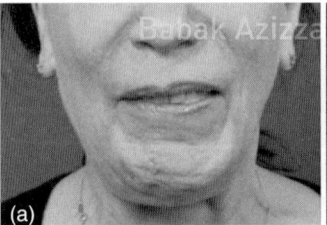
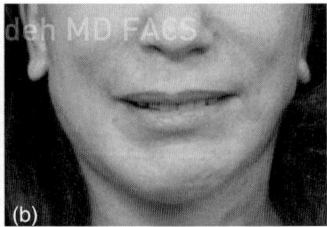

Figure 32.5 Synkenesis surgery: selective neurolysis for treatment of Bell's Palsy. (a) Before synkenesis surgery; (b) after synkenesis surgery. Reprinted from www .facialparalysisinstitute.com/treat ments/surgery-for-synkinesis-partial-facial-paralysis with permission from Dr. Babak Azizzadeh, the Facial Paralysis Institute. 2019.

In Bell's palsy, in addition to surgical options, there are other forms of noninvasive cosmetic procedures. At the Facial Paralysis Institute, Dr. Babak Azizzadeh performs a ground-breaking procedure for permanent treatment of Bell's palsy, known as synkenesis surgery or selective neurolysis, which is a selective neurectomy [33]. Figure 32.5 shows a patient before and after synkenesis surgery performed by Dr. Azizzadeh.

Botox injections are another effective treatment to achieve facial symmetry in patients with Bell's palsy [33]. Figure 32.6 shows a patient with Bell's palsy before and after Botox treatment, also performed by Dr. Azizzadeh.

Advanced tools are now being utilized to predict the outcome of cosmetic procedures. Innovative methods of digital facial analysis, such as Analyze My Face, are available online

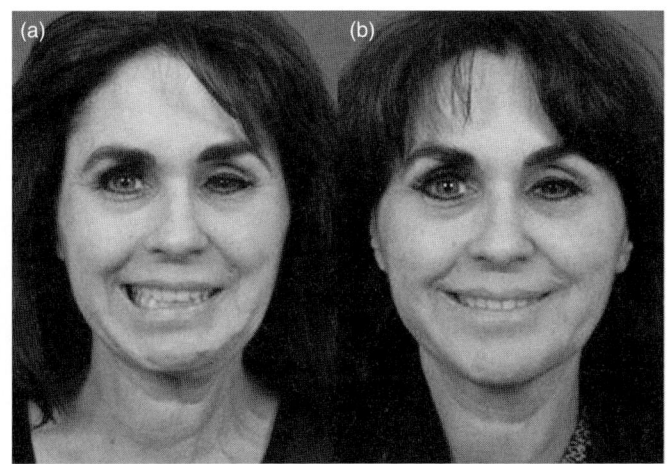

Figure 32.6 Botox injections for treatment of facial asymmetry. (a) Before Botox; (b) after Botox. Reprinted from www.facialparaly sisinstitute.com/treatments/sur gery-for-synkinesis-partial-facial-p aralysis with permission from Dr. Babak Azizzadeh, the Facial Paralysis Institute. 2019.

to provide detailed analysis to patients prior to undergoing facial cosmetic procedures [34]. These procedures contribute tremendously to improvement in the patient's overall well-being.

Styling and Wellness

Surgical cosmetic procedures and minimally invasive cosmetic procedures are not the only form of aesthetics that can affect wellness; for example, temporary aesthetic procedures such as make-up and clothing have been investigated in relation to wellness and its maintenance.

Make-Up

Although make-up provides a very temporary adjustment to our physical appearance as observed by those around us, it has been determined to have long-lasting effects on our well-being. Our physical appearance affects how we feel and our achievement of success in this world: results dating back to a 1989 study involving female college students indicated more positive body-image cognitions in cosmetic-present women than cosmetic-absent women [35]. Interestingly, a greater amount of make-up on the female correlated to a greater body-image difference between the cosmetic-present women and the cosmetic-absent women. In 2004, Richetin et al. found associations of make-up with positive traits and high-status professions at the implicit level after examining psychology, business, and aesthetics students [36]. Make-up has also been suggested to relate to academic performance, in a 2017 Palumbo et al. study that divided 186 female undergraduate students into three groups: wearing make-up, listening to positive music, and face coloring [37]. The results showed that female students who had put on make-up before a simulated university examination received higher grades compared to those who listened to music and those who face-colored. Make-up has also been used to improve wellness in medical conditions such as Bell's palsy. In a 2019 study, 70 female facial-nerve-palsy patients received specialized make-up therapy to adjust for their asymmetrical facial appearances [38]. As a result, there were substantial improvements in symptoms of depression and in overall score for the Facial Clinimetric Evaluation (FaCE) scale.

Clothing

While most people think of aesthetics as related to the cosmetic enhancements discussed earlier, the simple act of wearing the right look can have a comparable effect. In fact, the term "ensemble empowerment" has been used to describe this concept – feeling confident in what one wears [39]. While more rigorous research needs to be performed to examine clothing's impact on wellness, anecdotal evidence (via internet blogs, magazines, talk shows, and our own personal experiences) reflects the importance of how styling, fitting, and our own feelings about what we wear affect self-perception and thus the mental aspect of wellness. One article suggests that the clothing we wear may worsen anxiety due to being uncomfortable, ill-suiting, and generally not making us feel positive about ourselves; wearing clothes like this, we create a façade that allows for misinterpretation of character and later discontent with oneself [40].

While the avenues for fashion advice continue to grow as popular culture changes, the Internet has introduced multiple opportunities for individuals to improve their wellness through clothing. An essential part of wellness is destressing one's mind and efficiently allocating time in our schedules for important/non-urgent tasks, such as picking out and wearing clothing that makes us feel better about ourselves. Personal styling available online, and through apps such as Stitch Fix [41] and The Stïl Trust [42], may soon prove to be an accepted method of improving overall wellness by helping individuals look their best while having time to focus on other aspects of wellness that are important to them.

Conclusion

Although popular culture emphasizes the importance of innate personality traits for the accomplishment of goals and living well, there is a lack of knowledge in regard to wellness and its relationship to aesthetics – a term encompassing anything capable of maintaining or improving physical appearance. No matter how hard we try as individuals to remain unbiased, it remains clear that physical appearance will continue to play a huge role in our daily lives and overall sense of well-being and general life satisfaction. Our physical appearance and how it relates to the societal definition of attractiveness is closely connected to wellness. Due in part to the wellness benefits, aesthetic techniques such as cosmetic procedures and styling have gained tremendous popularity throughout the years, not only during and after illness to improve function, but also to improve the overall sense of well-being. With innovations and technological advancements constantly being made in aesthetic, cosmetic, and styling techniques, they could also be utilized as a therapy to improve wellness.

References

1. HL Dunn. *High Level Wellness*. Arlington, VA, Beatty Press; 1961.

2. Boston University Center for Psychiatric Rehabilitation. Eight dimensions of wellness. 2019. https://cpr.bu.edu/living-well/eight-dimensions-of-wellness (accessed September 5, 2019).

3. E Berscheid, E Walster. Physical attractiveness. *Adv. Exp. Social Psychol.* 1974; 7: 157–215.

4. DB Yarosh. Perception and deception: human beauty and the brain. *Behav Sci (Basel)* 2019; **29**: pii: E34.

5. American Society of Plastic Surgeons. Cosmetic Procedures. 2019. www.plasticsurgery.org/cosmetic-procedures (accessed September 5, 2019).

6. Zion Research. Global cosmetic products market share expected to reach $863 billion by 2024: ZMR. 2019. www.globenewswire

.com/news-release/2019/01/31/1708263/0/
en/Global-Cosmetic-Products-Market-Sha
re-Expected-To-Reach-863-Billion-by-202
4-ZMR.html (accessed September 5, 2019).

7. H Hojjat, R Raad, J Lucas, et al. Public
perception of facial fillers. *Facial Plast Surg*
2019; **35**: 204–209.

8. JC Bensoussan, MA Bolton, S Pi, et al.
Quality of life before and after cosmetic
surgery. *CNS Spectr* 2014; **19**: 282–292.

9. T von Soest, IL Kvalem, KC Skolleborg, HE
Roald. Psychosocial changes after cosmetic
surgery: a 5-year follow-up study. *Plast
Reconstr Surg* 2011; **128**: 765–772.

10. B Ristow. Facial rejuvenation included
maintaining all the patient's natural fat
(except under the chin), elevation of low
eyebrows, eyelid operations and
restoration of the natural fullness of the
lips. 2019. https://commons.wikimedia
.org/wiki/File:Face_Lift_01_Dr._Ristow.jpg
(accessed September 1, 2019).

11. D Scharschmidt, U Mirastschijski, S Preiss,
et al. Body image, personality traits, and
quality of life in botulinum toxin A and
dermal filler patients. *Aesthetic Plast Surg*
2018; 42(4): 1119–1125.

12. A Roche, PM Sedgwick, CC Harland. Laser
treatment for female facial hirsutism: are
quality-of-life benefits sustainable? *Clin
Exp Dermatol* 2016; **41**: 248–252.

13. American Society of Plastic Surgeons.
Rhytidectomy. 2019. www.plasticsurgery
.org/cosmetic-procedures/facelift
(accessed September 1, 2019).

14. American Society of Plastic Surgeons.
Rhinoplasty. 2019. www.plasticsurgery
.org/cosmetic-procedures/rhinoplasty
(accessed September 1, 2019).

15. American Society of Plastic Surgeons.
Tummy tuck, 2019. www.plasticsurgery
.org/cosmetic-procedures/tummy-tuck
(accessed September 1, 2019).

16. American Society of Plastic Surgeons.
Liposuction. 2019. www.plasticsurgery
.org/cosmetic-procedures/liposuction
(accessed September 1, 2019).

17. American Society of Plastic Surgeons.
Breast. 2019. www.plasticsurgery.org/

cosmetic-procedures (accessed September
1, 2019).

18. M Delgado. Mommy makeover. 2019.
https://commons.wikimedia.org/wiki/File:
Mommy_Makeover_Patient_3_periopera
tive_photo.jpg; https://commons.wikime
dia.org/wiki/File:Mommy_Makeover_Pati
ent_3_post-op_photo.jpg (accessed
September 1, 2019).

19. RJ Honigman, KA Phillips, DJ Castle. A
review of psychosocial outcomes for
patients seeking cosmetic surgery. *Plast
Reconstr Surg* 2004; **113**: 1229–1237.

20. MC Alves, LE Abla, A Santos Rde, LM
Ferreira. Quality of life and self-esteem
outcomes following rhytidoplasty. *Ann
Plast Surg* 2005; **54**: 511–514.

21. E Floyd, SW Perkins. The past, present and
future of facial plastic and reconstructive
surgery: facelift. *Facial Plast Surg* 2019; **35**:
353–357.

22. AK Alderman, J Bauer, D Fardo, et al.
Understanding the effect of breast
augmentation on quality of life:
prospective analysis using the BREAST-Q.
Plast Reconstr Surg 2014; **133**: 787–795.

23. Y Kececi, E Sir, M Gungor. Patient-reported
quality-of-life outcomes of breast reduction
evaluated with generic questionnaires and
the breast reduction assessed severity scale.
Aesthet Surg J 2015; **35**: 48–54.

24. N Bertozzi, M Pesce, P Santi, E Raposio.
One-stage immediate breast
reconstruction: a concise review. *BioMed
Res Int* 2017; **20**: 5058–5066.

25. M Sollie. Management of gynecomastia:
changes in psychological aspects after
surgery – a systematic review. *Gland Surg*
2018; 7: S70–S76.

26. C Rudolph, C Hladik, DF Stroup, et al. Are
cosmetic procedures comparable to
antidepressive medication for quality-of-
life improvements? A systematic review
and controlled meta-analysis. *Facial Plast
Surg* 2019; **35**: 549–558.

27. CN Kraus, LW Chapman, DZ Korta, CB
Zachary. Quality of life outcomes
associated with treatment of human
immunodeficiency virus (HIV) facial

lipoatrophy. *Int J Dermatol* 2016; 55: 1311–1320.

28. TH Osaki, MH Osaki. Eyelid make-up to manage transient blepharoptosis after botulinum toxin injection. *Aesthet Surg J* 2018; **38**(1): NP16–NP18.

29. N Roche, R Zory, A Sauthier, et al. Effect of rehabilitation and botulinum toxin injection on gait in chronic stroke patients: a randomized controlled study. *J Rehabil Med* 2015; **47**: 31–37.

30. F Kuroda, C Urban, G Zucca, et al. Evaluation of aesthetic and quality-of-life results after immediate breast reconstruction with definitive form-stable anatomical implants. *Plast Reconstr Surg* 2016; **137**(2): 278e–286e.

31. T Zhong, J Hu, S Bagher, A Vo, et al. A comparison of psychological response, body image, sexuality, and quality of life between immediate and delayed autologous tissue breast reconstruction: a prospective long-term outcome study. *Plast Reconstr Surg* 2016; **138**: 772–780.

32. MK Kim, T Kim, HG Moon, et al. Effect of cosmetic outcome on quality of life after breast cancer surgery. *Eur J Surg Oncol* 2015; **41**: 426–432.

33. B Azizzadeh. Photo gallery before and after undergoing facial paralysis surgery in with Babak Azizzadeh, MD, FACS. 2019. www.facialparalysisinstitute.com/photo-gallery (accessed September 5, 2019).

34. V Quinzi, ET Scibetta, E Marchetti, et al. Analyze my face. *J Biol Regul Homeost Agents* 2018; **32**: 149–158.

35. TF Cash, K Dawson, P Davis, M Bowen, C Galumbeck. Effects of cosmetics use on the physical attractiveness and body image of American college women. *J Social Psychol* 1989; **129**(3): 349–355.

36. J Richetin, J Croizet, P Huguet. Facial make-up elicits positive attitudes at the implicit level: evidence from the implicit association test. *Curr Res Social Psychol* 2004; **9**(11): 145–164.

37. R Palumbo, B Fairfield, N Mammarella, A Di Domenico. Does make-up make you feel smarter? The "lipstick effect" extended to academic achievement. *Cogent Psychol* 2017; **4**(1): 1327635.

38. K Fujiwara, Y Furuta, W Aoki, et al. Make-up therapy for patients with facial nerve palsy. *Ann Otol Rhinol Laryngol* 2019; **128** (8): 721–727.

39. K Hoffman. Amazing results of feeling confident in what you wear – otherwise known as ensemble empowerment. 2015. www.bustle.com/articles/64781–6-amazing-results-of-feeling-confident-in-what-you-wear-otherwise-known-as-ensemble-empowerment (accessed September 5, 2019).

40. V Leblanc. How what you're wearing can affect your anxiety. 2018. www.calmclinic.com/anxiety/clothing-matters (accessed September 5, 2019).

41. Stich Fix. Home page. 2019. www.stitchfix.com (accessed September 5, 2019).

42. A Mikhail. The Stīl Trust. 2019. www.thestiltrust.com (accessed September 5, 2019).

Massage, Humor, and Music

Soo Liang Ooi and Sok Cheon Pak

Massage

Massage is the therapeutic manipulation of the body's soft tissue in a patterned and purposeful way [1]. It is a form of healing, with various ancient civilizations, including Egyptian, Chinese, Indian, and Greek, developing different systems of massage throughout history. Modern Western massage therapy can trace its roots to two Europeans, Pehr Henrik Ling (1776–1839) of Sweden, who developed Swedish massage techniques, and Johann Mezger (1838–1909) of Amsterdam, who invented a system of soft tissue manipulation known as remedial massage [2].

Today, massage is one of the most commonly used complementary therapies worldwide [3]. Approximately 12.8 percent of American adults have visited massage therapists at least once, and 6.8 percent of them visited a massage therapist in the past 12 months, not only for wellness and general disease prevention, but also to address specific health problems. A majority of users (69.4 percent) believed that massage can be combined with medical treatment to help their health conditions [4].

Effects and Mechanisms of Massage

Current evidence points toward four main beneficial effects of massage: to reduce stress and anxiety; to alleviate pain; to aid in tissue repair; and to enhance immunity. Although the underlying mechanisms of how massage achieves these health effects have not been fully understood, there is enough research to support some informed suppositions.

Reduce stress and anxiety. Massage is believed to promote relaxation by stimulating the parasympathetic branch of the autonomic nervous system, which facilitates the return to homeostasis from a stressful "fight-or-flight" state. A single treatment of massage can significantly lower salivary cortisol and heart rate, whereas multiple treatments of massage appear to lower diastolic blood pressure [5]. Massage also elevates levels of serotonin and dopamine. This explains why one generally feels "good" immediately after a massage, and multiple massage treatments help to alleviate anxiety and depressive symptoms [6].

Alleviate pain. The nerve "gates" to painful input can be suppressed by stimulation of non-painful sensations transmitted through the large nerve fibers to the spinal cord. Massage is a potent mechanical stimulus and an effective trigger to "close the gates" of pain sensations [7]. The mechanical force from massage also initiates a cascade of neurophysiological responses from the peripheral and central nervous systems, such as the release of β-endorphin and anandamide, lessening of temporal summation, alteration of inflammatory mediators, as well as stimulation of autonomic responses [8]. Such complex interactions lead to observed clinical outcomes of pain reduction.

Aid in tissue repair. Damage to skeletal muscle triggers an injury–repair–regeneration cascade that is associated with inflammatory processes. Massage initiates a mechanical transduction to reduce cellular infiltration by mast cells and subsequent inflammation and edema. It influences a phenotypic change in which the M1 macrophage transitions to the M2 macrophage that secretes anti-inflammatory products which in turn facilitate tissue regeneration and increased recovery of function [9].

Enhance immunity. Beyond alteration of the inflammatory signaling pathway, massage also affects innate immunity, especially the activity of natural killer cells [10]. Natural killer cell activity increases after a series of massage treatments, even though the number of natural killer cells remains the same [10]. The greater natural killer cell activity plays a role in enhancing the body's ability to ward off pathogens and malignancies.

Massage for Different Populations and Conditions

Massage is generally safe when it is applied by a qualified practitioner. Besides general wellness, research has shown it to be beneficial in many different groups of populations and conditions. Table 33.1 summarizes some of these benefits.

Summary

Massage is one of the most commonly used complementary therapies worldwide. Besides helping to reduce stress and manage pain, massage can also promote tissue healing and enhance immunity. It is widely utilized in diverse populations ranging from infants to older adults, not only for wellness and disease prevention purposes, but also for treatment of specific conditions such as chronic pain and cancer.

Humor

Humor is defined in the *Oxford Dictionary* to be either "the quality of being amusing or comic" or "a state of mind." Humor has been in the human behavioral repertoire for thousands or even millions of years. It is an extension to language and is considered the most complex cognitive function of humans that augments social abilities [20]. Humor often leads to laughter but does not equate to laughter, since laughter can also be elicited in the absence of humor, such as through tickling or intentional simulation. Nevertheless, humor and laughter are often inseparable when applied in health and wellness practices.

The healing power of humor has been recognized since ancient times, as referenced in the Bible, "A joyful heart is a good medicine, but a crushed spirit dries up the bones" (Proverbs 17:22). However, the interest in applying humor as an intervention in modern medicine is only a recent phenomenon. The personal account of how Norman Cousins "laughed his way out" of ankylosing spondylitis, a crippling and irreversible disease, was published in 1976. Cousins claimed laughter to be a reliable painkiller and episodes of laughter resulted in the reduction of inflammatory biomarkers [21]. Since the early 1970s, Hunter "Patch" Adams has devoted his life to bringing love and humor into hospital settings. His unique approach has seen the development of clown therapy, which has become an important aspect of hospital pediatric care [22]. Madan Kataria, an Indian

Table 33.1 Beneficial effects of massage in different populations and conditions

Population/condition	Beneficial effects of massage
Infants	Massage helps to improve weight gain in preterm infants. Massaging newborns with tender touch also has the positive effects of better sleep–wake patterns, enhanced neuromotor development, better emotional bonding, and reduced rates of infection in hospitals [11].
Children and adolescents	Massage appears to be beneficial in addressing emotional distress and reducing pain and side effects of chemotherapy treatment in children with cancer [12]. Massage also demonstrated benefits for children/adolescents with autistic spectrum disorders, attention-deficit/hyperactivity disorder, anxiety and depression, asthma, and aggression [13].
Pregnancy and labor	Women who received massage during pregnancy reported less depression, anxiety, leg pain, and back pain. The rates of premature birth and low birth weight were also lowered. During labor, massage significantly reduces pain and the need for pain medication [14].
Older adults	Older adults often seek massage to manage pain and improve function. Improvement of arthritis, constipation, loss of balance, insomnia, and depression has also been reported. Massage also potentially assists in reducing agitated behaviors associated with dementia. It is a popular palliative care treatment to improve quality of life [15].
Sports	Massage is extensively utilized in sport medicine to assist athletes in event preparation to reduce pre-game anxiety as well as improve strength and flexibility to enhance performance. It aids recovery after competition through preventing or decreasing the impact of delayed onset muscle soreness. Theoretically, massage can help to increase blood flow and the clearance of lactic acid to accelerate recovery. Massage is also used in sport injuries and rehabilitation to achieve better treatment outcomes [16].
Chronic pain	Massage is strongly recommended as a pain management option for many chronic pain conditions, notably lower back, neck and shoulder pain, headache, fibromyalgia, and arthritis. Evidence suggests massage helps to reduce pain intensity/severity and anxiety, as well as to improve function and quality of life when compared to no treatment [17].
Cancer	Massage therapy complements conventional cancer treatment by offering a human touch to ease the emotional distress of cancer patients. Increasingly, massage therapy is being integrated into protocols at cancer treatment centers [18]. Positive effects of massage in cancer care include relieving fatigue, pain, anxiety, and nausea while promoting relaxation, improving sleep, and enhancing immune responses [19].

physician, created laughter yoga, which uses simulated laughing exercise to eventually generate real laughter in an individual or a group. Since 1995, laughter Yoga has spawned the creation of laughter clubs worldwide [23].

Effects and Mechanisms of Humor

Despite its popular application in healthcare settings, research into the therapeutic effects of humor and its mechanisms remains sparse. Rod Martin postulated that humor and laughter may exert positive effects through four potential mechanisms [24].

Beneficial physiological changes. A hearty laugh improves muscle tone. It elevates heart rate and disrupts the normal breathing pattern, which increases blood oxygenation as seen with aerobic exercise. Laughter also impacts the immune system via changes to the circulating catecholamines and cortisol levels. After laughter, relaxation is experienced, and the effect can last up to 45 minutes [25].

Positive emotional state. The health significance of positive emotions is well recognized. The positive emotions, as accompanied by humor and laughter, not only dispel low moods but also have analgesic, immune-enhancing effects, as well as an antagonistic effect on the cardiovascular sequelae of negative emotions [24].

Stress modulating effect. Humor, or a humorous outlook on life, moderates the degree to which individuals appraise threatening and stressful conditions and thus has the effect of reducing the degree to which stress would normally affect health adversely [24].

Social support. Humor can foster satisfying social relationships. The greater levels of social support resulting from these relationships may confer stress-buffering and health-enhancing effects [24].

Humor for Different Populations and Conditions

Humor in healthcare settings is well appreciated by patients [26] and may facilitate a social connection between doctors and patients to allow easier discussions of difficult topics [27]. Humor and laughter can also be readily embraced as a complementary therapy without the concerns of dose, side effects, interactions, or allergies, as per other medical therapies [28]. The health benefits of humor have been examined in various population settings to address different conditions, as listed in Table 33.2.

Summary

As the saying goes, "laughter is the best medicine." Even though empirical studies to support the use of humor and laughter as an intervention for specific conditions remain scarce, with limited adverse effects and easy prescription, humor should be a part of any wellness program to promote joy and its healing effects.

Music

Music is linked to emotions. When we listen to mellow tunes that move us, we feel happy or relaxed due to an increase in neurochemical levels and activation of brain regions that respond to pleasure and rewards. Conversely, sad music has been shown to invoke regions

Table 33.2 Beneficial effects of humor in different populations and conditions

Population/condition	Beneficial effects of humor
Children	A 2016 systematic review found clown therapy played a significant role in reducing anxiety in hospitalized children and their parents [29]. A newer study also reported that humor therapy had beneficial effects in lowering stress levels in hospitalized children compared to no intervention [30].
Older adults	Laughter yoga, laughter qigong, and laughter exercise are interventions that can enhance the well-being of older adults aged 60 and above, as reported by a systematic review of five studies [31]. A cross-sectional study of 20,934 older Japanese adults found a higher daily frequency of laughter to be associated with a lower prevalence of heart diseases and stroke [32].
Palliative care	Humor is essential in palliative care, with the key functions of building relationships, managing circumstances, and expressing sensitivity. Humor produces relaxation, reduces pain, and helps cope with symptoms. However, there are situations in which the use of humor is to be avoided, such as during coma or near death [33].
Mental health	Laughter yoga helps to improve depressive moods but its effects on stress, anxiety, and general well-being remain unclear [34]. Even though empirical studies are still lacking, humor and laughter have been used as both individual and group psychotherapy for serious mental illnesses such as major depression or schizophrenia [35].
Cancer	Laughter therapy in cancer patients was found to be beneficial to reduce the stress, anxiety, and depression that affects cancer patients. The use of laughter therapy reportedly helps to improve the quality of life of cancer patients [36].

of the brain implicated in negative affective states and anxiety [37]. Because music has such an impact on one's emotions, it has been used clinically in managing psychological and physiological conditions.

Even though music is an old cure, with its use for therapeutic purposes probably dating to the Paleolithic period [38], the interest in music therapy research is only a recent phenomenon. In a pioneering article published in 1977, Marian Palmer described a variety of music therapy techniques aimed to improve physical and mental functioning in elderly residents, implying the potential medical effectiveness of those techniques [39].

Today, music therapy is widely utilized in many sectors, including hospital, mental care, aged care, early childhood, and home care.

Effects and Mechanisms of Music

As the knowledge base of scientific evidence supporting music therapy for well-being is expanding, it is becoming clear that these effects impact different aspects of the human organism, notwithstanding that the underlying mechanisms are still poorly understood.

Reduce anxiety. A meta-analysis of 19 studies found listening to music decreased self-reported anxiety in a non-clinical population with a medium effect size (Cohen's $d = 0.3$) [40]. Relaxing music has the ability to relieve patients' anxiety levels before surgery, with significant reductions in heart rate variability and mean heart rate [41].

Reduce pain. Music is widely used during dressing changes and debridement to help pain and anxiety in burn patients. A recent systematic review found a positive correlation between music interventions and pain alleviation in burn patients [42]. It is suggested that music can positively modify the release of cortisol [43], which is beneficial for healing.

Increase muscle force. Most research findings report positive effects of music on athletes' perceived exertion and performance. High-tempo music for high-intensity exercise increased muscle peak power and mean power [44], providing additional evidence for the importance of including music during warm-up before a major competition.

Synchronize with cerebral rhythms. Music can cause immediate emotional responses by stimulating different sensory pathways. By tracking physiological variables such as heart rate, respiration, blood pressure, middle cerebral artery flow velocity, and skin vasomotor tone with music emphasis and rhythmic phrases, autonomic responses were found to synchronize with music, which might therefore convey emotions through autonomic arousal during crescendos or rhythmic phrases [45].

Music for Different Conditions

With contemporary pharmacotherapy options merely providing symptomatic alleviation, presenting with undesirable side effects, and increasing burden on the public healthcare system, the professional practice of music therapy has gained momentum as a treatment approach for many conditions, especially for mental care, in recent years. We present the latest evidence-based information of music therapy drawn from the scientific literature (Table 33.3).

Summary

Music itself is potentially healing. The application of music therapy as an adjunct to address many conditions such as dementia and depression is promising. Providing music to patients suffering from medical conditions can be a cost-effective and feasible strategy to improve unpleasant symptoms. Music can be more widely applied to enhance the health and wellness of patients.

Conclusion

Massage, humor, and music are wellness medicines applied through different sensory inputs, but impacting the body and mind in many similar ways. Reducing stress, anxiety, and pain, elevating mood, enhancing the immune system, and promoting a better quality of life are some of their common benefits. They have been shown to improve the physical, emotional, and mental well-being of patients of different ages and conditions. With limited or no side effects and wide accessibility, they should be incorporated into a range of wellness treatment plans.

Table 33.3 Beneficial effects of music in different conditions

Condition	Beneficial effects of music
Dementia	Receptive music therapy is found be more effective than interactive music therapy in reducing agitation, behavioral problems, and anxiety in patients with dementia. The use of receptive music therapy is recommended in nursing homes, daycare centers, and home care, given its easy and convenient implementation [46].
Depression	A Cochrane review found music therapy to provide short-term beneficial effects for people with depression. Music therapy added to usual treatment seems to improve depressive symptoms better compared to usual treatment alone. Music therapy also shows efficacy in decreasing anxiety levels and improving the functioning of depressed individuals [47].
Alzheimer's disease	Music therapy has beneficial impacts on cognition (memory, attention, language) and behavior (anxiety, depression, and agitation) in patients with Alzheimer's disease [48]. A community-based music therapy support group was found to improve memory, movement, language, and socialization for Alzheimer's disease patients. Through the increase of meaningful interactions with loved ones with disease, music therapy was reported to relieve some of the strain on caregivers [49].
Parkinson's disease	Music therapy has beneficial effects for motor/non-motor symptoms and quality of life of people with Parkinson's disease [50]. A meta-analysis of six studies found music-based movement therapy to be a promising intervention to improve gait and gait-related activities in Parkinson's disease [51].
Schizophrenia	A longitudinal study assessed the effects of listening to Mozart on insular functional connectivity in patients with schizophrenia. Patients who received a one-month music intervention with antipsychotic drugs showed increased functional connectivity in the dorsal anterior insula and posterior insular networks compared to those with no music intervention [52].
Cancer	A randomized trial on the effects of music therapy in women with breast or gynecological cancer found it to be effective to reduce radiotherapy-induced fatigue as well as to improve quality of life [53].
Fibromyalgia	Music has been found to control pain in fibromyalgia patients [54]. When combined with imagery or with low-impact aerobic exercise, music was found to reduce anxiety, depression, and general discomfort while improving well-being and quality of life in patients with fibromyalgia [55, 56].

References

1. AB Kennedy, JA Cambron, PA Sharpe, RS Travillian, RP Saunders. Clarifying definitions for the massage therapy profession: the results of the best practices symposium. *Int J Ther Massage Bodyw Res Educ Pract* 2016; **9** (3): 15–26.

2. PJ Benjamin. Historical overview. In: T Dryden, CA Moyer, eds., *Massage Therapy: Integrating Research and Practice.* Champaign, IL, Human Kinetics; 2012; 3–13.

3. PE Harris, KL Cooper, C Relton, KJ Thomas. Prevalence of visits to massage therapists by the general population:

a systematic review. *Complement Ther Clin Pract* 2014; **20**(1): 16–20.

4. T Sundberg, H Cramer, D Sibbritt, J Adams, R Lauche. Prevalence, patterns, and predictors of massage practitioner utilization: results of a US nationally representative survey. *Musculoskelet Sci Pract* 2017; **32**: 31–37.

5. A Moraska, RA Pollini, K Boulanger, MZ Brooks, L Teitlebaum. Physiological adjustments to stress measures following massage therapy: a review of the literature. *Evidence-Based Complement Altern Med* 2010; **7**(4): 409–418.

6. T Field, M Hernandez-Reif, M Diego, S Schanberg, C Kuhn. Cortisol decreases and serotonin and dopamine increase following massage therapy. *Int J Neurosci* 2005; **115**(10): 1397–1413.

7. GC Goats. Massage: the scientific basis of an ancient art: Part 2. Physiological and therapeutic effects. *Br J Sports Med* 1994; **28**(3): 153–156.

8. JE Bialosky, MD Bishop, DD Price, ME Robinson, SZ George. The mechanisms of manual therapy in the treatment of musculoskeletal pain: a comprehensive model. *Man Ther* 2009; **14**(5): 531–538.

9. C Waters-Banker, EE Dupont-Versteegden, PH Kitzman, TA Butterfield. Investigating the mechanisms of massage efficacy: the role of mechanical immunomodulation. *J Athl Train* 2014; **49**(2): 266–273.

10. T Field. Massage therapy research review. *Complement Ther Clin Pract* 2016; **24**: 19–31.

11. A Kulkarni, JS Kaushik, P Gupta, H Sharma, RK Agrawal. Massage and touch therapy in neonates: the current evidence. *Indian Pediatr* 2010; **47**(9): 771–776.

12. J Rodríguez-Mansilla, B González-Sánchez, S Torres-Piles, et al. Effects of the application of therapeutic massage in children with cancer: a systematic review. *Rev Lat Am Enfermagem* 2017 **8**(25): e2903.

13. S Shipwright. Pediatrics. In: T Dryden CA Moyer, eds., *Massage Therapy: Integrating Research and Practice.* Champaign, IL, Human Kinetics; 2012; 90–101.

14. T Field. Pregnancy and labor massage. *Expert Rev Obstet Gynecol* 2010; **5**(2): 177–181.

15. DL Thompson. Massage and older adults. In: T Dryden, CA Moyer, eds., *Massage Therapy: Integrating Research and Practice.* Champaign, IL, Human Kinetics; 2012. 130–143.

16. J Brummitt. The role of massage in sports performance and rehabilitation: current evidence and future direction. *N Am J Sports Phys Ther* 2008; **3**(1): 7–21.

17. C Crawford, C Boyd, CF Paat, et al. The impact of massage therapy on function in pain populations: a systematic review and meta-analysis of randomized controlled trials. Part I, patients experiencing pain in the general population. *Pain Med* 2016; **17**(7): 1353–1375.

18. VS Cowen, B Tafuto. Integration of massage therapy in outpatient cancer care. *Int J Ther Massage Bodywork* 2018; **11**(1): 4–10.

19. NC Russell, S-S Sumler, CM Beinhorn, MA Frenkel. Role of massage therapy in cancer care. *J Altern Complement Med* 2008; **14**(2): 209–214.

20. R Polimeni. The first joke: exploring the evolutionary origins of humor. *Evol Psychol* 2006; **4**: 347–366.

21. N Cousins. Anatomy of an illness (as perceived by the patient). *N Engl J Med* 1976; **295**(26): 1458–1463.

22. A Boscarelli. Clown therapy: not only a pediatric matter. *Transl Pediatr* 2017; **6**(2): 111–112.

23. MA Woodbury-Fariña, MM Rodríguez Schwabe. Laughter yoga: benefits of mixing laughter and yoga. *J Yoga Phys Ther* 2015; **5**(4). DOI:10.4172/2157-7595.1000209.

24. RA Martin. Humor, laughter, and physical health: methodological issues and research findings. *Psychol Bull* 2001; **127**: 504–519.

25. MP Bennett, C Lengacher. Humor and laughter may influence health: III. Laughter and health outcomes. *Evidence-based Complement Altern Med* 2008; **5**(1): 37–40.

26. M Mccreaddie, S Payne. Humour in health-care interactions: a risk worth taking. *Heal Expect* 2014; **17**(3): 332–344.

27. KA Phillips, N Singh Ospina, R Rodriguez-Gutierrez, et al. Humor during clinical practice: analysis of recorded clinical encounters. *J Am Board Fam Med* 2018; **31** (2): 270–278.

28. WB Strean, C Chaplin. Laughter prescription. *Can Fam Physician* 2009; **55**: 965–967.

29. K Sridharan, G Sivaramakrishnan. Therapeutic clowns in pediatrics: a systematic review and meta-analysis of randomized controlled trials. *Eur J Pediatr* 2016; **175**(10): 1353–1360.

30. JC Sánchez, LF Echeverri, MJ Londoño, et al. Effects of a humor therapy program on stress levels in pediatric inpatients. *Hosp Pediatr* 2017; **7**(1): 46–53.

31. FN Gonot-Schoupinsky, G Garip. Laughter and humour interventions for well-being in older adults: a systematic review and intervention classification. *Complement Ther Med* 2018; **38**: 85–91.

32. K Hayashi, I Kawachi, T Ohira, et al. Laughter is the best medicine? A cross-sectional study of cardiovascular disease among older Japanese adults. *J Epidemiol* 2016; **26**(10): 546–552.

33. C Pinna, V Mahtani-chugani. The use of humor in palliative care: a systematic literature review. *Am J Hosp Palliat Med* 2018; **35**(10): 1342–1354.

34. D Bressington, C Yu, W Wong, TC Ng, WT Chien. The effects of group-based laughter yoga interventions on mental health in adults: a systematic review. *J Psychiatr Mental Health Nurs* 2018; **25**(8): 517–527.

35. M Gelkopf. The use of humor in serious mental illness: a review. *Evidence-based Complement Altern Med* 2011. DOI:10.1093/ecam/nep106.

36. M Demir. Effects of laughter therapy on anxiety, stress, depression and quality of life in cancer patients. *J Cancer Sci Ther* 2015; **7**(9): 272–273.

37. P Vuilleumier, W Trost. Music and emotions: from enchantment to entrainment. *Ann N Y Acad Sci* 2015; **1337**(1): 212–222.

38. MR Montinari, S Giardina, P Minelli, S Minelli. History of music therapy and its contemporary applications in cardiovascular diseases. *South Med J* 2018; **111**(2): 98–102.

39. MD Palmer. Music therapy in a comprehensive program of treatment and rehabilitation for the geriatric resident. *J Music Ther* 1977; **14**(4): 190–197.

40. Y Panteleeva, G Ceschi, D Glowinski, DS Courvoisier, D Grandjean. Music for anxiety? Meta-analysis of anxiety reduction in non-clinical samples. *Psychol Music* 2018; **46**(4): 473–487.

41. K-C Lee, Y-H Chao, J-J Yiin, et al. Evidence that music listening reduces preoperative patients' anxiety. *Biol Res Nurs* 2012; **14**(1): 78–84.

42. J Li, L Zhou, Y Wang. The effects of music intervention on burn patients during treatment procedures: a systematic review and meta-analysis of randomized controlled trials. *BMC Complement Altern Med* 2017; **17**(1): 158.

43. R Rahimi, M Ghaderi, MA Azarbayjani. The effect of motivational and relaxation music on aerobic performance, rating perceived exertion and salivary cortisol in athlete males. *South African J Res Sport Phys Educ Recreat* 2009; **31**(2): 29–38.

44. M Jarraya, H Chtourou, A Aloui, et al. The effects of music on high-intensity short-term exercise in well trained athletes. *Asian J Sport Med* 2012; **3**(4): 233–238.

45. B Luciano, P Cesare, C Gaia, B Rossella, et al. Dynamic interactions between musical, cardiovascular, and cerebral rhythms in humans. *Circulation* 2009; **119** (25): 3171–3180.

46. KKF Tsoi, JYC Chan, Y-M Ng, et al. Receptive music therapy is more effective

than interactive music therapy to relieve behavioral and psychological symptoms of dementia: a systematic review and meta-analysis. *J Am Med Dir Assoc* 2018; **19** (7): 568–576.e3.

47. S Aalbers, L Fusar-Poli, RE Freeman, et al. Music therapy for depression. *Cochrane Database Syst Rev* 2017. DOI:10.1002/14651858.CD004517.pub3.

48. N García-Casares, RM Moreno-Leiva, JA García-Arnés. Music therapy as a non-pharmacological treatment in Alzheimer's disease: a systematic review. *Rev Neurol* 2017; **65**(12): 529–538.

49. R Rio. A community-based music therapy support group for people with Alzheimer's disease and their caregivers: a sustainable partnership model. *Front Med* 2018. DOI:10.3389/fmed.2018.00293.

50. N García-Casares, JE Martín-Colom, JA García-Arnés. Music therapy in Parkinson's disease. *J Am Med Dir Assoc* 2018; **19**(12): 1054–1062.

51. MJ de Dreu, ASD van der Wilk, E Poppe, G Kwakkel, EEH van Wegen. Rehabilitation, exercise therapy and music in patients with Parkinson's disease: a meta-analysis of the effects of music-based movement therapy on walking ability, balance and quality of life. *Parkinsonism Relat Disord* 2012; **18**: S114–S119.

52. H He, M Yang, M Duan, et al. Music intervention leads to increased insular connectivity and improved clinical symptoms in schizophrenia. *Front Neurosci* 2018; **23**(11): 744.

53. TR Alcântara-Silva, R de Freitas-Junior, NMA Freitas, et al. Music therapy reduces radiotherapy-induced fatigue in patients with breast or gynecological cancer: a randomized trial. *Integr Cancer Ther* 2018; **17**(3): 628–635.

54. G Alparslan, B Babadağ, A Özkaraman, et al. Effects of music on pain in patients with fibromyalgia. *Clin Rheumatol* 2016; **35** (5): 1317–1321.

55. GV Espí-López, M Inglés, M-A Ruescas-Nicolau, N Moreno-Segura. Effect of low-impact aerobic exercise combined with music therapy on patients with fibromyalgia: a pilot study. *Complement Ther Med* 2016; **28**: 1–7.

56. E Torres, IN Pedersen, JI Pérez-Fernández. Randomized trial of a group music and imagery method (GrpMI) for women with fibromyalgia. *J Music Ther* 2018; **55**(2): 186–220.

Nature and Pets

Vinathe Sharma-Brymer, Katherine Dashper, and Eric Brymer

Introduction

In recent years, research has shown that nature and pets have a profound impact on positive wellness outcomes and lifestyle behaviors. In this chapter, we provide evidence for the importance of nature and pets, otherwise referred to as companion animals, in facilitating human wellness, and point to the implications of this evidence for the development of policy and practice initiatives. Specifically, we argue that nature and pets have important roles in the initiation and enhancement of wellness lifestyle habits and outcomes across multiple wellness domains. Evidence indicates that interacting with nature and pets positively influences emotional, intellectual, spiritual, physical, occupational, and social wellness [1]. Viewing pictures and videos of nature, being active in the presence of nature, and immersive experiences in nature have proven to have resulted in enhanced levels of wellness. Equally, interacting with pets in various contexts, such as hospitals and homes, supports wellness in ways that cannot be replicated by other means. A better understanding of the implications of the outcomes gained from interacting with nature and pets has tremendous potential for improving current policies and professional practice in fields such as healthcare, education, and the built environment/architecture, and the potential to support new developments that are inclusive of nature and pets.

Nature

The idea of nature is often associated with images of wide-open spaces, tree covered landscapes, savannas, or mountain ranges. However, in a wellness context, nature is often defined more broadly to allow for multiple interpretations of how nature is experienced and to encompass multiple ways of being in or with nature. In a wellness context, "nature could be a plant sitting on an apartment ledge in midtown New York city, the pristine Olympic National Park in Washington, or a community park on the outskirts of San Diego" [2]. For the most part, research indicates two broad mechanisms that underpin how human–nature relationships enhance wellness. The first, feelings of connection to nature, has been associated with high wellness behaviors and outcomes. The second mechanism, physical activity in nature, encompasses a range of activities from being active indoors while viewing videos or pictures of nature to multi-day immersive experiences in nature. Activity in the presence of nature, such as walking in a park or gardening, has been linked to high level of wellness outcomes.

A review carried out in 2010 [1] determined that human interactions with nonhuman nature and feeling connected to nature have profound impact on holistic wellness that stem from a sense of belonging facilitated by the restoration of the human–nature relationship.

Humans are understood as part of nature and nature experiences are opportunities for restoring mental fatigue, nurturing, and for facilitating deep reflection. The growing evidence base for the acceptance of nature as important for human wellness is reflected internationally through policy initiatives such as the United Nations Sustainable Development Goals (Goal 3), the UK government's 25-year plan for the environment (which focuses on human wellness from nature interactions), and the Australian government's 2018–2030 draft plan for the environment, which also focuses on the wellness outcomes from more effective human–nature relationships. The growing evidence base has also triggered practitioner involvement and increases in the intensity of calls from a variety of sectors (such as psychology, sports science, tourism, health, forestry, wildlife, and conservation) for normalizing engagement with nature as a singular, incomparable, fundamental factor in the development of positive health and wellness lifestyles and wellness outcomes. For example, Reece and Myers [3] advocated for the integration of eco-wellness in counseling. They observed that despite the plethora of research supporting the importance of nature in the development of holistic human wellness, models of wellness rarely integrated nature-based experiences in counseling contexts. They argued that nature experiences should be integral to counseling practice, especially as they had the potential to influence lifelong wellness behaviors in a meaningful manner. The American Public Health Association [4], in its policy statement on the beneficial influence of nature on human health and wellness, stated that public health professionals should advise patients and the broader public on the benefits of green exercise (physical activity in natural spaces such as urban or near-urban parks), gardening, nature play, and nature-based recreational activities (e.g., bird watching, fishing, and outdoor and adventure activities). Nature has even been promoted as important for effectiveness in high-performance settings such as hospitals. For example, research on staff at a post-surgical unit [5] recommended increased opportunities for contact with indoor, outdoor, and indirect nature features to reduce the impact of the high stress experienced at work. These recommendations, at both practitioner and policy levels within the health sector, illuminate the importance of nature contact for human wellness and the importance of evidence-based research and policy recommendations for the promotion of good practice.

There is now a considerable sound research base evidencing that feeling connected to nature enhances holistic wellness. This is the case even if opportunities to interact with nature are not immediately apparent [6]. According to Nisbet et al. [7], nature connection describes the experience of cognitive, affective, and experiential connection with the rest of nature. An individual who feels part of nature, who feels that nature is part of their self-identity, and who feels comfortable in natural settings is more likely to experience high levels of wellness [6]. Chawla [8] reviewed research emerging in the last four decades on nature connection and its impact on children's health and well-being. She determined that opportunities to interact with nature improved connection to nature which in turn improved holistic wellness. Nature features, natural landscape, green areas, parks, and rough ground for creative play are essential components of children's overall wellness. An evaluation of a supported nature play program for young children in Australia [9] found that the program enhanced interpersonal relationships and emotional wellness. Immersion in and with nature in childhood years may have beneficial effects on overall wellness in adulthood.

A multidisciplinary synthesis of the literature undertaken by Russell et al. [10] confirmed that interacting with nature had improved physical and mental wellness. The evidence reported highlighted that human wellness was impacted most profoundly through personal experiences of being in nature and interacting with nature. The influence of nature on human wellness seems greater when nature is perceived as providing opportunities for actions rather than when nature is perceived purely as an aesthetic reflection of beauty. For example, Fiskum and Jacobsen [11] found that a number of affordances (opportunities for action) in nature benefited psychological and emotional wellness in childhood. Watching a river flow, or doing hands-on activities like constructing a shelter with fallen twigs, branches, and rocks, can influence relaxation, calmness, togetherness, joy, and satisfaction, adding to holistic wellness. Sandseter [12] found that early childhood experiences with nature provided important affordances for resolving challenges, emotional health, and learning which had a long-term impact on wellness into adulthood. In summary, the natural environment provides rich affordances for experiencing connection, motivating physical activity, and promoting activities directly linked to holistic wellness, not available in contexts void of nature [13]. The education sector would benefit from incorporating programs of nature connection in school curricula for holistic wellness in childhood, which might continue into adulthood as positive experiences.

While not extensively studied, promotion of close interaction with any form of nature (plants in office settings, urban green spaces, extensive natural landscapes, specific features of the natural world such as trees, rivers, mountains, fresh air, birds, and animals), and activities in nature result in improved social interactions and relationships, better community bonds, reduced work stress, and enhanced harmony among humans from all backgrounds, ages, and cultures [1]. A review of the social benefits of contact with nonhuman nature determined that nature-based environments also improved connection between disparate communities, increased social support, and reduced crime [14]. Explanations for these findings include the notion that humans are a part of the natural world akin to all other forms, which is reflected in the beliefs and spiritual practices of many of the world's wisdom traditions and ancient cultures. Nature's impact on the development of cooperative, peaceful, calm, and empathetic individuals may potentially also change the current trajectory for competitive approaches to economic activities, and at the same time foster global togetherness [15]. However, care must be taken when promoting nature for wellness as evidence also indicates that some nature-based contexts – for example, unlit or unkempt urban parks – can also trigger experiences of fear, anxiety, and stress.

In summary, frequent and regular contact with nature is important for all population groups irrespective of socioeconomic or cultural backgrounds. Engagement with nature improves wellness in the workplace, improves social relationships, sustains emotional and physical wellness, and adds spiritual depth in everyday life contexts. Direct and indirect contact with nature in any form can be a positive source of wellness for all population groups, irrespective of factors such as age, gender, ethnicity, class, race, and health background. Even short bouts of nature-based activities enhance confidence, resilience, and self-awareness more effectively than contexts and interventions void of nature.

Sustaining wellness across individual and global levels requires enhanced human–nature relationships. As is often evident in many indigenous cultures [15], self-esteem, cooperation, empathy, and contentment based on non-materialistic values are deeply connected to nature-oriented lifestyles. Everyday practices of interacting with nature might also prove beneficial for the planet, which in turn will enhance human wellness. For example, pro-nature activities, such as sustainable behaviors, will enhance individual wellness and potentially facilitate equality, inclusion, acceptance, and meaningful relationships between humans and the rest of nature. A close relationship with nature and opportunities for being with nature, whether in wilderness, urban green spaces, or indoor contexts, encourages attitudes and values that are pro-environment and conservation-oriented, such as efforts to contain carbon emissions and practice equality principles. In turn, this enhanced human–nature relationship might also result in improvement in the overall health of the planet.

Pets

Nonhuman animals are an important part of both natural and human worlds, and interactions between humans and nonhumans can contribute toward increased wellness lifestyles and outcomes and facilitate mutual understanding. Companion animals, or pets as they are called in everyday language, offer a particularly important and potentially powerful connection between people and the rest of the natural world. Pets play important roles in many people's lives, sharing a home and consequently a high level of routine intimacy and interaction. A variety of nonhuman animals occupy the status of pets in human households, but cats and dogs are perhaps the most common species to share the day-to-day closeness of the pet–caretaker relationship. Human–pet interactions have been linked to positive wellness behaviors across a multitude of wellness domains, including physical, emotional, social, and spiritual wellness. Although limited in scope, research is also pointing to the importance of pets for intellectual and occupational wellness.

Caring for a pet is believed to result in multiple positive outcomes for the human partner, from lowered stress to increased self-confidence and awareness of the value of others and the natural world [16]. Although the evidence to support such claims about the physical and mental benefits of pet ownership is not clear-cut [17], those who do share their lives and homes with pets consider these animals as their close companions, friends, and often even as family members [18]. Humans and pets develop close relationships, similar in many ways to those between people, based around feelings of trust and affection, forming bonds, and providing social support. Human–pet relationships are often similar to human–human family relationships, but pets are not just surrogate humans, standing in for a parent, child, or partner. Rather, as Sanders [19] argued, people often come to define pets as "persons" with whom they form lasting, intimate, and emotional relationships. The pet is incorporated into the owner's network of relationships, and is seen as an individual with distinct likes and dislikes, moods and feelings which are unique to that animal, and to that human–pet relationship, and humans often grieve deeply when a pet dies. While there is clearly some anthropomorphism occurring in how people construct the "personhood" of their pet, animals are also valued for their differences to humans and are sometimes seen as better, more supportive and affectionate, and less judgmental than human family and friends [20]. This helps explain why people value their pets so highly, expending large resources of money, time, and emotion on their well-being and on forming and sustaining a productive relationship.

Pets also act as social facilitators between people, providing them with something to talk about, a form of connection and mutual interest. Whether this be between dog owners who meet on their regular walks [21] or horse owners who meet daily to care for their equine charges at a shared livery boarding facility [22], companion animals act as a social lubricant for human–human interactions and so can help combat feelings of loneliness and isolation.

The benefits of human–companion animal interactions, as experienced through pet–owner relationships, are mirrored and developed further through animal-assisted therapy, which builds on the perceived power of interspecies connections to overcome a range of mental, physical, and psychological issues people may be experiencing. The UK-based humanitarian charity Pets as Therapy (PAT) has exemplified this approach. The PAT dogs and PAT cats, along with their owners, visit hospices, hospitals, nursing and care homes, and special needs schools to "enhance health and wellbeing in the community," by providing companionship and developing confidence and enjoyment [23]. Through this and other animal-assisted therapy interventions, the power of human–companion animal interactions is harnessed and transmitted beyond individual owner–pet dyads.

However, although owner–pet relationships can be wonderful, empowering, and mutually rewarding, these interspecies encounters are not always positive for both parties. Fox [24] argued that pets occupy a liminal position in families; appreciated as friends, loved as family, yet also treated as objects or possessions to be discarded if they fail to live up to human expectations. Pets are valued for their "animalness" while also being subject to practices, such as training, neutering, and selective breeding, which attempt to make them more like "little humans." While this poses serious questions about the ethics of pet-keeping, and the responsibilities and duties humans owe to animals in their care, it may also entail a certain degree of guilt and anxiety about the animal's behavior and well-being, particularly where the relationship is seen to be unsuccessful. Failing to "gel" with a pet may be experienced as a personal failing on the part of the human, amplifying feelings of self-doubt and loneliness.

Most humans may well acquire a pet with good intentions to care for that animal, and treat him or her with compassion and fairness, but there is widespread evidence of deliberate abuse and cruelty to companion animals. While some studies argue that cruelty to animals may be a precursor to violence against humans, Arluke and Irvine [25] suggested that low-level violence against animals may be seen by many as just a normal part of interspecies interactions, and not a sign of future aggressive behavior. Violence against animals, including pets and other companion species, is pervasive and, when at a relatively low level, is not seen by many people as particularly worrying and troublesome, indicative of the liminal status of animals in a human-centric world.

Relationships between people and their pets are thus complex and multifaceted; at times providing sources of happiness and enjoyment, and at others, guilt, indifference, or even outright cruelty. As one of the closest links between humans and the natural world in contemporary societies, pets provide an important lens through which to consider relationships between nature and human wellness.

Future Implications

While the specific means by which humans relate to pets and the natural world might be different across social, cultural, and economic variables, the wellness outcomes seem profound. Interactions with nature and pets have proven beneficial for human wellness in educational settings, hospitals, therapeutic environments, and homes, to name but a few. An individual's age, gender, income, health status, and dwelling space factors might influence the type of pet or the way that they interact with nature. For example, cats and dogs are the most common pets for people living in urban areas; however, people living outside urban areas and in the countryside tend to own a range of animal companions. Certain pets in urban contexts are associated with owners using the outdoors more, such as to walk their dogs. Even tending to other types of pets such as chickens, guinea pigs, ducks, fish, and birds is associated with human–nature connection in a wellness context. Although pet ownership and interactions with nature are strongly linked with positive mental health benefits and social interactions, the capacity for improved physical wellness benefits is often linked to practical involvement with pets in outdoor and natural spaces. In these cases, pets and the outdoors might be more beneficial in strengthening human–nature contact for wellness through direct physical, emotional, and psychological attachment, connection, and relationship.

Accompanying pets in the outdoors provides humans with many diverse opportunities, not only encouraging physical exercise and improvement in health but also initiating and sustaining social interactions, possibly breaking the barriers of language, race, and class. A community of people interacting with each other in nature enhances connectedness and social harmony, reflecting good levels of social and spiritual wellness. However, to support this, resources and opportunities need to be readily available:

1. Policy-makers from across a range of sectors (e.g., health, sport, education, social care, and planning) need to work together to achieve a joined-up approach to green space and the potential for interactions in green spaces, especially in urban contexts, and policies that support wellness at national and local levels.

2. Green spaces in the public domain need to be more effectively resourced and managed at a local level. The challenge of balancing financial needs at local government level means that the utilization or design of public green spaces for wellness needs careful thought. However, poorly managed green space is likely to adversely affect wellness.

3. Public green spaces must be thoughtfully designed to emphasize quality rather than quantity. To reap the greatest benefits for human and planetary wellness, green spaces will need to consider accessibility, appropriate resources, biodiversity, and landscape diversity, and be well maintained and designed to attract diverse population groups with an intention of interacting in and with nature.

4. Practitioners and practitioner training need to better reflect the importance of interacting with nature and pets. Rather than interactions with nature and pets being seen as on the periphery, or as an extra activity, practice should embrace nature connection in all possibly ways. This might mean a possible sociocultural and economic shift.

5. A number of resources and activities could be initiated and adopted in different everyday human environments for optimum wellness through nature connection. Table 34.1 provides a few suggested resources and activities.

Summary

Nature and pets are fundamental to the development of effective holistic wellness lifestyles and outcomes. Interacting with nature and pets as part of everyday wellness habits has the potential to enhance wellness in ways that cannot be achieved by other means. While there is an emerging shift toward the acceptance of the importance of nature and pets for wellness, more is needed to make the most of the potential impact of nature and pets. Shifting the

Table 34.1 Examples of including nature and pets in everyday life for holistic wellness

Type of location	Features of animal life forms	Features of plant life forms	Activities/engagement/practice for nature interaction, inclusion and participation
Educational settings	Fish tanks/bowls, aquariums, frog ponds, guinea pigs, chickens, ducks, turtles and tortoises, bird visitors, nesting birds, butterfly gardens, bug hotels, chicken coops, duck ponds, bird feeders	Vegetable gardens, herb patches, flower beds, fruit trees, flower plants, indoor plants, running water features, sensory gardens, fairy gardens, nature patches, ample amount of sun and natural light	Age-appropriate nature-related physical activities, eating lunch outside, enhanced nature contact during meetings, school lessons, school activities, nature music, nature baskets, nature-based curricula, nature pedagogy; Forest Schools, green schools, ecology tours, orienteering within the school setting, nature-based mindfulness meditation; multi-themed mini-landscapes and nature hubs attracting different sociocultural populations for inclusion
Healthcare units	Fish tanks/bowls, aquariums, frog ponds, guinea pigs, guide dogs, cat visitors, turtles and tortoises, bird visitors, nesting birds, butterfly gardens, bug hotels	Vegetable gardens, herb patches, flower beds, fruit trees, flower plants, indoor plants, running water features, sensory gardens, fairy gardens, nature patches, butterfly gardens, aviaries, bird feeders, duck ponds, ample amount of sun/natural light	Age-appropriate and gender-sensitive nature-related physical activities, walking, nature immersion, yoga, meditation in nature, eating lunch outside, enhanced nature contact during meetings, using pets in therapy, recovery and rehabilitation; nature music, Forest Schools, nature hubs, and nature retreats for children and adult patients, ecology tours for patients within the setting; multi-themed mini-landscapes attracting different sociocultural populations for inclusion

Table 34.1 (cont.)

Type of location	Features of animal life forms	Features of plant life forms	Activities/engagement/practice for nature interaction, inclusion and participation
Work environments	Fish tanks/bowls, aquariums, indoor frog ponds, guinea pigs, turtles and tortoises, butterfly gardens, aviaries, bird feeders, duck pond	Flower beds, flower plants, indoor plants, running water features, sensory gardens, fairy gardens, nature patches, ample amount of sun and natural light	Nature-related physical activities, nature music, walking, orienteering in nearby parks, yoga, meditation/mindfulness in nature, eating lunch outside, outdoor café, outdoor food carts, enhanced nature contact during meetings, using pets in the reception areas, multi-themed mini-landscapes and nature hubs attracting different sociocultural populations for inclusion; employee retreats at outdoor and adventure education centers
Public spaces	Aquariums, frog ponds, duck ponds, lakes and ponds, wildlife areas, vegetation attracting insects and birds, developing locations as safe houses for animals and birds, edible gardens, fruit trees, aviaries, bird feeders, sensory gardens, running water features, den and shelter building spots, nature hubs		Any number of nature-based activities suiting various age groups and genders; promotion of nature connection, interacting with animals, engaging with wildlife (observation, protection, conservation), outdoor picnics, free access to aviaries, sensory gardens, duck ponds; outdoor adventure points; multi-themed landscapes attracting different sociocultural populations for inclusion

focus to one where humans are once again recognized as part of nature will partially resolve this issue. However, there also needs to be a greater emphasis placed on providing the resources and training to facilitate interactions between humans, nature, and pets. Research is pointing to the importance of nature and pets, and practitioners are calling for more resources; the last step is the thoughtful provision of resources to support human wellness. The ramifications of this shift might also mean a better outcome for the planet, not just humans.

References

1. E Brymer, TF Cuddihy, V Sharma-Brymer. The role of nature-based experiences in the development and maintenance of wellness. *Asia-Pacific J Health Sport Phys Educ* 2010; 1(2): 21–28.

2. RF Reese, TF Lewis, JE Myers, E Wahesh, R Iversen. Relationship between nature relatedness and holistic wellness: an exploratory study. *J Humanist Couns* 2014; 53: 63–79.

3. RF Reese, JE Myers. EcoWellness: the missing factor in holistic wellness models. *J Counsel Dev* 2012; 90: 400–406.

4. American Public Health Association. Improving health and wellness through access to nature: policy number: 20137. 2013. www.apha.org/policies-and-advocacy /public-health-policy-statements/policy-database/2014/07/08/09/18/improving-health-and-wellness-through-access-to-nature (accessed January 22, 2019).

5. D Trau, KA Keenan, M Goforth, et al. Nature contacts: employee wellness in healthcare. *HERD* 2016; 9(3): 47–62.

6. P Martyn, E Brymer. The relationship between nature relatedness and anxiety. *J Health Psychol* 2016; 21(7): 1436–1445.

7. EK Nisbet, JM Zelenski, SA Murphy. Happiness is in our nature: exploring nature relatedness as a contributor to subjective well-being. *J Happiness Stud* 2011; 12: 303–322.

8. L Chawla. Benefits of nature contact for children. *J Plan Lit* 2015; 30(4): 433–452.

9. T Ward, S Goldingay, J Parson. Evaluating a supported nature play programme, parents' perspectives. *Early Child Dev Care* 2019; 189(2): 270–283.

10. R Russell, AD Guerry, P Balvanera, et al. Humans and nature: how knowing and experiencing nature affect well-being. *Annu Rev Environ Resour* 2013; 38(1): 473–502.

11. A Fiskum, K Jacobsen. Outdoor education gives fewer demands for action regulation and an increased variability of affordances. *JAEOL* 2013; 13(1): 76–99.

12. EBH Sandseter. Affordances for risky play in preschool: the importance of features in the play environment. *Early Child Educ J* 2009; 36: 439–446.

13. D Araujo, E Brymer, R Withagen, H Brito, K Davids. The empowering variability of affordances of nature: why do exercisers feel better after performing the same exercise in natural environments than in indoor environments? *Psychol Sport Exerc* 2019; 42: 138–145.

14. M Heinsch. Getting down to earth: finding a place for nature in social work practice. *Int J Soc Welfare* 2012; 21: 309–318.

15. M Gratani, SG Sutton, J Butler, E Bohensky, S Foale. Indigenous environmental values as human values. *Cogent Soc Sci* 2016; 2. DOI:10.1080/ 23311886.2016.1185811.

16. M O'Haire. Companion animals and human health: benefits, challenges, and the road ahead. *J Vet Behav* 2010; 5(5): 226–234.

17. H Herzog. The impact of pets on human health and psychological well-being: fact, fiction, or hypothesis? *Curr Dir Psychol Sci* 2011; 20(4): 236–239.

18. N Charles, CA Davies. My family and other animals: pets as kin. *Sociol Res Online* 2008; 13(5). DOI:10.5153/sro.1798.

19. CR Sanders. The animal "other": self-definition, social identity and companion animals. *Adv Consum Res* 1990; **17**: 662–668.

20. N Charles. Animals just love you as you are: experiencing kinship across the species barrier. *Sociology* 2014; **48**(4): 715–730.

21. T Fletcher, L Platt. (Just) a walk with the dog? Animal geographies and negotiating walking spaces. *Soc Cultur Geogr* 2018; **19** (2): 211–229.

22. K Dashper. *Human–Animal Relationships in Equestrian Sport and Leisure*. Abingdon, Routledge; 2017.

23. Pets as Therapy. About pets as therapy. 2019. https://petsastherapy.org/about-us (accessed March 11, 2019).

24. R Fox. Animal behaviours, post-human lives: everyday negotiations of the animal–human divide in pet-keeping. *Soc Cultur Geogr* 2006; 7(4): 525–537.

25. A Arluke, L Irvine. Physical cruelty of companion animals. In: J Maher H Pierpoint, P Beirne, eds., *The Palgrave International Handbook of Animal Abuse Studies*. London, Palgrave Macmillan; 2017; 39–57.

Circadian Rhythm in the Digital Age

Mona Ezzat-Velinov and Mimi Guarneri

Introduction

It is early morning and the sun is just starting to rise, showering the land with light and warmth from the cold night (Figure 35.1). As we start to move outside in the fresh air the light gently stimulates our eyes. Taking deep breaths, we feel the energy of the day building. With bare feet on the ground, we feel at one with the planet. How many of us start our day like this? What would happen if we did? Within our body is a beautiful system, in tune with nature, that knows just what we need and at what time. The circadian system streamlines production of all the essentials for life. With astonishing accuracy and precision, our circadian cues direct our hormones, enzymes, and molecular signals to keep us buzzing healthily throughout the day.

We all want health, happiness, peace, and love in our lives, and so pursue the things that stoke our joy. To feel alive and powerful, we drink caffeine and energy drinks or take other substances to support these feelings. We push our bodies to do more, multitasking at the highest level and often beyond sunset, not acknowledging the transition of day to night. What if, instead, we used the power of the sun and light in the day to support our health and healing? What if we paid much closer attention to a rhythm and pattern to time our lives? What if the day would start to wind down after sunset? This is the beauty of the rhythm of the day. Just as music leads us to sway to the beat and keep a rhythm in the body. The pulse of our lives could be set to the elegance lying within our cells. Let's explore this grand system and how we can return to this beneficial design to maintain health.

Circadian Rhythm Defined

Circadian comes from the Latin words *circa*, or around, and *dian*, meaning day. This daily rhythm is present in all biological species. As the Earth rotates around the Sun, the circadian cycle is approximately 24 hours. Sunrise stimulates a cascade of pathways through the brain out into the body in a harmonious symphony. As we progress through the day, all the activities we do – eating, exercising, working, studying, giving lectures, reading – have an optimal time for peak performance. As darkness approaches, our brain and body are signaled to rest. Light plays a huge role in how we feel through the day and how it works is fascinating.

In 1974 an area of the brain called the hippocampus was found to have designated cells which set the cycle of day and night. The superchiasmatic nucleus (SCN) is a bundle of approximately 20,000 cells sitting just above the region where the information from the eyes crosses, called the optic chiasm. Within the nuclei of the cells are genes that are transcribed in an oscillating rhythm. As daylight is perceived, the genes *CLOCK* and *BMAL1* are turned

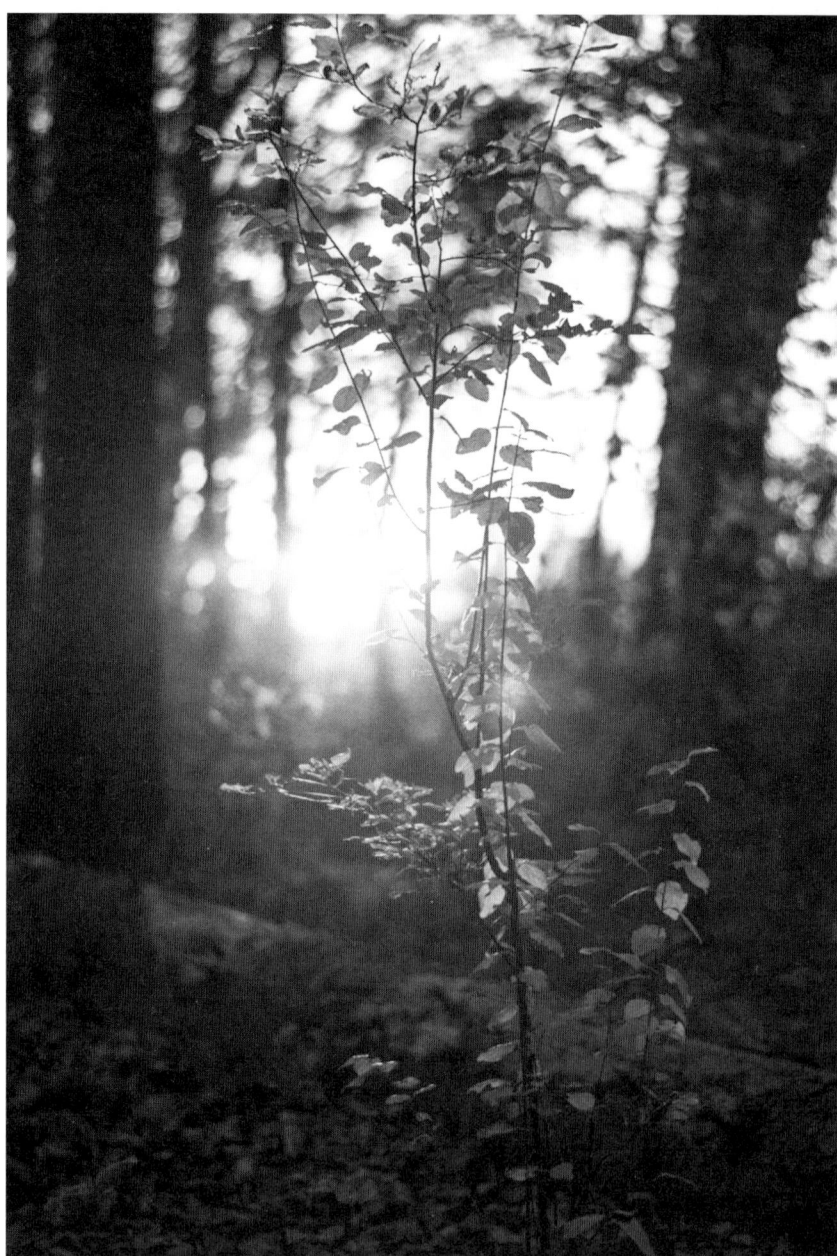

Figure 35.1 Starting the day.

on, sending a signal within the cytoplasm of the cell. The cells are instructed on which hormones, proteins, or neurochemicals to produce. There is a feedback loop from another set of genes to downregulate the production of *CLOCK* and *BMAL1*. This feedback loop is like the bell ringing at recess, alerting us that we have had enough running around and that its time to settle down. For many years, it was a mystery as to how the information of light was translated by the SCN. It was thought the eyes only contained rod and cone cells to code for vision. It was not until the 1990s that the light-sensitive photopigment melanopsin was discovered. When retinal cells are stimulated, melanopsin is released, giving the SCN the signal to act as the master clock. A wave of activity in response to daytime needs is set in motion [1, 2].

What exactly is regulated by the SCN? It influences many systems, including regulation of the heart rate, which needs to rise in the morning to prepare for the day. The digestive system is awakened to prepare for breakfast. Muscles are energized to move and even the thirst center is awakened after a night of sleep, to reset hydration status. When the light begins to wane toward the end of the day, the SCN sends signals to the pineal gland to start making melatonin and to prepare the body for sleep. What do we tend to do when dusk sets in? Turn the lights on of course! Sleep and daily rhythm of life have changed drastically in our most recent history because of the luxury of light being available at all times – but at what price? In the past, the day would have ended with sunset. What happens to our hormones, our organ systems, and our ability to restore when the day is ending much later than naturally intended?

Circadian Rhythm and Sleep

While the best time to slow down in the evening is an individual matter, most of us are doing far more in the evening hours than our body is prepared for, resulting in profound sleep disturbance (Figure 35.2). According to the American Sleep Association, 50–70 million US adults have a sleep disorder. Of these, insomnia is the most common issue: 30 percent of adults note an acute issue with insomnia, and 10 percent have chronic insomnia. Sleep deprivation is a common concern as well. Thirty-seven percent of 20–39-year-olds have sleep disturbance, while 40 percent of 40–59-year-olds report the same issues. How much sleep do you need? According to the Institute of Medicine, adults will need 7–9 hours, teens 8–10 hours, and children vary by age, but in general need 10–14 hours overall. If you watch television or read a magazine article, the most common recommendation is to use a pill, supplement, tea, or tincture to enhance your sleep. What if we just started living with rhythm? We

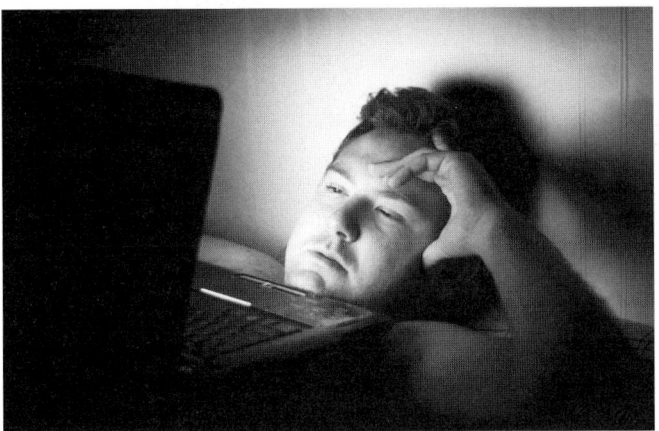

Figure 35.2 Circadian rhythm and sleep.

can go out in the morning, getting a boost of natural light. We can turn our lights down in the evening, allowing for a decrease in natural light. We can pace our lives to flow more with the day and respect the night for rest. Jet lag is a great example of what happens when you are out of sync.

As devices are ubiquitous in homes around the world, so is exposure to LED light that is predominantly in the blue spectrum. The LED light technology is fantastic for illumination of a small screen, but when we are exposed at night it tends to lower our peak of melatonin. Researchers investigated the difference between reading an e-book with light versus a regular book with light from a lamp. The participants were instructed to turn off the lights by 10 p.m. even if they did not feel sleepy. They found that the group who used electronic devices had less melatonin and took more time to fall asleep. They shortened their sleep cycle and did not attain as much REM sleep. You can add a change to your screen, blocking blue light, or wear blue-blocking glasses to decrease the stimulus. In a study of 14 individuals with insomnia, those wearing amber-colored glasses two hours prior to sleep, to decrease exposure to blue light, demonstrated improved sleep parameters. The ultimate solution would be to curb the time spent using a screen at night. You can use low light to read a book before bed or do some gentle stretching or moon salutations. All of these suggestions allow the SCN to stimulate production of melatonin at the proper time to achieve deeper, more restorative sleep [3–5].

Influencing the Clock

The SCN is considered the master clock of the body, but we also have peripheral clocks that take input from food intake, exercise, stress, alcohol, and caffeine (Figure 35.3). Peripheral clocks are like the local news, giving the status of what is happening in the neighborhood, while at the same time being in sync with the SCN. The challenge occurs when the peripheral clocks are receiving inputs that are not in sync with our light–dark cycle. Food intake, for example, is an important clock-setter. With the ability to acquire food easily with no set mealtimes, we are often eating all day. Snacks and late-night meals happen at a time

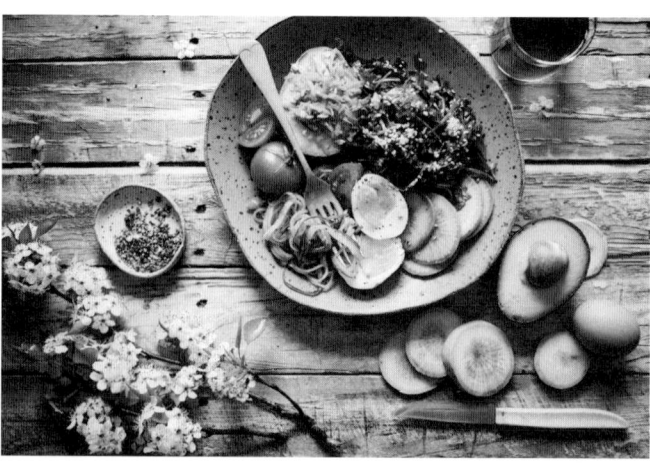

Figure 35.3 Food intake: a clock-setter.

we are not designed to digest. Establishing eating patterns is important as it improves digestion and metabolism. When the liver and pancreas are in sync with food breakdown, the proper enzymes, storage of nutrients, and metabolism are more efficient. For many years the focus has been on what we eat. Should we follow a Paleo, vegetarian, or ketogenic diet to lose or manage body weight? What is the best combination of macronutrients, what proteins, fats, and carbohydrates should we consume? What we have neglected is *when* we eat. According to the World Health organization (WHO), as of 2016 1.9 billion adults were overweight, and of this group, 650 million were obese. In addition, the WHO reported that 41 million children under the age of five years were overweight or obese in 2016. Being overweight or obese increases the risk of heart disease, diabetes, joint disease, and cognitive decline. Consuming a healthy plant-diverse diet with lean proteins and healthy fats has been shown to prevent most chronic diseases. What if we take the next step and time our food? Just as there is no one diet for everyone, the timing of food is also important and unique to the individual. For most, eating during sunlight hours enables the body to handle and use the calories. Having a nighttime fast in which your digestion is quiet and has time to repair can enhance health [6, 7].

A recent study evaluated the oral and gut microbiomes of individuals eating at different times of the day [8, 9]. The main objective of the study was to evaluate the difference in bacterial composition in saliva and gut bacteria based on the timing of food. This study divided participants into two groups: one having their main meal at 2 p.m., the other having their main meal at 5:30 p.m. They collected saliva samples at four points in the day and collected stool as well. The study demonstrated for the first time that there is a daily rhythm in human saliva microbiota, and diversity of the type of bacteria present at different times of the day. These results suggest that eating late in the day drives changes in salivary microbial diversity in a similar way as that observed in obesity and inflammation. Since inflammation is the source of most chronic disease, even eating late may trigger an inflammatory response.

The pancreas, responsible for enzymes that digest food and insulin to break down carbohydrate sources, has its own rhythm. The pancreas is regulated by the SCN and a peripheral clock that prepares it for the day. The pancreatic peripheral clock tends to be more active earlier in the day, ready with insulin to respond to food intake. For most people the ability to digest meals slows down later in the day, making it more difficult to respond to a late meal or snack. If you start to notice what your eating pattern is, metabolism can be optimized to have a better balance in your day. Are you someone who needs to have breakfast when you wake up, or are you more comfortable starting your meal much later in the day? Do you tend toward late-night eating or a lot of snacking after dinner? As you start to pay attention to the timing of your meals, you will tap into what is being termed chrononutrition. Chrononutrition is an area of research focused on three elements of eating behavior: timing, frequency, and regularity [10, 11]. When we eat at different times of the day that do not align with a sleep–wake, fast–feed, light–dark cycle, this affects our glucose metabolism, lipid metabolism, and blood pressure control. From a 2018 review of scientific papers looking at chrononutrition, it was found that glucose tolerance tends to decline over the day and reaches a low in the evening. This rhythm comes from changes over the course of the day in insulin sensitivity, insulin secretion, and glucose utilization. What the trend of these studies showed is that if you are having your meals later in the day, you tend to have fewer fruits and vegetables in your diet. You may be prone to take in more energy drinks, alcohol, sugar, caffeine, and more fat. Your pancreatic clock has its own timing, and if you can have your main meals when your body is most ready to digest, absorb, and make nutrients available, it can play a great role in balancing your energy through the day.

Metabolism on the Clock

Potter and colleagues [7] demonstrated that circadian disruption resulting in sleep disturbance also triggers metabolism changes. When sleep is disturbed, it changes the ratio of ghrelin to leptin production. Ghrelin, the hunger hormone, tends to encourage seeking of food. Leptin signals satiety. These hormones then communicate with adiponectin, which is made by fat cells. Adiponectin regulates the storage or release of fat for energy. If these hormonal signals are out of balance, it is much easier to overeat, choose the wrong foods, or have trouble using fat for fuel. Over time, this dysregulation may lead to insulin resistance and diabetes. By considering the timing of meals, you may gain the advantage of better food choices and improved hormonal signaling. Improved insulin secretion and response from the cells will lower your chance for diabetes and blood sugar imbalance.

Time-restricted eating is gaining a lot of popularity as people look for ways to lose weight, improve their blood sugar levels, and feel better. The theory is that if you limit the time that you take in calories to an 8- or 12-hour window during the day, blood sugar and weight will improve. Research has shown that even without changing the diet and just altering the timing of food, body weight is improved. One of the lead researchers in this area, Dr. Satchin Panda of the Salk Institute [12], shared a story recently at a conference. He was in San Francisco, taking a taxi, when he decided to ask the taxi driver how he feels, being awake at odd hours of the day. The taxi driver graciously shared his secret with Dr. Panda: time-restricted eating. Unbeknownst to him, the taxi driver was speaking to one of the foremost researchers in this field! Intermittent fasting or time-restricted eating is not for everyone; if you are someone who has a lot of stress and fatigue, fasting can be an added stress to your body. In this case, learning to transform your stress response would be the first step before fasting. Even our stress response is under circadian control.

Stress: To Be or Not To Be

Cortisol, one of the main stress hormones, produced by the adrenal glands, has a diurnal production. The pituitary gland sends a signal to the adrenal gland to peak cortisol in the morning with what is called the cortisol-awakening response. Having our highest cortisol in the morning gets us ready for the day. Cortisol will slowly raise our body temperature and prepare us to wake up. By noon, the cortisol level starts to come down and continues to decrease until evening, when it elegantly gives way to hormones such as melatonin. Melatonin is produced in the pineal gland in response to the light–dark cycle. The timing of melatonin production helps to guide the brain into restful sleep. When we stay up late and keep our lights on full brightness, the balance of these hormones shifts. The body and brain get the signal that it is not dark, and we are stimulated to stay awake. You may have experienced this when you feel a little sleepy around 9 or 10 p.m., but you stay awake and eventually get a "second wind." You may even find that you have difficulty falling asleep. Insomnia may be related to high cortisol level at night, when the body should be making melatonin. Melatonin not only helps to

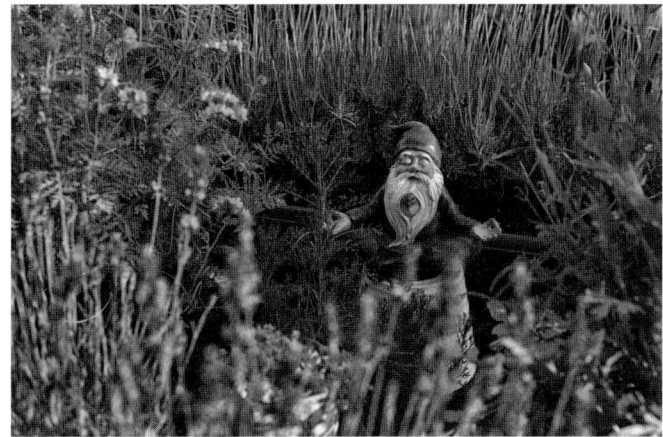

Figure 35.4 Rebalancing the autonomic nervous system.

induce sleep, it is also a powerful antioxidant that helps the cells of our body to heal and clean house from a day of activities. Having enough melatonin is an important part of our natural rhythm and it is a key hormone in maintaining health.

The peripheral clock of the adrenal gland is affected by inputs from the nervous system. When you are stressed, a release of cortisol above the normal amount is produced. Your body believes it needs to be on alert and ready to go! Often with stress you consume too much coffee or sugar in an attempt to keep up with life. These substances also stimulate the adrenal glands, but end up throwing you out of balance as you come down from the caffeine or sugar high and your body is even more depleted than before. Excessive exercise can also affect your adrenal glands, making you feel sluggish and cause you difficulty performing at an optimal level. How do you know if this is happening? Check your heart rate variability. The timing between heart beats varies from beat to beat and is a reflection of the autonomic nervous system. The autonomic nervous system has both parasympathetic and sympathetic input. The parasympathetic system controls the rest-and-digest response, while the sympathetic system is the fight-flight-or-freeze response. When your heart is well trained and balanced, your heart rate is low but you have a high heart rate variability. When individuals are overtrained or overstressed, heart rate variability is decreased. Low heart rate variability is an independent risk factor for cardiovascular disease [13]. There are a number of devices or apps to help determine heart rate variability. Meditation and breath work are two of the best ways to help rebalance the autonomic nervous system (Figure 35.4). Explore what feels right to you and take that first step to start a practice.

Systems under Circadian Control

Another important hormone with a circadian rhythm is testosterone. Testosterone, like cortisol, peaks in the morning and slowly decreases throughout the day. It is best to check testosterone levels in the early morning to determine the highest physiologic level. Testosterone levels respond to the sleep cycle, weight, diet, and stress. Lifestyle change should be the first step in improving testosterone levels.

Caring for your heart with circadian biology is just as important. Your heart expresses 13 percent of the genes and 8 percent of the proteins in a rhythmic fashion. These genes and proteins mainly control growth, metabolism, and repair of myocytes. When light is present, it signals the active phase for the heart. Myocytes, the muscular cells of the heart, exhibit more metabolic activity to make energy and contract. The rest phase occurs at night to repair and store nutrients for the following active phase.

Blood vessels also exhibit a circadian rhythm. In daylight hours, the amount of resistance and flow of nutrients in blood vessels increases to maintain proper blood pressure. At night, blood pressure should go down to allow for restoration and clean-up of the blood vessel lining. Clinical trials have demonstrated the importance of controlling blood pressure at night [14]. There is ongoing research to evaluate the timing of medication and how using the circadian system can optimize the performance of a medication.

There is also a peripheral clock within the heart that is tightly regulated by the nervous system. If the sympathetic nervous system is stimulated by a stressful event, the heart responds with increased activity. Transcendental meditation is associated with a 48 percent reduction in cardiovascular events [15–17]. Perhaps meditation keeps the peripheral cardiac clock in tune with the SCN, allowing for rest of the cardiovascular system.

The immune system also oscillates throughout the day and has a profound response to sleep cycles. Circadian factors play a predominant role in regulating the distribution of immune cells. Regardless of nocturnal sleep, the number of T and B cells reaches a maximum in the evening or early night, and then declines throughout the remaining night to reach a minimum in the morning hours. In humans, this circadian rhythm of T cells in the blood is independent of sleep and is coupled to the rhythm of cortisol. The peak in cortisol at the beginning of the awake period precedes a decrease in blood T cell number by about three hours.

In contrast to circadian factors, nocturnal sleep plays a predominant role in the regulation of adaptive immune responses [18, 19]. When nocturnal sleep is disturbed, the stress hormones released block the production of antibodies in the body. In one study by Spiegel et al., [20], when sleep was disrupted there was a loss of immune system response to the flu vaccine. Another study by Lange et al. [21] demonstrated a similar response to the hepatitis A vaccine when sleep was disturbed. Think of when you were last under stress and cutting down on sleep for a deadline. How often do you get sick after the completion of a project? Operating on epinephrine for the deadline pushes the body to do more than it was designed to do. Loss of circadian rhythm affects the immune system and your ability to avoid infection. Many studies have looked at shift-work and demonstrated that working at night increases the risk for chronic diseases, mood disorders, and even cancer. This is an extreme example of loss of circadian rhythm. Switching your time to work, eat, and move around when we are designed to sleep can be detrimental to the body. If the immune system signaling malfunctions, you may be more prone to illness.

Getting in Your Rhythm

An excellent way to apply circadian biology to your everyday life is to understand your chronotype. Your chronotype is your propensity for sleep and activity during the day. The two extremes of chronotype are the morning or evening type. Morning chronotypes wake early and are more active at the beginning of the day; evening types are later risers and are more productive in the later hours. Most people are one or the other; the rest will fall somewhere closer to the middle. Understanding how your type manifests can have a powerful impact on how you structure your day.

The Munich morning/evening type questionnaire helps to assess an individual's morning, evening, or neutral tendency. When you are in rhythm with your chronotype, you can move more smoothly through your day and be more productive. You will find the energy to focus on the work you want to accomplish. You will feel more energetic in your exercise and be more creative at the optimal time [22–28].

For example, a morning person would do best to wake up, exercise, and get to the most difficult tasks right away. By the afternoon, most morning types have a decrease in energy and focus.

This may take the form of needing some booster to get through the rest of the day. What if we were to take a short nap or a leisure walk, instead of trying to power through? How might that change our outlook on life and decision-making?

If you are an evening type, perhaps failing to wake up early is not a character flaw, but just your natural circadian rhythm.

It is postulated that as primal human beings we evolved to be individuals with different circadian rhythms. The morning type can gather food and the evening type can protect the tribe at night. Is there one type that is better than another? Not necessarily, but modern life is geared toward the morning type. Work, school, and even play are regimented to happen during certain times. People tend to gravitate toward jobs or schedules at school that allow for the most flexibility, but it can still be a struggle. If you are an evening chronotype it may be difficult to fit into society when your biological clock is different to most. On the flip side, when you are a morning type, technology makes it easy to stay up late, causing you to go well beyond the timing your chronotype thrives on.

Social jet lag sets in when we are active outside of our natural chronotype. As an evening type, your job may require you to wake up early during the week, but since this is not your normal time to be up, you sleep later on the weekends. There is a discrepancy between what is expected of you socially versus what you manifest biologically. As you accumulate sleep debt, the body feels like it is changing time zones over and over. Over the years, the strain on your brain without proper rest is immense.

Teens who are afraid of missing out on social news or activity frequently ignore their need for rest, spending many hours on their devices. This form of social jet lag comes with a high price to a developing young brain and body.

Social jet lag plays out now in many scenarios. With access to online shopping, movies, video games, television, news, and social platforms, we end up spilling from one day to the next. Technology and social media can easily capture our attention. Social jet lag is a real and concerning trend. The more awareness we have of it, the better we can guide our lives in a more fulfilling way.

Steps to Living in Tune with Nature

The circadian system throughout our body is dedicated to helping us thrive in the world. By knowing your chronotype, you can begin to make conscious choices toward a rhythmic life (Figure 35.5). Start your day by stepping outside and letting natural light stimulate your eyes. Sit for a few minutes in meditation or quiet contemplation. Gently stretch to stimulate your muscles. Meditation and yoga can train you to transform the stress response and modulate your emotions. There are many ways to incorporate meditation into your day. Attend a group meditation or download an app; use technology to transform your autonomic nervous system

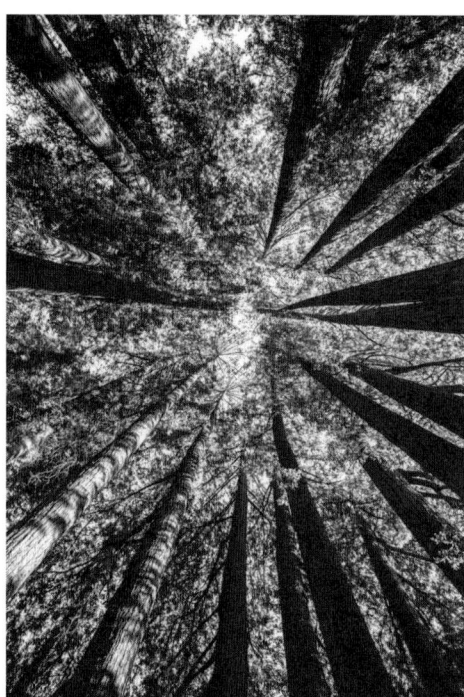

Figure 35.5 Living in tune with nature.

response to stress. Heartmath and Muse are examples of technology that can train individuals in biofeedback and meditation.

Nature deficit disorder is a term used to describe the negative impact on children raised without time in nature. In his book *Last Child in the Woods*, Richard Louv describes the importance of nature for children: "In nature, a child finds freedom, fantasy, and privacy: a place distant from the adult world, a separate peace." Forest bathing, the Japanese tradition of Shinrin-Yoku, implores you to go to the forest and take it in through your senses. Being outdoors, surrounded by trees, the ocean, meadows, and fields can help to reset the body and decrease stress. Your body relaxes, your mind is in sync with nature, and you find a pulse of life frequently missing in urban settings.

Pay close attention to the lights in your home and turn them down later in the day. Use glass that blocks blue light and the setting on your computer or phone that does the same. Have time away from devices, especially at night.

We have more convenience in our lives, which limits heavy manual labor and physical activity. We have watches to tell us to walk or stand throughout the day. Activities that were once part of our daily lives, such as climbing, chopping, and gathering, have virtually disappeared. Look at your daily activity outside of exercise class or gym time. See if you can increase your physical activity by walking and lifting more.

Determine the best time for your main meal. When do you have your first meal? How late are you eating? Try timing your food intake to an 8–12-hour window to optimize your metabolism and give your digestive system a rest. Being mindful of what we eat and when can help maintain optimal weight and blood sugar. Seasonal eating mimics circadian rhythm as you enjoy the foods nature has provided with the proper nutrients for the season.

Gather, share, and cook together; create the memories and love for healthy food as a family and as a community.

In ancient cultures there is a deep reverence toward the day and night and toward the change of seasons. For example, on a Navajo reservation it is encouraged to greet the first snow and introduce oneself to winter. For many, winter signifies cold days, slippery roads, and darkness. But in Navajo Nation, winter is not greeted as an inconvenience; it is about nature and ushering in a phase of life with special reverence.

In many cultures, the start of a new season can signal a new year. In the Persian tradition, Nooroz, the first day of spring, is a new year. The table is set with symbols of health, wealth, love, and family. To think of the first day of spring as a new beginning filled with life and rebirth connects life directly to nature.

For jet lag, reset your system by getting out into the light in your new location. Stay physically active and get your body tired enough to sleep. Avoid a lot of bright lights when you want to rest – this includes on the flight as well!

Social jet lag is just as taxing to your body as actual jet lag. Learn to bring more balance to when you turn to social media, chat online, or spend late nights streaming the popular shows and movies. Once again, it is up to you to choose when your day ends, and how it ends. Experiment with a nighttime routine that matches your chronotype and supports your mind, body, and spirit toward its best.

As research continues in the fascinating field of circadian biology, we believe it will further support the importance of humans living as nature intended. Live with the day and rest in the night and you will see your health improve in numerous ways.

> When you arise in the morning, think of what a precious privilege it is to be alive – to breathe, to think, to enjoy, to love.
>
> Marcus Aurelius

References

1. TA LeGates, DC Fernandez, S Hattar. Light as a central modulator of circadian rhythms, sleep and affect. *Nat Rev Neurosci* 2014; **15**(7): 443–454.

2. AS Fisk, SKE Tam, LA Brown, et al. Light and cognition: roles for circadian rhythms, sleep, and arousal. *Front Neurol* 2018; **9**: 56.

3. G Tosini, I Ferguson, K Tsubota. Effects of blue light on the circadian system and eye physiology. *Mol Vis* 2016; **22**: 61–72.

4. A Shechter, EW Kim, MP St-Onge, AJ Westwood. Blocking nocturnal blue light for insomnia: a randomized controlled trial. *J Psychiatr Res* 2018; **96**: 196–202.

5. Y Esaki, T Kitajima, Y Ito, et al. Wearing blue light-blocking glasses in the evening advances circadian rhythms in the patients with delayed sleep phase disorder: an open-label trial. *Chronobiol Int* 2016; **33**(8): 1037–1044.

6. GDME Potter, JE Cade, PJ Grant, LJ Hardie. Nutrition and the circadian system. *Br J Nutr* 2016; **116**(3): 434–442.

7. GDME Potter, DJ Skene, J Arendt, et al. Circadian rhythm and sleep disruption: causes, metabolic consequences, and countermeasures. *Endocr Rev* 2016; **37**(6): 584–608.

8. NG Nikitakis, W Papaioannou, LI Sakkas, E Kousvelari. The autoimmunity–oral microbiome connection. *Oral Dis* 2017; **23**(7): 828–839.

9. MC Collado, PA Engen, C Bandín, et al. Timing of food intake impacts daily rhythms of human salivary microbiota: a randomized, crossover study. *FASEB J* 2018; **32**(4): 2060–2072.

10. GK Pot. Sleep and dietary habits in the urban environment: the role of chrono-nutrition. *Proc Nutr Soc* 2018; **77** (3): 189–198.

11. J Lopez-Minguez, P Gómez-Abellán, M Garaulet. Circadian rhythms, food timing and obesity. *Proc Nutr Soc* 2016; **75** (4): 501–511.

12. K Gabel, KK Hoddy, N Haggerty, et al. Effects of 8-hour time restricted feeding on body weight and metabolic disease risk factors in obese adults: a pilot study. *Nutr Healthy Aging* 2018; **4**(4): 345–353.

13. AT Hutchison, P Regmi, ENC Manoogian, et al. Time-restricted feeding improves glucose tolerance in men at risk for type 2 diabetes: a randomized crossover trial. *Obesity (Silver Spring)* 2019; **27**(5): 724–732.

14. SS Thosar, MP Butler, SA Shea. Role of the circadian system in cardiovascular disease *J Clin Invest* 2018; **128**(6): 2157–2167.

15. AH Zohar, CR Cloninger, R McCraty. Personality and heart rate variability: exploring pathways from personality to cardiac coherence and health. *Open J Soc Sci* 2013; **1**(6): 32–39.

16. C Dunster. Treatment of anxiety and stress with biofeedback. *Global Adv Health Med* 2012; **1**(4): 76–83.

17. SI Nidich, MV Rainforth, DA Haaga, et al. A randomized controlled trial on effects of the Transcendental Meditation program on blood pressure, psychological distress, and coping in young adults. *Am J Hypertens* 2009; **22**(12): 1326–1331.

18. MR Iron. Why sleep is important for health: psychoneuroimmunology perspective. *Annu Rev Psychol* 2015; **66**: 143–172.

19. N Labrecque, N Cermakian. Circadian clocks in the immune system. *J Biol Rhythms* 2015; **30**(4): 277–290.

20. K Spiegel, JF Sheridan, E Van Cauter. Effect of sleep deprivation on response to immunization. *JAMA* 2002; **288**(12): 1471–1472.

21. L Besedovsky, T Lange, J Born. Sleep and immune function. *Pflugers Arch* 2012; **463** (1): 121–137.

22 T Roenneberg, M Merrow. The circadian clock and human health. *Curr Biol* 2016; **26** (10): R432-43.

23. M Maukonen, N Kanerva, T Partonen, et al. The associations between chronotype, a healthy diet and obesity. *Chronobiol Int* 2016; **33**(8): 972–981.

24. AS Panev, TA Tserne, AS Polugrudov, et al. Association of chronotype and social jetlag with human non-verbal intelligence. *Chronobiol Int* 2017; **34**(7): 977–980.

25. JSG Muñoz, R Cañavate, CM Hernández, V Cara-Salmerón, JJH Morante. The association among chronotype, timing of food intake and food preferences depends on body mass status. *Eur J Clin Nutr* 2017; **71**(6): 736–742.

26. JA Vitale, E Roveda, A Montaruli, et al. Chronotype influences activity circadian rhythm and sleep: differences in sleep quality between weekdays and weekend. *Chronobiol Int* 2015; **32**(3): 405–415.

27. M Juda, C Vetter, T Roenneberg. Chronotype modulates sleep duration, sleep quality, and social jet lag in shift-workers. *J Biol Rhythms* 2013; **28**(2): 141–51.

28. AM Schroeder, CS Colwell. How to fix a broken clock. *Trends Pharmacol Sci* 2013; **34**(11): 605–619.

The Arts in Health Settings
Inspirational, Educational, and Therapeutic Approaches to Wellness

Amy Bucciarelli, Gail K. Ellison, Eleanor K. Sommer, and Heather Spooner

Introduction

Evidence shows that the arts have been part of human society from as early as the Paleolithic period, which stretches across more than two million years of human existence [1, 2]. Cave paintings are among the earliest discovered art forms, and archeological research notes that visual and performing arts were integrated into human culture tens of thousands of years ago [3]. Anthropologists agree that artistic expressions such as painting, chanting, dancing, music-making, and storytelling have provided important societal, psychological, and health functions in human groups throughout time [4–6].

The significance of art used for health and well-being is recorded throughout millennia and across cultures. For example, classical era Greece used satire theater to treat depression [7]; Australian aborigines decoratively painted their bodies in preparation for healing ceremonies [5]; and dance was linked to fertility rituals in African cultures [4]. Dissanayake [5] proposed that there is a bioevolutionary importance to aesthetic expression beyond societal and cultural functions:

> Art is said to be both pleasurable and advantageous because it is therapeutic: it integrates powerful contradictory and disturbing feelings (Stokes, 1972; Fuller, 1980); it allows for escape from tedium or permits temporary participation in a more desirable alternative world (Nietzsche, 1872); it provides consoling illusions (Rank, 1932); it promotes catharsis of disturbing emotions (Aristotle, Poetics 6.2), and so forth.

The arts and health, for example, are mentioned in the writings of Greek philosophers [4] and ancient Egyptians [6]; in the observations of Benjamin Franklin that patients benefited from creative activities, in this case specifically writing [4]; and in a detailed essay by physician Richard Browne about the healing effects of music, specifically singing [8, 9]. As Western medicine formalized, the use of arts within healthcare continued.

Professionalization of the arts in medical settings emerged at the beginning of the twentieth century. Bibliotherapy was the first to be formalized in the early 1900s [10]. Creative arts therapies such as music therapy and art therapy established governing organizations, codes of ethics, and education and credentialing standards during the 1940s–1970s [11, 12]. Medical humanities emerged around the 1960s and are now institutionalized within many medical education programs [13]. Arts in health began to formalize in the early 1990s [14] and continues to be defined as a field. A code of ethics was established in 2018 [15] and formalized training programs in arts in health are growing.

Through professionalization, three distinct areas of arts practice are relevant to healthcare today. Each discipline has unique characteristics and purpose:

- *Arts in health* engages artists in clinical or community health settings. Practitioners, called artists in healthcare, volunteer or work as professional artist-staff [16]. They have excellent proficiency in their artistic discipline and have training to safely navigate healthcare environments [17]. Artists in healthcare facilitate arts activities or performances one-on-one or in workshops with patients, families, and/or staff and clinicians. They provide positive creative experiences that enhance well-being [18]. Additionally, there are arts administrators who manage artists in healthcare, design health spaces, curate exhibits, and/or host performances within health settings [16]. Recently, arts in community and public health have been included within the field of arts in health [19].

- *Medical humanities* is an interdisciplinary field in medical education and practice that incorporates literary works, films, plays, visual arts, music, and popular media as a framework to explore the interface between medicine and history, philosophy, ethics, religion, the arts, and the social sciences. Medical humanities programs are reported to be in place in many universities in the USA and other countries [20].

- *Creative arts therapies* use arts processes and materials to work toward specific mental health or rehabilitation goals within a therapeutic relationship led by a creative arts therapist [21]. Creative arts therapists' education and credentials meet standards established by their individual discipline, and include arts, human development, and psychotherapeutic training [22]. Their credentials include an advanced degree and postgraduate registration, board certification, and/or licensure. The National Coalition for Creative Arts Therapists (NCCATA) in the USA includes art therapy, music therapy, dance/movement therapy, drama therapy, poetry therapy, and psychodrama. Additionally, some people include expressive arts therapy and bibliotherapy.

Evidence-based studies beginning in the later twentieth century show the efficacy of using arts within health contexts. Qualitative and quantitative research on the impact of the arts in health have increased over the past 15 years. These studies include, for example, how the arts are used in hospitals, with aging populations (particularly dementia), with oncology patients, and in community and public health settings [23, 24], as well as studies that focus on biomarkers and psychological behavior in relation to creative activities [6, 25]. As the pace of research accelerates, studies are also addressing professionalism and scope of practice, as well as definitions for and differences in arts in health and the creative arts therapies [24, 26, 27]. The following are some examples of specific research:

- Live preferential music can decrease the amount of pain medication requested in emergency rooms [28].
- Creative writing can increase empathy and decrease stress for medical students [29].
- Dance classes for people living with Parkinson's disease can improve functional mobility, quality of life, and self-efficacy [30].
- Group art therapy supports active duty service members to better understand their medical conditions and reduces isolation [31].

- Music therapy can reduce anxiety, depression, and pain for people undergoing cancer treatment [32].
- Documented health benefits in 11 studies of using the arts with older adults were supported in a systematic literature review [33].

Arts in health research is predominantly, but not entirely, qualitative and can sometimes be limited by the implausibility of strictly controlled and double-blind interventions. Nevertheless, arts in health research, especially in the UK and the USA, is increasingly incorporating biomarkers and other testing to measure physiological responses to arts encounters, as well as implementing quantitative study design [6, 23–25, 34].

The arts have also established an increasingly solid position in medical education. In addition to reflective writing as described in this chapter, many medical schools promote theatrical performances, visits to art museums, and reading and discussion of literature [35–38]. Further studies are needed to explore and validate the impact of arts education on the communication skills of physicians and longitudinal effects on the clinical care they provide; research results are more significant in confirming the role of the arts in improving skills in observation and description [39, 40].

In the field of creative arts therapies, the National Endowment for the Arts is supporting research, particularly focused on active duty military service members, veterans, and families. An initiative of the National Endowment for the Arts, Creative Forces®: The NEA Military Healing Arts Network, is a partnership with the US Departments of Defense and Veterans Affairs and the state and local arts agencies, with administrative support provided by Americans for the Arts. In addition to hosting a database of research studies (www.arts.gov /national-initiatives/creative-forces/research), Creative Forces includes a five-year research agenda (2018–2022) that will provide significant contributions to creative arts therapies research. Initial research has focused on service members with posttraumatic stress disorder (PTSD) and traumatic brain injury (TBI), including retrospective analysis of clinical data, case studies, and program evaluation. This research provides preliminary support that the creative arts therapies may enhance overall treatment satisfaction and be helpful in expressing emotions and managing trauma symptoms [41]. Several additional studies explore the relationship between visual images and other sources of information, such as standardized measures and clinical notes [31, 42]. The Creative Forces research agenda works toward increasingly robust levels of evidence.

In other areas of creative arts therapies, systematic reviews have found that art therapy participants often report positive experiences, but research has historically consisted of small sample sizes and provided mostly anecdotal support [43–45]. There is growing evidence that art therapy positively impacts the quality of life and psychological coping for patients undergoing cancer treatment [46, 47]; however, research with other medical populations is less persuasive. Art therapists working in community mental health clinics or private practice often lack funding and collaboration opportunities that can contribute to more robust research studies that are possible in larger healthcare facilities or universities, often limiting the size and scope of art therapy research. The Creative Forces initiative is an excellent model for strategic, cross-disciplinary research efforts essential to advancing application and implementation of arts and wellness programs.

The remainder of this chapter uses examples to explore how these arts-based approaches are used in healthcare. The subheadings "inspirational," "educational," and "therapeutic" distinguish overarching aspects of each area:

- arts in health focuses on providing *inspiration* and hope while humanizing healthcare experiences and environments;
- medical humanities uses the arts to inform health sciences *education* and improve holistic, empathetic medical training; and
- creative arts therapies work to achieve *therapeutic* goals that support medical and mental health treatment and rehabilitation.

The authors acknowledge that these subheadings may seem reductive by implying divisions among the disciplines that are not always exclusive, yet these categories help conceptualize the overarching purpose of each approach. Overlap exists in that, at various times, all three of these disciplines could be described as inspirational, educational, and therapeutic.

Arts in Health: *Inspirational*

Arts in health brings arts engagement and performance into health settings with the intention of enhancing overall well-being through the creative process and aesthetic experience. Artists in healthcare might facilitate activities for participants to engage in or they might perform their art while participants watch or listen. Inspiration is a key component to arts in health. Framed by theorists Thrash and Elliot [48], inspiration elicits motivation and energy through a trigger (in this case participating in or witnessing the arts) that allows a person to transcend a current state or limitation (such as physical illness or poor quality of life). The creative process inherent in art [18] stimulates inspiration that supports wellness within healthcare settings, for example:

- during a creative writing workshop, a patient with cancer might write a poem about nature recalling the simple beauties of life while experiencing the joy of social connection by sharing it with the group;
- a hospital musician might play a favorite uplifting song upon request of a patient waiting for a transplant; or
- a dancer might help a patient with sickle cell disease move her arms and breathe like the waves of the ocean, initiating a momentary "vacation" from the pain.

Beyond the creative process, these experiences become inspirational and transformative because they are unexpected within the Western medical setting. Contemporary medicine focuses on physical health concerns. Yet, patients experience vulnerability and loss of control, and struggle to find meaning within the health crisis. Complex themes of identity and control surface even at the point of admission to a healthcare facility. Tina Mullen, director of UF Health Shands Arts in Medicine, described the process in an essay by Dylan Klempner [49]:

> We take your clothes first. We hand them back to your loved one in a bag. You don't get to choose your room. We assign you a room. You don't get to choose who comes in and out of that room. You don't get to choose when they come in and out of that room. You barely get to choose what you eat, and you certainly don't get to choose when you eat it. You don't even really get to choose when people visit you ... But what we've taken away in that process ... is your ability to navigate yourself.

The arts can shift this experience by adding a more personalized focus to the patient journey, establishing identity beyond a diagnosis, and helping maintain control while undergoing treatment. Instead of idly watching TV or sleeping, patients can actively

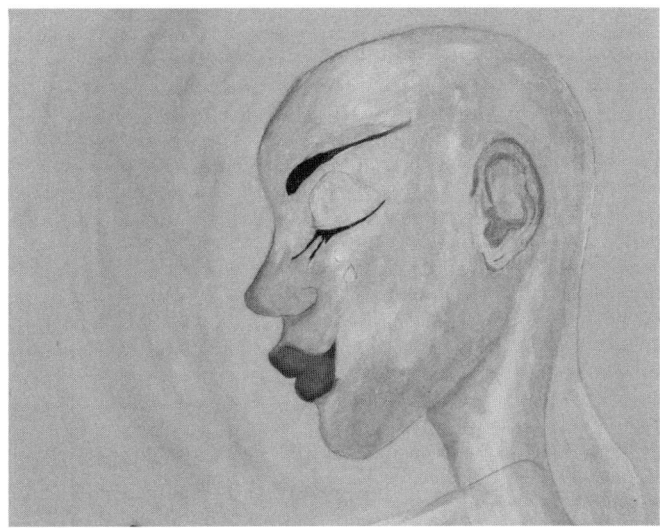

Figure 36.1 Painting by Khandice.

experience art that is both aesthetically pleasing and purposeful. Furthermore, art can elicit empathy from the healthcare staff toward the challenges of the medical situation [18].

For example, Figure 36.1 was created by a young woman undergoing cancer treatment. The viewer might empathize – sensing sadness and humility, yet also, power and strength.

The painting communicates an inner viewpoint and simultaneously taps into universal human experiences of suffering and optimism. This example illustrates how artwork can build a bridge for relationships between patients and healthcare staff:

> She was no longer the Osteosarcoma patient in room 203. She was Khandice, who bravely continued treatment when mouth sores, exhaustion, and hair loss were devastating. She painted this image while she was taking college courses from her hospital bed and rediscovering the inner-artist, poet, and songwriter that was forgotten in childhood. [Joanne Lagmay, UF hematologist/oncologist, personal communication]

When the medical team acknowledges a patient's creative work, like with Khandice, the identity shifts from "patient" to "person," resulting in a more successful relationship. A sense of partnership between the patient and medical team can enhance medical compliance and improve perceived quality of care [50, 51]. Within the medical journey, the patient experiences a sense of accomplishment that offers purpose and hope, bringing optimism that has been linked to enhanced recovery outcomes [52, 53] and better medical compliance [54, 55].

This is just one illustration of how arts in health provides unique opportunities for patients that can have favorable impacts on medical outcomes. Arts in health can help patients in various ways:

- regain a sense of control by making decisions about art materials, processes, and levels of participation;
- engage in something pleasurable amid treatment that might be unpleasant or painful;
- provide satisfaction, accomplishment, and empowerment by participating in productive activities, making something that is tangible, and building artistic skill;

- share connections when art is created and/or viewed;
- promote empathy and compassion by tapping into universal expressions that evoke understanding;
- elicit hope and joy through beauty, imagination, idealization, and the creative process;
- feel more relaxed by offering activities that calm the nervous system, offer distraction from stressors, and are soothing; and
- make legacy through narrative work that is tangible and lasting, and documents memories.

As illustrated in this section, arts in health activities promote well-being and are inspirational for patients. The arts can enhance the healthcare environment, with benefits both to patients and to healthcare staff. Arts in health programs contribute to positive outcomes and also improve the overall perception of healthcare facilities [56].

Medical Humanities: *Educational*

Medical humanities exist within health training programs and aim to introduce students to social sciences and the arts in ways that are relevant to medicine. In recent years, the Accreditation Council for Graduate Medical Education (ACGME) has called for competencies that include demonstration of "interpersonal and communication skills that result in the effective exchange of information and collaboration with patients, their families, and health professionals" [57]. The Association of American Medical Colleges (AAMC) also identified "communications-related goals for medical students," in such areas as extracting, processing, and responding to information; recognizing emotions; drawing inferences; interpreting non-verbal cues; and clarifying unclear communication [58].

Those goals can be addressed through the medical humanities, with courses that include reflective writing, as well as reading and discussion of poetry, patient narratives, and physician reflections [59]. Programs that include visual thinking strategies are another approach whereby viewing artwork, often in a museum, promotes visual literacy, communication, and critical thinking [60].

Pennebaker and Charon [61, 62] highlight the following values of writing for medical students by correlating skills that both writers and physicians need:

- Observe detail and the big picture. Learning to see takes practice and is self-reinforcing.
- Listen to stories with interest and empathy. Genuinely listening – with heart – comes naturally to some people; others can develop the capacity with practice.
- Encourage narratives that have personal meaning. This offers a sense of control over life events, requires self-reflection, and rehearses possible outcomes.
- Engage in stress reduction and healthy living. Professionals must develop lifelong practices to prevent burnout, emotional breakdown, depression, and suicide. Writing and other forms of art contribute to resiliency and wellness.

The University of Florida College of Medicine, for example, established an elective reflective writing course that invited medical students to engage in creative writing, reading, journaling, and critical discussions about issues such as death and dying, cultural competency, allocation of health resources, stress management, and physicians as patients. Instead of focusing on technical writing, the course aimed to develop three primary skills:

1. observation to accurately perceive and describe experiences that impact practice, including mood of self and others, cultural differences, and the effects medical environments have on patients and staff;
2. reflection and communication, leading to compassionate listening, effective responses to challenging situations, and physician–patient/physician–colleague communication strategies; and
3. self-awareness and personal development to understand personal values, articulate fears and concerns, notice sources of pride, develop supportive communities to prevent burnout, and understand the habits that lead to being healthy, competent, and compassionate physicians.

Throughout the course, students wrote descriptions, stories, or poems about (1) patients observed in public areas of the hospital; (2) noteworthy interactions with fellow students or faculty members; (3) experiences encountered in training, including coming to terms with their own reactions to illness, death, and dying; and (4) social and ethical issues in medicine. At the conclusion of the course, students were surveyed about the effectiveness of creative writing in medical education (Box 36.1). Of 80 respondents, the majority believed that reflective writing helped them enhance their ability to practice medicine (77.8 percent), increase listening skills (80.0 percent), increase awareness of details, which can improve patient interaction and diagnosis (86.7 percent), increase perceived empathy (75.6 percent), and reduce stress levels (60 percent). Furthermore, 91.1 percent of the students reported "enjoying" the course and 88.9 percent reported they would "recommend" it to other students [63].

When asked what was particularly valuable or transformative about the creative writing process, four educational themes emerged that impact both personal and professional performance:

1. Personal reflection and growth. Feeling overwhelmed, questioning one's professional choice, and regretting distance from family and friends are common challenges for medical students. The course helped students survive the early years of medical school by exploring personal values, direction, and the capacity to articulate perspectives and emotions while hearing and respecting those of colleagues.
2. Professional development. Participants developed a writing practice useful in meeting day-to-day demands of medicine, which include listening to stories and perceiving, recording, and transmitting issues and information. They also learned

---

Box 36.1   Student Responses to Reflective Writing Course Survey [63]

- "Occasionally pieces of writing I reflected on in class were able to be developed into well-polished poems, short stories, etc. Often these pieces helped me sort out how I felt about complex issues dealt with in the medical education process. I still cling to those pieces after emotionally charged days/experiences."
- "For many, the first two years of medical school can be a grueling time, one in which we are absorbed in textbooks and labs – stuck as we are in the windowless corridors. By participating in this course, I had the opportunity to step both inside my own head and then outside of myself as I listened to others. This course truly allowed me to grow as a person and a physician."

strategies to cope with stressors associated with being a physician through private journaling, reading literature, and/or publishing stories.

3. Stress reduction. Students felt that the course activities such as reflective writing, class discussion, and arts engagement promoted positive coping for the chronic pressures of medical education.

4. Reflective writing as valuable to medical education. The course developed a reputation among medical students for enhancing study and professional development. One student wrote: "[This was] perhaps the most valuable course of my medical education."

These qualitative findings suggest that engagement in the creative process through reflective writing is a valuable and efficient tool for developing self-expression, introspective reflection, and skill building within arts-based education. Medical humanities counterbalance the rigorous scientific memorization and examination legendary in medical school experiences by humanizing the educational experience and training humane, compassionate, self-expressive, and healthy physicians.

Creative Arts Therapies: *Therapeutic*

The creative arts therapies are mental health and rehabilitation professions that integrate the arts into treatment within the context of a therapeutic relationship. Creative arts therapists work in a variety of educational, mental health, and healthcare settings. Due to variation in each discipline and setting, this section will focus on art therapy in healthcare as one example of the creative arts therapies.

Art Therapy in Healthcare

In recent years, healthcare facilities have begun to place greater focus on whole health or multidimensional models of healthcare that consider emotional, social, and even spiritual wellness as having a role in healing and recovery [64]. These models lend themselves to the work of art therapists in healthcare settings. Already a stressful experience, medical care is exacerbated by the events that lead to hospitalization, including accidents, abuse, physical illness, or even mental health conditions that cause physical problems [65]. People receiving medical treatment may have layered experiences of trauma, health issues, and mental health challenges. The whole-person model encourages patients to develop areas of strength and holistic support while dealing with complex physical and emotional health issues.

Art therapy uses visual art processes and media combined with psychological theory and understanding of human development to support therapeutic goals [66]. Within healthcare settings, art therapists are integrated members of the clinical team and work collaboratively with medical staff to support treatment [67]. Art therapy can be used in healthcare settings to support the following:

- stabilization from symptoms of anxiety, stress, and trauma by providing therapeutic safety, emotional containment, and trauma debriefing [65];
- adjustment to the medical situation by developing coping skills, managing environmental stressors, and navigating the social and cultural structures of healthcare [68];
- cognitive and motor–sensory rehabilitation, including visuospatial functions [48], decision-making abilities, sensory stimulation, and art-based assessments to monitor progress over time;

- self-regulation through body-based responses elicited during the art-making process that focus on present moment awareness, regulating physical symptoms, and self-soothing;
- effective communication by using nonverbal self-expression to access thoughts and feelings, convey important messages, and decrease isolation;
- emotional resilience by using the symbolic and expressive qualities of art to elicit emotional awareness and provide tools for effectively processing feelings;
- self-esteem through activities that promote personal insight, address body image issues, and increase independence and motivation;
- meaning-making through documentary and narrative artwork that brings understanding and value to difficult circumstances; and
- coping with grief by using artwork to process fears and losses or as a transitional object/ memory after someone has died.

Case Example

Valerie is a veteran who began art therapy following heart surgery [69]. She was in a serious accident more than 10 years prior that resulted in a traumatic brain injury (TBI) and ongoing symptoms of posttraumatic stress, causing her challenges in neurocognitive organization. Her surgery reactivated feelings of powerlessness related to her trauma and left her physically isolated from her usual support systems. For patients with complex medical issues, like Valerie, it can be difficult to put words to their experiences. Especially with trauma, the brain's occipital lobe, which is responsible for visual processing, becomes activated during times of intense stress, while the Broca's area, which is responsible for language, is impaired [70]. As such, it is often easier for patients to process traumatic experiences nonverbally through art images than to communicate through words [71].

Early in art therapy, Valerie began to utilize detailed pen drawings for relaxation and stress reduction. The process gave her a meaningful and meditative activity that allowed her to reflect on her complex emotions. Additionally, the detailed drawings helped her work on pattern recognition and spatial interpretation, which are key brain processes for effective decision-making [72]. Figure 36.2 shows a pen drawing created by Valerie at a particularly stressful time in her treatment. The process served as a form of mindfulness to help Valerie reduce her anxiety.

Valerie remained in art therapy throughout her recovery and continued even after she regained mobility and independence. She created art on her own between therapy sessions and found that it relaxed her and helped her cope with stress. Working with an art therapist helped Valerie push through frustrations, taught her new cognitive processes, and showed her tools that she could use to safely contain difficult emotions. As with Valerie, art therapy in healthcare focuses on the whole person and allows patients who have layered physical and mental health needs to safely manage the disease process, contextualize self-identity, explore intense emotions, and make meaning out of difficult experiences through art.

Summary

When health organizations integrate arts into healthcare delivery, exponential effects are possible. Benefits span from improved perception of patient care, to enhanced clinician self-care and burnout prevention, and physical and psychological therapeutic gains. The arts are a unique entry point that supports healthcare goals through inspirational, educational, and

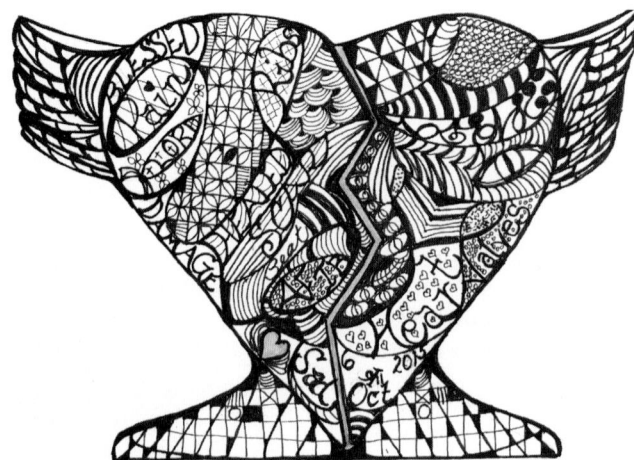

Figure 36.2 Valerie's reflective pen drawing.

therapeutic means. Arts-based approaches are accessible, approachable, and supportive. The impact of arts-care moves beyond individual recipients and has a positive influence on family members, other patients, students, and medical professionals. Whether delivered by an artist in healthcare, an educator-artist, or by a creative arts therapist, arts-based activities enhance the medical environment, support the goals of medical staff, and engage the healthcare community in well-being through the arts.

References

1. AW Pike, DL Hoffmann, M Garcia-Diez, et al. U-series dating of Paleolithic art in 11 caves in Spain. *Science* 2012; **336**(6087): 1409–1413.

2. M Samuels, N Samuels. *Seeing with the Mind's Eye: The History, Techniques, and Uses of Visualization.* New York, Random House; 1975.

3. RG Bednarik, G Kumar, RG Watchman, A Roberts. Preliminary results of the EIP project. 2004. https://ro.uow.edu.au/scipapers/3611 (accessed April 21, 2020).

4. J Sonke-Henderson. History of the arts and health across cultures. In J Sonke-Henderson, R Brandman, I Serlin, J Graham-Pole, eds., *Whole Person Health Care, Volume 3: The Arts and Health.* Westport, CT, Praeger; 2007; 23–42.

5. E Dissanayake. *What Is Art For?* Seattle, WA, University of Washington; 1998.

6. D Fancourt. *Arts in Health: Designing and Researching Interventions.* Oxford, Oxford University Press; 2017.

7. E Belfiore. The arts and healing: the power of an idea. In: S Clift, P Camic, eds., *Oxford Text of Creative Arts, Health, and Wellbeing.* Oxford, Oxford University Press; 2016; 11–17.

8. R Browne. *Medicina Musica: Or, A Mechanical Essay on the Effects of Singing, Musick, and Dancing, on Human Bodies. Revis'd and Corrected. To which is Annex'd a New Essay on the Nature and Cure of the Spleen and Vapours Vapours.* J. Cooke; 1729.

9. P Gouk. Raising spirits and restoring souls: early modern medical explanations for music's effects. *Hearing Cultures* 2004; **3**: 87.

10. DT Ouzts. The emergence of bibliotherapy as a discipline. *Reading Horizons* 1991;**31** (3): 3.

11. American Society of Group Psychotherapy and Psychodrama. About. 2014. https://asgpp.org/about-asgpp.php (accessed April 21, 2020).

12. M Junge. History of art therapy. In D Gussak, M Rosal, eds., *The Wiley*

Handbook of Art Therapy. Chichester, Wiley Blackwell; 2016; 7–16.

13. T Adachi. Medical humanities. In: H ten Have, ed., *Encyclopedia of Global Bioethics.* New York, Springer; 2015.

14. R Brandman. The development of the contemporary international arts in healthcare field. In: I. Serline, ed., *Whole Person Healthcare.* Westport, CT, Prager; 2007; 43–65.

15. NOAH (National Organization for Arts in Health). Code of ethics for arts in health professionals and standards of practice for arts in health professionals. https://the noah.net/wp-content/uploads/2018/10/N OAH-Code-of-Ethics-and-Standards-for-Arts-in-Health-Professionals.pdf (accessed April 21, 2020).

16. J Sonke, JB Lee, M Helgemo Rollins, et al. Arts in health: considering language from an educational perspective in the United States. *Arts Health* 2018; 10:2, 151–164.

17. J Sonke, R Rollins, R Brandman, J Graham-Pole. The state of the arts in healthcare in the United States. *Arts Health* 2009; **1**: 107–135.

18. J Sonke, R Brandman. The hospital artist in residence program: narratives of healing. In: I Serlin, ed., *Whole Person Healthcare: The Arts in Health.* Westport, CT, Prager; 2007; 67–86.

19. E Byrne, E Elliott, R Saltus, J Angharad. The creative turn in evidence for public health: community and arts-based methodologies. *J Publ Health* 2018; **40** (suppl. 1): i24–i30.

20. Stanford Center for Bioethics. Other health humanities programs. https://med .stanford.edu/medicineandthemuse/Progr amLinks/OtherPrograms.html (accessed April 21, 2020).

21. C Malchiodi. Expressive therapies: history, theory, and practice. In: C. Malchiodi, ed., *Expressive Therapies.* New York, Guilford Press; 2005.

22. National Coalition of Creative Arts Therapies Associations. April 2019 About. www.nccata.org/aboutnccata.

23. J Sonke, J Rollins, J Graham-Pole. Arts in healthcare settings in the United States. In:

Oxford Textbook of Creative Arts, Health, and Wellbeing: International Perspectives on Practice, Policy, and Research. Oxford, Oxford University Press; 2016: 113–121.

24. C Dileo, J Bradt. On creating the discipline, profession, and evidence in the field of arts and healthcare. *Arts Health* 2009; **1**(2): 168–182.

25. G Kaimal, K Ray, J Muniz. Reduction of cortisol levels and participants' responses following art making. *Art Ther* 2016; **33**(2): 74–80.

26. T Van Lith, H Spooner. Art therapy and arts in health: identifying shared values but different goals using a framework analysis. *Art Ther* 2018; **35**(2): 88–93.

27. A Bucciarelli. Art therapy: a transdisciplinary approach. *Art Ther* 2016; **33**(3): 151–155.

28. J Tyndall, M Kerrigan, MA Baker Chowdhury, et al. Music in emergent settings: a randomized controlled trial. *Ann Emerg Med* 2017; **70**(4): S167.

29. G Ellison. Reflective writing: providing a useful tool to medical students. *San Francisco Med* 2008; **July–August**: 26–27.

30. C McRae, D Leventhal, O Westheimer, et al. Long-term effects of dance for PD on self-efficacy among persons with Parkinson's disease. *Arts Health* 2018; **10** (1): 85–96.

31. M Berberian, MS Walker, G Kaimal "Master my demons": art therapy montage paintings by active-duty military service members with traumatic brain injury and post-traumatic stress. *Medical Humanities* 2018; **45**(4): 353–360.

32. C Gramaglia, E Gambaro, C Vecchi, et al. Outcomes of music therapy interventions in cancer patients: a review of the literature. *Crit Rev Oncol Hematol* 2019; **138**: 251–254.

33. M Castora-Binkley, L Noelker, T Prohaska, W Satariano. Impact of arts participation on health outcomes for older adults. *J Aging Humanities Arts* 2010; **4**(4): 352–367.

34. S Clift. Creative arts as a public health resource: moving from practice-based

research to evidence-based practice. *Perspect Publ Health* 2012; **132**(3): 120–127.

35. PC Ünalan, A Uzuner, S Çifçili, et al. Using theatre in education in a traditional lecture oriented medical curriculum. *BMC Med Educ* 2009; **9**(1): 73.

36. J Shapiro, L Hunt. All the world's a stage: the use of theatrical performance in medical education. *Med Educ* 2003; **37**(10): 922–927.

37. MM Milota, GJ van Thiel, JJ van Delden. Narrative medicine as a medical education tool: a systematic review. *Med Teacher* 2019; **9**: 1–9.

38. SL Arntfield, K Slesar, J Dickson, R Charon. Narrative medicine as a means of training medical students toward residency competencies. *Patient Educ Couns* 2013; **91**(3): 280–286.

39. P Haidet, J Jarecke, NE Adams, et al. A guiding framework to maximise the power of the arts in medical education: a systematic review and metasynthesis. *Med Educ* 2016; **50**(3): 320–331.

40. S Naghshineh, JP Hafler, AR Miller, et al. Formal art observation training improves medical students' visual diagnostic skills. *J Gen Intern Med* 2008; **23**(7): 991–997.

41. G Kaimal, J Jones, R Dieterich-Hartwell, B Acharya, X Wang. Evaluation of long-and short-term art therapy interventions in an integrative care setting for military service members with post-traumatic stress and traumatic brain injury. *Arts Psychother* 2019; **62**: 28–36.

42. G Kaimal, MS Walker, J Herres, LM French, TJ DeGraba. Observational study of associations between visual imagery and measures of depression, anxiety and post-traumatic stress among active-duty military service members with traumatic brain injury at the Walter Reed National Military Medical Center. *BMJ Open* 2018; **8**(6): e021448.

43. A Maujean, CA Pepping, E Kendall. A systematic review of randomized controlled studies of art therapy. *Art Ther* 2014; **31**(1): 37–44.

44. RL Beard. Art therapies and dementia care: a systematic review. *Dementia* 2012; **11**(5): 633–656.

45. LA Clapp, EP Taylor, S Di Folco, VL Mackinnon. Effectiveness of art therapy with pediatric populations affected by medical health conditions: a systematic review. *Arts Health* 2018; **4**: 1–9.

46. D Regev, L Cohen-Yatziv. Effectiveness of art therapy with adult clients in 2018: what progress has been made? A systematic review. *Front Psychol* 2018; **9**: 1531.

47. MJ Wood, A Molassiotis, S Payne. What research evidence is there for the use of art therapy in the management of symptoms in adults with cancer? A systematic review. *Psycho-Oncology* 2011; **20**(2): 135–145.

48. T Thrash, A Elliot. Inspiration as psychological construct. *J Pers Soc Psychol* 2003; **84**(4): 871–889.

49. D Klempner. Music and art have impact in hospital. 2017, February17. *Gainesville Sun*. www.gainesville.com/opinion/20170217/dylan-klempner-music-and-art-have-impact-in-hospital (accessed April 21, 2020).

50. J Archer, L Stevenson, A Coulter, AM Breen. Connecting patient experience, leadership, and the importance of involvement, information, and empathy in the care process. *Healthcare Manage Forum* 2018; **31**(6): 252–255.

51. CL Roumie, R Greevy, KA Wallston, et al. Patient centered primary care is associated with patient hypertension medication adherence. *J Behav Med* 2011; **34**(4): 244–253.

52. S Parkin, J Swift. Utilizing patient hope and outcome expectations to facilitate treatment gains. *Med Res Arch* 2017; **5** (6): 1–9.

53. K Kortte, J Stevenson, R Hosey, R Castillo, S Wegener. Hope predicts positive functional role outcomes in acute rehabilitation populations. *Rehabil Psychol* 2012; **57**(3): 248–255.

54. C Berg, M Rapoff, C Snyder, J Belmont. The relationship of children's hope to pediatric asthma treatment adherence. *J Posit Psychol* 2007; **2**: 176–184.

55. J Van Allen, R Steele, M Nelson. A longitudinal examination of hope and optimism and their role in type 1 diabetes in youths. *J Pediatr Psychol* 2016; **41**: 741–749.

56. HL Stuckey, J Nobel. The connection between art, healing, and public health: a review of current literature. *Am J Publ Health* 2010; **100**(2): 254–263.

57. Accreditation Council for Graduate Medical Education (ACGME). Common Program Requirements. www.acgme.org/What-We-Do/Accreditation/Common-Program-Requirements (accessed April 21, 2020).

58. Association of American Medical Colleges. *Contemporary Issues in Medicine: Communication in Medicine*. Washington, DC, AAMC; 1999.

59. GK Ellison. Reflective writing: providing a useful tool to medical students. *San Francisco Med* 2008; **81**(6).

60. N Mukunda, N Moghbeli, A Rizzo, et al. Visual art instruction in medical education: a narrative review. *Med Educ Online* 2019; **24**(1). DOI:10.1080/10872981.2018.1558657.

61. JW Pennebaker. Telling stories: the health benefits of narrative. *Lit Med* 2000; **19**(1): 3–18.

62. R Charon. *Narrative Medicine: Honoring the Stories of Illness*. Oxford, Oxford University Press; 2008.

63. GK Ellison. Evaluation of the UF College of Medicine reflective writing elective, supported by a grant from the Arnold P. Gold Foundation. Unpublished manuscript.

64. T Gaudet, B Kligler. Whole health in the whole system of the Veterans Administration: how will we know we have reached this future state? *J Altern Complement Med* 2019; **25**(S1): S7–S11.

65. C Ghetti, A Whitehead-Pleaux. Sounds of strength: music therapy for hospitalized children at risk for traumatization. In: C. Malchiodi, ed., *Creative Interventions with Traumatized Children* (2nd ed.) New York, Guilford Press; 2015.

66. American Art Therapy Association. About art therapy. 2017. https://arttherapy.org/about-art-therapy (accessed April 21, 2020).

67. SA Anand. Dimensions of art therapy in medical illness. In: DE Gussak, ML Rosal, eds., *The Wiley Handbook of Art Therapy*. New York: Wiley; 2016.

68. T Councill. Medical art therapy with children. In: C. Malchiodi, ed. *Handbook of Art Therapy*. New York, Guildford Press; 2003.

69. H Spooner, JB Lee, DG Langston, et al. Using distance technology to deliver the creative arts therapies to veterans: case studies in art, dance/movement and music therapy. *Arts Psychother* 2019; **62**: 12–18.

70. C Bourne, CE Mackay, EA Holmes. The neural basis of flashback formation: the impact of viewing trauma. *Psychol Med* 2012; **43**(7): 1521–1532.

71. K Coleman, HB Macintosh. Art and evidence: balancing the discussion on arts- and evidence- based practices with traumatized children. *Journ Child Adol Trauma* 2015; **8**(21). DOI:10.1007/s40653-015-0036.

72. F Reynolds. Art therapy after stroke: evidence and a need for further research. *Arts Psychother* 2012; 39(4): 239–244.

Engaging the Five Senses

Taste, Smell, See, Listen, and Touch

Vladimir Bokarius

Original illustrations in this chapter by Andrew V. Bokarius

We live on the leash of our senses. There is no way in which to understand the world without first detecting it through the radar-net of our senses.

Diane Ackerman

Introduction

A Google search for the definition of "wellness" returns 348,000,000 results. The first one is simple and makes sense: "Wellness is an active process of becoming aware of and making choices toward a healthy and fulfilling life" [1].

The World Health Organization (WHO) defines wellness as "a state of complete physical, mental, and social well-being and not merely the absence of disease or infirmity" [2]. Mental, physical, and social domains interact bidirectionally, and health across all domains is integral to a holistic picture of wellness. This understanding of wellness guides this chapter.

The senses have been addressed in philosophy and medicine since ancient times, from the Vedas of ancient India to *The Yellow Emperor's Classic of Internal Medicine* in ancient China and the works of pre-Aristotelian Greek philosophers. In ancient Egypt, the five senses were illustrated in pictograms (Figure 37.1).

Senses were utilized both in treatment and for promoting joy of life by improving its quality. In the biblical Genesis, Eve heard the snake, saw the fruit, picked it, and tasted it. Although no mention is made of smell, she was likely influenced by the apple's aroma.

In ancient civilizations, feasts were held to stimulate taste. Aromatic oils were used to engage scent. Sculpture, pictures, dance, and reverence for nature relied on well-honed human vision. Elaborate bodywork and sex guides attest to the universal import of touch. Finally, people enjoyed the sounds of nature, created music, and sang to stimulate hearing, just as they do today.

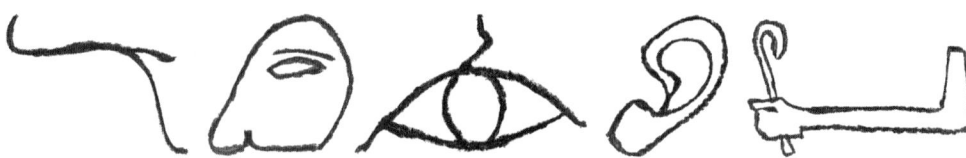

Figure 37.1 Egyptian pictograms of senses.

Table 37.1 Functions of the senses

	Learning	Self-protection	Appetite stimulation	Sexual behavior	Recognition	Orientation	Communication	Locomotion	Sleep–wake cycle
Taste	×	×	×	×	×				
Smell	×	×	×	×	×	×			
Sight	×	×	×	×	×	×	×	×	×
Hearing	×	×	×	×	×	×	×	×	×
Touch	×	×	×	×	×	×	×	×	×

With the advent of civilization, use of the senses became more sophisticated, with the development of visual art, music, perfumes, bodywork, and sensual techniques, and the rise of new flavors:

- The exponential growth of gourmet restaurants and ethnic food isles in supermarkets has given rise to "foodie" culture, and the birth of a neurogastronomy nation, as celebrated by the International Society of Neurogastronomy [3].
- A multitude of fragrances have hit the market, not just as personal cosmetics but for homes, offices, and cars, with and without claims of therapeutic effects. Likewise, foods and beverages have been artificially colored and flavored to enhance palatability, sometimes at the cost of nutritional integrity.
- Developments in audiovisual technology provide constant and instant access to information, permeating gaming and social media. The resulting sensory overload has some seeking refuge in "sensory diets."
- Bodywork has become much more elaborate and widespread. Spas and massage parlors use an increasingly diverse array of techniques, including ethnic modalities, stones, muds, salts, and beverages.

Contrary to popular belief, the human senses are more advanced than those of many other mammals. We are believed to be capable of distinguishing over one trillion different compounds by scent, at thresholds that mimic or surpass those of other animals [4]. Human vision has been tested and found to be superior to that of all but a few animals [5]. Although we are not able to detect high and/or low frequencies like some aquatic and land animals, our ability to differentiate between frequencies is unrivaled [6]. Supremacy of human sense of touch does not need any comment. The senses play an important role in multiple domains of functioning, both physical and psychological. Table 37.1 illustrates their involvement.

Psychological Effects

Each of the five senses is capable of triggering positive or negative emotions, pleasant or unpleasant memories, excitation or relaxation, or causing psychiatric symptoms like anxiety, panic attacks, flashbacks, anger, depression, psychotic outbreaks, and phobias:

- Some Native American tribes used scent to evoke memories by carrying around boxes containing fragrant substances, which they smelled on auspicious occasions to summon up the associated feelings at will.

Table 37.2 Sensory overstimulation

	Arousal	Sedation	Pain	Nausea/vomiting	Dizziness	Seizure	Fainting	Hypertension	Itching/tickling	Sneezing
Taste	×			×						
Smell	×	×		×						×
Sight	×	×	×	×	×	×	×			
Hearing	×	×	×	×	×		×	×		
Touch	×	×	×	×	×				×	×

- Medicinal music was integral to traditional shamanic practices worldwide. Contemporary research shows that certain keys of music are more relaxing or stimulating than others [7].
- The possibility of music triggering suicidality has long been discussed, but never scientifically confirmed. Nevertheless, the "Hungarian suicide song" portrayed in the movie *Gloomy Sunday* was banned by the BBC from the 1930s through 2002 due to multiple suicides that allegedly occurred after listening to the song [8].
- Auditory stimulation by means of spoken words can have striking physiological consequences. Consider not only the psychological but the bodily effects (including brain remodeling, cardiovascular changes, and endocrine alterations) of hearing speech in the context of psychotherapy, juxtaposed with the shock of hearing that a loved one has died or the humiliation at being insulted and cursed at!

When overstimulated, sensory overload may damage the mind and body (Table 37.2):

- Seizures can be induced by cartoons and video games [9, 10].
- Stendhal syndrome is a striking disorder that exemplifies visual overstimulation. Symptoms include dizzy spells, palpitations, hallucinations, and confusion. They are triggered by "art that is perceived as particularly beautiful or when the individual is exposed to large quantities of art that are concentrated in a single place," such as a museum or gallery [11]. It is also called Florence syndrome, so named after over 100 visitors to Florence were stretchered to hospital from the city's art galleries and museums during the 1980s [12].

Senses in Diagnosing

In ancient Greece and China, physicians were taught to observe patients' movement and skin color, touch patients to determine body temperature and pulse, listen to lung and abdominal sounds, smell breath or feces, and even taste sweat or urine. In contemporary medicine, physicians' senses are still important, but are frequently enhanced or supplanted by various devices, including computerized imaging, scopes, electronic devices for evaluation of movement and strength, animals (including service dogs for diabetics), and electronic noses [13].

The use of smell in diagnosis may sound odd or outdated, but there are several examples of rare genetic diseases with associated bodily smells:

- trimethylaminuria, which produces a distinctive fish-like body odor
- maple syrup urine disease, named after the hallmark maple syrup smell of the urine

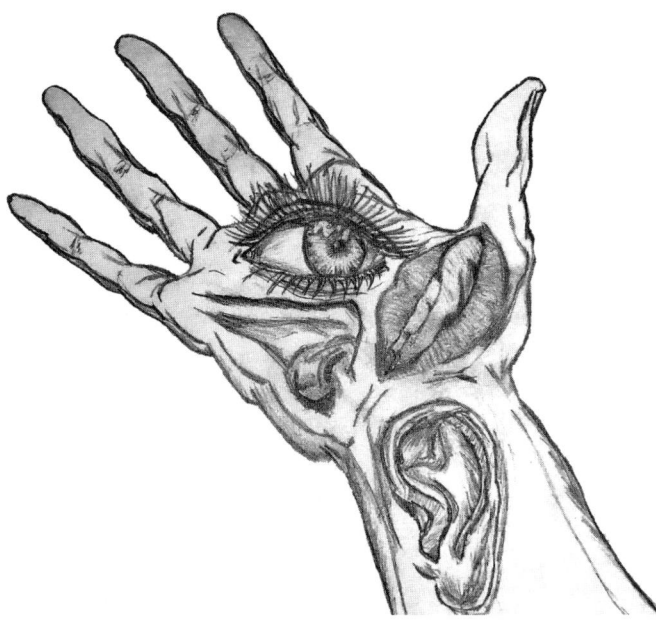

Figure 37.2 The five senses.

- phenylketonuria, frequently responsible for a "mousy" or "musty" odor
- isovaleric acidemia, with the presence of a "sweaty foot" body odor

The following sections will explore the role of each sense (Figure 37.2) in promoting wellness, review associated pathologies, and suggest how they can be addressed both medically and through lifestyle modification. It should be noted that wellness can be derived from any sense by exposing it to pleasurable stimuli. This aspect will not be discussed in each individual sense.

Taste

Our ability to taste obviously guides food selection. However, human taste preferences have outgrown evolutionary functions like tasting bitterness to detect toxic compounds in vegetables, sourness to detect spoiled or rotting plant matter, and selection of salty and sweet foods for their nutritive value. We have trained the palate through cooking and food preparation and tolerate bitter compounds if we know they are medicinal or beneficial to health, such as stimulant compounds in tea or coffee. Adults learn to enjoy combinations of tastes that are off-putting to most infants. In addition to the four conventional tastes, *umami* was recently confirmed to be a taste in its own right. It bespeaks our ability to detect glutamate, felt as the "meatiness" in foods like mushrooms, meats, and seafoods [14]. Retronasal olfactory receptors located at the back of the throat aid in flavor recognition.

Promoting Wellness

- Use of taste (e.g., menthol) in relieving anxiety or panic.
- Addition of flavoring to medications.
- Use of oral candies or sprays and flavored lubricants to enhance sexual experience.

Pathological States

Taste and smell are interdependent, and difficulty with one is sometimes interpreted as a problem with the other. Pathology of taste includes:

- hypogeusia – diminished taste
- dysgeusia/aliageusia – distorted/altered taste
- ageusia – no taste
- phantogeusia – persistent abnormal taste in the absence of a stimulus

A multitude of medical and psychiatric conditions, surgical interventions, medications, environmental exposure, and aging may lead to pathological states of taste.

Addressing Pathology

Initial treatment of gustatory dysfunction should seek to correct the causative pathology. Further treatment may include:

- Eliminate local irritants (e.g., mouthwashes, ill-fitting dentures).
- Artificial saliva or salivary stimulants and local anti-inflammatory medications may improve some taste dysfunction.
- Traditional Chinese medicine: Although taste plays an important part in diagnosis and choice of herbal medicines and diet, treatment of taste disorders is not common. Low-quality evidence for acupuncture's ability to improve taste has been found [15].
- Devices: electronic tongues are widely used in water safety, pharmaceutical, and food production industries to ensure consistency in taste across a product line. None are used in treatment or rehabilitation yet.
- Lifestyle/prevention:
  - Avoid excessive use of sugar, salt, acid, and spice, all of which can dull taste if unmoderated. Stay mindful of increasing diversity of food colors, textures, spices, and flavorings to enhance taste and enjoyment.
  - Abstain from heavy alcohol consumption and smoking [16, 17].
  - Maintain good oral hygiene.
  - Prevent trauma to the head and mouth.
  - Avoid toxic exposure, oral or inhaled.
  - Yoga: although yoga techniques to improve taste can be found online, no evidence-based treatment has been found.

More information on research and treatment of taste disorders can be found at:

- the Taste and Smell Clinic at University of Connecticut (https://health.uconn.edu/tasteandsmell)
- the Association for Chemoreception Sciences (https://achems.org/web)

Smell

Humans are able to detect odor both intranasally and retronasally. The olfactory bulb is unique among sensory systems in communicating directly with the cerebral cortex, bypassing subcortical structures. While seemingly not as useful to our immediate survival as the other senses, smell is unique in its immediate and potent ability to evoke emotional and behavioral responses.

Promoting Wellness

- Use of odors to evoke positive memories, increase positive emotions, decrease negative affect, disrupt cravings, facilitate learning, and reduce physiological indices of stress, including systemic markers of inflammation [18].
- Evidence-based use of aromatherapy has become more robust over the past two decades [19]. The following link is a good reference for aromatherapy databases: http://info .achs.edu/blog/credible-essential-oil-databases-for-research.

Pathological States

Deficiencies in smell function can lead to malnutrition, marital discord, social alienation, depression, and other problems. Patients with compromised smell may expose themselves and others to danger because they cannot detect spoiled food, leaking gas, or smoke. Smell deficits warrant treatment.

Pathology of smell includes:

- hyposmia – diminished sense of smell
- parosmia – aberrant odor perception, either with an odor stimulus (distortion) or without (phantosmia)
- anosmia – total loss of smell

Multiple medical and psychiatric conditions, medications, and environmental exposures affect olfaction. About 25 percent of individuals over age 50 experience some olfactory loss.

Addressing Pathology

Many disorders of olfaction improve over time. Treatment of olfactory pathology is contingent on its etiology. Surgical and pharmacological treatments are well established in contemporary medicine. Other treatment approaches include the following:

- Smell training – clinical studies assessing efficacy of olfactory training have been promising [20].
- Traditional Chinese medicine [21].
- Devices: electronic olfactory devices, or e-noses, are used as gas detection devices in home and workplace safety. They are also promising in diagnosis of a variety of medical conditions. While e-nose technology is not yet widely available in the mass-market, it is currently being pursued.
- Lifestyle/prevention:
  - Although olfactory loss can be caused by zinc deficiency, treatment with zinc supplementation is not effective and may worsen the condition [22]. Anecdotal improvement in olfaction through use of vitamins A, B12, and supplemental ATP has been reported [23].
  - Avoid excessive alcohol use and smoking [24, 25].
  - Limit or avoid use of opioids [26].

- Avoid allergens that may cause nasal inflammation.
- Engage in cardiovascular exercise [27, 28].
- For trauma prevention, avoid prolonged exposure to toxic chemicals and strong odors through the use of masks, respirators, and fume hoods. Also, use protective gear while engaged in sports, cycling, or other activities with potential for head trauma.

More information on contemporary research and treatment of smell disorders can be found at:

- the Taste and Smell Clinic at the University of Connecticut (https://health.uconn.edu/tasteandsmell)
- the Association for Chemoreception Sciences (https://achems.org/web)
- the University of Florida Center for Smell and Taste (http://cst.ufl.edu)

Sight

Vision is the predominant sense in humans. Although urban legend has it that visual input accounts for over 90 percent of all sensory data reaching the brain, there is no research confirming this number. It *is* known that around 50 percent of our neural tissue is related to visual processing [29]. The visual system has been honed by millions of years of evolution to aid in our survival by enhancing our abilities of food acquisition, self-defense from predators, tribe affiliation, and mate selection.

Promoting Wellness

- Light therapy for depression and sexual dysfunction.
- Art therapy as a part of psychotherapy.
- Dark therapy for mania, insomnia, and migraines.
- Eye movement desensitization and reprocessing for treatment of posttraumatic stress disorder.
- Mirror therapy for treatment of phantom pain and complex regional pain syndrome.
- Visual input to enhance learning, e.g., use of Prezi to help retain taught information (using cue images to make key points).
- Photo stimulation (to enhance seizures during electroencephalography).

Pathological States

Visual impairment is caused by the pathology of eye structures, visual pathways, and visual cortical fields, alone or in combination. Blindness is the total loss of visual acuity.

Causes of sight impairment are numerous and include medical and psychiatric conditions, medications, sleep deprivation, trauma, and environmental exposure.

Visual impairments other than blindness include:

- peripheral vision loss
- blurring of vision
- blind spots
- dyschromatopsia (color-blindness)

- photopsia (seeing flashing lights)
- dimness of vision

Addressing Pathology

Loss of vision should not be ignored nor accepted as a part of aging. It can be a manifestation of another underlying disease that needs to be treated. Furthermore, visual impairment may be partially or completely reversible.

Acquired vision loss has an enormous impact on the well-being of the afflicted. Acceptance of the condition and a positive attitude facilitate successful psychosocial adjustment. Equally important is social support from family, friends, and peers.

As with others, the underlying causative pathology should be identified and addressed first. Multiple treatment options are available for impaired vision:

- devices, including lenses and conventional eyeglasses
- corrective surgeries
- peripheral electrical stimulation [30]
- transcranial direct current stimulation [31]
- transcranial magnetic stimulation [32, 33]
- gene therapy [34]
- nanotherapy is widely discussed but has no approved use yet
- traditional Chinese medicine [35–38]
- biofeedback training to improve vision [39]
- vision rehabilitation, to improve functional ability and quality of life when correction is not possible, including:
  - Video magnifiers/closed-circuit television [40].
  - Peripheral prism glasses [41].
  - Retinal prosthesis (bionic eye) [42].
  - Mobility training, including white canes, service animals, smart wheelchairs, electronic badges with emergency alert systems, the 3D sound virtual reality system, talking braille, and radiofrequency identification devices and floors.
  - Balini Naidoo developed a line of clothing with braille embroidery for recognition of garments.
  - Regulations related to websites which are classified as places of public accommodation require ADA compliance for accommodation of screen readers with text-to-speech for the web visitor; refreshable braille text for touchscreens or refreshable braille terminals can also be used to consume content from the web.
- lifestyle/prevention:
  - At least seven hours of nightly sleep is recommended for prevention of miokimia, dryness and eye pain, burning, blurring, and possible eventual vision loss.
  - Diet: vitamin A, lutein, zeaxanthin, vitamin E, vitamin C, essential fatty acids, and zinc are contributors to optimal eye health [43].

- Eye exercises: William Bates, MD, attributed nearly all vision problems to habitual eye strain, coming up with a set of relaxation exercises aimed at improving sight [44]. While not supported by any body of scientific evidence, there are anecdotal benefits to this method, which is still used by some alternative medicine practitioners.
- Yoga: although evidence is low, some practitioners have claimed benefits to vision [45, 46].
- Trauma prevention: UV protection, goggles as protection from mechanical injury, optimizing brightness and contrast on electronic displays.

Hearing

Humans respond well to the sounds of nature and have over the centuries developed ways to reproduce sounds at will, which have been elaborated and turned into music. Human auditory processing is second only to vision for its use in guiding our actions, orienting us to where we are, communicating, and altering our physical and psychological well-being.

Promoting Wellness

- Psychotherapy, including music therapy.
- Use of nature sounds for relaxation and promotion of sleep.
- Hypnosis.

Pathological States

Hearing loss, temporary or permanent, is a common medical condition. Causes are numerous and include medical and psychiatric conditions, medications, environmental exposure, and the natural aging process.

There are four major types of hearing loss:

- conductive
- sensorineural
- mixed
- auditory processing disorders

Treatment should be guided based on etiology and type of loss. Auditory problems should not be accepted as an unavoidable part of aging.

Addressing Pathology

Many disorders of hearing are temporary and apt to improve. Surgical and pharmacological treatments are used to treat the underlying pathology. Additional options include:

- Devices:
  - Hearing aids, listening devices, cochlear implants, and alerting devices connected to doorbells, telephones, or alarms. Specialized devices may enhance telephonic and in-person communication through use of amplifiers and TTY/TTD technology [47].

- Speech-to-text technology converts spoken words to written.

- Captions are available on mainstream video and streaming platforms, including cable television and services such as Amazon Video and Netflix.

- White-noise machines, hearing aids, and masking devices relieve tinnitus. Masking devices are worn in the ear and produce continuous white noise. Tinnitus retraining devices deliver individually programmed tonal music that masks the endogenous frequencies, facilitating eventual habitation [48].

- Gene therapy trials for hearing loss are ongoing [49].
- Biofeedback has been used with some success in treating tinnitus [50].
- Traditional Chinese medicine: both herbs and acupuncture have been used for centuries to improve hearing and increase cochlear blood flow. Antioxidant, anti-inflammatory, anti-apoptotic, and neuroprotective mechanisms are relevant in reducing hearing loss [51].
- Lifestyle/prevention:
  - Diet:
    - Nutritional status is important in maintenance of auditory capacity. Obesity, diabetes, abnormal cholesterol, and dietary insufficiency are implicated in age-related hearing loss [52]. Strategies that prevent obesity and dyslipidemia are inherently preventive of age-related hearing decline.
    - Auditory function may improve with intake of polyunsaturated lipids, including omega-3 fatty acids, with consumption of two or more servings of fish per week.
    - Vitamin A, folic acid, and iron intake may slow down hearing loss.
  - Yoga and Ayurveda: although both techniques have been claimed to improve hearing, no evidence-based treatment has been found. The same is true of physical exercise.
  - Trauma prevention:
    - Avoid extensive periods of excessive noise, including television and music players, especially if using headphones or ear buds.
    - Wear noise filters or noise-canceling headphones if exposure to loud noise is unavoidable.
    - Avoid damage from foreign objects.
    - Don't use cotton swabs to clean your ears.
    - Avoid washing with unclean water to prevent ear infections.
    - Prevent head injury by using protective headgear and avoiding injury-causing activities when possible.

Touch

Touch is the first sense to develop *in utero*, at an early stage of gestation. It is conveyed through skin sensors all over the body, tongue, and the oral, vaginal, and rectal mucosa. It can be divided into two subsystems. Discriminative touch facilitates perception of pressure, vibration, slip, texture, and temperature. This is also called haptic touch and provides information about handled objects and during exploratory procedures. In contrast, affective touch describes the ability to sense gentle, low-force stroking of the skin, squeezing of body parts, hugging, and tickling. Oxytocin, opioids, serotonin, and dopamine mediate and modulate our affective and behavioral responses to touch, including in sexual, therapeutic, and social contexts.

Promoting Wellness

- Affective touch plays crucial roles in interpersonal communication and the formation and maintenance of social bonds. These social ties in turn impact mental, emotional, and physical well-being.
- Sex – stimulation of erogenous zones.
- Vibration therapy.
- Touching animals (pets, equine therapy, dolphins).
- Gentle stroking touch can lower heart rate and blood pressure.
- Manual therapy for fractures, dislocations, visceral manipulation, hernia reduction, musculoskeletal/myofascial techniques, lymphatic drainage, and acupressure.

Pathological States

- Anesthesia – insensitivity to pain.
- Hypo/hyperesthesia – reduced or increased sensitivity to sensory stimuli.
- Dysesthesia – unpleasant sensory sensation, including but not limited to pain.

Addressing Pathology

Pathology of touch perception is multileveled and may happen in any relay from nerve periphery to cortex. Treatment is aimed toward the underlying cause. Additional treatment may include [53]:

- physical therapy
- pneumatic cuff
- mirror therapy
- stimulus-specific training
- electrical stimulation
- local anesthetics
- Traditional Chinese medicine: no strong evidence-based treatment has been found.
- Devices: voice recognition technologies for typing and ADA-compliant websites may be navigated via voice input. Voice-driven commands in smart homes include virtual assistants like Alexa or Google, which are widely available and no longer expensive.
- Research on somatosensory function is promising, both in restoring sense of touch and in utilizing the somatosensory interface to improve prosthetic limbs [54].
- Lifestyle/prevention:
  - Control diabetes to prevent neuropathy.
  - Avoid gluten if there is evidence of sensitivity to prevent neuropathy.
  - Avoid alcohol and other sedatives.

– Yoga and Ayurveda: no evidence-based treatment has been found.
– Trauma prevention: avoid mechanical, temperature, and chemical trauma by utilizing protective gear.

Closure

Although each of the senses is unique, they are often enjoyed in combination, such as when:

- admiring bel canto and the costumes of singers at the opera
- savoring the aroma (smell and taste) and color of wine
- reveling in a massage on the beach with ocean views and the smell and sound of waves

A blend of all five senses may culminate in extraordinary sensations:

- At a Catholic Mass, observing the rich decor, listening to powerful music, smelling incense, receiving the eucharist, and kissing the priest's hands may crest in an apogee of religious feeling.
- At a chef's tasting, one appreciates the appearance, flavor, texture, and accompanying sounds (crunching, poured beverages) of degustation, rendering the experience "orgasmic."
- During the sexual act, leading to an orgasm.

These capacities may be harnessed in grounding techniques to quell acute anxiety. One such method is to distract yourself by looking around and identifying:

- five things you can see
- four things you can touch
- three things you can hear
- two things you can smell
- one thing you can taste

Beyond the Five Senses

The conventional five senses are used in communication and interpretation of the outer world (Figure 37.3). Additional human senses are, with a few exceptions, used to connect with the internal milieu, and include:

- nociception
- pruriception
- proprioception
- equilibrioception
- hunger and thirst
- visceral distention, fullness, passage of solids and liquids
- numerous internal specific chemical receptors (CO_2, opioids, etc.).

Acknowledgments

A special thank-you to my son and colleague, Andrew V. Bokarius, MD, for creating the illustrations for this chapter.

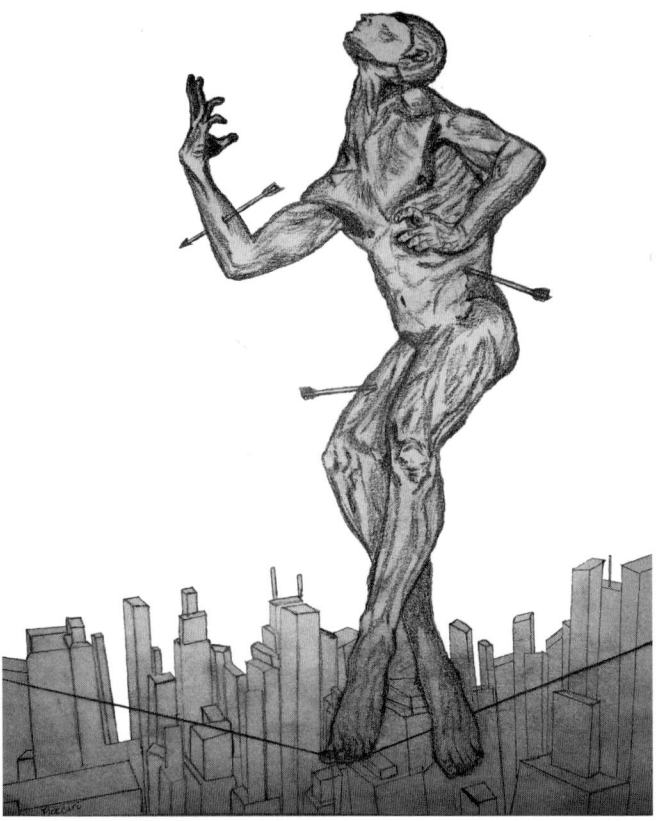

Figure 37.3 Beyond five senses.

References

1. Student Health and Counseling Services. What is wellness? 2019. https://shcs .ucdavis.edu/wellness/what-is-wellness (accessed April 21, 2020).

2. World Health Organization. Constitution of the World Health Organization. *Am J Publ Health* 1946; **36**(11): 1315–1323.

3. R Herz. Birth of a neurogastronomy nation: the inaugural symposium of the International Society of Neurogastronomy. *Chem Senses* 2015; **41**: 101–103.

4. C Bushdid, M Magnasco, L Vosshall, A Keller. Humans can discriminate more than 1 trillion olfactory stimuli. *Science* 2014; **343**(6177): 1370–1372.

5. E Caves, N Brandley, S Johnsen. Visual acuity and the evolution of signals. *Trends Ecol Evol* 2018; **33**(5): 358–372.

6. Science Daily. Humans have more distinctive hearing than animals, study shows. 2008. www.sciencedaily.com/relea ses/2008/04/080401095216 .htm (accessed April 21, 2020).

7. H Schaefer. Music-evoked emotions: current studies. *Front Neurosci* 2017; **11**: 600.

8. S Stack, K Krysinska, D Lester. Gloomy Sunday: did the "Hungarian Suicide Song" really create a suicide epidemic?. *OMEGA J Death Dying* 2008; **56**(4): 349–358.

9. H Takada, K Aso, K Watanabe, et al. Epileptic seizures induced by animated cartoon, "pocket monster." *Epilepsia* 1999; **40**(7): 997–1002.

10. X Yang, Y Fu, Q Zhan, et al. Clinical features of patients with game-induced

seizures in the Chinese population. *Seizure* 2016; **41**: 51–55.

11. MDC Correll, MDB Stetka, MDA Harsinay. Rare and unusual psychiatric syndromes: a primer. 2018. www.medscape.com/viewarticle/8 99520 (accessed April 21, 2020).

12. I Bamforth. Stendhal's syndrome. *Br J Gen Pract* 2010; **60**(581): 945–946.

13. L Bijland, M Bomers, Y Smulders. Smelling the diagnosis: a review on the use of scent in diagnosing disease. *Netherlands J Med* 2013; **71**(6); 300–308.

14. DR Reed, A Knaapila. Genetics of taste and smell: poisons and pleasures. *Prog Mol Bio Transl Sci* 2012; **94**; 213–240.

15. S Kumbargere Nagraj, S Naresh, K Srinivas, et al. Interventions for the management of taste disturbances. *Cochrane Database Syst Rev* 2014; **12**: CD010470.

16. C Silva, V Dias, J Almeida, et al. Effect of heavy consumption of alcoholic beverages on the perception of sweet and salty taste. *Alcohol Alcoholism* 2015; **51**(3): 302–306.

17. S Glennon, T Huedo-Medina, S Rawal, et al. Chronic cigarette smoking associates directly and indirectly with self-reported olfactory alterations: analysis of the 2011–2014 National Health and Nutrition Examination Survey. *Nicotine Tob Res* 2017; **21**: 818–827.

18. R Herz. The role of odor-evoked memory in psychological and physiological health. *Brain Sci* 2016; **6**(3): 22.

19. M Koo. A bibliometric analysis of two decades of aromatherapy research. *BMC Res Notes* 2017; **10**(1): 1–9.

20. K Pekala, R Chandra, J Turner. Efficacy of olfactory training in patients with olfactory loss: a systematic review and meta-analysis. *Int Forum Allerg Rhinol* 2015; **6**(3): 299–307.

21. Q Dai, Z Pang, H Yu. Recovery of olfactory function in postviral olfactory dysfunction patients after acupuncture treatment. *Evidence-Based Complement Altern Med* 2016; **2016**: 1–6.

22. RM Henkin, P Schecter, W Friedewald, D Demets, M Raff. A double blind study of the effects of zinc sulfate on taste and smell dysfunction. *Am J Med Sci* 1976; **272**(3): 285–299.

23. A Welge-Lüssen. Re-establishment of olfactory and taste functions. *GMS Curr Top Otorhinolaryngol Head Neck Surg* 2005; **4**: Doc06.

24. P Maurage, P Rombaux, P de Timary. Olfaction in alcohol dependence: a neglected yet promising research field. *Front Psychol* 2014; **4**: 1007.

25. M Katotomichelakis, D Balatsouras, G Tripsianis, et al. The effect of smoking on the olfactory function. *Rhinology* 2007; **45** (4): 273–280.

26. L Mizera, G Gossrau, T Hummel, A Haehner. Effects of analgesics on olfactory function and the perception of intranasal trigeminal stimuli. *Eur J Pain* 2016; **21**(1): 92–100.

27. C Schubert, K Cruickshanks, D Nondahl, et al. Association of exercise with lower long-term risk of olfactory impairment in older adults. *JAMA Otolaryngol Head Neck Surg* 2013; **139**(10): 1061.

28. A Rosenfeldt, T Dey, J Alberts. Aerobic exercise preserves olfaction function in individuals with Parkinson's disease. *Parkinson's Dis* 2016; **2016**: 1–6.

29. S Sells, R Fixott. Evaluation of research on effects of visual training on visual functions. *Am J Ophthalmol* 1957; **44**(2): 230–236.

30. A Sehic, S Guo, K Cho, et al. Electrical stimulation as a means for improving vision. *Am J Pathol* 2016; **186**(11): 2783–2797.

31. J Behrens, A Kraft, K Irlbacher, et al. Long-lasting enhancement of visual perception with repetitive noninvasive transcranial direct current stimulation. *Front Cell Neurosci* 2017; **11**(238): 1–10.

32. P Maurice, K Ron. Transcranial magnetic stimulation of the visual cortex in congenital blindness. *Front Neurosci* 2016; **10**(13).

33. M Mulckhuyse, T Kelley, J Theeuwes, V Walsh, N Lavie. Enhanced visual perception with occipital transcranial

magnetic stimulation. *Eur J Neurosci* 2011; **34**(8): 1320–1325.

34. R Voelker. Gene therapy for vision loss. *JAMA* 2018; **319**(5): 434.

35. S Wang, K Cunnusamy. Traditional Chinese medicine (TCM) for the treatment of age-related macular degeneration – evaluation of WO2012079419. *Expert Opin Ther Pat* 2013; **3**(2): 269–272.

36. Y Yang, Q Ma, Y Yang, et al. Evidence-based practice guideline of Chinese herbal medicine for primary open-angle glaucoma (qingfeng-neizhang). *Medicine* 2018; **97**(13): e0126.

37. T Blechschmidt, M Krumsiek, M Todorova. The effect of acupuncture on visual function in patients with congenital and acquired nystagmus. *Medicines* 2017; **4**(2): 33.

38. B Kim, M Kim, S Kang, H Nam. Optimizing acupuncture treatment for dry eye syndrome: a systematic review. *BMC Complement Altern Med* 2018; **18**(1): 145.

39. B Gilmartin, L Gray, B Winni. The amelioration of myopia using biofeedback of accommodation: a review. *Ophthalmic Physiol Opt* 1991; **11**(4): 304–313.

40. GE Legge. Reading digital with low vision. *Visible Lang* 2016; **50**(2): 102–125.

41. A Bowers. Community-based trial of a peripheral prism visual field expansion device for hemianopia. *Arch Ophthalmol* 2008; **126**(5): 657.

42. E Bloch, Y Luo, L da Cruz. Advances in retinal prosthesis systems. *Ther Adv Ophthalmol* 2019; **11**: 251584141881750.

43. S Richer, S Newman. Diet & nutrition. 2019 www.aoa.org/patients-and-public/caring-for-your-vision/diet-and-nutrition (accessed April 21, 2020).

44. W Bates. *Perfect Sight Without Glasses*. The Central Fixation Publishing Company; 1920.

45. S Kim. Effects of yogic eye exercises on eye fatigue in undergraduate nursing students. *J Phys Ther Sci* 2016; **28**(6): 1813–1815.

46. C Bansal. Comparative study on the effect of Saptamrita Lauha and Yoga therapy in myopia. *AYU* 2014; **35**(1): 22.

47. NIDCD. Assistive devices for people with hearing, voice, speech, or language disorders. 2011. www.nidcd.nih.gov/health/assistive-devices-people-hearing-voice-speech-or-language-disorders (accessed April 21, 2020).

48. Mayo Clinic. Tinnitus: diagnosis and treatment. 2019. www.mayoclinic.org/diseases-conditions/tinnitus/diagnosis-treatment/drc-20350162 (accessed April 21, 2020).

49. Columbia University Irving Medical Center. World's first gene therapy trial for hearing loss. www.entcolumbia.org/world-s-first-gene-therapy-trial-hearing-loss (accessed April 21, 2020).

50. ZQ Zhao, GX Lei, YL Li, et al. Neurofeedback therapy in the treatment of tinnitus. *Lin Chuang er bi yan hou tou hing wai ke za zhi [Journal of Clinical Otorhinolaryngology, Head, and Neck Surgery]* 2018; **32**(3): 233–236.

51. R Castañeda, S Natarajan, S Jeong, B Hong, T Kang. Traditional oriental medicine for sensorineural hearing loss: can ethnopharmacology contribute to potential drug discovery? *J Ethnopharmacol* 2019; **231**: 409–428.

52. A Puga, M Pajares, G Varela-Moreiras, T Partearroyo. Interplay between nutrition and hearing loss: state of art. *Nutrients* 2018; **11**(1): 35.

53. M Auld, R Russo, G Moseley, L Johnston. Determination of interventions for upper extremity tactile impairment in children with cerebral palsy: a systematic review. *Dev Med Child Neurol* 2014; **56**(9): 815–832.

54. V de Lafuente. Regaining the senses of touch and movement. *eLife* 2018; **7**: e32904.

Chapter

38

Emotional Intelligence and Its Role in Sustaining Fulfillment in Life

Harry C. Sax and Bruce L. Gewertz

Introduction

Irrespective of our life paths, the ability to initiate and sustain effective interactions with others is a key determinant of success and fulfillment. Conflicts occur on a regular basis, hence a level of personal insight is vital. As physicians and healthcare professionals, we can help our patients by better understanding the components of emotional intelligence (EQ) and suggesting how they can incorporate the best attitudes and behaviors into their lives. We can be far more effective in this mission if we model the desired traits in our professional and personal actions. This standard is a challenge, given the often-demanding nature of our clinical responsibilities and the need to achieve balance with family and friends. Yet, it is vital if we are to maintain fulfillment throughout our lives.

The importance of EQ is supported by a strong set of data that demonstrates that enhanced social interactions improve personal performance in a wide range of settings. Boyatzis studied 2000 supervisors and executives and found that 14 of 16 distinguishing traits for success were emotional not cognitive [1]. Spencer and Spencer defined job competencies in 286 organizations and noted that 18 of 21 competencies associated with high performance were emotionally based [2]. Comparing "star" performers to average performers in diverse industries, Goleman found that emotional insight and skills were noted twice as frequently in high performers and were a much better predictor of achievement than cognitive superiority [3].

In this chapter we will quantify the traits associated with EQ and examine the role of EQ in a variety of settings, including the environment of medical practice. We will also provide insights into the neurobiology of human emotion, address how experiences shape our ability to interact with others, and describe how emotional intelligence can be measured and quantified. Finally, and most importantly, we will suggest what we each can do to improve our EQ and enhance both professional performance and personal satisfaction.

The Scope of Emotional Intelligence

The term "emotional intelligence" describes the set of personal attributes that enhance social and professional relationships. As developed by Goleman and others, the elements of emotional intelligence span the full range of interactions between individuals and society, including self-awareness, self-regulation, social awareness, and relationship management [4, 5].

Self-awareness encompasses one's openness to their own emotional experience. This includes our ability to appraise realistically our own skills and abilities and to integrate feedback for self-improvement. It requires higher levels of functioning to see our emotions from the perspective of distance – to recognize that we are feeling anger, frustration, unbridled joy, or sorrow. With this insight we learn not to react immediately to those emotions (Goleman uses "emotional hijacking") [4]. Rather, we recognize what we are feeling and integrate how those feelings can affect our perception of reality. In sum, those with insight into their emotions develop appropriate levels of confidence and self-esteem. They recognize anger triggers that lead to impulsive, negative reactions. With such self-regulation, they can often remain above the fray, both limiting emotional trauma and making more reasoned decisions.

An important component of self-awareness is the inherent property of "grit." Although resilience is vital in our response to setbacks, grit takes it one step further. Those with grit are able to work hard and stay focused on a goal despite distraction. They appreciate that life is not always fair, but that perseverance can overcome failures. This is manifest in the next element, self-regulation.

Self-regulation is the ability to modulate and manage emotions within the context of any situation. Self-regulation is about balance; it is not appropriate to suppress all emotion any more than it is to be carried away into the extremes of paralyzing darkness or manic heights. Regardless of our circumstances, we cycle through emotions throughout the day, albeit to varying degrees. Those with strong self-management skills better organize their thoughts and actions. They can remain rationally optimistic in the face of challenges and even failure. This maturity allows them to view the setbacks not as "disasters," but rather as learning experiences contributing to later success. In sum, they are relentlessly positive and adaptable. If sustained levels of performance are the measure, self-regulation is perhaps the most important skill to master. Impulsivity in response to a difficult situation, driven by anger or strong emotion, has derailed many.

Understanding ourselves is vital. We are fundamentally highly social animals, characterized by the need to interact with others. That said, while we can appreciate internally how we may be feeling at the moment, these feelings are not always put into words. Up to 85 percent of communication comes from nonverbal cues – facial expression, tone of voice, subtle body language [4–6]. In medical practice, it has been shown that a soothing tone of voice and projected empathy positively correlates with patient satisfaction and influences outcomes such as the risk of medical–legal entanglements [7]. Indeed, the ability to project and read these nonverbal cues predicts success in a wide range of human interactions. Behaviors associated with *social awareness* include compassion, political acumen, organizational dynamics, and openness to contrary points of view. This level of attunement ideally begins in childhood and is facilitated by parents who are able to accept their children's feelings, creating an empathic environment. Most simply, those with strong skills in social awareness are seen as good "listeners," although in truth the "listening" extends well beyond the words per se and targets the feelings and motivations behind them.

The final competency is the ability to *manage relationships* over time. This requires a consistent ability to connect and relate despite the expected differences of opinions and conflict that exist within groups. In *Tipping Point*, Malcolm Gladwell identifies those with special skills in these areas as *connectors* [8]. Because of their adaptability, they know large numbers of people and are in the habit of making introductions. They typically cross a wide array of social, cultural, professional, and economic circles, and have the skill set to see potential affinities among people who work in different fields.

Those skilled in relationship management are able to respond to others in a way that creates a connection, mindful of both verbal and nonverbal modes of communication. In his book

Flourish, Seligman describes four ways to react to any situation: active constructive, passive constructive, active destructive, and passive destructive [9]. For example, on hearing of a raise and promotion, the *active constructive* response will show enthusiasm and interest, maintain eye contact, and ask questions to draw the teller out. Both parties are thereby uplifted by the good fortune. A more *passive constructive* response is to say "congratulations, you deserved it," with little or no emotion. Although not overtly hostile, the chance to bond over the good fortune is lost; the teller will often be sorry she brought it up. *Active destructive* responses will remind the teller of increased responsibility, time away from home, and higher taxes. Negativity is often conveyed through a dismissive tone of voice or facial expression. The *passive destructive* person won't even acknowledge the news, and may bring up an unrelated topic.

Nature versus Nurture: The Biology of Emotion

Early studies on the brain and emotion centered on observed changes in personality after stroke, trauma, or surgical resection. More primitive organisms required near instantaneous responses to threats in order to survive. Further basic regulation of physiologic function and movement was required. The brainstem and amygdala serve these functions, with the olfactory lobe as the main interaction with the surrounding environment. As our brains evolved, emotions developed before the recognition of emotions. Fight-or-flight was reflexive [10]. With the emergence of the limbic system came the ability to remember previous experiences and feel wider ranges of emotion. It remains our pleasure center. In psychopathology, the amygdala and limbic region have been implicated as a key neural region in emotional regulation.

With evolution and the specialized functions of the ever-enlarging neocortex, humans could now experience wide ranges of nuanced emotion. Concomitantly, neural pathways developed to modulate the primitive forebrain and the passionate amygdala. This region is essential to learning the emotional significance of cues in the environment. It is not static. The white matter of the frontal lobe grows through the end of adolescences and into early adulthood [11]. Liston and colleagues have shown that white matter tracts between pre-frontal–basal ganglia and posterior fiber tracts continue to develop across childhood into adulthood, but only tracts between the prefrontal cortex and basal ganglia are correlated with impulse control. This may also explain why childhood experiences in learning to deal with impulses are important while neural pathway development catches up [12]. In some individuals, these pathways that lead to higher levels of control do not develop and, taken to extreme, can lead to sociopathic behavior.

Functional magnetic resonance imaging (MRI) has given us even greater insight into the nuances of where emotional intelligence may lie. It is clear that the ability to recognize nonverbal cues (facial expression, tone of voice, word versus non-word sound) requires integration of disparate stimuli. Kreifelts et al. examined functional MRI in a series of healthy adults who presented with various words or non-word sounds, and human versus inanimate pictures [13]. In some cases, the words were presented in either a happy or angry tone. Degree of activation in multiple areas of the brain was correlated with results from pre-study EQ testing. Subjects with higher EQ showed more activity in the right posterior middle temporal gyrus during periods in which integration of voice and facial expression was required. Of interest, in all subjects the amygdala responded strongly to images of human faces but not voice. What remains undecided is how well brain plasticity through life allows these pathways to be enhanced with training [14].

Traumatic events of childhood clearly are correlated with later depression, yet not everyone with early life stress (ELS) develops depression. Cisler et al. mapped the emotion regulation network in a group of women who had ELS, some of whom subsequently became clinically depressed and others of whom had no history [15]. Higher activity in the prefrontal cortex was seen in the resilient group, while more activation was seen in the primitive amygdala in those with depression.

Emotional Intelligence in Medical Practice

There is much supporting information that would argue that physicians are experiencing heightened emotional stress ("burn out") due to a host of financial and other pressures that are dramatically changing both the practice of medicine and how doctors perceive their role in society. A survey of 1951 full-time physicians and scientists from four geographically separated medical schools noted that 20 percent had significant depressive symptoms [16]. Depression and anxiety scores were higher in young physicians (<35 years of age) than in their more senior colleagues. Relevant to this discussion, the very highest depression and anxiety levels were noted in surgeons; the lowest scores were recorded in emergency medicine physicians, who had high acuity challenges but "controllable lifestyles." This suggests that the context in which the stress occurs (e.g., the degree of personalization, total work hours) has more to do with adverse emotional effects than the level of stress itself, since both groups deal with critical illnesses and occasional bad outcomes.

These differences are apparent in medical students and residents. Indeed, deficiencies may be exacerbated during training. Chew et al. administered the Mayer–Salovey–Caruso Emotional Intelligence Test (MSCEIT) to 163 first- and final-year medical students at the University Putra in Malaysia [17]. They correlated EQ with performance on standardized exams as well as clinical performance during rotations. There was a stronger correlation of higher EQ and performance in final-year students than first-years, perhaps reflecting the importance of resilience and humanism in successfully completing medical school. First-year students were more focused on standardized knowledge testing, and many came into medical school with some ambivalence toward a career in medicine, given their relative immaturity (entering school at age 18).

In a related study of American medical students, optimism, which is measured in the self-awareness realm, was correlated with higher satisfaction in course work and eventual National Board of Medical Examiners shelf examinations [18]. In a classic longitudinal study from the University of California, San Francisco, students with behavioral or emotional issues during medical school were much more likely to have subsequent malpractice cases or censure from medical boards [19].

In a study of nursing students, Beauvis et al. correlated several realms of EQ, spirituality, and resilience to academic success [20]. A similar pattern emerged to that of the Chew et al. study. For younger undergraduate students, the only component of EQ that correlated to success was perceiving emotions, and that effect was moderate. In contrast, high-performing graduate nursing students had overall higher total EQ with significant strength in facilitating thoughts and managing emotions. Finally, an overall strong association with academic success was seen with spirituality; however, there may be selection bias as the nursing school studied was supported by a religious order.

Although surgeons have been accused of having poor social skills, in fact they are strong in many realms. In a study by Stanton et al., 148 British psychiatrists and surgeons were assessed for EQ [21]. Overall scores were similar. Psychiatrists scored strongly in the subsets of empathy, self-awareness, and impulse control. Surgeons had higher subscores in areas of self-regard, stress tolerance, and optimism. These traits inspire patient confidence, as no one wants to hear their surgeon say, "I hope I can help you . . . "

While it is obvious that developing an improved understanding of one's emotions is the ideal first step in this process, achieving personal insight is often difficult. In designing a recent study of 43 highly successful business leaders, Bennis and Thomas postulated that the "more modern" leader would have fundamentally different skills and tactics then CEOs of a more traditional era [22]. In fact, their subsequent research demonstrated that the views of both sets of leaders were remarkably similar. One common experience was particularly revealing. A majority of those interviewed described an unplanned and usually traumatic incident in mid-life which caused them to reformat their personal views of achievement and develop a higher level of empathy for others. In nearly every instance, they credited this specific response for their improved leadership performance.

Organizations can create a culture in which team dynamics support EQ. In a recent article in the *Harvard Business Review*, Lee and Duckworth take the grit analogy one step further [23]. Although certain individuals are inherently "gritty," institutions can instill grittiness as a culture. In medicine, highly motivated, individualistic practitioners are required to function as teams for the good of the patient. Without an alignment focusing on the patient, discord can ensue. Yet done correctly, teams of highly trained and motivated individuals can excel in rapidly changing environments. McChrystal's description of the creation of a SEAL in *Team of Teams* clearly highlights this concept. He emphasizes that it is not about individual performance, but the ability to develop trust and adaptability within small units [24]. As a baseline, you may wish to gauge your own "grittiness" at Duckworth's website: http://angeladuckworth.com/gritscale.

Can I Improve My EQ?

Most workers in the field believe EQ is not static but is a set of skills that can be learned with commitment and behavioral modeling [6, 25]. Those identified as true leaders tend to have developed these skills well, including conflict management, open communication, persuasiveness, and change management. The ability to inspire through public speaking is coupled with drawing out others' opinions and building consensus. Of these, the key constituents of EQ are self-assessment and empathy.

Irrespective of the potential for all of us to develop higher EQ, many of the skills seen in high-EQ individuals are an inherent part of their personalities. What can be most clearly improved through socialization and role-modeling are the specific constructive behaviors associated with EQ. The prepared learner sees opportunities for growth through observation of others who perform well, but also is able to profit from the witnessed mistakes of others.

With that in mind, we have employed three processes with our colleagues and patients in assessing EQ and identifying specific areas of strength and weakness. These are the MSCEIT [5]; the Thomas–Kilmann Conflict Mode Analysis (TKI) [26]; and the 360 evaluation. Taken together, and with appropriate interpretation and coaching, we have observed growth in their performances.

The MSCEIT analyzes specific tasks in each of the four areas of EQ: self-awareness; self-management; social awareness; and relationship management. Test-takers are assessed on

Table 38.1 Eight sections of the MSCEIT

Ability	Test sections	Question types
Identifying	Faces	Identify subtle emotions in faces.
	Pictures	Identify emotions in complex landscapes and designs.
Using	Facilitation	Knowledge of how moods impact thinking.
	Sensations	Relate various feeling sensations to emotions.
Understanding	Changes	Multiple-choice questions about how emotions change over time.
	Blends	Multiple-choice emotion vocabulary definitions.
Managing	Emotion management	Indicate effectiveness of various solutions to internal problems.
	Emotional relations	Indicate effectiveness of various solutions to problems involving other people.

their ability to identify emotions expressed by faces or pictures, appreciate the effects of mood on problem-solving, and define how emotions are generated. Finally, the interaction of emotions in analyzing situations in ourselves and others is quantified by presentation of various scenarios. As in any test of this type, validation questions will reveal whether the subject is attempting to present themselves in a favorable light. The eight specific sections are outlined in Table 38.1 [5].

In our own assessment of emerging physician leaders at our institution, we generally found strong self-management skills at baseline accompanied by a much wider variation in social awareness and relationship management. This is not surprising, given the selection bias of those who go into medicine, are trained to be self-reliant, and are taught to be stoically objective in the face of pain and suffering. This baseline helped us focus training in the important aspects of social skills in influencing group behaviors.

Although there are four realms to EQ, success many times rests on the ability to resolve conflict. Conflict is not necessarily negative; opposing viewpoints may bring clarity to a situation. The TKI (Figure 38.1) was an outgrowth of work in the 1960s on managerial styles [26]. It recognizes that there are gradations of assertiveness and cooperativeness in any conflict negotiation. Assertiveness is the degree to which you try to satisfy your own needs; cooperativeness is the degree to which you try to satisfy others' needs and be receptive to their ideas. These are not mutually exclusive. Depending on the situation, each style may be appropriate.

Being both unassertive and uncooperative is consistent with an *avoiding* style. This may be appropriate in conflicts with low impact that are in the process of resolving themselves, or for which you may need to buy time to become more prepared. The risks include declining workplace relationships as people become uncomfortable working through differences.

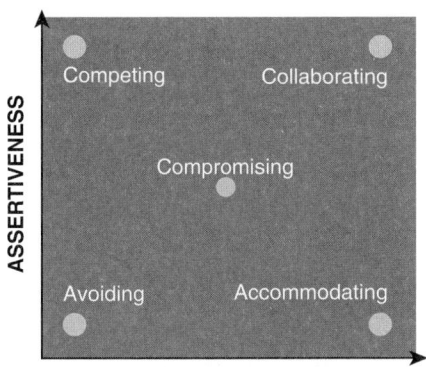

Figure 38.1 Conflict resolution styles. Used with permission from Kilmann Diagnostics. Copyright © 2009–2018 by Kilmann Diagnostics. All rights reserved. Original figure is available at: www.kilmanndiagnostics.com/overview-thomas-kilmann-conflict-mode-instrument-tki.

Those who *accommodate* are high in cooperativeness, but low in assertiveness. They are willing to concede their own needs for the good of others. This can support others and smooth ruffled feathers, but if done excessively causes loss of self-respect and motivation.

Being highly assertive and uncooperative can lead to rapid victories and protection of self-interest. This *competitive* style forces active debate of one's own position and the need to justify it. Appropriate in highly time-constrained negotiations, it can also lead to escalation and deadlock as well as poor decisions and resentment by the loser.

Those favoring a *compromising* style try to find "middle ground." Both parties give up something as well as retain key components that are of value to them. Compromise maintains relationships and fairness, but the solution can too often be suboptimal ("no one is happy"). In this setting, the hard work of hammering out the best result is traded for less conflict and expediency.

The most time-consuming negotiation style is *collaboration*. Parties strive for a "win–win." Through a structure of understanding that both likely share many common values and goals, early agreement is sought. With openness and trust, the areas of disagreement are dissected, and both parties challenged to create innovative solutions that are better than each's initial proposal. Done well, collaborative negotiations increase team cohesiveness and mutual respect. That said, if not facilitated tactfully, exposed vulnerabilities may lead to exploitation and hurt feelings around sensitive issues.

Over the years we have been surprised to find that our colleagues most commonly dealt with conflict by accommodation or avoidance. While compromise was occasionally chosen, few physicians scored strongly in collaboration. Importantly, with purposeful discussion and mentoring, we saw a shift in avoidance behavior, with increases in compromise and collaboration. The key lesson is that conflict is unavoidable, but when channeled properly it can lead to innovation and increased performance.

Perhaps one of the greatest innovative disruptions in performance management is 360-degree feedback. Gone are the days when subordinates were evaluated only by their supervisors, who themselves were responsible to a level higher in the organizational chart. Personal success was narrowly defined, and corporate cultures focused on shareholder value or for academic medical centers on grants, patient care dollars, and charitable giving. A true understanding of mission, vision, and core values was lacking. Personal growth and the ability to manage and supervise to the mission required a far greater understanding of one's own style, strengths, and areas of opportunity. The 360 also requires high levels of trust and self-awareness to yield meaningful behavioral change. Selection of the feedback tool, the raters, the method of feedback, and the integration into the culture are key decision points to be considered. In general, the more feedback from multiple sources, the better [27]. The ability to lead teams that are multigenerational and multidisciplinary is an increasingly important skill.

Done well, 360-degree evaluations not only enhance personal performance, but can also guide an organization to develop programs in areas consistently identified as high impact. The risk of the 360 is to focus on deficiencies and then not have the resources in place to optimize individuals' performances. It is also vital to tie the evaluations of the individual to clear understanding of the organization's goals. If the mission is the service of the local urban community, cultural awareness should be included; if it is to compete in a highly specialized technology transfer environment, the ability to understand big data and communicate that clearly is paramount.

As with any form of evaluation, standardized testing is but one component of an overall program of personal and professional development. You can be coached, read self-help books, and do exercises to better read facial expressions. But finding joy in one's life comes from within. Success is expanded by dispassionately comparing your interactions with others to your inner values. It is genuine human connections, forged through both adversity and success, that are the greatest tool in understanding our own emotions and how we are perceived.

These insights have been useful in assisting the "difficult" physician who disparages and turns over associates repeatedly. These poor working relationships were rarely the result of the skill level of the new colleague. Far more often they reflected some other issue entirely, such as the senior surgeon's discontent over perceived status in the organization. While it was rarely easy to initiate, a frank discussion that identified the key driver and addressed it has been a far more efficient tactic than recycling yet another young physician into an adverse environment. In addition to exploring the obvious (i.e., what the senior physician could do to improve the comfort and performance level of his juniors), on a number of occasions deeper personal insight was gained. Quite often, this self-knowledge translated to more collegial behavior in other areas.

Such successful "teaching" of EQ requires an immediate and real-life context to both stimulate and reward skill acquisition. Personal insight is an important element, but it is useful to remember that efforts are most effective when directed toward modification of *behavior* not *personality*. The goal is a practical one – minimization of poor personal interactions by recognition and self-correction of non-productive behavior. While motivated learners can occasionally gain these skills by self-study, the presence of role models and mentors can greatly facilitate the process. As a consequence, surgical leaders must always be aware that their personal conduct and equanimity sends a strong signal to the entire group [28].

How Can I Improve My Own EQ?

Although old patterns of behavior and interactions may be hard to break, with insight and some specific exercises, EQ skills and new neural pathways can be developed [22]. Becoming *self-aware* requires the ability to recognize one's emotional state and how perceptions are altered. Journaling creates a dedicated time to review the day and forcibly reflect on emotions felt and triggers that were recognized. In addition to looking within, asking for feedback from trusted friends and colleagues can help frame your actions and feelings within a broader and more objective context. As you become more aware of your physiologic response to stress, you will be able to slow down, before your primitive brainstem takes over. *Self-management* feeds on the recognition of impulsivity and the ability to put a temporary hard stop on a proposed action.

Social awareness cannot occur if you are "in your own head," fail to truly appreciate the importance of body language, or anticipate what the other person is saying, leading to premature and often inaccurate conclusions. The key is to listen and assess, sometimes a difficult feat for high achievers who are often geared to being proactive with imperfect or incomplete information. Perhaps the greatest skill is to put yourself in the other person's position. We have found this useful when counseling other physicians while in our leadership roles. Sometimes a simple, "what would you do, if you were sitting in my chair?" brings clarity.

One simple measure of one's listening capacity is paying attention to the fraction of time you speak rather than listen during a meeting. For example, if there are four people participating, in general you shouldn't speak more than 25 percent of the time. We are most effective when we understand that, often "less is more." For example, when all relevant points have been raised and the consensus favors your position, it is best to gracefully end the meeting rather than wandering on to extraneous territory. We have all seen effective decision-making undermined by a poorly considered or mis-interpreted remark well after the substantive work has been done.

Relationship management coalesces around the other three skills. Being available to those you lead and setting a strong example of drawing in diverse opinions sets a tone of collaboration and respect. It is important to acknowledge and praise those who have contributed to a goal and take personal responsibility when there are missteps of those you lead. It involves humor and strength . . . and sometimes luck and good timing.

Self-esteem is not the same as self-compassion. Although it is important to recognize one's strengths, it is also vital to treat failures and mistakes objectively and as learning opportunities [29]. Although this may seem like the rhetoric of a self-help book, there are distinct differences. As noted, if all we do after failure and disappointment is look to other rewards to bolster our self-esteem, we are ignoring basic flaws and vulnerabilities that will again manifest themselves and prevent our growth. There is little correlation with high self-esteem and strong leadership skills. This is not to say we should catastrophize and become despondent and stuck; rather, we should treat ourselves as humans with inherent flaws and recognize our compensatory strengths. Failure and disappointment are part of the human experience, not a measure of our self-worth. In a study of college undergraduates, Neff showed that higher levels of self-compassion were associated with happiness, optimism, positive affect, and initiative [30]. Not surprisingly, they were also inversely associated with neuroticism. Self-compassion is a learnable skill, although it may require dismantling of well ingrained but less useful responses.

Conclusion

Experiencing and improving our EQ takes place every day if we allow ourselves to be aware and present. We can see it in the body language of physicians who were residents together, when they are recounting their internship days over a coffee at a national meeting; we experience the sense of flow during a presentation when we are connecting with our audience, or we relish it in a spontaneous sharing of advice with our teenage daughter during a trip to Starbucks. And perhaps we feel it most poignantly when we watch a friend, colleague, or mentor self-destruct a long and distinguished career because of their lack of EQ, self-awareness, and self-control.

In the highly demanding environment of modern medical practice, positive interpersonal interactions are necessary to optimize clinical and academic productivity. Searching for a better understanding of others has the additional value of enhancing insights into our own actions and reactions, and improving personal satisfaction [31, 32]. As the value of EQ becomes even more evident, it is quite likely that more formal assessments of these skills will be used in selecting and training the surgical leaders of tomorrow.

References

1. R Boyatzis. *The Competent Manager: A Model for Effective Performance.* New York, Wiley; 1982.

2. L Spencer, S Spencer. *Competence at Work.* New York, Wiley; 1993.

3. D Goleman. What makes a leader? *Harvard Business Review.* 1998.

4. D Goleman. *Emotional Intelligence.* New York, Bantam Books; 1995.

5. JD Mayer, D Caruso, P Salovey. Emotional intelligence meets traditional standards for intelligence. *Intelligence* 2000; **27**: 267–298.

6. GJ Taylor, JD Parker, RM Bagby. Emotional intelligence and the emotional brain: points of convergence and implications for psychoanalysis. *J Am Acad Psychoanal* 1999; **27**: 339–354.

7. N Ambady, M LaPlante D Nguyen, et al. Surgeons' tone of voice: a clue to malpractice history. *Surgery* 2002; **132**: 5–9.

8. M Gladwell. *The Tipping Point: How Little Things Can Make a Big Difference.* New York, Little Brown and Company; 2002.

9. M Seligman. *Flourish: A Visionary New Understanding of Happiness and Well-Being.* New York, Simon and Schuster; 2011.

10. S Maren, GJ Quirk. Neuronal signaling of fear memory. *Nat Rev Neurosci* 2004; **5**: 844–852.

11. RK Lenroot, JN Giedd. Brain development in children and adolescents: insights from anatomical magnetic resonance imaging. *Neurosci Biobehav Rev* 2006; **30**: 718–729.

12. C Liston, R Watts, N Tottenham, et al. Frontostriatal microstructure modulates efficient recruitment of cognitive control. *Cereb Cortex* 2006; **16**: 553–560.

13. B Kreifelts, T Ethofer, E Huberle, W Grodd, D Wildgruber. Association of trait emotional intelligence and individual fMRI-activation patterns during the perception of social signals from voice and face. *Hum Brain Mapp* 2010; **31**: 979–991.

14. JM Schwartz, S Begley. *The Mind and the Brain: Neuroplasticity and the Power of Mental Force.* New York, Regan Books/Harper Collins Publishers; 2002.

15. JM Cisler, GA James, S Tripath, et al. Differential functional connectivity within and emotion regulation neural network among individuals resilient and susceptible to the depressogenic effects of early life stress. *Psychological Med* 2013; **43**: 507–518.

16. BA Schindler, DH Novack, DG Cohen et al. The impact of the changing health care environment on the health and well-being of faculty at four medical schools. *Acad Med* 2006; **81**: 27–34.

17. BH Chew, AM Zain, F Hassan. Emotional intelligence and academic performance in first and final year medical students: a cross-sectional study. *BMC Med Educ* 2013; **13**: 44–50.

18. AR Artino, JS LaRochelle, SJ Durning. Second year medical students' motivational beliefs, emotions, and achievement. *Med Educ* 2010; **13**: 1203–1212.

19. MA Papadakis, A Teherani, MA Banach, et al. Disciplinary action by medical boards

and prior behavior in medical school. *NEJM* 2005; **353**: 2673–2682.

20. AM Beauvais, JG Stewart, S Denisco, JE Beauvais. Factors related to academic success among nursing students: a descriptive correlational research study. *Nursing Educ Today*. DOI:10.1016/j.nedt.2013.12.005.

21. C Stanton, FN Sethi, O Dale, et al. Comparison of emotional intelligence between psychiatrists and surgeons. *Psychiatrist* 2011; **35**: 125–129.

22. WG Bennis, RJ Thomas. Crucibles of leadership. *Harvard Business Review* 2002: 39–45.

23. TH Lee, AL Duckworth. Organizational grit. *Harvard Business Review* September/October 2018: 99–105.

24. S McChrystal. *Team of Teams: New Rules of Engagement for a Complex World*. New York, Penguin Publishing; 2015.

25. T Bradberry, J Greaves. *Emotional Intelligence 2.0*. San Diego, CA, Talent Smart Press; 2009.

26. KW Thomas, RH Kilmann. *Thomas–Kilmann Conflict Mode Instrument*. Mountain View, CA, Xicom, a subsidiary of CPP, Inc; 1974.

27. MA Peiperl. Getting 360 degree feedback right. *Harvard Business Review* 2001; **79**: 142–147.

28. WW Souba. The inward journey of leadership. *J Surg Research* 2006; **131**: 159–167.

29. H Grant. To succeed, forget self-esteem. 2012, September 20. https://hbr.org/2012/09/to-succeed-forget-self-esteem. (accessed April 21, 2020)

30. KD Neff, SS Rude, K Kirkpatrick. An examination of self-compassion in relationship to positive psychological functioning and personality traits. *J Res Pers* 2007; **4**: 908–916.

31. P Taylor, C Funk, P Craighill. *Are We Happy Yet?* Washington, DC, Pew Research Center; 2006.

32. M Csikszentmihalyi. *Flow: The Psychology of Optimal Experience*. New York, Harper & Row; 1990.

Psychotherapy and Positive Psychology

Andrea Svicher and Eva-Lotta Brakemeier

Do you want to live happy? Travel with two bags, one to give, the other to receive.
Attributed to Johann Wolfgang von Goethe (translation by the authors)

Introduction: The Role of Positive Affects and Positive Emotions in Psychotherapy

Alice Aisen's work was pioneering in the domain of positive psychology as she provided the first empirical evidence on the beneficial role of positive affect (happy feelings) in cognitive processes [1, 2]. She suggested that the three basic components of cognitive processes (cognition, motivation, and affection) are integrated into common networks [3] and mediated neurotically by similar brain circuits [4]. She observed that positive affect promotes cognitive flexibility between the three components, enabling a flexible, open-minded, and creative thinking oriented to problem-solving [5].

In this context, Barbara Fredrickson formulated the broaden-and-build theory of positive emotions. She outlined that positive emotions (e.g., joy, interest, contentment, pride, and love) increase people's momentary thought–action repertoires and develop their personal resources, ranging from physical and intellectual resources to social and psychological resources [6, 7]. Fredrickson conceived a theory in which the experience of positive emotions has also long-lasting consequences, leading to enduring personal resources [7]. In turn, by building these enduring personal resoucres, positive emotions should enhance people's subsequent resilience [7].

Isen and Fredrickson's findings laid the foundation for further studies on positive psychological dimensions [8], but the birth of positive psychology as a scientific movement is historically attributed to Martin E.P. Seligman [9]. Seligman and Csikszentmihalyi questioned the point of view of traditional psychology research, as a science characterized by a focus on pathology, disease, weakness, and damage [9]. They outlined a new mission for psychological research: the study of positive psychological dimensions such as strength, virtue, work, education, insight, love, growth, and play [9]. From these premises, Seligman and Csikszentmihalyi have proposed to change the focus of clinical psychological interventions, from preoccupation with the repair of the worst aspects in patients' lives, to the building of positive dimensions of patient functioning, such as hope, wisdom, creativity, future mindedness, courage, spirituality, responsibility, and perseverance [9].

Over the past two decades, research in positive psychology has increased, mostly investigating psychotherapeutic protocols such as the positive psychotherapy of Seligman

[10, 11], the quality of life therapy and coaching by Frisch [12], as well as a large variety of single activities and exercises aimed to promote a specific positive emotion or character strength (i.e., positive psychology interventions) [13]. Another innovative psychotherapeutic protocol developed in the context of positive psychology is the four-step strengths-based cognitive-behavioral therapy (CBT) by Mooney and Padesky [14]. This latter intervention intersects the classical CBT approach with the positive psychology framework in order to build resilient beliefs and behaviors [15]. However, as there are only a few pilot studies on the effectiveness of this therapy in the literature [16] and it is not a manualized psychotherapy, it is not described in detail in this chapter.

The first part of the present chapter aims to provide clinicians with a toolkit concerning positive psychology strategies that have been developed and tested in clinical trials: positive psychotherapy as well as quality of life therapy and coaching. The last part of the chapter provides information on another evidence-based psychotherapy intervention that is based on a new concept of positive mental health (i.e., both stressors and positive resources are assessed): well-being therapy by Giovanni Fava [17].

Psychotherapy Approaches within the Context of Positive Psychology

Positive Psychotherapy

Positive psychotherapy (PPT) [10] was developed by Martin Seligman and Tayyab Rashid, and aims to alleviate symptomatic distress by increasing well-being [11].

Seligman described well-being as composed by five elements, denoted by the acronym PERMA: *positive emotions, engagement, relationship, meaning,* and *accomplishment* [18].

Rashid and Seligman postulated that PPT should not be considered a new genre of psychotherapy, but rather a therapeutic reorientation from a "fix what's wrong" model to a "build what's strong" model [11]. Therefore, within the context of PPT patients are called clients. In line with this, the goal of PPT interventions is to "help clients learn concrete, applicable, personally relevant skills that best use their strength to strive for engaged, satisfying, and meaningful lives" [11]. According to this principle, Rashid and Seligman suggested conducting the assessment of personality toward a hybrid process that explores strengths as well as weaknesses [11]. They encouraged therapists to conduct a systematic assessment of character strengths according to the character strengths and virtues (CSV) model of Peterson and Seligman [19]. This model classifies six virtues and 24 strengths [19]. For example, the virtue of wisdom and knowledge subsumes the strengths creativity, curiosity, open-mindedness, love of learning, and perspective, while the virtue courage includes bravery, persistence, integrity, speaking, vitality, and zest strengths. The other virtues reported by Peterson and Seligman are: humanity, justice, temperance, and transcendence [19].

Seligman and Rashid suggest clinicians conduct the assessment of the abovementioned strengths following a *comprehensive strengths assessment* approach that should cover [11]:

1. a brief description of each core strength based on the CSV [11];
2. an identification (not rank) of up to five strengths, i.e., the *signature strengths* that best illustrate the client's personality [19]; and
3. a choice of specific, attainable, and measurable goals that target the client's concerns and identify adaptive uses of signature strengths [11].

Table 39.1 The three phases of positive psychotherapy

Phase	Content	Mechanism of change involved
Phase 1 Sessions 1 to 4	Clients create a personal narrative that "brought out the client's best." They assess their strengths, set realistic goals, and develop master strengths that enable ability to regulate emotions and reconfigure cognitions	Reeducation of attention to notice and remember positive experience
Phase 2 Sessions 5 to 8	Clients discuss open (unresolved) and negative memories that continue to trouble them. They learn specific positive and meaning-based coping strategies	Positive reappraisal i.e., reinterpreting negative memories to promote a balanced perspective
Phase 3 Sessions 9 to 15	Clients seek meaning and goals through their strengths. They focus on recovering or promoting positive relationships. Clients are encouraged to experience happiness as given by interpersonal relationships, generativity, altruism, social activism, spirituality	Identification of character strengths, balanced use of strengths, and exploration of meaning and purpose

Data from T Rashid, MEP Seligman. *Positive Psychotherapy: Clinician Manual*. New York, Oxford University Press; 2018. PP Victor, T Teismann, U Willutzki. A pilot evaluation of a strengths-based CBT intervention module with college students. *Behav Cogn Psychother* 2017; **45**(4): 427–431.

Concerning the concrete conduct of therapy, Seligman and Rashid suggest that each PPT session should begin with a 3–5-minute relaxation exercise [11]. Throughout the course of therapy, clinicians should support clients to keep a *gratitude journal* to describe three good things that have happened to them in everyday life [11].

In total, PPT consists of three phases across 15 sessions that comprise the generic session structure, which is applicable for both individual and group settings [11]. Table 39.1 summarizes the three phases.

In the past 10 years, a growing body of research has analyzed the literature on the efficacy of PPT interventions [20–22].

A meta-analysis of 51 clinical studies underlined that PPT interventions increased the levels of well-being and decreased the levels of depressive symptoms [20]. In line with this, a follow-up meta-analysis including 39 randomized control trials showed that PPT is effective in increasing subjective well-being [21]. In contrast, a recent systematic PRISMA review showed that the efficacy of the PPT could only be confirmed for a few of the core components of PPT (i.e., the gratitude journal and the character strengths) [22]. Moreover, Walsh et al. noticed that the protocols applied in the studies are different, not corresponding to the standard sessions described in the PPT manual [22]. Rashid summarized that the efficacy of PPT was tested for the treatment of depression, anxiety, psychosis, borderline personality, and to support smoking cessation, covering different settings (e.g., inpatient settings, mental health clinics, or college students) and comparing PPT with other treatments (i.e., vs. cognitive-behavioral therapy and dialectical–behavioral therapy) [23].

However, as Boiler et al. noted, the data on PPT come mainly from pilot studies with small samples and methodological limitations, so the efficacy should be investigated through further high-quality studies with different (clinical) populations, different active control arms, and outcome measures in order to assess the efficacy of PPT [21].

Quality of Life Therapy and Coaching

Quality of life therapy (QOLT) and quality of life therapy and coaching (QOLTC) are manualized therapies developed by another pioneer in positive psychology: Michael B. Frisch [12]. Quality of life therapy and coaching is aimed at clients who have not been diagnosed with mental disorders but wish to grow their well-being, whereas QOLT involves patients with mental and physical disorders [24]. As reported by Frisch, QOLT should be integrated into other clinical interventions (e.g., psychotherapies or pharmacotherapies) and not be seen as a substitute for other clinical interventions [24].

He suggests motivating clients to use two strategies: one for "boosting positive affect experience" and another strategy "for the control of negative affects and feelings" [24].

In light of this principle, QOLT interventions aim to gain clients' well-being according to a "life satisfaction approach" that defines happiness as the result of cognitive processes based on life satisfaction assessments [12]. Thus, the degree of customer satisfaction or dissatisfaction is determined by the perceived gap between what clients have and what clients want to have in the relevant areas of life [12].

Frisch identified 16 relevant areas of life and labeled them "the sweet 16": health, self-esteem, goals and values, money, work, play, learning, creativity, helping, love, friends, children, relatives, home, neighborhood, and community [12]. As a result, the QOLT protocol usually begins by assessing clients' satisfaction in the "sweet 16" using the 16-item self-report Quality of Life Inventory (QOLI) [22]. The areas of life that are classified as areas of dissatisfaction become the target for QOLT interventions. Moreover, Frisch recommends assessing general "life goals" that are considered key points for setting appropriate goals for QOLT sessions [12].

The framework for QOLT interventions is the CASIO model, which identifies "five paths to happiness" [12]. The CASIO model offers clinicians five different "basic strategies" for each path, which include skills and exercises for solving or managing problems in order to increase the satisfaction in the "sweet 16" areas of life. They can be used both as homework and in-session exercise [12]. The five paths and related strategies are reported in Table 39.2.

The QOLT considers three daily practices for well-being, which Frisch refers to as the "three pillars" to be shared with clients and assigned as homework: *inner abundance, quality time,* and *find a meaning* [12, 24]. In addition to the three pillars, Frisch offers "the tenets of contentment," a list of 30 positive schemes or beliefs designed to promote well-being, as opposed to negative or "irrational beliefs" (e.g., the emotional honesty principle, the we are family principle, the happiness habits principle) [12].

Quality of life therapy also teaches clients basic mood control exercises and life management skills to control negative affect so that this does not offset the increases in positive affective experiences [24].

Three randomized controlled trials were conducted to test the efficacy of QOLT: first, in 58 patients awaiting lung transplantation [25]; second, in 62 adults with end-stage renal disease awaiting kidney transplantation [26]; and third, in 60 patients with implantable cardioverter defibrillators [27]. The results showed that QOLT groups differ significantly from supportive therapy groups or health education groups in follow-up assessments

Table 39.2 The five paths and related strategies of the QOLT

Path	Content	Basic strategy
Path C	Change the client's objective *circumstances* of an area of life	Problem-solving to improve the situation
Path A	Change client's personal *attitude* to an area of life	Find out what is really happening and what it means for you and your future
Path S	Change client's *standards* or fulfillment for the area of life	Set realistic goals and experiment with raising and lowering standards
Path I	Change the client's importance or the priority given to this area of life	Reevaluate life priorities and emphasize what is most important and controllable
Path O	Increase the overall satisfaction in other areas of life not previously considered by clients	Increasing satisfaction in all areas that are important to you for a general increase in happiness

Data from MB Frisch. *Quality of Life Therapy*. Hoboken NJ, Wiley; 2006. MB Frisch. Quality of life therapy. In: AM Wood, J Johnson, eds., *The Wiley Handbook of Positive Clinical Psychology*. Oxford, Wiley; 2016; 409–425.

(ranging from one week to three months) in terms of greater quality of life and lower mood disturbance, indicating that QOLT might be effective in increasing well-being [25–27]. The effectiveness of QOLT in promoting a higher quality of life was also observed in other three studies with different clinical populations: patients with major depressive disorder [28], mothers of children with obsessive-compulsive disorders [29], and caregivers of lung transplant candidates [30].

In summary, the results on the efficacy and effectiveness of QOLT appear promising as they were obtained in clinical populations with serious, chronic diseases and low well-being and quality of life [24]. However, only three randomized controlled trials were run, without involving groups of subjects with mental disorders. Thus, the efficacy should be tested through further high-quality studies, particularly on different clinical populations.

Well-Being Therapy

Giovanni Andrea Fava is the founder of well-being therapy (WBT), a manualized evidence-based short-term psychotherapeutic strategy aimed to increase psychological well-being and resilience [17]. Fava stresses that WBT was not developed as a general cure for mental disorders, but as a therapeutic tool to be integrated into a therapy plan, suitable for second- or third-line treatments [31]. Fava developed the WBT starting from a practical clinical point of view, highlighting that standard treatments for mood and anxiety disorders were not sufficiently effective in determining full recovery and prevention of relapse in patients who were assessed to be remitted in accordance with DSM standard criteria [31, 32]. Conversely, the author observed that these patients frequently showed a substantial residual symptomatology that in turn may progress to become prodromes of relapse [32]. Based on these findings, he noted that the optimal balance of positive and negative cognitions and affects could protect patients from relapses and recurrences, more than the absence of illness or the presence of wellness [32]. Thus, Fava introduced a new rationale for well-being interventions: the achievement of an optimal balance between psychological well-being and distress [32].

Well-being therapy considers a cognitive model that was originally developed by Marie Jahoda [33]. She identified six dimensions of positive mental health or well-being:

1. autonomy (regulation of behavior from within);
2. environmental mastery;
3. satisfactory interactions with other people and the milieu;
4. the individual's style and degree of growth, development, or self-actualization;
5. the attitudes of an individual toward his/her own self (self-perception/acceptance); and
6. the individual's balance and integration of psychic forces [33].

Moreover, WBT considers the model of Carol Ryff, which further elaborated the first five dimensions of Jahoda's positive functioning and introduced a method for its assessment, the psychological well-being scales [34].

According to this latter model, the aim of WBT is to lead the patient from an impaired level of well-being to an optimal balanced functioning in the six dimensions of psychological well-being [31, 35].

Well-being therapy consists of 8–12 sessions, which may take place every week or every other week, and the duration of each session may range from 45 to 60 minutes [31]. In the case that WBT is used as the only psychotherapeutic strategy, Fava suggested that the number of sessions may reach 16 or 20 [31]. If WBT is used in sequential combination with other psychotherapeutic strategies, in particular CBT, he indicated that the number of sessions may be abridged to four or six [31].

Fava describes WBT as a technique that emphasizes the concept of self-therapy and involves self-observation, use of a structured diary, homework, as well as interaction between patients and therapists [32]. The basic mechanism of WBT is similar to the search for automatic thoughts in Ellis's rational–emotional and behavioral therapy and in Beck's cognitive therapy [32]. However, in WBT the trigger for self-observation is different, being based on well-being instead of distress [32]. Thus, WBT is focused on the search for automatic thoughts and dysfunctional behavior that interrupted well-being moments [32]. The sessions of WBT are reported in Table 39.3.

Well-being therapy has been employed in 10 randomized controlled trials, mostly as an adjunctive treatment ingredient [31]. A CBT package that contains as a specific ingredient the WBT (CBT-WBT) was tested in 40 patients with recurrent major depression, who had been successfully treated with antidepressant drugs [36]. The group that received the CBT-WBT condition had a significantly lower level of residual symptoms after drug discontinuation, in comparison with the clinical management group; in both groups, antidepressant drugs were tapered and discontinued [33]. The findings were replicated by three independent and larger studies [37–39]. Significant advantages of WBT-CBT sequential combination (four sessions of CBT followed by other four sessions of WBT) were observed over CBT in 20 patients with generalized anxiety disorder [40]. Similarly, the CBT-WBT group was found to yield significant and persistent benefits in cyclothymic disorder with respect to the clinical management group [41]. Moreover, the WBT group showed a significant advantage over the cognitive-behavioral strategies group in patients with affective disorders who had been successfully treated by behavioral or pharmacological methods [42]. Lastly, three randomized controlled studies on middle- and high-school student populations showed

Table 39.3 The sessions of well-being therapy

Session	Content
Initial sessions (couple of sessions)	Patients are encouraged to identify episodes of well-being and to list the associated activities or situations. Patients are asked to report in a structured diary the circumstances surrounding their episodes of well-being, rated on a 0–100 scale, with 0 being absence of well-being and 100 the most intense well-being that could be experienced.
Intermediate sessions (two or three sessions)	Patients are encouraged to identify thoughts and beliefs leading to premature interruption of well-being as well as in searching and engaging in optimal experiences and pleasant activities. In addition, specific dimensions of psychological well-being are gradually introduced to the patient, depending on which areas appear in his or her diary.
Final sessions	The relevant dimensions of psychological well-being as well as errors in thinking and alternative interpretations are discussed. At this time, the patient is expected to be able to readily identify moments of well-being, be aware of cognitions that lead to interruptions to well-being, utilize cognitive-behavioral techniques to address these interruptions, and pursue optimal experiences.

Adapted from GA Fava. *Well-Being Therapy: Treatment Manual and Clinical Applications.* Basel, Karger; 2016.

that WBT-based interventions produced significantly greater benefits compared to clinical management [43] or improvement in symptoms and psychological well-being comparable to CBT [44, 45]. Moreover, in a large number of the controlled trials, the changes induced by WBT tend to persist at follow-up, underlining that WBT increased resilience and entailed less relapse in the face of current events [32].

In conclusion, results showed that WBT appears efficacious in combination with different therapeutic strategies, and unlike standard cognitive therapy, which is based on rigid specific assumptions (e.g., the cognitive triad in depression), WBT is characterized by flexibility and an individualized approach, completely in line with the positive clinical psychology approach that calls for a number of different interventions to be selected based on individual specific needs [32].

Summary

Since the late 1990s, positive psychology has experienced a broad upswing in many areas of psychology, including clinical psychology. As a result of this development, the first programs for the treatment of mental disorders exist using positive psychology methods. In this chapter, three specific psychotherapy approaches were presented and results on their effectiveness were reported and discussed.

The approaches presented have in common the following aspects:

- Patients are evaluated toward a process involving a multidimensional assessment of well-being.
- Ill-being or symptoms are assessed and considered in the development of psychotherapeutic strategies.

Well-being interventions are not considered as a substitute for evidence-based interventions such as CBT or pharmacotherapy.

On the contrary, they differ in terms of the following points:

- They applied different concepts of well-being: PPT and QOLT involved the provision of psychotherapeutic strategies to increase subjective experiences of well-being, whereas WBT applied psychotherapeutic strategies to provide patients an optimal balance of positive and negative affects and cognitions.
- They apply different psychotherapeutic strategies: QOLT and WBT apply intervention based on standard cognitive psychotherapy (e.g., Ellis or Beck approach), whereas PPT applies intervention derived from Fredrickson's and Seligman's theories.

Regarding effectiveness, the results concerning PPT and WBT are well established: PPT was evaluated in more than 30 randomized controlled trials; WBT was evaluated in 10 randomized controlled trials. In contrast, the results on the effectiveness of QOLT should be considered preliminary, since it was tested in only three randomized controlled trials.

Exploring what treatment works for whom in improving levels of well-being and decreasing levels of psychological symptoms, the results of randomized controlled trials indicated that:

- PPT appears efficacious in patients with major depressive disorder, patients with passive or active suicidal ideation or suicide attempt, patients with diagnosis of schizophrenia or schizoaffective disorder, and patients with type-2 diabetes and depression [22];
- WBT shows efficacy (mostly as an adjunctive treatment ingredient) in patients with recurrent major depression [36–39], affective disorders [42], cyclothymic disorder [41], and generalized anxiety disorder [40];
- QOLT is found to be efficacious in patients awaiting lung transplantation [25], in patients with end-stage renal disease awaiting kidney transplantation [26], and in patients with implantable cardioverter defibrillators [27].

More research on positive psychology and psychotherapy is worth striving for to gain a deeper understanding of how focusing on the positive and well-being side can better minimize the disease side in the patient – in the sense of the continuous and dynamic transition from disease to health/well-being in the biopsychosocial model of Georg Engel [46] and the clinimetric approach [47].

References

1. AM Isen. Positive affect, cognitive processes, and social behavior. *Adv Exp Soc Psychol* 1987; **20**: 203–253.

2. AM Isen. Positive affect and decision making. In: M Lewis, JM Haviland-Jones, eds., *Handbook of Emotions* (2nd ed.) New York, Guilford Press; 2000; 417–435.

3. AM Isen. Positive affect, systematic cognitive processing, and behavior: toward integration of affect, cognition, and motivation. In: F Dansereau,

FJ Yammarino, eds., *Multi-Level Issues in Organizational Behavior and Strategy*. Bingley, Emerald International Publishing; 2003; 55–62.

4. FG Ashby, AM Isen, AU Turken. A neuropsychological theory of positive affect and its influence on cognition. *Psychol Rev* 1999; **106**(3): 529–550.

5. AM Isen. Positive affect as a source of human strength. In: UM Staudinger, LG Aspinwall, eds., *A Psychology of Human Strengths: Fundamental Questions and*

Future Directions for a Positive Psychology. Washington, DC, American Psychological Association; 2003; 179–195.

6. BL Fredrickson. What good are positive emotions? *Rev Gen Psychol* 1998; **2**(3): 300–319.

7. BL Fredrickson. The role of positive emotions in positive psychology: the broaden-and-build theory of positive emotions. *Am Psychol* 2001; **56**(3): 218–226.

8. CR Snyder, SJ López. *Handbook of Positive Psychology.* New York, Oxford University Press; 2002.

9. MEP Seligman, M Csikszentmihalyi. Positive psychology: an introduction. *Am Psychol* 2000; **55**(1): 5–14.

10. MEP Seligman, T Rashid, AC Parks. Positive psychotherapy. *Am Psychol* 2006; **61**(8): 774–788.

11. T Rashid, MEP Seligman. *Positive Psychotherapy: Clinician Manual.* New York, Oxford University Press; 2018.

12. MB Frisch. *Quality of Life Therapy.* Hoboken, NJ, Wiley; 2006.

13. AC Parks, S Schueller, eds. *The Wiley Blackwell Handbook of Positive Psychological Interventions.* Oxford, Wiley; 2014.

14. KA Mooney, CA Padesky. Applying client creativity to recurrent problems: constructing possibilities and tolerating doubt. *J Cogn Psychother* 2000; **14**(2): 149–161.

15. CA Padesky, KA Mooney. Strengths-based cognitive-behavioural therapy: a four-step model to build resilience. *Clin Psychol Psychother* 2012; **19**(4): 283–290.

16. PP Victor, T Teismann, U Willutzki. A pilot evaluation of a strengths-based CBT intervention module with college students. *Behav Cogn Psychother* 2017; **45**(4): 427–431.

17. GA Fava. *Well-Being Therapy: Treatment Manual and Clinical Applications.* Basel, Karger; 2016.

18. MEP Seligman. Positive psychology: a personal history. *Annu Rev Clin Psychol* 2018; **15**(1): 1–23.

19. C Peterson, MEP Seligman. *Character Strengths and Virtues: A Handbook and Classification.* New York, Oxford University Press; 2004.

20. NL Sin, S Lyubomirsky. Enhancing well-being and alleviating depressive symptoms with positive psychology interventions: a practice-friendly meta-analysis. *J Clin Psychol* 2009; **65**(5): 467–487.

21. L Bolier, M Haverman, GJ Westerhof, et al. Positive psychology interventions: a meta-analysis of randomized controlled studies. *BMC Publ Health* 2013; **13**(119): 1–20.

22. S Walsh, M Cassidy, S Priebe. The application of positive psychotherapy in mental health care: a systematic review. *J Clin Psychol* 2017; **73**(6): 638–651.

23. T Rashid. Positive psychotherapy: a strength-based approach. *J Posit Psychol* 2015; **10**(1): 25–40.

24. MB Frisch. Quality of life therapy. In: AM Wood, J Johnson, eds., *The Wiley Handbook of Positive Clinical Psychology.* Oxford, Wiley; 2016; 409–425.

25. JR Rodrigue, MA Baz, MR Widows, et al. A randomized evaluation of quality-of-life therapy with patients awaiting lung transplantation. *Am J Transplant* 2005; **5**(10): 2425–2432.

26. JR Rodrigue, DA Mandelbrot, M Pavlakis. A psychological intervention to improve quality of life and reduce psychological distress in adults awaiting kidney transplantation. *Nephrol Dia Transplant* 2010; **26**(2): 709–715.

27. ER Serber, JL Fava, LM Christon, et al. Positive psychotherapy to improve autonomic function and mood in ICD patients (PAM-ICD): rationale and design of an RCT currently underway. *Pacing Clin Electrophysiol* 2016; **39**(5): 458–470.

28. GM Grant, V Salcedo, LS Hynan, et al. Effectiveness of quality of life therapy for depression. *Psychol Rep* 1995; **76**(3 pt 2): 1203–1208.

29. MR Abedi, P Vostanis. Evaluation of quality of life therapy for parents of

children with obsessive-compulsive disorders in Iran. *Eur Child Adolesc Psychiatry* 2010; **19**(7): 605–613.

30. JR Rodrigue, MR Widows, MA Baz. Caregivers of lung transplant candidates: do they benefit when the patient is receiving psychological services? *Prog Transplant* 2006; **16**(4): 336–342.

31. J Guidi, C Rafanelli, GA Fava. The clinical role of well-being therapy. *Nord J Psychiatry* 2018; **72**(6): 447–453.

32. GA Fava. Well-being therapy. In: AM Wood, J Johnson, eds., *The Wiley Handbook of Positive Clinical Psychology*. Oxford, Wiley; 2016; 409–425.

33. M Jahoda. *Current Concepts of Positive Mental Health*. New York, Basic Books; 1958.

34. CD Ryff. Psychological well-being revisited: advances in the science and practice of eudaimonia. *Psychother Psychosom* 2014, **83**(1): 10–28.

35. GA Fava, P Bech. The concept of euthymia. *Psychother Psychosom* 2015; **85**(1): 1–5.

36. GA Fava, C Rafanelli, S Grandi, et al. Prevention of recurrent depression with cognitive behavioral therapy: preliminary findings. *Arch Gen Psychiatry*; 1998; **55**(9): 816–820.

37. U Stangier, C Hilling, T Heidenreich, et al. Maintenance cognitive-behavioral therapy and manualized psychoeducation in the treatment of recurrent depression. *Am J Psychiatry* 2013; **170**(6): 624–632.

38. BD Kennard, GJ Emslie, TL Mayes, et al. Sequential treatment with fluoxetine and relapse-prevention CBT to improve outcomes in pediatric depression. *Am J Psychiatry* 2014; **171**(10): 1083–1090.

39. M Moeenizadeh, KKK Salagame. The impact of well-being therapy on symptoms of depression. *Int J Psychol Stud* 2010; **2**(2): 223–230.

40. GA Fava, C Ruini, C Rafanelli, et al. Well-being therapy of generalized anxiety disorder. *Psychother Psychosom* 2005; **74**(1): 26–30.

41. GA Fava, C Rafanelli, E Tomba, et al. The sequential combination of cognitive behavioral treatment and well-being therapy in cyclothymic disorder. *Psychother Psychosom* 2011; **80**(3): 136–143.

42. GA Fava, C Rafanelli, M Cazzaro et al. Well-being therapy: a novel psychotherapeutic approach for residual symptoms of affective disorders. *Psychol Med* 1998; **28**(2): 475–480.

43. C Ruini, F Ottolini, E Tomba, et al. School intervention for promoting psychological well-being in adolescence. *J Behav Ther Exp Psychiatry* 2009; **40**(4): 522–532.

44. C Ruini, C Belaise, C Brombin, et al. Well-being therapy in school settings. *Psychother Psychosom* 2006; **75**(6): 331–336.

45. E Tomba, C Belaise, F Ottolini, et al. Differential effects of well-being promoting and anxiety-management strategies in a non-clinical school setting. *J Anxiety Disord* 2010; **24**(3): 326–324.

46. GL Engel. A unified concept of health and disease. *Perspect Biol Med* 1960; **3**: 459–485.

47. GA Fava, D Carrozzino, L Lindberg, et al. The clinimetric approach to psychological assessment: a tribute to Per Bech, MD (1942–2018). *Psychother Psychosom* 2018; **87**(6): 321–326.

Resilience and Wellness

Nathalie Herrera and Waguih William IsHak

Introduction

How do people face challenging events that impact, and sometimes change, their lives? Adversity is ordinary, not extraordinary. Most of us at some point will experience a major trauma: the death of a loved one, debilitating illness, loss of a job, a natural disaster, or other traumatic events. It is estimated that up to 90 percent of us will experience at least one serious traumatic event during our lifetime [1]. The ability to cope, respond to change, and return to a degree of normal functioning following a crisis is known as resilience [2]; this process may have not only a genetic basis and neurobiological substrate, but also factors and actions that can be learned and developed [3]. As physicians and healthcare providers, we can make a difference by better understanding the coping mechanisms proven to be effective at enhancing resilience and its role in fostering wellness. With a better understanding of the process, we can develop interventions suggesting how patients can incorporate the best behaviors in their lives.

In this chapter we discuss the definition of resilience, its neurobiological basis, and the recent advances on understanding its genetic background. We also provide insights into the most common coping mechanisms that have been associated with resilient individuals, describe which instruments have the best psychometric ratings and strongest measurement qualities, and explore the cyclic relationship between resilience and wellness.

Defining Resilience

Most people at some point will be exposed to a very challenging and stressful life experience: natural disasters, accidents, catastrophic illnesses, the death of a loved one, or war, among others. It is estimated that up to 90 percent of us will experience at least one serious traumatic event during our lives [1].

There are different styles in which people cope with these life-changing situations. The majority react acutely to such circumstances, with overwhelming emotions accompanied usually by a strong physiological response; despite this, many find a way to overcome adversity, and even become stronger in the process.

Unfortunately, for some people the acute stress response will become chronic, diminishing their well-being and increasing their risk of developing mental illnesses such as posttraumatic stress disorder (PTSD) and depressive disorders.

These differences in adaptation to stress and the consequences of different styles of coping with adversity have gained increasing attention over the past decade, and have significantly shaped queries on resilience and how its understanding will provide guidance for intervention in high-risk people.

Discourse about resilience arose in the 1970s in the context of ecological studies as a description of how systems respond to disaster. Environmental sociologist Raven Cretney has traced the development of resilience through time and concluded that it is currently a "popularly understood concept that distinguishes the ability to cope, respond to change and return to a degree of normal functioning following a crisis" [2]. The American Psychological Association defines it as "the process of adapting well in the face of adversity, trauma, tragedy, threats and even significant sources of stress – such as family and relationship problems, serious health problems or workplace and financial stresses" [3].

Prior research substantiates the belief that the style to coping with stress depends not only on the individual, but also on available resources through family, friends, a variety of organizations, and on the characteristics of specific cultures and religions, communities, societies, and governments – all of which in themselves may be more or less resilient [4].

Despite the existence of numerous, discipline-specific definitions for the term, at its core resilience embodies a vision of healthy individuals and thriving communities opening the door for a resilience-centered framework that could provide concrete actions to promote the sustainable and long-term well-being of communities in the face of adversity and disaster [5].

Genetics and Physiology of Resilience

The ability to maintain normal psychological and physiological functioning despite exposure to stress and adversity most likely reflects active processes that contribute to maintaining homeostasis within a broad range of environmental circumstances [6]. These processes may have a genetic basis and contribute to the resilient phenotype through a cascade of molecular and cellular events that subsequently regulate neural, physiological, and endocrine systems; these ultimately converge to the maintenance of what we consider adaptive behavior [7].

The diathesis-stress model, which postulates that cumulative environmental adversity eventually will lead to dysfunction and that genetic variables determine the individual threshold of adversity necessary for dysfunction to occur, has critically influenced academic dialog on gene-by-environment interactions; this model, however, fails to enclose the phenomenon of genetic resilience within a more general theory of environmental sensitivity that is independent of the environment's valence [8]. The match–mismatch and differential susceptibility frameworks that embed susceptibility and resilience genotypes have propelled to the forefront in investigations a unifying theory of general programming susceptibility to environmental influences, be they adverse or positive [7]. Recent studies have focused on common variants in three candidate genes that may moderate the effect of adverse life events on psychiatric disorders and related intermediate phenotypes: the corticotropin-releasing hormone receptor 1 gene (*CRHR1*), the FK506 binding protein 5 gene (*FKBP5*), and the serotonin transporter gene (*SLC6A4*) [7, 9].

Several anatomical structures (Table 40.1), neurotransmitters, and hormones (Table 40.2) are implicated in the stress response. Its adequate functioning and interaction regulate an optimal and rapid response to threat – high enough to react appropriately to danger, but not so high as to cause incapacitating anxiety and fear. Hyperactive or hypoactive neurobiological stress systems tend to be maladaptive [10, 11].

Table 40.1 Anatomical structures implicated in the stress response

Structure/system	Function
Amygdala	Central role in fear conditioning Triggers the "fight-or-flight" response
Prefrontal cortex	Facilitates planning and rational decision-making Acts to keep the amygdala in check
Anterior cingulate cortex	Important role in our ability to focus attention Detects and monitors errors and conflict Assesses the importance of emotional information and regulates emotions Connected to both the prefrontal cortex and amygdala Associated with the pleasurable effects of social attachment, food, sex, and other positive stimuli
Anterior insula	Marks the boundary between the frontal and temporal lobes Involved in many functions related to emotions Aids the sense of self-awareness
Nucleus accumbens	Also referred as the "pleasure center" Central role in the brain's reward circuit In association with the *ventral tegmental area*, mediates the experience of reward and punishment Associated with the pleasurable effects of food, sex, and drug abuse
Limbic system	Includes the amygdala, hippocampus, and other structures and regions Involved in emotion and memory
Sympathetic nervous system	Mobilizes the body under conditions of stress
Parasympathetic nervous system	Conserves resources and maintains functioning under normal non-stressful conditions
Hypothalamic–pituitary–adrenal axis	Responds to stress with a complex set of reactions that involves communication between the hypothalamus, the pituitary gland, and the adrenal glands.

As can be seen, the understanding of the key anatomical structures that play an important role in the maintenance of physiological homeostasis and the complex and dynamic processes between systems in the human body and the environment when faced with adversity can positively influence the design of effective resilience interventions.

The nervous system has the ability to respond to intrinsic or extrinsic stimuli by reorganizing its structure, function, and connections; this capacity is known as neuroplasticity [12]. This means that each person, to some degree, has the power to change the structure and function of his or her brain. The key is activity. By repeatedly activating specific areas of the central nervous system (CNS), those areas can be strengthened; in other words, resilience is a multidimensional and complex skill that can be enhanced [11].

Table 40.2 Neurotransmitters and hormones implicated in the stress response

Neurotransmitter/hormone	Function
Cortisol	Stress hormone released through activation of the HPA axis Produces energy by converting food into fat and glucose Temporarily bolsters the immune system
Epinephrine (adrenaline)	Released by the adrenal glands under conditions of stress and accelerates heart rate Constricts blood vessels and dilates air passages as part of the sympathetic nervous system fight-or-flight response
Norepinephrine	Facilitates alerting and alarm reactions in the brain Critical for responding to danger and remembering emotional and fearful events
Serotonin	Involved in the regulation of mood as well as sleep, appetite, and other functions
Dopamine	Associated with pleasurable feelings Plays a key role in the reward systems of the brain Important factor in cravings and addictive behaviors
Neuropeptide Y (NPY)	Associated with decreasing anxiety and hastening return to baseline after the nervous system reacts to stress
Oxytocin	Associated with maternal behaviors, pair bonding, social communication, trust, social support, and anxiety reduction
Brain-derived neurotrophic factor (BDNF)	Acts to support the nervous system through the repair of existing neurons and growth of new ones

Building Resilience

Resilience is not rare; on the contrary, it is common and can be witnessed all around us. For most people it can be enhanced through learning and training. Nevertheless, developing resilience is a personal journey; we need to acknowledge that building resilience and "bouncing back" is easier for some than for others; for this reason, when designing strategies to build resilience we must approach from multiple perspectives and use a number of different lenses [3, 11].

Ten Factors to Build Resilience

To truly understand resilience Southwick and Charney [11] conducted in-depth interviews with a large number of highly resilient individuals who had clearly demonstrated an admirable response when faced with extreme stress. They turned to three groups: former Vietnam prisoners of war (POWs), Special Forces instructors, and civilian men and women who survived enormous stress and trauma, and somehow endured and even thrived. Although their circumstances differed greatly, the three groups tended to use the same or similar coping strategies when confronted with high levels of stress.

The authors identified 10 coping mechanisms that proved to be effective for dealing with trauma (Figure 40.1).

Realistic optimism. Future-oriented attitude involving hope and confidence that things will turn out well, paying close attention to negative information that is relevant to the situation. Assessing obstacles realistically helps to surmount them.

Optimism increases resilience, reducing physiological arousal, broadening visual focus, thoughts, and behavior, which helps to become more creative, inclusive, flexible, and integrative. One practical approach to enhancing optimism involves learning to recognize and modify the individual's typical explanatory style.

Facing fear. Fear is a normal adaptive response that prepares us to react to danger; nonetheless, when fear, stress, or hypervigilance continue without changes for a long period of time, triggered by neutral stimuli, the effects can be serious. Prior research substantiates the belief that prolonged stress can damage the prefrontal cortex and the hippocampus [11, 13].

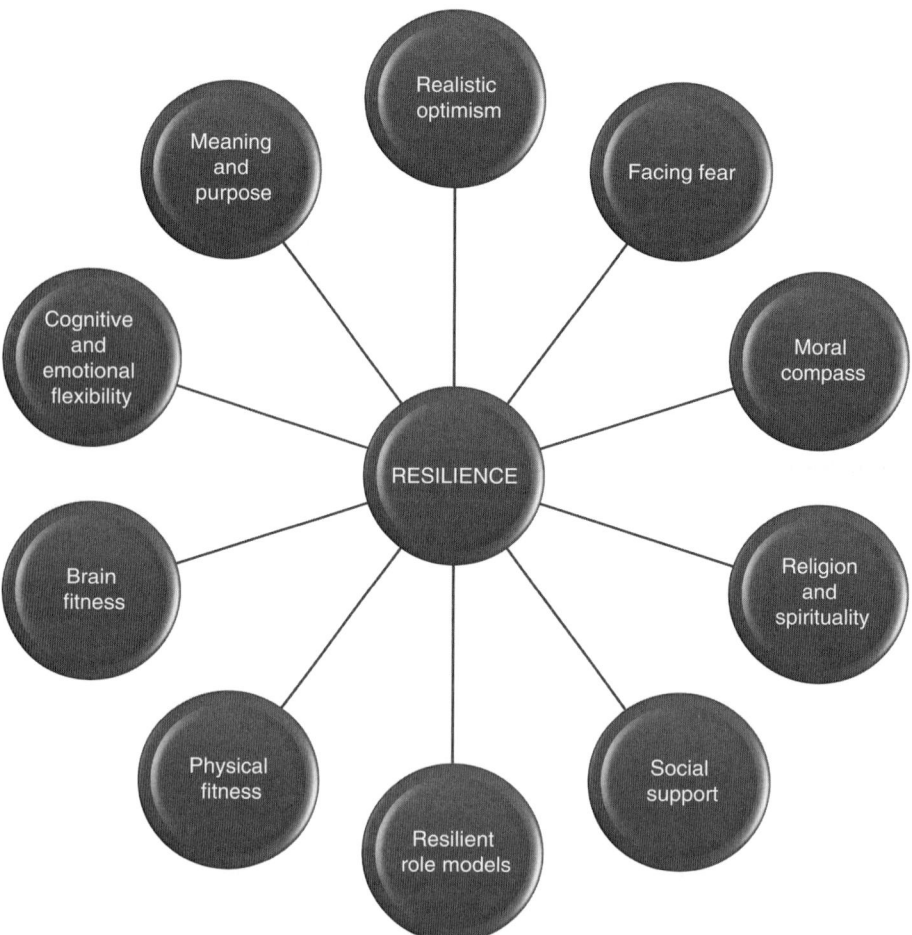

Figure 40.1 Ten coping mechanisms for dealing with trauma.

Therefore, learning to face fear is essential; some techniques to face fear include viewing it as a guide and as an opportunity, acquiring information about what is feared, and facing the fear with social and spiritual support.

Moral compass. Actively identifying personal core values, assessing the degree to which these core values are being lived, and accepting the challenge to adopt a higher standard can strengthen character and build resilience [11].

Religion and spirituality. Religion and spirituality are deeply personal matters. As a potential source of strength and resilience, religion, spirituality, mindfulness, and meditation may foster a number of factors, including optimism, altruism, empathy, and a sense of meaning and purpose. Prior research suggests that practicing religion is associated with physical and emotional well-being among healthy individuals, and with better coping among people who are suffering medical illnesses [11, 13].

Social support. Social isolation and low levels of social support are associated with high levels of stress, depressive disorders, and PTSD [11]. Isolation can affect physical health, and studies have shown that a small social network or inadequate emotional support is associated with a threefold increase in subsequent cardiac events [14]. Accepting help and support from close family members, friends, or others strengthens resilience; some people find that being active in civic groups or other local organizations provides hope as well as assisting others in their time of need [3].

Resilient role models. Studies have shown that resilient individuals have role models whose beliefs, attitudes, and behaviors inspire them [11]. Imitation is a powerful form of learning and plays an important role in shaping human behavior; role-modeling depends, in part, on observational learning, but also involves learning rules of behavior that then serve as a guide for future actions [11, 15].

Physical fitness. Mastering physical challenges can improve mood, cognition, and emotional resilience. Exercise increases the concentration of endorphins, serotonin, and dopamine, and also helps to protect against the hormonal effects of chronic stress – for example, the stress hormone cortisol, which over time can damage neurons in the hippocampus. Aerobic exercise enhances the growth of neurons by increasing production of neurotrophic factors such as BDNF [11].

Brain fitness. Resilient people tend to be lifelong learners, continually seeking opportunities to become more mentally fit. There exists a considerable body of literature over the past decade on the ability of individuals to improve cognitive abilities through a series of brain exercises [11]. Neurons that are actively used tend to make more connections with other cells and transmit messages more efficiently [11, 16].

Cognitive and emotional flexibility. Resilience involves maintaining flexibility and balance in life, even in stressful situations and traumatic events. As a dynamic process, resilience implies a shift from one coping strategy to another, depending on the circumstances. Resilient individuals are able to accept what they cannot change, learn from failure, and use negative emotions to look for opportunity and meaning in adversity [3, 11]. Jerry White outlines five steps to overcoming a life crisis: face facts, choose life, reach out, get moving, and give back [17].

Meaning and purpose. Previous psychological research has showed that having a clear and valued purpose and committing fully to a mission can dramatically strengthen resilience [11].

Measuring Resilience

Tools designed to measure resilience are based on the common characteristics aligned with the definitions of the term. A comprehensive review of resilience scales suggested that the Brief Resilience Scale, Connor–Davidson Resilience Scale (CD-RISC), and Resilience Scale for Adults (RSA) potentially have the best psychometric ratings and strongest measurement qualities of those studied [18, 19].

Resilience and Wellness

The term *wellness* is a relatively common, everyday concept that has been appropriated by academics, particularly in the medical field, concerning disease prevention and health promotion [20].

Wellness has been defined as "a holistic and multidimensional state of being that guides one to achieve one's full potential" [21]. The wellness paradigm incorporates numerous domains of personhood (social, spiritual, psychological, and physical) as well as stressing the importance of holistic integration of them. Similarly, a study conducted by Gallup scientists proposed five universal elements of well-being: career, social, financial, physical, and community [22].

A wellness approach supports shared decision-making between patients and healthcare providers, effectively increasing patient engagement and treatment adherence [23].

An essential part of the wellness process emphasizes several aspects of person-in-environment functioning, which has critically influenced academic dialog on the necessity of building new models involving the promotion of healthy habits, since healthy individuals cultivate healthy communities and in turn healthy communities foster healthy individuals. The public health implications of fostering greater levels of well-being in individuals who experience adversity are diverse and significant [24].

With regard to the link between resilience and wellness, several studies agree that both individual characteristics (such as competence and resilience) and environmental characteristics (such as empowerment and social systems) are "blueprints" for building and fostering wellness [20]. Resilience is a personal characteristic that allows a person to persist when there is an imbalance in any of the five elements of well-being proposed by Gallup [22, 25]. Previous research demonstrates that resilience buffers the development of disability in those with chronic disease [23].

Theories of reserve suggest that individuals accrue resources over time to combat challenges in life. Given the multidimensional nature of resilience, there are many domains in which individuals can build reserve. For instance, in the life course model of multimorbidity resilience, it is proposed that there are three areas that work in concert to foster resilience in the face of adversity: individual, social, and environmental resources [24].

Populations around the world are rapidly aging; this increase in longevity represents a great achievement for mankind and a challenge for individuals reaching older ages, as the likelihood of encountering some form of adversity increases proportionally with age. Traditional models of "successful aging" do not actively include components of adversity; in contrast, models of resilience actively incorporate them; the addition of adversity to the healthy aging model via resilience makes this concept much more accessible to the aging population [24].

Fullen et al.'s research underlines the importance for healthcare professionals of acknowledging the heterogeneity of older adults, since the data suggest that within-group differences affect constructs like wellness and resilience [23]; they invite others to use these differences as a guide for future research on effective assessment, diagnosis, and treatment of mental and physical well-being in older adults. As a consequence, if we are able to foster greater well-being in this specific population, there is the potential to decrease the burden on caregivers, clinicians, and aging individuals themselves [24].

In this context of building resilience as a tool to foster wellness, it is worthwhile to consider the importance of provider wellness in patient health outcomes and satisfaction. Resilient leadership suggests that the modern workplace is a complex system and that each person's interactions have a ripple effect in that system [25].

Saeed et al. created a 60-minute interactive workshop aimed only at faculty members. It is designed such that it can be used across health professions; it serves as an introduction to the five elements of well-being and to the importance of resilience in achieving well-being, and at the same time helps to outline some of the specific stressors in health professions and the effect these stressors have on providers and educators [25].

Increasing attention has been devoted to the study of resilience as a multifaceted construct with relevance in many domains, making it a valuable public health objective and tool [20]. The cyclical and synergistic pattern between resilience and wellness corroborates the necessity of developing new types of interventions and models aimed to promote resilience, since greater well-being has been associated with reduced monetary burden and increased economic contributions. There is evidence that employment outcomes in individuals with greater levels of well-being include lower healthcare costs, fewer unscheduled employment absences, and greater productivity [24].

The discussion of resilience is often inspired by examples of when it has emerged, sometimes by accident, sometimes in response to adversity, and sometimes through the intentional actions of determined individuals and organizations [5]. These arguments suggest that engagement of individual, social, and environmental resources may enable people to face challenges in the best possible way, fostering greater well-being in their own lives. Accordingly, these types of asset approaches to resilience emphasize the contributions of resources beyond the individual (e.g., social and environmental) that have strong potential for policy intervention [24].

Conclusion

Resilience is, interestingly, a term taken from the physical sciences: materials and objects are termed resilient if they resume their original shape upon being bent or stretched [11]. These characteristics have subsequently been applied to individuals. Despite, since the inception of the notion of resilience, there having been many conceptualizations, they all share the common idea that resilience is the ability to adapt to, cope with, and even be strengthened by adverse circumstances.

Research concerning resilience aims to attain a deeper understanding of the concept as a state, condition, and practice. As noted earlier, prior research has agreed on the presence of a neurobiological substrate based on genetics, which correlates with personal traits, and its interplay with risk and protective factors at individual, family, and social levels. The same logic underlies the fact that resilience is a dynamic process that lasts a lifetime.

On the other hand, the notion of wellness has been seen as very much attached to health building, this approach is in keeping with the World Health Organization's conceptualization of health [20].

The central issue addressed in this chapter is the relationship between resilience and wellness; there is agreement that challenges in the personal, professional, financial, family, and emotional reality of individuals are on the rise; evidence has proven that resilience allows the person to adapt and cope when there is an imbalance in any of the elements of well-being, consequently building and fostering wellness. Similarly, previous research demonstrates that resilience buffers the development of disability in those individuals with a chronic disease [23].

Although the notion of resilience grew out of the study of developmental psychopathology and the concern with identifying risk factors in the lives of children that are associated with psychiatric disorders in adulthood, discussions regarding the relationships between aging, resilience, and well-being have dominated research in recent years, and theories of resilience have been integrated into models of healthy aging [24]. Fostering well-being in the context of increasing exposure to challenges and adversity has significant implications for aging individuals and society as a whole.

It can be concluded that resilience is a multidimensional construct that actively includes the challenges and adversities that individuals face, making it a much more accessible public health tool. The contribution of multiple resources beyond the individual sphere (e.g., environmental and social), has strong potential and should motive new model designs and policy interventions in health, education, and social fields, fostering wellness at a population level.

References

1. FH Norris, LB Sloane. The epidemiology of trauma and PTSD. In: MJ Friedman, TM Keane, PA Resick, eds., *Handbook of PTSD*. New York, Guilford Press; 2007; 78–98.

2. R Cretney. Resilience for whom? Emerging critical geographies of socio-ecological resilience. *Geogr Compass* 2014; **8**(9); 627–640.

3. American Psychological Association. Help center. www.apa.org/helpcenter/road-resilience (accessed June 21, 2019).

4. SM Southwick, B Litz, DS Charney, MJ Friedman, eds., *Resilience and Mental Health: Challenges Across the Lifespan*. Cambridge, Cambridge University Press; 2011.

5. K Wulff, D Donato, N Lurie, et al. What is health resilience and how can we build it?. *Annu Rev Publ Health* 2015; **36**: 361–374.

6. SJ Russo, JW Murrough, MH Han, DS Charney, EJ Nestler. Neurobiology of resilience. *Nat Neurosci* 2012; **15**: 1475–1484.

7. IG Elbau, C Cruceanu, EB Binder. Genetics of resilience: gene-by-environment interaction studies as a tool to dissect mechanisms of resilience. *Biol Psychiatry* 2019. DOI:10.1016/j. biopsych.2019.04.025.

8. E Assary, JP Vincent, R Keers, M Pluess. Gene–enviroment interaction and psychiatric disorders: review and future directions. *Semin Cell Dev Biol* 2018; 77: 133–143.

9. T Halldorsdottir, EB Binder. Gene × enviroment interactions: from molecular mechanisms to behavior. *Annu Rev Psychol* 2017; **68**: 215–241.

10. A Feder, EJ Nestler, D Charney. Psychobiology and molecular genetics of resilience. *Nature Rev* 2009; **10**: 446–466.

11. SM Southwick, DS Charney. *Resilience: The Science of Mastering Life's Greatest Challenges*. Cambridge, Cambridge University Press; 2012.

12. SC Cramer, M Sur, BH Dobkin, et al. Harnessing neuroplasticity for clinical

applications. *Brain* 2011; **134**(6): 1591–1601.

13. AFT Arnsten. Stress signaling pathways that impair prefrontal cortex structure and function. *Nature* 2009; 10: 410–422.

14. A Rozanski, JA Blumenthal, J Kaplan. Impact of psychological factors on the pathogenesis of cardiovascular disease and implications for therapy. *Circulation* 1999; **99**: 2192–2217.

15. A Bandura. *Social Learning Theory.* Englewood Cliffs, NJ, Prentice-Hall; 1977.

16. A Pascual-Leone. The brain that plays music and is changed by it. *Ann NY Acad Sci* 2001; **930**: 315–329.

17. J White. *I Will Not be Broken: Five Steps to Overcoming a Life Crisis.* New York, St. Martin's Press; 2008.

18. G Windle, KM Bennett, J Noyes. A methodological review of resilience measurement scales. *Health Qual Life Outcomes* 2011; **9**: 8.

19. S MacLeod, S Musich, K Hawkins, et al. The impact of resilience among older adults. *Geriatr Nurs* 2016; **37**: 266–272.

20. S Cadell, J Karabanow, M Sanchez. Community, empowerment, and resilience: paths to wellness. *Can J Community Mental Health* 2001; **20**(1): 21–35.

21. KA Strout, DJ Dyer, RC Gray, RH Robnett, EP Howard. Behavioral interventions in six dimensions of wellness that protect the cognitive health of community-dwelling older adults: a systematic review. *J Am Geriatr Soc* 2016; **64**: 944–958.

22. T Rath, J Harter. *Wellbeing: The Five Essential Elements.* New York, Gallup Press; 2010.

23. MC Fullen, DH Granello. Holistic wellness in older adulthood: group differences based on age and mental health. *J Holistic Nurs* 2018; **36**(4): 395–407.

24. TD Cosco, K Howse, C Brayne. Healthy ageing, resilience and wellbeing. *Epidemiol Psychiatr Sci* 2017; **26**: 579–583.

25. S Saeed, R Quock, J Lott, N Kashani, W Woodall. Building resilience for wellness: a faculty development resource. *Med Ed Portal* 2017; **13**: 10629.

Developing Purpose, Meaning, and Achievements

Jennice Vilhauer

Introduction

As the humanistic perspective would tell us, life is all about the journey of becoming who you want to be. But in order to move in the direction of your idealized self, you must first know where you want to go and, just as importantly, how to get there. Not having direction is like going through life without a road map. Purpose and meaning give you direction, while your achievements in life are the result of the actions that you take toward closing the gap between who you are and who you are becoming.

This chapter focuses on clinical skills and interventions that can help one develop purpose, meaning, and achievement. The discussion will begin with identifying the activities that research has demonstrated are known to promote the development of purpose, and then specifically four therapy models are highlighted with a brief review of their theory and application. Logotherapy and meaning therapy focus on the development of meaning, while hope therapy and future-directed therapy focus on the mindset and skill development necessary for achievement.

Purpose

While definitions of purpose vary, it is commonly accepted that purpose in life represents a stable and generalized intention to accomplish something that is both personally meaningful and leads to productive engagement with some aspect of the world beyond the self [1]. This definition encompasses three important aspects. First, purpose represents an intentional goal with a long-term aim that directs more proximal behaviors, generated by the motivational self, the aspect of our being that can identify preferences for what we want [2]. Next, purpose must be personally meaningful so that an individual will feel compelled to actively pursue his/her purpose by investing time, energy, and resources to accomplish it. Lastly, purpose is inspired by a desire to contribute one's efforts and talents to the world in some way. Purpose is not always moral or prosocial in nature. Hitler was driven by his purpose. It is the perception one has about his or her own contribution that gives meaning to one's goals.

Having a purpose has positive psychological benefits. People who report having higher levels of purpose tend to be emotionally and physically healthier than those who do not. They also tend to report higher levels of optimism, life satisfaction, self-esteem, and self-efficacy [3–5]. Younger people with purpose often perform better academically. Those with less purpose are more likely to report depression, boredom, loneliness, anxiety, and substance abuse [6–10]. Due to the positive relationship between purpose and positive psychological states, purpose is a central component of most theories of optimal human development and well-being [11].

The Development of Purpose

Despite the benefits of having purpose, only one in five high-school students and one in three college students reports having a clear purpose in life; rates decline somewhat into midlife, with steeper drops in later adulthood [11]. Purpose can be developed and maintained over one's lifetime, but it is something that for many requires conscious pursuit.

While the seeds of purpose can be developed in children by teaching values and gratitude, as well as being allowed to pursue enjoyable activities [11], adolescence is the period in life during which individuals become actively engaged in discovering purpose. As one establishes meaningful interests and dreams, then commits to long-term goals, a sense of identity becomes more defined. While how adolescents develop purpose is not a well-studied area, exposure to a wide variety of activities (e.g., volunteering, science club) peer groups, and personal experiences (e.g., domestic violence or a school shooting) tend to be the most common avenues [11, 12].

In early adulthood, searching for purpose is associated with life satisfaction; however, by midlife this search is a less comfortable experience and those without purpose can feel they are in a crisis [5]. For many at this stage, the parenting of children and caregiving for older parents can provide an important source of purpose [13], though it often comes at the cost of happiness as these can be stressful experiences [14]. These findings underscore the nuanced experience of purpose. Work is another common source of purpose among midlife adults [13]. Perhaps not surprisingly, individuals who find purpose in their work report feeling more satisfied. How people perceive their work is more important than the actual tasks they perform; for example, cleaning staff in a hospital who perceive their job as thankless were less happy than those who viewed what they were doing as a valuable contribution to the process [15].

The final stage of life begins in the sixties. Compared to others, older adults with high levels of purpose tend to be more social and have more positive relationships. They are more likely to live in private homes than in institutional settings [16]. Older adults with purpose are also more likely to be employed, have better health, have a higher level of education, and be married. Interestingly, regular contact with family, more so than friends, is a stronger predictor of purpose among older adults [17].

Therapeutic settings can be effective places for nurturing the growth of purpose. There are several empirically based strategies that mental health professionals can use to help people develop more purpose and greater overall meaning in life. The rest of this chapter focuses on established therapeutic models that can be used specifically for the development and achievement of a purposeful life.

Meaning

The term "meaning" has somewhat different definitions, depending on the school of thought. Behaviorists tend to view it an expressed action, while cognitive psychologists see it as the valued narrative that we mentally attach to a subject. In terms of this discussion, meaning is more generally defined as the mental construct of attaching significance or value to an experience. A part of the humanistic/existential movement, psychiatrist Victor Frankl believed that human beings are motivated by a desire to find meaning in life and that the motivation for living comes from finding that meaning.

Logotherapy

Logotherapy, developed by Victor Frankl, is the first psychological intervention specifically intended to help individuals develop more personal meaning in their lives. Highly influenced by his time in a concentration camp during World War II, Frankl believed people were driven by a "will to meaning" as opposed to the "will to pleasure" postulated by Sigmund Freud or a "will to power" highlighted by Alfed Adler [18, 19]. The main premise of logotherapy is that lack of meaning is a source of distress that is so significant it can cause anxiety, emptiness, hopelessness, or despair, and that in order to help others find their emotional stability it is necessary to help them identify meaning in their lives [20].

Frankl believed that all people had a healthy core, and that if you could help them to recognize that life offers meaning but does not promise fulfillment or happiness, and provide them with the tools to access their own inner resources, they would be able to find their way to mental health. According to Frankl, this could be done by helping people identify values about being creative, open to experience, and having choice in the attitude one takes toward life's experiences such as suffering. Frankl viewed logotherapy as a collaborative approach that could be combined with other psychotherapy orientations [18].

Techniques of Logotherapy

Logotherapists use a Socratic type of questioning process with their patients to get them to elicit their own responses. The three primary techniques used in logotherapy include dereflection, paradoxical intention, and attitude modification.

1. **Dereflection.** This technique is aimed at helping someone be less self-absorbed about a problem by getting them to focus their attention outward. For example, if someone is depressed because they hate their job, dereflection could be used to help them focus their attention on why they go to work and the people they support with the money they earn.

2. **Paradoxical intention.** With this technique, the patient wishes for the things that are feared most. Paradoxical intention uses humor to help clients get over their greatest fear, and is similar to exposure therapy. For example, someone who worries constantly about embarrassing themselves might humorously imagine themselves doing lots of embarrassing things to distance themselves from the anxiety. Paradoxically, the fear would dissipate when the intention involved the thing that was feared most.

3. **Attitude modification.** Attitude modification focuses on modifying one's attitude toward a situation. Similar to cognitive therapy, which asks people to modify their thinking about a situation, Frankl used the term attitude to encompass a set way of thinking about a situation. For example, if a client is upset about a divorce, they can be asked to identify and adopt an alternative attitude about the situation. Perhaps now the client will have time to pursue goals and dreams that have been put on hold.

These techniques highlight the emphasis on meaning by helping clients identify what gives their lives meaning, and what they should focus on in turn.

Research

There have been over 1700 empirical and theoretical papers published on logotherapy. A review of the research shows positive correlations between having meaning and life satisfaction, happiness, resilience, and marital satisfaction. An inverse relationship exists between lower levels of meaning and higher levels of mental health problems, suicidal thoughts, and job burnout.

Meaning Therapy

Meaning therapy, developed by Paul Wong, evolved from logotherapy and focuses on using a positive psychology approach to help individuals make life worth living despite suffering and limitations. Meaning therapy also incorporates other therapeutic modalities, such as CBT, existential-humanistic therapy, and narrative psychotherapy, with meaning as its central, organizing construct [21, 22].

Similar to logotherapy, meaning therapy focuses on existential meaning but also places a very high emphasis on the relationship context of psychotherapy; similar to Carl Roger's person-centered therapy, it places a high value on cultivating unconditional positive regard for the client. The motto "meaning is all we have, relationship is all we need" captures the essence of this intervention. Meaning therapy can be incorporated in an adjunctive way into other modalities of therapy.

Techniques of Meaning Therapy

Meaning therapy centers around five interventions based on major theoretical concepts [23]:

1. **Cultivation of intrinsic self-worth.** In order to help clients develop an understanding and appreciation of the value of every life, they are asked to explore intrinsic worth across several domains. In the area of relationships, one technique involves having the client identify who they matter to most in the world (e.g., their spouse, children, parents). To identify a client's own singularity they may also be asked to identify what unique contributions they are capable of making. In the domain of spirituality, clients may be asked to explore their own core beliefs and view of the world, as well as what they would like their life to stand for. A growth mindset is encouraged in all domains as clients are taught to value their own development. Other techniques to cultivate a positive self-identity include guided life review, expressive disclosive writing, and exercises to develop one's signature strengths. The mirror test can also be used by looking into a mirror and asking what you like about yourself and which aspects you want to change.

2. **The double-vision strategy.** The objective of this strategy is to encourage clients to have a larger perspective on life and to look beyond immediate concerns. The intention is to normalize a problem by showing a client that what often seems personal is instead universal. Some strategies to help clients develop double-vision include taking a long-range view to provide a proper perspective for the present predicament, looking at personal problems from the perspective of universal problems (existential givens), looking at relevant macro forces such as global economic recession and systemic discrimination, stepping out of the situation and lifting one's eyes to the sky and the horizon, and looking at the problem from a historical perspective.

3. **The PURE intervention.** This strategy gives a conceptual framework for goal-setting and striving. It incorporates four major aspects of meaning: purpose, understanding, responsibility, and enjoyment. There are skills that clients can learn in order to develop these aspects in their own lives. For example, the following techniques can be used to enhance clients' awareness of their true purpose: (a) For each situation ask: "What purpose does this serve?" If it doesn't serve any useful function, then don't proceed.

(b) Reflect on the big questions: "What should I do with my life?" "What really matters in life?" (c) Behavioral experiments: Have you ever unfairly blamed your friend in order to get out of a difficult situation? Have you ever sacrificed your self-interest in order to help others or serve society? Have you found something for which you are willing to work hard and sacrifice? The following are some techniques to activate awareness of responsibility: (a) Ask yourself how your action will affect your loved ones and friends. (b) Write down instances when you have broken a promise and let people down in the past month. (c) Describe an instance in which you assumed personal responsibility at great cost.

4. **The ABCDE intervention.** This strategy provides a conceptual framework for coping with existential anxieties. ABCDE stands for acceptance, belief, commitment, discovery, and evaluation. Each component represents an important existential theme and helps clients to develop meaning around difficult life events. For example, acceptance is an important coping strategy in dealing with death and bereavement or a natural disaster.

5. **The dual-systems strategy** [23]. PURE and ABCDE in a dual-process approach can be symbolized by Yin and Yang. These strategies effectively integrate the negatives and positives that are present in life and negotiate a dialectic balance between opposing forces.

Conclusions

Meaning therapy has evolved to merge the world of existential psychotherapy with that of positive psychology. While it is a nascent intervention, with limited research, it is grounded in established psychological theories and models, and Dr. Wong has developed numerous assessment tools and authored several theoretical papers that support its utility.

Achievement

Achievement is the accomplishment of intentional goal-directed behavior. It signifies the outcome of a series of sequenced steps that begins with initial desire, then a calculated decision to pursue, followed by a deliberate planning process, and an execution of action that results in a manifested experience. Each of these steps is necessary for any goal to become a reality. It is the movement toward these end goals that gives purpose and meaning to our lives, yet the accomplishments themselves require distinct mental states and cognitive processes that must be successfully navigated for an individual to achieve a desire. This next section covers two interventions designed to facilitate optimal mental process and behavior that leads to achievement.

Hope Therapy

C.R. Snyder and his colleagues defined hope as the synthesis of thinking that one can imagine moving from the present into a desired future state via one or more pathways. Hope is seen as a cognitive construct that reflects people's motivation and capacity to strive toward personally relevant goals. Snyder and his colleagues believe that hope depends on agency thinking and pathways thinking. Agency thinking refers to one's perceived ability to pursue goals despite obstacles and is evident in self-statements such as "I can do this." Pathways thinking refers to one's perceived ability to generate plausible paths toward goals and is evident in self-statements such as "I can find a way to get this done."

In hope therapy, goals are viewed as the mental endpoint of hopeful thought. Snyder et al. perceived emotions to be the outcome of goal pursuit. The successful pursuit of goals leads to positive emotion, while the unsuccessful pursuit of goals leads to negative emotion. One's level of trait hope can develop overtime as one develops a history of successful or unsuccessful experiences [24].

Techniques of Hope Therapy

Hope therapy was designed to increase one's hopeful thought regardless of the presenting problem. Snyder believed hope was a common factor of all psychotherapies and proposed that therapy works specifically because it enables people to identify goals that represent solutions to their problems. Interventions designed on Snyder's hope theory have several components in common.

1. **Psychoeducation about hope.** The basic principles of hope theory are presented to the client, including a description of hope as a cognitive construct related to goal pursuit, an illustration of agency and pathways thinking, and a discussion of barriers and the negative emotions they can elicit.
2. **Goal-setting.** The client identifies meaningful goals. Goal identification can be accomplished by encouraging the client to explore his or her satisfaction in various areas of life such as school, work, and relationships. After a personally relevant goal has been identified, the next step would be for the client to generate multiple pathways toward its accomplishment. Pathways cognitions can be increased by breaking goals into smaller steps, anticipating obstacles, and planning alternative routes in case of setbacks.
3. **Agentic cognitions.** Next, the client would identify thoughts about perceived agency related to the desired goal. Ways to identify and modify thoughts may include use of personal narratives and storytelling. For example, clients might be encouraged to relate and transcribe stories about events in their childhood that illustrate their capacity to face specific challenges. Clients may identify low-hope elements of these narratives and replace them with positive, hopeful thoughts.

Research

A meta-analysis of 27 studies utilizing hope interventions and involving 2154 participants showed significant but small effect sizes for hopefulness and life satisfaction, and no overall relationship between hope-enhancement strategies and decreased psychological distress. It also appears that briefer interventions in structured settings are better at improving hope [25]. Hope therapy is likely to be most useful when integrated with other empirical forms of psychotherapy and treatment.

Future-Directed Therapy

Future-directed therapy (FDT) was developed as an evolved form of cognitive therapy, to map onto the cognitive and biological knowledge that has emerged regarding future thinking. The "future" in FDT is not necessarily far off in time; it can refer to any point in time beyond the present moment, near or far. Rather, FDT is about under-standing that because we can only move forward, most of our thinking and behavior is anticipatory or future-oriented. We constantly speculate about what will happen, whether it is in the very next moment, tomorrow, or five years from now, and that speculation has a huge impact on how we process information, how we feel about different situations and, ultimately, how we create our lives.

Future-directed therapy was originally designed as a full clinical intervention intended to reduce symptoms of depression and improve well-being by promoting a paradigm shift from dwelling on the past, or highlighting one's limitations in the present, toward creating more positive expectancies about the future, by developing and employing a comprehensive and well-defined set of skills. It is based on a positive psychology model, and the skills in FDT are applicable to any individual interested in developing skills for creating positive future experiences.

The theoretical premise behind FDT is based on humanistic models of behavior and posits that human beings live in a continuous state of wanting to close the gap between where they are in the present and where they want to be in the future. Each time a desired want is attained, a new want is born. When individuals perceive they can move toward a desired state, they feel they are able to thrive and grow, which is experienced as positive emotion. However, when movement toward desired states is inhibited, it generates negative emotions. The more unable to thrive one feels, the more emotional distress he or she will experience. Improved thriving is achieved by actions taken to close the gap between present states and future desired states [26].

Techniques of Future-Directed Therapy

Unlike traditional cognitive therapy, in FDT the focus is on the anticipatory part of the human experience, both in understanding the patient's problem as well as where primary interventions occur. The interventions in FDT center around the FDT anticipatory cognitive model of human experience (Figure 41.1), in which a distinction is made between anticipatory beliefs and the present or past beliefs on which anticipatory assessments are based. It highlights the anticipatory response process of choice calculation, in which people decide what actions they will take based on what they anticipate will happen in any given situation. If a patient is aware of what his/her faulty thoughts are about a future situation,

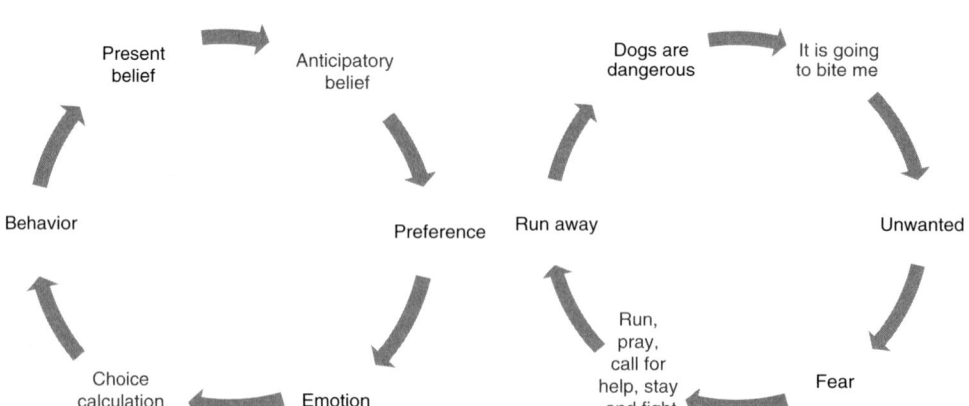

Figure 41.1 FDT anticipatory cognitive model of human experience.

then they can be changed before the situation occurs and, potentially, a different outcome can be created.

The interventions in FDT also integrate knowledge about attentional and cognitive biases in reward processing and are incorporated into what is referred to as the 4-A (anticipate, activate, assess, act) achievement model, which represents the sequential set of skills the individual is taught to use to improve their ability to create more positive future experiences.

1. **Anticipate.** In the *anticipation* phase, the individual identifies what they want, what steps are necessary to achieve it, what the obstacles are, and what their current beliefs are about their ability to achieve their goal. During this initial phase, there is a significant education process around the anticipatory model and about the relationship between anticipatory thought and action that creates lived experiences.
2. **Activate.** This is the phase where there is a significant effort to shift biased thinking away from the unwanted to the more wanted aspects of a situation. In this phase, individuals *activate* attention to benefits of a desired goal (e.g., journal exercises, worksheets) to increase a goal's value, which increases motivation to act. They also decrease attention to costs by giving more attention to implementation plans to overcome perceived obstacles. This shifts belief in one's ability to achieve the desired goal by increasing the focus on why and how it can be done. This phase highlights another unique component of FDT in that it uses affect-biased attention as a direct emotion regulation strategy, by training patients to self-monitor attentional process and to redirect attention to rewards.
3. **Assess.** Cost–benefit ratios of action to outcome are the basis of all decisions to engage in behavior that will lead to any desired goal. In this phase the individual *assesses* the planned steps toward their goal, along with their plans to overcome any obstacles, and makes a determination as to whether they are likely to achieve an outcome that is worth the cost of their actions.
4. **Act.** In this phase the mental process and planning to engage in the desired goal has been achieved, and mental barriers have been removed so the focus is on implementing the action plans developed at earlier stages.

Research

Two non-randomized clinical studies have been completed using FDT. The first study involved comparing 16 patients in an FDT group with 17 patients treated simultaneously in traditional CBT groups. All patients had a confirmed diagnosis of DSM-IV major depressive disorder. Patients treated with FDT demonstrated significant improvements from baseline to posttreatment, with a reduction of symptoms of depression ($p = 0.001$) and anxiety ($p = 0.021$) and reported improvement in quality of life ($p = 0.035$). Additionally, they reported high satisfaction with the therapy [27].

In a follow-up study that again compared FDT to group-based CBT, the Beck Hopelessness Scale (BHS) was added to assess positive and negative anticipation. In one year, 42 patients completed a 10-week, 20-session group therapy program (FDT [$n = 22$] and CBT [$n = 20$]). Key findings from baseline to posttreatment showed that FDT improved depression ($p = 0.001$), positive anticipation (BHS-subfactor) ($p = 0.001$), and quality of life ($p = 0.001$); FDT was significantly better than CBT at reducing anhedonia. Regression analysis indicated that change in positive anticipation (BHS) predicted change in anhedonia ($p = 0.038$) and overall depression ($p = 0.008$) in the FDT group, but not the CBT control group. Even with small sample sizes and non-randomized assignment to condition, these findings suggest that FDT is uniquely changing depressive symptoms via alteration of cognitions regarding positive expectations [28].

References

1. W Damon, J Menon, KC Bronk. The development of purpose during adolescence. *Appl Dev Sci* 2003; 7: 119–128.

2. A Fishbach. The motivational self is more than the sum of its goals. *Behav Brain Sci* 2014; **37**: 143–144.

3. R Friedman, J Leserman, M Caudill, PC Zuttermeister, H Benson. An inventory of positive psychological attitudes with potential relevance to health outcomes: validation and preliminary testing. *Behav Med* 1991; **17**: 121–129.

4. MF Steger, P Frazier. Meaning in life: one link in the chain from religiousness to well-being. *J Couns Psychol* 2005; **52**(4): 574–582.

5. KC Bronk, P Hill, D Lapsley, T Talib, WH Finch. Purpose, hope and life satisfaction in three age groups. *J Posit Psychol* 2009; **4**: 500–510.

6. M Bigler, GJ Neimeyer, E Brown. The divided self revisited: effects of self-concept clarity and self-concept differentiation on psychological adjustment. *J Soc Clin Psychol* 2001; **20**: 396–415.

7. Bronk, K. C., Hill, P., Lapsley, D., Talib, T., & Finch, W. H. (2009). Purpose, hope, and life satisfaction in three age groups. Journal of Positive Psychology 4(6),500–510. well-being. Journal of Counseling Psychology, 52, 574.

8. LL Harlow, MD Newcomb, PM Bentler. Depression, self-derogation, substance use, and suicide ideation: lack of purpose in life as a mediational factor. *J Clin Psychol* 1986; **42**: 5–21.

9. T Nicholson, W Higgins, P Turner, et al. The relation between meaning in life and occurrence of drug abuse: a retrospective study. *Psychol Addict Behav* 1994; **8**: 24–28.

10. CR Roos, M Kirouac, MR Pearson, BC Fink, K Witkiewitz. Examining temptation to drink from an existential perspective: associations among

temptation, purpose in life, and drinking outcomes. *Psychol Addict Behav* 2015; **29**: 716–724.

11. KC Bronk. *Purpose in Life: A Component of Optimal Youth Development*. New York, Springer; 2013.

12. PL Hill, AL Burrow, KC Bronk. Persevering with positivity and purpose: an examination of purpose commitment and positive affect as predictors of grit. *J Happiness Stud* 2014; **17**: 257–269.

13. W Damon. *The Path to Purpose: Helping Our Children Find Their Calling in Life*. New York, Free Press; 2008.

14. M Hughes. Affect, meaning, and quality of life. *Social Forces* 2006; **85**: 611–629.

15. JM Berg, A Wrzesniewski, JE Dutton. Perceiving and responding to challenges in job crafting at different ranks: when proactivity requires adaptivity. *J Org Behav* 2010; **31**: 158–186.

16. WS Laufer, EA Laufer, LS Laufer. Purpose in life and occupational interest in a gerontological sheltered workshop. *J Clin Psychol* 1981; **37**(4): 424–426.

17. M Pinquart. Creating and maintaining purpose in life in old age: a meta-analysis. *Ageing Int* 2002; **27**(2): 90–114.

18. M Ameli, FM Dattilio. Enhancing cognitive behavior therapy with logotherapy: techniques for clinical practice. *Psychotherapy* 2013; **50**(3): 387–391.

19. VE Frankl. On logotherapy and existential analysis. *Am J Psychoanal* 1958; **18**(1): 28–37.

20. S Faramarzi, F Bavali. The effectiveness of group logotherapy to improve psychological well-being of mothers with intellectually disabled children. *Int J Dev Disabil* 2017; **63**(1): 45–41.

21. PTP Wong. Towards an integrative model of meaning-centered counselling and therapy. *Int Forum Logother* 1999; **22**(1): 47–55.

22. PTP Wong. From logotherapy to meaning-centered counseling and therapy. In PTP Wong, ed., *The Human Quest for Meaning: Theories, Research, and Applications* (2nd ed.). New York, Routledge; 2012; 619–647.

23. PTP Wong. Meaning therapy: assessments and interventions. *Existential Analysis* 2015; **26**(1): 154–167.

24. CR Snyder: *The Psychology of Hope.* New York, Free Press; 1994.

25. R Weis, E Speridakos. A Meta-analysis of hope enhancement strategies in clinical and community settings. *Psychol Well-Being* 2011: 5. DOI:10.1186/2211-1522-1-5.

26. J Vilhauer (2014). *Think Forward to Thrive: How to Use the Mind's Power of Anticipation to Transcend Your Past and Transform Your Life.* Novato, CA, New World Library.

27. J Vilhauer, S Young, C Kealoha, et al. Treating major depression by creating positive expectations for the future: a pilot study for the effectiveness of Future Directed Therapy (FDT) on symptom severity and quality of life. *CNS Neurosci Ther* 2012; **18**: 102–109.

28. J Vilhauer, J Cortes, S Chung, et al. Improving quality of life for patients with major depressive disorder by increasing hope and positive expectations with Future Directed Therapy (FDT). *Innov Clin Neurosci* 2013; **10**: 3.

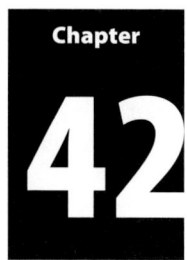

Chapter

42

Healing and Wellness

Paul Dieppe, Sarah Goldingay, and Sara L. Warber

The conceptual problem at the center of contemporary healthcare is the confusion between disease processes and disease origins. Instead of asking why an illness occurs and trying to remove the conditions that led to it, medical researchers try to understand the mechanisms through which the disease operates, so that they can then interfere with them. . . . In the process of reducing illness to disease, the attention of physicians has moved away from the patient as a whole person. By concentrating on smaller and smaller fragments of the body – shifting its perspective from the study of bodily organs and their functions to that of cells and, finally, to the study of molecules – modern medicine often loses sight of the human being, and having reduced health to mechanical functioning, it is no longer able to deal with the phenomenon of healing.

F. Capra, The Systems View of Life: a Unifying Vision, *2014*

Introduction

Fritjof Capra and others have pointed out that contemporary healthcare often has difficulty with the phenomena of healing. However, as we shall see, this is not always the case.

In biomedical discourses, healing is generally used to describe the body's intrinsic ability to mend a wound or a broken bone. But when complementary and alternative medicine (CAM) practitioners or the general public use the word they often mean something different and much more "holistic"; it may involve mending again, but mending of our whole selves, including concepts such as the (re)integration of body, mind, and soul [1].

The word "healing" can be used as a noun (e.g., "I have had healing"), a verb (e.g., "I am healing you"), or an adjective (e.g., "this is a healing environment"). Furthermore, it can be used to refer to individuals, to groups and communities, to animals and plants, to the environment, or the whole world.

In this chapter we concentrate on the healing of individual humans, and we put most of our emphasis on widely used contemporary healing practices in high-income countries such as the UK and USA.

We first look at healing as a noun (healed states), then we discuss different healing practices (adjective), and, finally, we consider healing as a verb (healing processes). It is important to note that each of these section titles is presented in the plural: There are many types of healed state, and a plethora of different healing practices and processes; no attempt will or should be made to claim that any one of these is superior to another – healing is an individual, experiential issue, not a "thing" that can be defined in reductionist language. Furthermore, what allows one person to "mend" has to be the right thing for them, even if it makes no sense and does not "work" for somebody else.

Box 42.1 Some Definitions of the Healed State

1. Wellness, or a feeling of wellness
2. Being whole
3. Wholeness in physical, emotional, intellectual, social, and spiritual aspects of self
4. Transcendence of suffering
5. Finding meaning beyond the illness experience
6. Being able to function well in spite of disease or illness
7. A sense of balance and peace
8. A sense of integrity
9. Flourishing, or being able to thrive

Healed States

There is much discussion of healed states for individuals in the literature, with a variety of different definitions being offered (Box 42.1). The point that these definitions emphasize is that you can be healed while still having a disease or illness. Indeed, we and others believe that you can die healed [2].

But a healed state is unlikely to be a permanent thing. We are all evolving and changing continuously; life does not stand still, and nor do our "states" of wellness, happiness or healing. We live in our stories of ourselves, and those stories change as we live them and tell them.

The word healing comes from the old English word "haelan," which literally means wholeness. So we should, perhaps, consider what might be the differences between wellness and wholeness. Cartesian dualism has resulted in our thinking of the body and mind as separate entities; even though we know that this is nonsense from a scientific and biological point of view, we still find this mindset hard to escape. This was not always the case. Some of the ancient Greeks differentiated the single entity of physical body/mind from the more ethereal, spiritual, or metaphysical concept of heart/soul. In our view, healing should be thought about in this way, as being about the integrity of body/mind with heart/soul. This is an alien idea to modern biomedical thinking, which is restricted to a materialistic, reductionist view of the world, and therefore to "matter" alone. However, it is more in line with the biopsychosocial-spiritual model [3] embraced by family physicians, and aligns with some concepts included in the increasingly used outcome "well-being" [4].

When we have asked people to provide us with one word that epitomizes healing for them, commonly used terms that fit the concept of a noun (healed states) include: integrity, balance, peace, hope, and warmth (Figure 42.1). However, the words that are used most often, many of which are not nouns, include love, compassion, acceptance, and nature, which lead us on to consider healing practices and processes.

Healing Practices

We all have the intrinsic ability to "self-heal" – that is, to reach our optimum state of flourishing (or functioning fully) across the life course, and to "mend" ourselves if broken. However, many things get in the way of that ability, fragmenting us, holding us back, and

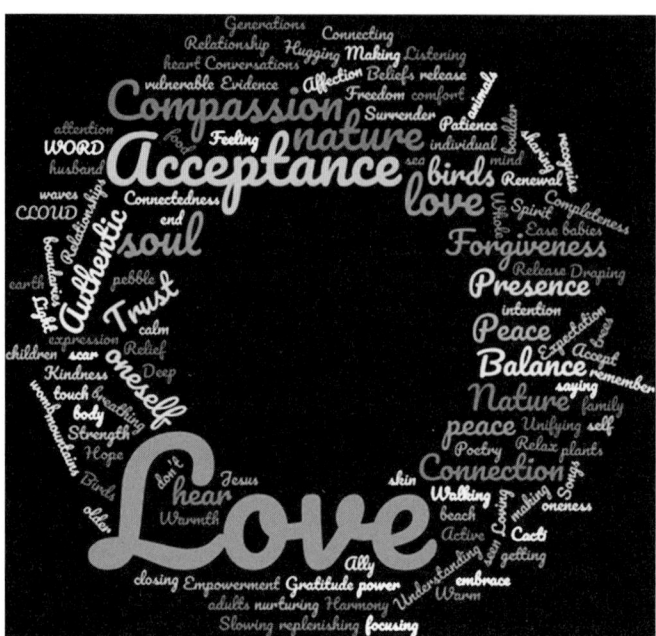

Figure 42.1 This word cloud is derived from the answers respondents have given us to the question "write down the one word that is most important to you in relation to healing." Audiences asked this question have included both healthcare professionals and members of the public, and in each case the word "love" has been the one used most often.

causing distress and suffering. Diseases can do this, but so can any number of social and environmental factors that medicine often cannot tackle. One consequence of this has been the development of a huge variety of different healing practices; people and rituals that are potent ways of giving us back our inherent ability to self-heal.

In addition to their designated medical professionals, all societies have other people working as self-proclaimed healers, using a variety of different practices, predicated on several different ontologies. We cannot address all of these, but we believe that there are common threads to most of those that are in widespread use in affluent countries today. After briefly discussing healing as ritual, we then consider how healing can be facilitated by conventional medical practitioners, before discussing the work of alternative healers in modern society.

Healing Practices and Rituals

There has always been a strong link between healing practices and religious belief systems. Shamanic and other healing practices that developed in ancient cultures were inextricably linked with the spiritual beliefs of their people. Cohen and others have written about the overlap between healing and religion in contemporary life [5]. Many modern churches perform healing services for their parishioners. There are several renowned Christian healing sites around the world, such as Lourdes in southwest France, where Catholic religious rituals become healing practices, and where we have carried out some of our own research on healing [6]. Similarly, Islam, Buddhism, and other world faiths have their healing beliefs and practices.

The importance of ritual in all healthcare interventions has been stressed by Kaptchuk [7], who has pointed out that the ways in which a modern doctor dresses in her white coat, uses tools such as the stethoscope, and follows a formulaic approach to gaining information and prescribing treatments for her patients has many similarities to shamanic and other healing rituals of old.

Biomedical Practitioners as Healers

An encounter with a doctor is usually a cause for anxiety. You (the powerless, supplicant "patient") come to the office of the powerful medical "man," who might be about to tell you that something terrible is wrong with you, or that you must take some dangerous pills, or have a surgical procedure. It is known that fear reduces our ability to communicate properly [8], and yet good communication is at the heart of healing. To be able to interact with another person in a meaningful way, you need to feel safe. Doctors often pay very little attention to the need to make their offices safe spaces to be in, or to establish enough safety and trust in their relationships with patients, so it is perhaps not surprising that healing processes are often missing from conventional medical encounters.

However, there is much more emphasis on the importance of healing, and the related process of caring, in nursing literature [9]; additionally some doctors have challenged the dismissive culture of biomedicine and written about healing. The publications of Cassell, Churchill and Schenk, Scott et al., and Egnew stand out for us [10–13]. Each of these authors recognizes that healing processes can take place in a doctor's office, and that relationships are key to this healing.

Conclusions as to how a doctor, nurse, or other healthcare professional might facilitate healing responses, through their practice, are summarized in Box 42.2. The contents of the box are derived from publications by Churchill and Schenck, Egnew, and Scott [11–13], as well as our own experiences and research.

Box 42.2 Advice for Medical Practitioners on How to Optimize Their Consultations with Patients, so That Healing Might Take Place

You
1. Prepare yourself well before seeing a patient, take time to focus
2. Be at peace with yourself
3. Make sure that your space is one in which the patient can feel safe
4. Be committed and trustworthy
5. Be prepared to be surprised, and be prepared to be wrong

The Consultation
1. Be open, establish a connection and rapport
2. Take time and listen to the story
3. Avoid being judgmental and avoid negative language
4. Be with the other person on the same level
5. Find something to like, and something to love about the person
6. Forget the protocols and charts, concentrate on the person
7. Share authority and negotiate a plan with the person
8. Laugh a little, and use the power of touch and compassion

Other Healers

Many individuals set up practices as healers. In the UK and USA (the societies we are familiar with), the majority of these people would describe themselves as one of the following: energy healer, biofield energy healer, Reiki healer, spiritual healer, or healing touch practitioner. For the remainder of the chapter we shall refer to these practices together, and use the generic term "energy healing."

We have observed and experienced the practices of many such healers, and we have also interviewed some of them, and some of their clients [6, 14–17]. Based on this data we have concluded that there are many similarities in what they do and believe, and we offer our brief generic summary of their practices.

A healing practice (treatment or intervention) given by one of these healers will usually start with the healer carefully preparing themselves and the room in which they are to work.

They will then generally establish a relationship with the client that involves trust, honesty, and mutual respect; most healers stress the central importance of the healer–client relationship to their work [14]. Varieties of different practices then take place, which may or may not include touch or talk, but are all designed to help change energy balance or flow. Central to many practitioners' working are the need for relaxation and making connections, both with the client and with the external source of energy. Both the healer and the client may appear to be in a transient altered state of consciousness during the process.

A shared belief in the potential for changing energy ("qi" or "prana") is the basis for most of these practices. When we asked energy healers to summarize what they thought were the most important components of their work – those that facilitated a healing response in a client – they stressed "unconditional love" and "focused attention with good intention."

The Effects of Healing Interventions

As already pointed out, many scientists, doctors, and others are skeptical about healing, often dismissing it as "just a placebo," although such an accusation neither explains nor devalues any benefits that might accrue for an individual. As far as we can ascertain, there has been very little research into the ability of healthcare professionals to facilitate healing, but other healers have been subject to rigorous scrutiny, perhaps driven by skepticism. But as it transpires, the evidence that the work of energy healers can be of great value is very strong.

The randomized controlled clinical trial (RCT) is currently considered to be the pinnacle of evidence of effectiveness for any intervention. Many RCTs have been carried out on energy healing practices, and they show positive results. Here we lean on a recent meta-analysis of all RCTs of "non-contact healing" (energy healing practices in which there is no physical contact made between practitioner and client) carried out by Roe and colleagues [18]. They found that there was a small but highly statistically significant positive effect of "healing intention." Furthermore, they found that this effect could be seen when healing intention was applied to plants, to the germination of seeds, and even to *in vitro* enzyme preparations, as well as intact animals including humans. This makes it difficult to dismiss it as a "placebo effect" within the current belief that such effects are mediated by expectation, suggestion, and conditioning. Furthermore, we have shown that the RCT will systematically underestimate the effect of any intervention in which the relationship between practitioner and client is a key component of the intervention (as with energy healing practices) [19], so we conclude that, according to the best modern "evidence," healing can be effective.

A different sort of evidence comes from surveys of the clients of healers [16, 20], which indicate that the clients usually report improvements, and in addition often experience abnormal sensory events (such as seeing colors or feeling tingling of the skin) while being treated by a healer [16]. Such data certainly support the contention of the healers that something is "happening."

Healing Processes

As noted above, it has been shown that healing practices can be effective and of value to individuals, resulting in changes and experiences that are different from those that accompany conventional medical practices. The explanations usually offered by healers are grounded in an energetic worldview [14], relating to concepts of energy change or flow, and connection with aspects of the universe that are not part of our materialistic, rational understandings.

So, as rational academics, we must ask ourselves: What is going on here?

From our work and interviews with healers themselves, we conclude that some of them have no interest in such questions. For such practitioners the value to their clients is obvious, and they describe "feeling" changes in energies and states, so have no need to search for any further understanding of explanations for what they do, or what is going on. But that is not enough for all energy healers, many of whom want more research to be done (particularly on the responses of their clients) [21], and it may not be enough for readers of this book, any more than it is for us, the authors of this chapter.

When thinking about what is going on, one option is to split the processes into those that are going on outside the individual, and those that go on within them. We briefly consider this split, before going on to think about the issue of time, and then emphasizing that what might matter most is the "space between" practitioner and client.

Outside Influences/Factors That Can Help Activate a Healing Response

As stated earlier, we think that there are many different relationships and activities or practices that can help us unblock barriers that prevent us from activating our natural healing abilities; there are many things, other than medical professionals or healers, that can help us mend (heal). A recent study by Scott et al. [22] explored the perspectives of 23 people identified by their general practitioner as having healed from trauma or illness. The authors describe an iterative "journey" from being wounded, fragmented, and suffering to being healed and intact; the disease or the trauma had not gone from these people, but they reached a stage at which they were able to function effectively again, and even flourish. The in-depth interviews carried out with these subjects were analyzed to ascertain what factors facilitated that healing journey. Some were things largely dependent on the person themselves, but many were external, and in addition to relationships with doctors and healers, these included love of family and friends, relationships with pets, expressive arts and culture, nature, and spirituality (Figure 42.2).

Safe, trusted relationships, connections with others, and connections with the environment seem to be key elements to healing processes. Looking back to our word cloud (Figure 42.1), we see the word "love" has the most prominence.

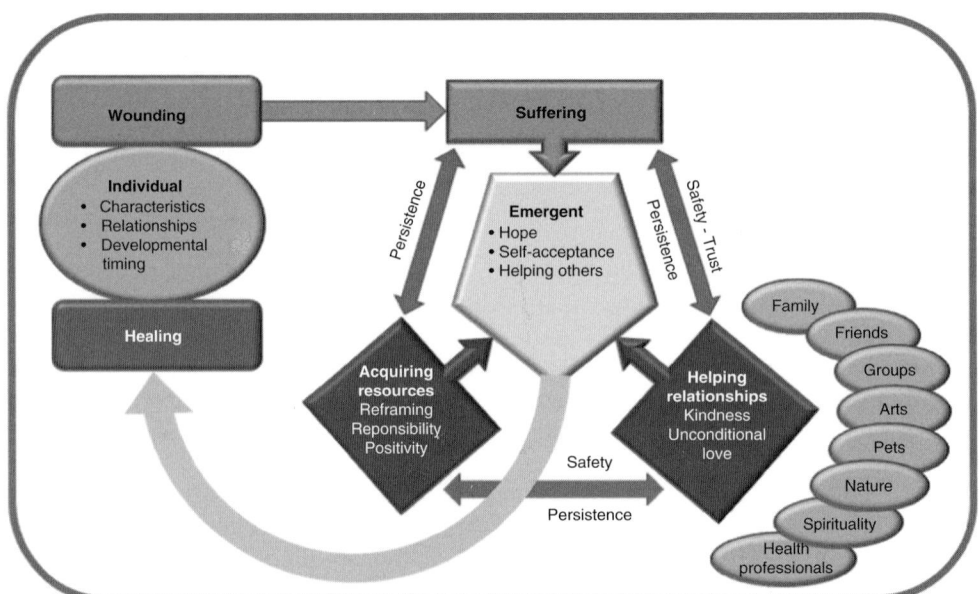

Figure 42.2 The healing journey. The model is based on the stories of 23 people who were thought to have healed from serious illness or trauma by their physicians. Their healing journeys were facilitated by the development of trust and a sense of safety, allowing meaningful relationships and connections to be made. This, along with the acquisition of resources, and reframing of the problem leads to the emergence of hope, self-acceptance, and the desire to help others, leading, in fits and starts, to a sense of integrity and wholeness that constituted their healing.

Processes within the Individual as Healing Progresses

We live in our stories of ourselves, and a part of the human condition is the need to find meaning within our lives, and explain what is going on within them. A key element to the healing process within an individual appears to be the "reframing" of the story, the change from victimhood to a state of acceptance and understanding of the problem, trauma, disease, or suffering that was previously overwhelming us [22].

Coming to terms with (accepting) who you are and what has happened to you in the past, being willing to let that go, persistence, the emergence of hope, and the developing realization that you can be of help to others also seem to be other key internal changes that people make on their healing journeys (Figure 42.2).

Healers also emphasize the importance of the client's state of "readiness to heal," which involves being open to energy, open to change, fully present and aware, motivated and ready to work on issues, ready to engage and release, as well as accepting the possibility of self-healing [21, 23].

Fast and Slow Healing Changes

The healing process is about change. The research summarized above centered on the long journey of healing undergone by many people. This is a journey that never ends, but instead is a part of life's story for that individual.

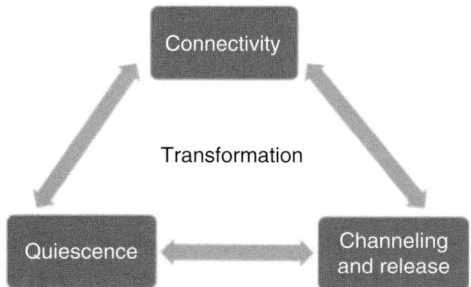

Figure 42.3 A model of key factors in sudden healing moments. Connectivity describes intense connections, experienced through touch, empathy, and love, which could provide reciprocal benefits for healers as well as clients. Quiescence captures the quiet, calm atmosphere that pervades many healing episodes. The contrasting aspects of control encompassed healers relinquishing control to channel healing, and clients seizing control to become empowered in their own healing process.

However, as described by Rhatz et al. [15], people can also experience rapid, sudden transformational changes in their health status and "wellness."

As Rhatz et al. write, in religious terms, dramatic change may take the form of spiritual or religious conversion, described by William James as a transformation from unhappiness and conflict to a unified, energized self, which can be gradual or sudden; a journey or a moment [24]. In psychotherapy, "quantum change" describes sudden transformations in someone's perception of themselves and their environment: transformations that have substantial beneficial effects on mental and physical health [25]. Unique moments of connection and change are also described in the nursing literature, and are said to depend on the interaction between nurse and client.

Rahtz et al. collected short stories of "healing moments" from 69 attendees at a conference for healing practitioners. From a thematic analysis of the data, she derived a model of how such sudden changes take place (Figure 42.3).

Reciprocity and Healing Processes: The Healer and the "Healee"

We note that Rhatz et al. [15] emphasized the reciprocal benefits experienced by healers and their clients when those essential moments of intense connection occurred between them. Others have also noted this, and it is talked about by healers, but it is a subject that appears to have attracted very little attention from the academic community. Some empirical work on reciprocal healing has been conducted in anthropology, psychiatry, and nursing, emphasizing caring [26], valuing feelings and outlook, attending to power differences, and forming abiding relationships [27]. The Institute of Medicine, Education, and Spirituality at Ochsner (IMESO) explicitly addresses the reciprocal nature of the healing relationship in their guiding statement [28]:

> Illness is a multifactorial mosaic experience because it affects the body, mind, and spirit. Any illness has the potential to change the patient, and the healing experience has the potential to change the healer. In this reciprocal relationship, both the patient and the healthcare professional can find meaning and wholeness through enlightenment, compassion, and wisdom.
>
> Establishing such a reciprocal healing relationship requires healthcare professionals to go beyond the sole consideration of the mechanisms of disease and illness and to see each patient as a person – a unique human being. When this reciprocity occurs, both the one seeking healing and the healer enter, consciously or not, into a spiritual – a self-transcendent – realm.
>
> Healthcare professionals play a major role in humanity's desire for wholeness and well-being. They apply the principles and practices of science tethered with understanding to

form the compassionate relationship ... of "treating individual human beings who are ill rather than treating a disease."

The Space Between

So, what is going on when healing processes take place?

There is a well-established trope in many traditional cultures and religions that we are all interconnected. Terms such as *web of life* have slipped into common discourse and become a shorthand for the interconnectedness of our material world. The scientific and mathematical theories that are often under the umbrella term *the butterfly effect*, which set out to understand the cause and effect of these unpredictable relationships, have also become commonplace. And, for some scientists and thinkers, the emergence of quantum mechanics has given a theoretical underpinning to this idea of interrelatedness via the theory of quantum entanglement. What is less clear, however, in this discourse is how the complex relationships and variables at play in the relationship of healer and healee work. They shift across time, culture, and the life course of an illness. They are a vehicle of interpretation. They are relative. At their best they offer a moment of mutuality when both parties feel benefit. Much has been written about the role of both "doctor" and "patient," but which suggests separation rather than connectedness.

The literature and our research suggest that deep, meaningful connections between people, and with all living things and the environment, are critical. As well as what is going on outside the person, or what is happening within them, it is the "space between" and the connectivity of all things that really matters. This is metaphysical language. But we should not be frightened of that. As Radin [29] and many others have pointed out, like it or not, paranormal events are a part of our lives, and "magic" is real. A physical explanation for magic, and for healing, is provided for us by the science of "non-locality," the idea that consciousness or information is the basis of our universe, and that physical things are a product of that – an idea first put forward by the developer of quantum theory, Max Planck. Some scientists think that the brain is the generator of consciousness; this is a relatively "new" idea. But recently, this belief is being challenged by neuroscientists, who, like many quantum physicists, see consciousness as the basic stuff of the universe, to which our brains can connect [30]. This, for us, helps make sense of the phenomenology of healing.

Conclusion

Humans have the ability to heal. Self-healing includes the body's physiologic capacity to mend and extends to the hard-won return to congruence and meaning found in seeking wholeness or wellness in the face of dis-ease. Healing, however, is not something that can be defined; rather, it is experiential, and involves a variety of practices leading to many different outcomes or healed states. We favor the concept of a return to integrity of body/mind with heart/soul as a description of those healed states we aspire to. There are no absolutes, or fixed time points for healing, we are all constantly in a state of change and healing experiences are a part of the ebb and flow of life as we seek the return to (re)integration.

Humans have the ability to facilitate another's self-healing. Culturally grounded rituals, energy healing practitioners, and healthcare practitioners of all stripes can enhance another's movement toward healing. Many healing practices depend on establishing meaningful relationships between people. Key elements to forming a healing relationship include:

- preparation of self and environment;
- creating safety and trust;
- being fully present and open with good intentions for the other; and
- caring, compassion, and love.

The complex processes involved in healing are not easily explained by materialistic science alone. Internal factors such as reframing one's story interact with external factors like deeply meaningful relationships with others, nature, or spiritual beliefs. Healing can happen in a twinkling or across a lifetime. With focused preparation, healing can go both ways across a relationship in a heightened moment of mutuality and connection with consciousness loose in the universe that we still do not fully understand.

We are both those who need healing and those who devote their professional lives to helping others. Expanding our understanding of healing offers hope that we may consciously create the possibility of healing in every encounter.

References

1. J Levin. What is healing? Reflections on diagnostic criteria, nosology and etiology. 2017. *Explore*; **13**: 244–256.

2. B Stuart, T Danaher, R Awdish, L Berry. Finding hope and healing when cure is not possible. *Mayo Clin Proc* 2019: **19**: 30039-4.

3. M Saad, R De Medeiros, AC Mosini. Are we ready for a true biopsychosocial-spiritual model? *Medicines (Basel)*; 2017; **4**: e79.

4. MJ Linton, P Dieppe, A Medina-Lara. Review of 99 self-report measures of assessing well-being in adults: exploring dimensions of well-being and developments over time. *BMJ Open* 2016; **6**: e010641.

5. MH Cohen. *Healing at the Borderland of Medicine and Religion.* Chapel Hill, NC, University of North Carolina Press; 2007.

6. S Goldingay, P Dieppe, M Farias. And the pain just disappeared into insignificance; the healing response in Lourdes. *Int Rev Psychiatry* 2014; **26**: 315–323.

7. TJ Kaptchuk. The placebo effect in alternative medicine: can the performance of a healing ritual have clinical significance? *Ann Intern Med* 2002; **136**: 817–825.

8. M Greville-Harris, P Dieppe. Bad is more powerful than good: the nocebo response in medical consultations. *Am J Med* 2015; **128**: 126–129.

9. J Watson. Caring science and human caring theory: transforming personal and professional practices of nursing and health care. *J Health Hum Serv Adm* 2009; **31**: 466–482.

10. EJ Cassell *Nature of Healing: The Modern Practice of Medicine.* Oxford, Oxford University Press; 2012.

11. LR Churchill, D Schenk. Healing skills in medical practice. *Ann Intern Med* 2008; **149**: 720–724.

12. JG Scott, D Cohen, B Dicicco-Bloom, et al. Understanding healing relationships in primary care. *Ann Fam Med* 2008; **6**: 315–322.

13. TR Egnew. The meaning of healing: transcending suffering. *Ann Fam Med* 2005; **3**: 255–262.

14. SL Warber, RL Bruyere, K Weintrub, P Dieppe. A consideration of the perspectives of healing practitioners on research into energy healing. *Global Adv Health Med* 2015; **4** (Suppl.): 72–78.

15. E Rhatz, S Bonell, S Goldingay, S Warber, P Dieppe. Transformational changes in health status: a qualitative exploration of healing moments. *Explore* 2017: **13**: 298–305.

16. E Rahtz, S Child, S Knight, S Warber, P Dieppe. Clients of UK healers: a mixed methods survey of their demography, health problems, and experiences of healing. *Complement Ther Clin Pract* 2019: **35**; 72–77.

17. P Dieppe, C Roe. Is healing an option to aid sustainable healthcare futures? *J Holistic Healthc* 2015; **12**(1): 22–25.

18. CA Roe, C Sonnex, EC Roxburgh. Two meta-analyses of noncontact healing studies. *Explore* 2015; **11**: 11–23.

19. C Paterson, P Dieppe. Characteristic and incidental (placebo) effects in complex interventions such as acupuncture. *BMJ* 2005; **330**: 1202–1205.

20. AE Kristoffersen, T Stub, O Knudsen-Baas, AH Udal, F Musial. Self-reported effects of energy healing: a prospective observational study with pre-post design. *Explore* 2019; **15**: 115–125.

21. SL Warber, D Cornello, J Straughn, G Kile Biofield energy healing from the inside. *J Altern Complement Med* 2004; **10**(6): 1107–1113.

22. JG Scott, SL Warber, P Dieppe, D Jones, KC Stange. Healing journey: a qualitative analysis of the healing experience of Americans suffering from trauma and illness. *BMJ Open* 2017; 7: e016771.

23. D Cornelio, S Warber. Social construction of CAM. *Mol Interv* 2003; **3**(4): 182–185.

24. W James. *The Varieties of Religious Experience*. New York, Longmans Green and Co., 1922.

25. WR Miller. The phenomenon of quantum change. *J Clin Psychol* 2004; **60**: 453–460.

26. P Dieppe, C Roe, S Warber. Caring and healing in health care: the evidence base. *Int J Nurs Studies* 2015; **52**: 1539–1541.

27. C Rogers. *Client Centred Therapy*. London, Constable and Robinson; 2003.

28. AJ De Conciliis. Reciprocal healing in healthcare. *Ochner J* 2014: **14**: 310–311.

29. D Radin. *Real Magic*. New York, Harmony Books; 2018.

30. GE Schwartz, M Woollacott, A Schwartz, et al. The Academy for the Advancement of Post Materialist Sciences: integrating consciousness into mainstream science. *Explore* 2018; **14**: 111–113.

Chapter 43

Connection, Compassion, and Community

Rebecca Hedrick and Kristina Jones

Of all the means which are procured by wisdom to ensure happiness throughout the whole of life, by far the most important is the acquisition of friends.

Epicurus

Introduction

Neuroscience reveals that human beings are interdependent creatures, hardwired for empathy and relationship. Natural selection has favored prosocial traits like empathy, kindness, sharing, cooperative play, mutual understanding, perspective taking, and trust [1, 2]. Social connection is central to both physical and mental well-being and increased survival [1, 3]. Conversely, social isolation is correlated with myriad deleterious consequences to health and longevity. Nervous system development, genetic expression, and health are integrally dependent on social connection [4, 5]. Children who are raised within secure environments with healthy bonds of presence, attunement, and resonance and trust will develop a neural framework that promotes receptivity, flexibility, self-understanding, mindful awareness, empathy (the ability to feel with others), and compassion (the feeling that arises when confronted with another's suffering and desire to alleviate that suffering). Conversely, children exposed to chaotic social systems of trauma, abuse, or insecure attachment face a lifetime of reactivity and dysregulation of mood, attention, physiology, impaired self-soothing, poor distress tolerance, and interpersonal conflict [5]. This chapter explores the health benefits of social connection and suggests interventions to enhance social ties and a sense of belonging through compassion-based interventions and community engagement.

Social Connection

Social connection has biological, psychological, and social benefits. These may be mediated by the release of oxytocin and endorphins, calming the nervous system and decreasing stress-induced cortisol levels [1]. Socially active people with fulfilling interpersonal relationships demonstrate a multitude of improved outcomes, including prosocial behaviors, happiness, quality of life, resilience, cognitive capacity, and wisdom [1, 3]. The quality of interpersonal relationships is more important to well-being than the quantity [1]. Having even just one trusted friend is linked to decreased recurrence in breast cancer survivors [1]. Positive-thinking friends are important since their thoughts and behaviors are contagious [6]. In fact, studies show that this contagion works with three degrees of influence; i.e., our actions and moods (positive or negative) may shape those of the friends of our friends'

friends [4]. In this way, we are interdependent; the interpersonal environment is dynamic in a positive feedback loop.

Health Risks of Social Isolation

Social isolation and loneliness are linked to poorer physical well-being, with increased risk of inflammation, infection, stroke, cardiovascular disease, and early mortality [1, 3, 6, 7]. Loneliness has health consequences on par with psychiatric illnesses and predicts earlier mortality in the elderly. Lacking social connection carries a risk that is comparable, and in many cases exceeds, that of other well-accepted risk factors, including smoking up to 15 cigarettes per day, obesity, physical inactivity, and air pollution [4]. Lack of social support also impacts mental health, with higher rates of hostility, jealousy, anxiety, depression, suicide, poor school performance, and dementia [1, 3]. Social exclusion and rejection activate the same brain centers as physical pain [1, 7]. Interventions for loneliness that have been shown to be superior to control groups include (1) improving social skills, (2) enhancing social support, (3) increasing opportunities for social contact, and (4) addressing maladaptive social cognition [8].

Interventions

Interventions that lead to wellness through connection, as well as healthier social bonds, include developing a compassionate relationship with oneself, either through developing a meditation practice of self-compassion, or via individual therapy. Studies show that mindfulness-based therapies decrease interpersonal conflict and stress, thereby enhancing connection and cooperation with immediate others, partners, children, family, and unknown others in the community via volunteer work and mentoring. In the following section we enumerate the benefits of each. To date there are no head-to-head comparisons of these types of therapies, but there is a strong indication in the literature that all of them contribute to prosocial attitudes and behaviors. Dan Buettner studied large communities across the world. In *Blue Zones of Happiness: Lessons from the World's Happiest People* he found that individuals with high degrees of social engagement and support reported not only greater levels of well-being but demonstrably increased longevity [6].

Self and Self (Psychotherapy)

Cognitive-behavioral therapy improves empathy and social relationships [7]. The quality of the therapeutic relationship with the provider is more important than the modality of therapy used. Therapy serves as a bridge to improved relationships with family, friends, and the wider community [3].

Self and Partner (Love Life)

Healthy partnerships can lead to a lifetime of well-being, while staying in an unhealthy relationship can negatively impact physical and mental health. It is important to find a compassionate partner who aligns with one's own values, interests, and sense of humor. Healthy partners listen well, speak freely, and foster independence, and learn how to deal with conflict in a healthy way [6].

Self and Children (Parenting)

While having children does not automatically bring greater happiness, with its added financial and relationship stressors, having *healthy* relationships with children is associated with well-being and longevity. Healthy parenting includes engaging in active pursuits with children, and prioritizing quality screen-free, face-to-face time (e.g., meals, reading, games, etc.) [6]. The American Academy of Pediatrics advises limiting children's screen time to two hours, removing screens and internet access from children's bedrooms at night, and monitoring their social media usage to ensure healthy development of social connection [9]. Early research indicates that mindfulness interventions for families with a child with chronic illness are an effective means to better (negative) emotion recognition, regulation, and expression, and decreases stress in all family members [10]. There are studies in development for parents and children with attention-deficit hyperactivity disorder.

Self and Family/Friends (Prioritize Quality Relationships)

It is important to gravitate toward happier people and limit the time spent with negative ones, as depression and pessimism are socially contagious. A healthy social network includes at least three happy, funny, trustworthy friends. The happiest people spend at least six hours a day socializing. This is best achieved with interactive activities such as communal meals, dancing, singing, and exercising, rather than passive activities such as watching TV, and by avoiding screen time during shared meals, opting instead for conversation [6].

Self and Community: Join

Joining a group that meets once a month increases happiness as much as doubling one's salary [6]! In fact, attending a weekly faith-based service of any denomination adds 4–14 years of life expectancy [6].

Self and Community: Volunteering and Mentoring

Empirical studies demonstrate that prosocial actions such as providing instrumental support (e.g., housekeeping, transportation, etc.) to friends, relatives, or neighbors decreases mortality, and increases happiness for those caregivers [1]. Elderly adults who volunteered to help underprivileged children to read demonstrated improved cognition, increased activity in the prefrontal cortex (responsible for executive function and expression of appropriate social behavior), and growth of the hippocampus (responsible for memory), instead of the expected age-related shrinkage of these brain regions [7]. Interestingly, research has shown that people's *perception* of their social support, rather than actual size of social support networks, is what influences their feelings of wellness and connection, and in turn shows that those with fewer social supports do not thrive, and have earlier mortality [11].

Mindfulness-Based Interventions

The last decade has seen a huge increase in using mindfulness-based interventions, including teaching meditation skills, as well as psychotherapy blending standard talk therapy with mindfulness ideas and techniques. The techniques have been used in both healthy and clinical populations, such as patients with schizophrenia and chronic pain. Mindfulness principles underlie the most successful therapy for borderline personality, developed by psychologist Marsha Linehan as dialectical behavior therapy (DBT). This therapy includes modules on self-compassion, identifying emotions without reacting, and decreasing anger and negative affect in all social relationships [12]. Mindfulness-based approaches are gaining ground in addiction treatment as well. Psychologists, psychiatrists, social workers, counselors, chaplains, yoga teachers, and meditation teachers all employ mindfulness concepts. Integrating mindfulness into stress management after heart attack, and for clinical disorders such as anxiety or panic, is an exciting tool beyond medication that is now becoming the standard of care.

Recently there have been attempts to study the effectiveness of these approaches. Unlike Western psychology, some of these mindfulness-based therapies focus on compassion for others and compassion for the self, and also these two things in combination. We will describe the central role of self-compassion in some approaches that may have a special role to play in combating professional burnout.

Compassion

If you want others to be happy practice compassion; and if you want yourself to be happy practice compassion.

His Holiness the Fourteenth Dalai Lama, Tenzin Gyatso

Definition

Compassion may be defined as the experience of being emotionally attuned to, or having empathy for, another's suffering, along with the desire to help alleviate that suffering and help them flourish [5, 13].

Self-Compassion

The construct of self-compassion and the Self-Compassion Scale (the primary measure of self-compassion in many outcome studies) were developed and formalized by psychologist Kristin Neff, PhD. The Self-Compassion Scale consists of three basic elements. The first element is self-kindness – the ability to respond to one's own weaknesses, failures, or distress with caring, warmth, and understanding, rather than harsh self-judgment and self-attack. The second element is the recognition of our common humanity – the recognition that one's suffering is part of the shared human condition rather than an isolating experience. The third element is mindfulness, taking a balanced perspective of equanimity – sometimes described as "detachment," "non-reactivity," or "balance" – rather than over-identification with thoughts or feelings by becoming lost in negative emotions and ideas [14]. Self-compassion is not about replacing negative feelings with positive ones. Instead, it promotes cognitive acceptance and integration of negative experiences [15].

There is extensive data correlating self-compassion with various aspects of well-being. Individuals with high self-compassion demonstrate lower levels of perceived stress, and increased resilience in the face of stressful situations, including chronic illness [16]. Research suggests that the mechanisms for this are related to improved coping, positive cognitive emotional reframing, acceptance, and decreased denial and less behavioral disengagement [16].

Self-compassion deactivates threat systems (e.g., fight, flight, or freeze) associated with the release of cortisol and epinephrine and activates the mammalian self-soothing system associated with the release of oxytocin and endorphins [17]. High self-compassion is correlated with life satisfaction, social connectedness, and family functioning, and decreased interpersonal problems and personality pathology [2, 18]. Low self-compassion is consistently associated with anxiety, depression, self-centeredness, self-criticism and avoidance [18].

Research on Compassion-Based Interventions

Kirby et al. conducted a meta-analysis of randomized controlled trials (RCTs) for empirically validated compassion-based interventions (CBIs), most notably mindful self-compassion, compassion-focused therapy, and loving kindness and compassion meditation [19]. They discovered strong evidence that CBIs improve compassion, self-compassion, mindfulness, depression, anxiety, psychological distress, emotion regulation, interpersonal relationships, physical and mental well-being, life satisfaction, and happiness.

Indeed, CBIs such as mindfulness-based stress reduction (MBSR) and mindfulness-based cognitive therapy (MBCT) have demonstrated improvements in compassion and self-compassion in a variety of clinical, community, and healthcare professional populations. Interestingly, evidence suggests that self-compassion appears to mediate the psychological benefits of CBIs on improving stress and depression and is a better predictor of psychological symptom severity and quality of life than mindfulness itself [14].

The CBIs aim to nurture the individual's compassion toward self and others, as well as their openness to receiving compassion from others by fostering empathy, kindness, and equanimity. All of the CBIs combine principles derived from both Western and Tibetan-Buddhist psychology, and embed in their foundation skills training in mindfulness (the non-judgmental awareness of the present moment) [19].

Mindful Self-Compassion

Mindful self-compassion (MSC; see Box 43.1) is an empirically supported CBI developed by Kristin Neff PhD, consisting of an eight-week program of two-hour weekly group sessions

---

Box 43.1 Exercise in Mindful Self-Compassion

During a moment of personal difficulty, find a quiet place. Bring the current circumstances and troubling emotions to mind. Give yourself a physical gesture of kindness and self-soothing, by placing a hand on your heart. Repeat the following phrases to yourself, or create your own personalized phrase:

"I am really suffering."

[This phrase uses mindfulness to bring awareness to the current experience.].

"We all struggle in our lives . . . " [common humanity].

"May I be gentle with myself . . . " or

"May I accept myself as I am in this moment . . . " [self-kindness].

If you find it difficult to access the self-kindness, imagine what a loved one might say to you, or you to a loved one in a similar circumstance, and then use that same language for yourself [14].

of didactics and experiential exercises. There have been multiple RCTs of MSC in community samples, demonstrating improvements in self-compassion, mindfulness, life satisfaction, depression, anxiety, and stress [18]. One RCT comparing diabetic patients with waiting-list controls showed that MSC led to statistically and clinically significant improvements in depression and hemoglobin A1C scores, which estimates the average blood sugar control over the past three months [17]. A more recent study demonstrated that a web-based MSC program led to improved functioning and decreased burnout in psychologists [20].

Compassion-Focused Therapy

Compassion-focused therapy (CFT) was created by psychologist Paul Gilbert, PhD and is the most evaluated CBI to date [21]. Rather than being a standalone school of therapy, CFT is proposed as a technique that may be incorporated into other psychotherapy frameworks, to help individuals in whom shame and self-criticism have made psychotherapy progress difficult [2]. It aims to mitigate the fight-or-flight response by enhancing self-soothing behaviors, using mindfulness techniques, compassionate visualizations, compassionate cognitive responding, and engaging in overt compassionate behaviors toward self and others [19]. Growing empirical evidence supports CFT's benefits in mood and anxiety disorders, trauma disorders, psychotic disorders (particularly persecutory auditory hallucinations), personality disorders with high self-criticism, eating disorders including bulimia/anorexia nervosa and binge-eating disorder, and smoking cessation [2, 19].

Loving Kindness Meditation and Compassion Meditation

Studies suggests that loving kindness meditation (LKM; see Box 43.2) and compassion meditation (CM) enhance affective processing, improve anger regulation (including in chronic pain sufferers), decrease depression, lower illness symptom severity, and can decrease stress-induced distress and impaired immune response [2, 13, 14]. They can be successfully applied to a range of ages (adolescents, students, and adults), and in a variety of settings (clinical, non-clinical, and healthy populations, including workplace wellness programs), with benefits demonstrated in even single-session trainings followed by self-practice [13].

Physicians, social workers, therapists, nurses, and community caretakers are chronically exposed to high levels of suffering and severe stress in their patients or clients. Many work and care for others at the expense of themselves, ignoring the familiar instruction from the flight attendant to place the oxygen mask on themselves before placing it on others. This can lead to empathic distress, sometimes called "compassion fatigue," which if left unchecked can lead to burnout. Burnout describes feelings of hopelessness, cynicism, detachment, isolation, irritability, low job satisfaction, and decreased effectiveness at work [20]. This is when the practice of self-compassion can give a healthier perspective and decrease the feelings of isolation and restore personal effectiveness in the role of clinician or caregiver. Buddhist psychologists caution that developing a compassion practice aimed only at others may be harmful without first training to develop a foundation of self-compassion [13]. Self-care is necessary for survival in all domains, whether medical, psychiatric, psychological, or social.

> **Box 43.2** Exercise in Combined Loving Kindness Meditation
>
> Take a moment to tune into your breathing, relaxing more with each out-breath. Imagine you are in the presence of someone you find loveable (a dear loved one, mentor, friend, or pet). Repeat these phrases (or your own):
>
> May you be happy, safe, and well.
>
> May you accept yourself lovingly just as you are in this moment.
>
> May you be free of emotional and physical pain.
>
> Allow yourself to connect with these wishes, and with any physical sensations that arise (e.g., warmth, openness, tenderness in your heart).
>
> Next, picture all of your loved ones together with you and repeat the same phrases toward them. Now visualize yourself among all your loved ones, repeating the phrases for yourself:
>
> May I be happy, safe, and well.
>
> May I accept myself lovingly, just as I am in this moment.
>
> May I be free of emotional and physical pain.
>
> If easier, imagine them saying this to you. Extend these wishes and phrases toward a neutral person or stranger, and then toward a person with whom you are experiencing mild difficulties.
>
> Lastly, expand the wishes toward all living beings: "May we all . . ." [22]

Community

If you want to go quickly, go alone. If you want to go far, go together.

African proverb

Defining Community

Defining community is not as straightforward as drawing a boundary around a neighborhood. Each person inside a community may define their inclusion boundaries differently. Communities are not a closed circle, but rather an overlapping Venn diagram of belonging and identification with many smaller groups. "Community" can include a partner, non-romantic cohabitants, children, animals, neighbors, friends, school, work, communities of faith, ethnic and racial groups, and communities of politically aligned people.

Wellness at Work

According to the Department of Labor and Statistics, Americans spend 8.59 hours per day at work. Attempts to study wellness interventions in the workplace are problematic. The majority of studies are observational and not sufficiently powered. Policy-makers struggle to contain epidemics of obesity, cardiovascular disease, and major depression, but without evidence for the most cost-effective measures.

A recent study published in *JAMA* conducted by Song and Baiker described a cluster-randomized trial involving 32,974 employees at a large US warehouse retail company. The study provided a wellness intervention with classes on nutrition, physical activity, and stress reduction and health prevention. Worksites with the wellness program had an 8.3 percentage point higher rate of employees who reported engaging in regular exercise and a 13.6 percentage point higher rate of employees who reported actively managing their weight, but there were no significant differences in other self-reported health and behaviors, clinical markers of health, healthcare spending or utilization, or absenteeism, tenure, or job performance after 18 months [23].

Here, the concept of wellness has been operationalized to mean maximizing the health of the workers to save on healthcare costs and increase work performance. This is a limited definition of wellness focusing on physically demonstrable health indicators and does not include psychological well-being. The study was not long enough to look at longevity among workers, such as retention at the same job.

Mindfulness at Work

Buddhist psychology and mindfulness meditation techniques are becoming accepted ways to cope with the stress and dysfunction of the office environment. In a meta-analysis of the effects of workplace mindfulness training using RCTs, results showed medium but definite positive effect sizes for mindfulness training decreasing stress, anxiety, and psychological distress, and increasing well-being but with less robust results for sleep. No conclusions could be drawn from pooled data for burnout due to mixed results, for depression due to publication bias, or for work performance due to insufficient data [24]. Mindfulness at work can involve time for breaks to meditate, use of apps, and group support meetings using Buddhist practices.

Modern American Tibetan-Buddhist psychologists add humor to classical mind-training techniques to help destress the culture of the office, including phrases such as "Work is a Mess" and "Welcome the Tyrant" for recognizing the power dynamics at work, and the pressures it puts on people that make them act in dysfunctional ways. These examples are from the Tibetan-rooted Shambhala tradition by Michael Carroll, called *Awake at Work* [25]. Lodro Rinzler, in *The Buddha Walks into the Office*, describes an even more contemporary approach with additional attitude-changing techniques [25].

Virtual Communities

Online communities that are unhealthy can have a seriously negative impact for young people being bullied, marginalized, or threatened. On a positive note, many people can connect to a community of like-minded or like-suffering people, who may not be part of their nearby physical community. Previously isolated people with rare diseases can now share information, advice, and get support from around the world via online communities [26]. For teens seeking support for being gay in an intolerant community, for depressed people not ready to speak to a practitioner, for someone in sobriety joining the recovery community, online interaction is a way to decrease isolation and make bonds around shared concerns. Though privacy concerns are still an issue, micro-communities form. Some examples are virtual communities for people with borderline personality; mothers who have lost a child to gun violence (Moms Demand Action for Gun Sense in America), formed after the Sandy Hook Elementary School shooting; Mothers Against Drunk Driving (MADD), and many groups for domestic violence survivors. This community of shared purpose and concerns is a valuable part of community, even if it can't be seen. Communities of faith also thrive online, connecting via push notifications to create a sense of connection, shared meaning, and decreased isolation.

> **Box 43.3** Exercise in Community Self-Assessment
>
> Whom do I consider part of my community?
>
> Where am I lacking in connection?
>
> Where am I over-connected or over-committed?
>
> If I am with a client or patient, how can I understand their community?
>
> Is there integration or rejection by the community?
>
> Is my community promoting or preventing my wellness?
>
> Where do I get the most support?
>
> Where do I need more support?
>
> Can I offer more to my immediate or global community?
>
> Is there balance between people and the environment?

Community wellness at a larger level occurs when social issues unite disparate parts of society. The "Indivisible" movement across cities in the USA aims to foster engagement in civil society and promote democracy. Only some states in the USA have a "right to shelter" law that protects homeless members of the community by funding sufficient shelter places. Only some countries have universal healthcare. Agencies like the United Nations try to connect countries into communities by promoting universal human rights, such as the Rights of the Child, Rights of Women, and a global code of Human Rights aimed at preventing persecution of minorities (whether based on ethnicity, race, gender, sexual orientation, or religion). This wellness intervention involves inviting a community to form around the idea of a universal humanity in all people, regardless of what geographical community or country they live in. Finally, the wellness of the planet united a global community across 185 countries when millions marched for the health of the planet on which we all live during the September 2019 Climate Strikes.

Conclusion

Compassion, connection, and community are powerful elements of wellness impacting the individual, and groups of people both small and large. Box 43.3 offers a brief exercise to evaluate "community" wellness.

References

1. E Seppala, T Rossomando, JR Doty. Social connection and compassion: important predictors of health and well-being. *Social Res* 2013; **80**(2): 411–430.

2. J Leaviss, L Uttley. Psychotherapeutic benefits of compassion-focused therapy: an early systematic review. *Psychol Med* 2015; **45**(5): 927–945.

3. R Walsh. Lifestyle and mental health. *Am Psychol* 2011; **66**(7): 579–592.

4. J Holt-Lunstad. Why social relationships are important for physical health: a systems approach to understanding and modifying risk and protection. *Annu Rev Psychol* 2018; **69**: 437–458.

5. D Siegel. Interpersonal connection, compassion, and well-being. In: J Loizzo, M Neale, E Wolf, eds., *Advances in Contemplative Psychotherapy: Accelerating Healing and Transformation*. New York, Routledge; 2017; 118–130.

6. D Buettner. *The Blue Zones of Happiness: Lessons from the World's Happiest People.* Washington, DC, National Geographic; 2017.

7. J Marchant. *Cure: A Journey into the Science of Mind over Body.* New York, Crown Publishers; 2016.

8. C Masi, H Chen, L Hawkley, J Cacioppo. A meta-analysis of interventions to reduce loneliness. *Pers Soc Psychol Rev* 2011; **15**(3): 219–266.

9. LM Cookingham, GL Ryan. The impact of social media on the sexual and social wellness of adolescents. *J Pediatr Adolesc Gynecol* 2015; **28**(1): 2–5.

10. SM Bögels, LM Emerson. The mindful family: a systemic approach to mindfulness, relational functioning, and somatic and mental health. *Curr Opin Psychol* 2019; **28**: 138–142.

11. B Uchino. Understanding the links between social support and physical health: a life-span perspective with emphasis on the separability of perceived and received support. *Perspect Psychol Sci* 2009; **4**(3): 236–255.

12. M Linehan. *Cognitive-Behavioral Treatment of Borderline Personality.* New York, Guilford Press; 1993.

13. E Shonin, W Van Gordon, A Compare, M Zangeneh, MD Griffiths. Buddhist-derived loving-kindness and compassion meditation for the treatment of psychopathology: a systematic review. *Mindfulness* 2014; **6**(5): 1161–1180.

14. KD Neff, CK Germer. A pilot study and randomized controlled trial of the mindful self-compassion program. *J Clin Psychol* 2013; **69**: 28–44.

15. U Zessin, O Dickhäuser, S Garbade. The relationship between self-compassion and well-being: a meta-analysis. *Appl Psychol Health Well Being* 2015; **7**(3): 340–364.

16. EM Sirois, DS Molnar, JK Hirsch. Self-compassion, stress, and coping in the context of chronic illness. *Self Identity* 2015; **14**(3): 334–347.

17. AM Friis, MH Johnson, RG Cutfield, NS Consedine. Kindness matters: a randomized controlled trial of a mindful self-compassion intervention improves depression, distress, and HbA1c among patients with diabetes. *Diabetes Care* 2016; **39**(11): 1963–1971.

18. E Inwood, M Ferrari. Mechanisms of change in the relationship between self-compassion, emotion regulation, and mental health: a systematic review. *Appl Psychol Health Well Being* 2018; **10**(2): 215–235.

19. JN Kirby, CL Tellegen, SR Steindl. A meta-analysis of compassion-based interventions: current state of knowledge and future directions. *Behav Ther* 2017; **48**(6): 778–792.

20. T Eriksson, L Germundsjö, E Åström, M Rönnlund. Mindful self-compassion training reduces stress and burnout symptoms among practicing psychologists: a randomized controlled trial of a brief web-based intervention. *Front Psychol* 2018; **9**: 2340.

21. P Gilbert, C Irons. Focused therapies and compassionate mind training for shame and self-attacking. In: P Gilbert, ed., *Compassion: Conceptualisations, Research and Use in Psychotherapy.* London, Routledge; 2005; 263–325.

22. P Chodron. *Awakening Loving-kindness.* Boulder, CO, Shambhala Publications; 2017.

23. Z Song, K Baicker. Effect of a workplace wellness program on employee health and economic outcomes: a randomized clinical trial. *JAMA* 2019; **321**(15): 1491–1501.

24. L Bartlett, A Martin, AL Neil, et al. A systematic review and meta-analysis of workplace mindfulness training randomized controlled trials. *J Occup Health Psychol* 2019; **24**(1): 108–126.

25. L Rinzler. *The Buddha Walks into the Office: A Guide to Livelihood for a New Generation.* Boulder, CO, Shambhala Publications; 2004.

26. X Zhu, RA Smith, RL Parrott. Living with a rare health condition: the influence of a support community and public stigma on communication, stress, and available support. *J Appl Commun Res* 2017; **45**(2): 179–198.

Wellness Interventions for Chronicity and Disability

Anna Klimowicz, Lorne Schussel,
and Waguih William IsHak

Introduction

According to the World Health Organization, chronic illnesses are responsible for 68 percent of global deaths, including more than 40 percent of premature deaths before the age of 70 [1]. In addition to psychological, social, and physical suffering caused by these conditions, the estimated economic losses for middle- and low-income countries in 2011–2025 are projected to be $7 trillion, which vastly outnumbers the annual $11.2 billion spent on implementing interventions aimed at reducing the chronic disease burden [1]. Given the personal, societal, and economic implications of chronic conditions, substantial research effort has been put into developing the best methods of care for the chronically ill population. Wellness medicine offers a unique perspective in advocating for positive well-being in addition to symptom alleviation. This chapter, drawing from evidence-based research and our own clinical experience, discusses how wellness can be fostered in the chronically ill by considering the biopsychosocial and spiritual approach. Additionally, we discuss the concept of demoralization – hopelessness as a result of a chronic illness – and the different approaches to combat it.

Psychological Considerations

Personal narratives of people affected by a chronic condition or disability are vastly heterogeneous: some might have been born with the condition (such as spina bifida, cerebral palsy, or cystic fibrosis), some may have had a traumatic event leading to a permanent loss of function (for example, a stroke or amputation), some may have experienced years of symptoms before being diagnosed (for example, people with multiple sclerosis [MS]), and some may have been surprised with a sudden devastating prognosis (such as brain cancer). There is a great diversity not only in the way people become chronically ill or disabled, but also in how they adapt to, cope with, and think about their condition. A serious, lasting, often progressive illness places substantial demand on the person's psyche – amid grief, loss, and existential uncertainty, the person needs to renegotiate their self-concept as well as their relatedness to others. In order to understand how to foster wellness in individuals living with disability or chronic illness, we must first address the psychological challenges that these conditions present.

Self-Concept

Incorporation of chronic illness into one's self-concept is a nonlinear process. When and how did the person learn about their diagnosis? What losses have they suffered due to their condition? What is their understanding of the illness and its prognosis? A young professional who was just diagnosed with terminal colon cancer after only a couple of episodes of rectal bleeding might not see herself as an ill person until her symptoms force her to resign from her job, or perhaps until she recognizes herself in other cancer patients she meets during chemotherapy sessions. Charmaz [2] identified four ways in which illness is defined: (1) having a crisis, (2) comparing self with sick people, (3) redefining feelings or behavior as symptoms, and (4) receiving test findings or medical pronouncements. During each of these experiences the patient may still challenge or otherwise renegotiate the diagnosis. For instance, a crisis might illuminate the illness severity but, once resolved, might challenge the permanence of the condition. The patient's relationship with their illness is thus fluid and periods of awareness and denial may be interwoven.

Disability

It is worth noting that not all patients with a functional impairment consider themselves disabled. Deafness is a commonly evoked example of an impairment that is recognized by able-bodied people as a disability but is often rejected as such by Deaf culture [3]. The proponents of Deaf culture may go so far as to reject cochlear implants in order to preserve their identity as a member of Deaf culture [3]. Even in conditions lacking such strong community identity, we increasingly hear phrases such as "differently abled" as opposed to "disabled." Such phrasing highlights the problem of ableism and cautions against making assumptions about a person's self-identification as disabled.

A factor at play in recognizing oneself as "disabled" is the visibility versus invisibility of the illness. In interviews with Gordon et al. [4], women affected by systemic lupus erythematosus (SLE) revealed that they initially did not consider themselves as disabled due to, for instance, not using a wheelchair, but as they came to terms with the permanence of their condition and impairments, they began to question their previous ideas about disability. Persons with visible medical conditions may struggle with stigma, discrimination, and being seen as disabled first, and as their own unique individuals second [5]. On the other hand, persons with an invisible illness (such as MS or SLE) may feel invalidated in their experience and need to justify their disability despite "looking healthy" (Figure 44.1). Such feelings of invalidation may lead to

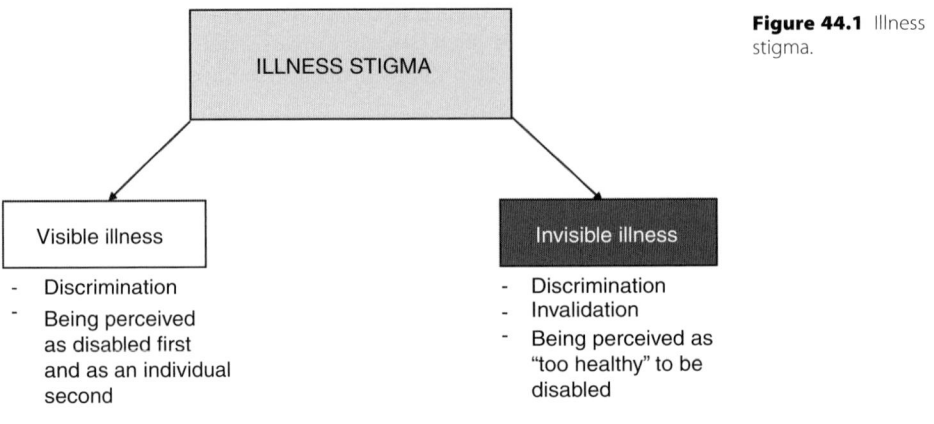

Figure 44.1 Illness stigma.

reluctance in utilizing accommodations such as reserved parking spots or disability payments [4]. Moreover, they may lead to loneliness and social isolation, and increased risk of suicidal ideation [6].

Independence

Living with a chronic condition comes with some degree of functional impairment. Abilities previously taken for granted, whether it is dressing oneself or going on a hike, may require adaptation or help from others. Loss of independence is a psychologically difficult situation to overcome, as it threatens the self-sufficiency we spend most of adulthood achieving. Gignac et al. [7] identified four main forms of adaptation to chronic illness and disability: (1) compensation, (2) efforts to optimize performance, (3) decisions to limit or forgo activities, and (4) utilization of help from others. They studied how each adaptation influences an individual's perception of independence. They found that reliance on others, especially for personal tasks such as hygiene, was most strongly associated with perceived loss of independence. It follows that, when possible, adaptations maximizing the person's ability to perform tasks themselves should be encouraged in order to foster subjective self-sufficiency. In instances when assistance from others is a necessity, retaining control over how and when the help occurs is important for the patient's sense of autonomy and dignity. Drawing from research on successful aging, wellness medicine would aim for "self-regulated dependency" [8], where control over receiving assistance becomes a positive part of coping with functional decline.

Fostering Wellness

In the previous section, we discussed the psychological impact of chronic illness and disability on an individual's identity. The renegotiation of self-concept in the light of an illness is clinically important, because the way a person sees themselves in relationship to their illness will affect how they relate to their wellness as well. Wellness medicine goes beyond the traditional allopathic model of medicine, which puts illness at the forefront – instead, it considers disease symptomatology as only one part of health. In a truly biopsychosocial and spiritual approach, wellness medicine aims to help people lead their best, most fulfilled lives. For persons living with long-lasting conditions requiring physical, psychological, and social adaptations, wellness medicine offers an approach that considers their illness in the greater context of their unique, individual lives. In this section, we will discuss the various wellness interventions according to the biopsychosocial and spiritual domains (Figure 44.2).

Biological Domain

In the accepted biopsychosocial model, physical symptoms are directly influenced by and in turn influence psychological and social well-being. Research has shown that persistent pain is related to increased psychological illness [9], while psychological well-being is a protective factor against pain [10]. Symptom alleviation through traditional medical methods as well as integrative medicine [11], psychology, and spirituality is one of the key components in approaching wellness in chronically ill populations. Additionally, care coordination to minimize confusion and illness burden is recommended.

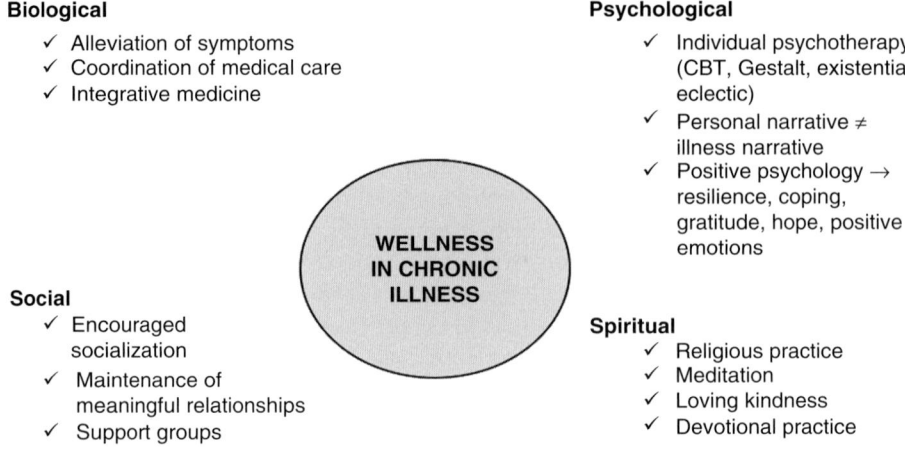

Biological
- ✓ Alleviation of symptoms
- ✓ Coordination of medical care
- ✓ Integrative medicine

Psychological
- ✓ Individual psychotherapy (CBT, Gestalt, existential, eclectic)
- ✓ Personal narrative ≠ illness narrative
- ✓ Positive psychology → resilience, coping, gratitude, hope, positive emotions

Social
- ✓ Encouraged socialization
- ✓ Maintenance of meaningful relationships
- ✓ Support groups

Spiritual
- ✓ Religious practice
- ✓ Meditation
- ✓ Loving kindness
- ✓ Devotional practice

WELLNESS IN CHRONIC ILLNESS

Figure 44.2 Wellness in chronic illness.

Psychological Domain

Personal Psychotherapy

Individual psychotherapy can be helpful in addressing the myriad psychological challenges that a chronic illness imposes on a self. Cognitive-behavioral therapy (CBT) is well validated in addressing maladaptive thought patterns such as perception of being a burden to others [12]. Existential psychotherapy explores the meaning that illness might bring into one's life, and aids in the understanding of the possibility of death [13]. Gestalt therapy brings awareness to one's feelings, beliefs, body sensations, reactions, and actions. By doing so, it reveals the person's inner conflicts, and aids in creating a healthy, congruent sense of self [13].

An important player in individual psychotherapy is personal narrative, i.e., the way a person construes her life experiences and interprets their impact on the different components of herself. In our clinical experience, for a chronically ill person the *illness* narrative might overtake their *personal* narrative. It can require a lot of psychological work and creativity to aid in deconstructing the illness from its dominant position in the person's sense of self. One of our patients, Jennifer, a 32-year-old female with chronic pelvic pain, engaged in excessive rumination over her symptoms, which she brought up regardless of the topic of the discussion. Her medical condition dominated all aspects of her life. Her therapist, Lorne Schussel, realized that traditional talk therapy – using the verbal/auditory pathway of communication – reached an impasse. He started bringing tarot cards to the sessions – thereby introducing a visual pathway – with the intention to evoke new themes in Jennifer's narrative. The archetypal imagery of the tarot cards aided in accessing the unconscious tropes in her life, ultimately helping her rebuild her *personal* narrative, of which the illness was only one part.

Positive Psychology

From a wellness perspective, positive psychology is a very suitable approach for the chronically ill and disabled populations, as it strongly focuses on *thriving*, as opposed to just *surviving*. It conceptualizes psychological well-being as the presence of positive psychological phenomena (happiness, joy, positive emotions, satisfaction, meaning, personal strengths and values, positive relationships, among others), rather than the absence of psychopathological symptoms. Positive psychology enlists and builds up an individual's internal resources to strengthen resilience, understood as the ability to flourish despite adversity, and to maximize positive psychological states. According to Fredrickson's broaden-and-build theory of positive emotions [14], positive emotions accumulate over time to increase a variety of favorable outcomes, such as increased satisfaction in life and resilience against adversity. The "broaden hypothesis" posits that positive emotions open up people's thinking, attention, and outlook, while the "build hypothesis" holds that positive emotions are cumulative over time [14]. There is a rich body of research on different methods of fostering positive emotions. Some examples include writing gratitude letters, practicing loving kindness, reliving positive experiences, and maintaining meaningful relationships.

For the chronically ill population, positive psychology brings not only mental health benefits but also improved physical health outcomes. Positive emotions such as curiosity and hope have a protective effect against respiratory tract infections, diabetes mellitus, or hypertension [15], while generally improved subjective well-being is associated with increased pain tolerance and stronger immune response [10].

Social Domain

Chronic illness can be an isolating experience. Whether it is canceling plans at the last minute due to a health crisis, giving up on athletic activities, not performing one's share of household tasks, or finding it difficult to relate to healthy friends, chronic conditions put a strain on the social lives of those affected by them. Socialization and maintenance of meaningful relationships with family, friends, coworkers, religious figures, etc. not only provides emotional and practical support when needed, but also helps retain and grow healthy parts of one's self.

For chronically ill patients, another source of social connection can be patient support groups. Such groups provide a unique community of individuals living a shared experience. One of us, Lorne Schussel, led support groups for patients with Parkinson's disease and other neurodegenerative diseases. Some of the positives of the support group mentioned by his participants were: a sense of understanding by others; a safe place to express emotions; increased agency and confidence; and development of self-compassion. Attending the group also strengthened participants' relationships with their loved ones. Some individuals chose to bring their loved one to the sessions, thereby increasing trust between them and allowing the loved one to gain a better understanding of the illness. On the other hand, some participants who chose to come alone stated that the group provided an additional emotional outlet for them, thereby decreasing their need to "burden" their loved ones with psychological struggles.

There are many ways to structure a support group, but some components that Schussel found helpful are: (1) meditation practice, such as loving kindness (he used the best self visualization method [16] described below); (2) emotional processing; (3) creation of a positive image of self; (4) psychoeducation; and (5) goal-setting. While each of these components is helpful on their own, their effectiveness is maximized when used as a composite practice. For example, loving kindness and creation of a positive image of self support the difficult work of emotional processing by increasing self-compassion and mobilizing resilience. Without these two positive psychology components, discussing emotional struggles and vulnerabilities would be much more challenging. Similarly, psychoeducation helps individuals gain confidence in their decision-making, which in turn potentiates their agency in goal-setting.

Although participants in his group were reluctant to provide any negative feedback, some researchers have found that excessive rumination over symptoms and medical advice provided by fellow patients can be counterproductive and provide a negative experience for the participants [17].

Spiritual Domain

Spirituality is now commonly recognized as the fourth pillar in the biopsychosocial approach to health. There is a robust and growing body of research demonstrating spirituality as a protective factor against mental illness, dementia, cardiovascular disease, hypertension, cerebrovascular events, and other health adversities [18]. For the chronically ill and disabled, who face both physical and psychological challenges, spirituality plays an important role in fostering wellness. There are many definitions of spirituality, but it may be broadly understood as a connection to something greater than oneself, which can be achieved through means such as religion, meditation, and mind–body or devotional practices. Here we will describe an example of a mind–body practice called the Best Self Visualization Method used in Schussel's support group for Parkinson's patients.

The Best Self Visualization Method

The Best Self Visualization Method (BSM) is a composite mind–body and meditation practice, partially drawn from the Buddhist tradition of loving kindness as well as *vedic* traditions of yogic breathing [16]. It comprises the following elements: (1) deep breathing (*pranayama*), (2) sound entrainment, (3) visualization of a best self, and (4) sending and receiving loving kindness [16]. Deep breathing and sound entrainment (with the use of a Tibetan singing bowl) prime the visualization aspect by helping induce a state of deep relaxation. During the visualization of a best self, participants form a positive self-image, drawing on their inner resilience and interpersonal and functional coping. The loving kindness component consists of sending and receiving love from the best self, the support group, and the world. For patients with somatic symptoms such as tremors in Parkinson's disease, the BSM allows a non-judgmental observation of symptoms in a state of relaxation, supported by self-compassion and the best self. Receiving loving kindness from the support group and the world further strengthens the positive image of self, who now accepts the symptoms in a compassionate, non-judgmental way. Notably, several patients remarked that the practice not only helped them cope with the symptoms, but also attenuated their tremors, possibly through the reduction of anxiety.

Demoralization

Psychiatrists are often consulted on medical and surgical wards to evaluate possible depression in patients who, in the face of an illness or a life-altering medical event, appear despondent, hopeless, withdrawn, and sometimes even lose the will to live. Upon a thorough psychiatric evaluation, what may transpire is that these patients had normative functioning prior to their illness, but over the course of their disease they developed a sense of futility and helplessness. However, when the circumstances of their health adversity change for the better, they return to their baseline functioning. The consulting psychiatrist may thus determine that such a patient is not depressed, but rather is *demoralized.*

Background

Demoralization emerged in the medical literature in the 1970s, when the psychiatrist Jerome Frank used the term to describe a state of mind in which patients with a psychiatric issue are most likely to seek psychotherapy [19]. In his observation, psychiatric patients rarely want help unless they are to some extent demoralized, i.e., exhibit "persistent failure to cope with internally or externally induced stresses" that they or others around them expect them to be able to manage [19]. It is this discrepancy between stress and coping reserves that, according to Frank, leads individuals to feel isolated and impotent, with a damaged self-esteem and a growing sense of life's meaninglessness [19]. There might be a sense of futility, especially in patients whose conditions are not likely to improve, as in a progressive or terminal disease. Given that chronic medical illness or a serious medical event are what we would commonly regard as overwhelming life stressors, it comes as no surprise that, over time, Frank's insights evolved to encompass individuals suffering from physical illnesses. Today's academic literature focuses on demoralization as related to individuals stricken by a medical condition. A recent systematic literature review [20] revealed that 13–18 percent of cancer patients suffer from demoralization.

Differential Diagnosis

Demoralization and depression share many potential clinical characteristics: sad mood, isolation, possible sleep and appetite disturbances, lack of energy, hopelessness, suicidal thinking. How can one differentiate between depression and demoralization? The key difference is that the former exhibits persistent anhedonia, while in the latter the patient can still experience joy and pleasure if some of the negative effects of his or her medical conditions are lifted [21] – for example, a patient with chronic pain achieves better pain control or a patient with MS enjoys a symptom-free day. In short, a person's demoralized state is tightly linked to their adversity, while depression is persistent regardless of circumstances. Another differential diagnosis is adjustment disorder, which shares with demoralization the difficulty in coping with the new situation. While it may indeed be the correct diagnosis in some patients with chronic illness, demoralization needs to be considered as a separate clinical possibility, given that it may have more severe manifestations such as suicidality. Lastly, medical etiologies of depressive symptoms always need to be ruled out, especially in patients with underlying chronic illness. Conditions such as hypothyroidism, Addison's disease, Cushing disease, neurodegenerative disorders, and nutritional deficiencies are just some of many examples of medically driven symptoms of depression.

Diagnosis

There is an ongoing debate about classifying demoralization as a psychiatric disorder [22]. Currently, demoralization is considered a clinically significant but non-pathological state. Medical practitioners might be more likely to learn about, recognize, and be able to treat a clinical state that has been given a diagnostic label. On the other hand, increased education among clinical staff can accomplish the same goal without the need to pathologize what might be a normative experience. More recently, Kissane et al. [23] advocated for the addition of demoralization as a specifier to the diagnosis of adjustment disorder or major depressive disorder, demonstrating through empirical studies that clinicians perceive such an addition as valuable in deepening their understanding of the condition, developing a plan of care, and communicating to other professionals about continuity of care.

Importance

Serious helplessness can dangerously lead to hopelessness – a powerful mediator of suicidality, as Beck famously showed [24]. A recent study on suicidal ideation in cancer patients found that demoralization was a stronger influencer of suicidal thinking compared to depression [25]. Given its clinical severity, recognizing early signs of demoralization is important for all clinicians involved in the patient's care.

Combating Demoralization

Griffith and Gaby [21], in their seminal paper "Brief psychotherapy at bedside: countering demoralization from medical illness," posit that demoralization is best fought with either (1) ameliorating physical or emotional stressors, or (2) strengthening a patient's resilience to stress. The use of methods mentioned in the previous section on fostering wellness is the backbone for improving overall well-being of demoralized patients. Additionally, elements of bedside psychotherapy as well as dignity therapy [26] are helpful in combating demoralization.

Griffith and Gaby [21] broke down demoralization into seven distinct existential components, which may guide the clinician's dialog with the patient toward resilience, strengths, and assertiveness. The components are: (1) coherence versus confusion (how does the patient make sense of their situation?); (2) communion versus isolation (who can the patient confide in?); (3) hope versus despair (what are the patient's sources of hope?); (4) purpose versus meaninglessness (what keeps the patient going?); (5) agency versus helplessness (what are the patient's priorities? What are some choices and decisions that the patient can make?); (6) courage versus cowardice (what are some examples of a time when the patient wanted to give up but didn't?); and (7) gratitude versus resentment (what is the patient grateful for?). The questions in parentheses are some examples that Griffith and Gaby provide that can be asked of the patient directly during bedside psychotherapy.

Chochinov's dignity therapy was studied in a terminally ill population and shown to increase sense of dignity, improve quality of life, increase spiritual well-being, and change how the family sees and appreciates the sick loved one [26]. Some questions guiding the therapy are: When did you feel most alive? What are your most important accomplishments, and what do you feel most proud of? What are your hopes and dreams for your loved ones? Are there words or perhaps even instructions that you would like to offer your family to help prepare them for the future? Similarly to Griffith's bedside psychotherapy, dignity therapy focuses on what is important in the patient's life, and additionally it gives the chance to reflect on how the patient might want to be remembered. This type of therapy may be especially well suited for patients with demoralization who suffer from a terminal illness.

Summary

- Consider the patient's self-concept: What is their understanding of their illness? Do they view themselves as ill/disabled and how does that affect their identity?
- Consider visible versus invisible illness: Does the patient struggle with social stigma and/or invalidation of their disability?

- Maximize the patient's agency by allowing them "self-regulated dependency."
- Aim for alleviation of physical symptoms, especially pain.
- Utilize psychotherapy to correct maladaptive cognition, aid in finding meaning, and strengthen coping and resilience.
- Peruse positive psychology techniques to build up positive emotions. According to the broaden-and-build theory, they accumulate over time to effectuate favorable psychological and physical outcomes.
- Encourage socialization and support groups.
- Foster spiritual practices; encourage a meditation practice such as loving kindness to increase self-compassion.
- Consider demoralization in an individual with a chronic or terminal illness who appears despondent, hopeless, and withdrawn, but whose mood improves when disease burden is alleviated.
- Utilize wellness medicine methods, in addition to bedside and dignity therapies for a demoralized patient.

References

1. World Health Organization. *Global Status Report on Noncommunicable Diseases 2014.* Washington, DC, World Health Organization; 2014.

2. K Charmaz. Experiencing chronic illness. In: GL Albrecht, R Fitzpatrick, SC Scrimshaw, eds., *Handbook of Social Studies in Health and Medicine.* New York, Sage; 2000; 277–292.

3. BP Tucker. Deaf culture, cochlear implants, and elective disability. *Hastings Center Rep* 1998; **28**(4): 6–14.

4. PA Gordon, D Feldman, R Crose. The meaning of disability: how women with chronic illness view their experiences. *J Rehabil* 1998; **64**(3): 5.

5. H Livneh, RF Antonak. Psychosocial adaptation to chronic illness and disability: a primer for counselors. *J Counsel Dev* 2005; **83**(1): 12–20.

6. CL Pederson, K Gorman-Ezell, G Hochstetler-Mayer. Invisible illness increases risk of suicidal ideation: the role of social workers in preventing suicide. *Health Soc Work* 2017; **42**(3): 183–186.

7. MA Gignac, C Cott, EM Badley. Adaptation to chronic illness and disability and its relationship to perceptions of independence and dependence. *J Gerontol B Psychol Sci Soc Sci* 2000; **55**(6): P362–P372.

8. MM Baltes, LL Carstensen. The process of successful ageing. *Ageing Soc* 1996; **16**(4): 397–422.

9. O Gureje, M Von Korff, GE Simon, R Gater. Persistent pain and well-being: a World Health Organization study in primary care. *JAMA* 1998; **280**(2): 147–151.

10. RT Howell, ML Kern, S Lyubomirsky. Health benefits: meta-analytically determining the impact of well-being on objective health outcomes. *Health Psychol Rev* 2007; **1**(1): 83–136.

11. JA Dusek, M Finch, G Plotnikoff, L Knutson. The impact of integrative medicine on pain management in a tertiary care hospital. *J Patient Saf* 2010; **6**(1): 48–51.

12. B Rybarczyk, D Gallagher-Thompson, J Rodman, et al. Applying cognitive-behavioral psychotherapy to the chronically ill elderly: treatment issues and case illustration. *Int Psychogeriatr* 1992; **4**(1): 127–140.

13. SA Imes, PR Clance, AT Gailis, E Atkeson. Mind's response to the body's betrayal: Gestalt/existential therapy for clients with chronic or life-threatening illnesses. *J Clin Psychol* 2002; **58**(11): 1361–1373.

14. BL Fredrickson, MA Cohn, KA Coffey, J Pek, SM Finkel. Open hearts build lives: positive emotions, induced through loving-kindness meditation, build consequential personal resources. *J Pers Soc Psychol* 2008; **95**(5): 1045.

15. LS Richman, L Kubzansky, J Maselko, et al. Positive emotion and health: going beyond the negative. *Health Psychol* 2005; **24** (4): 422.

16. L Schussel. *The Best Self Visualization Method: Clinical Implications and Physiological Correlates.* 2018. Doctoral dissertation, Columbia University.

17. KA Brennan, AM Creaven. Living with invisible illness: social support experiences of individuals with systemic lupus erythematosus. *Qual Life Res* 2016; **25**(5): 1227–1235.

18. HG Koenig. Religion, spirituality, and health: The research and clinical implications. *ISRN Psychiatry* 2012. DOI:10.5402/2012/278730.

19. JD Frank. Psychotherapy: the restoration of morale. *Am J Psychiatry* 1974; **131**(3): 271–274.

20. S Robinson, DW Kissane, J Brooker, S Burney. A systematic review of the demoralization syndrome in individuals with progressive disease and cancer: a decade of research. *J Pain Symptom Manage* 2015; **49**(3): 595–610.

21. JL Griffith, L Gaby. Brief psychotherapy at the bedside: countering demoralization from medical illness. *Psychosomatics* 2005; **46**(2): 109–116.

22. DW Kissane, DM Clarke, AF Street. Demoralization syndrome: a relevant psychiatric diagnosis for palliative care. *J Palliat Care* 2001; **17**(1): 12.

23. DW Kissane, I Bobevski, P Gaitanis, et al. Exploratory examination of the utility of demoralization as a diagnostic specifier for adjustment disorder and major depression. *Gen Hosp Psychiatr* 2017; **46**: 20–24.

24. AT Beck. Hopelessness as a predictor of eventual suicide. *Ann NY Acad Sci* 1986; **487**(1): 90–96.

25. CK Fang, MC Chang, PJ Chen, et al. A correlational study of suicidal ideation with psychological distress, depression, and demoralization in patients with cancer. *Support Care Cancer* 2014; **22**(12): 3165–3174.

26. HM Chochinov, LJ Kristjanson, W Breitbart, et al. Effect of dignity therapy on distress and end-of-life experience in terminally ill patients: a randomised controlled trial. *Lancet Oncol* 2011; **12**(8): 753–762.

Chapter

45

Work, Love, Play, and Joie de Vivre

Nicole Van Groningen, Waguih William IsHak, Shaina Ganjian, Michael Ong, and Wendelin Slusser

Introduction

In conceptualizing lifestyle approaches to promote health and well-being, most attention is paid toward physical rituals, including physical activity, dietary modification, and cessation of drugs and alcohol. Less discussed are the fundamental aspects of work, play, and love that have the potential to promote – or erode – overall health and wellness. These factors may, in certain cases, play an even more profound role in wellness than traditional physical practices. "Joie de vivre" is a term used to describe overall enjoyment of life, and in a sense, encompasses all three domains.

Work

Stress in the workplace is alarmingly prevalent in the USA. According to the American Psychological Association's Annual Stress in America Survey, two-thirds of all adults report that money and work are significant stressors [1]. The survey also found that the youngest working generation, Millennials, report the highest level of stress, and continue to report higher stress levels year after year. This finding suggests that workplace stress may continue to grow. Stress is also associated with over 70 percent regularly experiencing psychological and physical symptoms, and 54 percent reporting fighting with people close to them (http://safetymanagement.eku.edu/resour ces/infographics/work-related-stress-on-employees-health)

Current trends in employment conditions are likely contributing to this phenomenon. Employees are increasingly asked to work beyond their usual hours to meet tight deadlines and targets. Furthermore, rapid technological advancement has changed the nature of many jobs, making many tasks more automated and less flexible. This has given rise to a culture of short-term contracting or outsourcing, which can lead to feelings of job insecurity [2]. Furthermore, everyday risks like driving to work or heat waves are underestimated and less common risks not easily controlled by individuals are often overrated, like airline accidents or terrorism.

In this context, prioritizing occupational well-being is an increasingly important focus of efforts to enhance health and wellness. Occupational wellness refers to the ability to optimize the balance between work and personal life, reduce and prevent stress, and strive for satisfaction and meaning in life through working [3]. Indeed, although an abundance of evidence suggests work can be a major contributor to overall stress, a satisfying work life can also enhance wellness in a meaningful way.

Work offers individuals the opportunity to pursue economic security and financial well-being, become productive in their industry, utilize talents and develop skills, pursue their interests, connect with colleagues, and develop an identity in their field of work [3]. Work typically provides the most natural avenue through which humans strive for growth and self-actualization, which Maslow has identified as a fundamental human tendency [4]. Furthermore, work has the potential to challenge our senses, skills, and interests, frequently absorbing us in a state of consciousness that psychologist Mihaly Csikszentmihalyi calls "flow," in which one loses awareness of self and time while being highly engaged in a task [5].

Most major models of wellness emphasize the importance of occupational or workplace wellness:

- In the Wheel of Wellness model described by Sweeney and Witmer, "Work and Leisure" is the third life-task, and has the capacity to significantly influence psychological well-being [6].
- The National Wellness Institute's Six Dimensions of Wellness model includes occupational wellness as one of the six dimensions, and holds that work can provide personal satisfaction and enrichment [7].
- In the Eight Dimensions of Wellness model described by Swarbick, occupational wellness is included as one of the eight dimensions. The model also includes related concepts of intellectual and financial wellness [8].
- Based at the Centers for Disease Control and Prevention, the National Institute for Occupational Safety and Health has developed the Total Worker Health® model to advance the well-being of workers. A Total Worker Health approach is defined as policies, programs, and practices that integrate protection from work-related safety and health hazards with promotion of injury- and illness-prevention efforts to advance worker well-being (www.cdc.gov/niosh/docs/2017–112/pdfs/2017_112.pdf).

Numerous studies have explored the relationship between job or career satisfaction and health outcomes. Job satisfaction has been consistently shown to be correlated with multiple mental health measures, including burnout, depression, anxiety, and self-esteem [2]. There is also evidence that one's satisfaction with work life is linked with physical health. In a study of individuals from the National Longitudinal Survey of Youth 1979 Cohort, those with low levels of job satisfaction reported generally poorer physical health by age 40, and more commonly reported physical ailments such as back pain and frequent colds [9]. Job satisfaction has also been modestly inversely correlated with cardiovascular disease and musculoskeletal disorders [2].

Many jobs carry significant risks to workers. Job injuries are common in many settings. Increasing evidence links harmful or difficult working conditions to increased risks for cancer, heart disease, diabetes, depression, and other conditions. Obesity, tobacco use, and other substance-use disorders are more prevalent in certain industries and occupations than others, linking job demands and job environments with unhealthy behaviors and practices.

Given the significant association between job satisfaction and health, we must recognize job satisfaction as a central component of occupational wellness. Several instruments to measure job satisfaction have been developed in the research setting, but have not been widely deployed in clinical environments. However, the National Wellness Institute's wellness model proposes a broad framework for job satisfaction by offering two key tenets of a satisfying work life:

1. It is better to choose a career that is consistent with our personal values, interests, and beliefs than to select one that is unrewarding to us.
2. It is better to develop functional, transferable skills through structured involvement opportunities than to remain inactive and uninvolved.

More specifically, certain career aspects have been tied to increased job satisfaction [3, 10]. These are listed in Table 45.1.

Because of the increasing popularity of workplace wellness programs, a brief discussion of these programs and their potential impact is warranted. Although such programs have been widely deployed in a variety of industries, their effect on overall employee wellness remains unclear. This may be because workplace wellness programs are incredibly heterogeneous in their structure, focus, and scope. Some wellness programs have been shown to increase job satisfaction and decrease absenteeism [11], but the initial hope that they would cut organizational healthcare costs and improve physical health of employees, in objective terms, has not been proven. In fact, some data suggest that certain programs may inadvertently lead to worsening of some biometric measurements while trying to improve others, and may even lead to lower perceived well-being [12]. Therefore, to promote wellness at work, the focus should be on finding, modifying, or creating a role that has elements critical to job satisfaction. Working on policies and an environment that promote health and well-being would be as important, such as flexibility in work schedules and making the healthy choice the easy choice. Even the best workplace wellness program is unlikely to counteract low occupational well-being due to low job satisfaction.

Love

Although the health and wellness benefits of loving relationships are often overlooked in assessing overall health, the role that love plays in mental, emotional, and physical well-being is often even more significant than more commonly considered physical factors, such as diet and substance-use. The feeling of being loved and valued by others is the foundation

Table 45.1 Elements of job satisfaction

Element	Examples
Autonomy	• Ability to work independently • Sense of control over one's environment and assignments
Content	• Work is considered interesting • Role is clear
Communication	• Professional relationships • Clear feedback
Financial reward	• High income
Growth	• Clear advancement and promotion opportunities
Organization	• High level of perceived organizational support • Job security
Social	• Fulfilling relationships with coworkers and managers • Holding a valued social position at work

of social support, which has been repeatedly correlated with decreased morbidity and mortality through changes in cardiovascular, neuroendocrine, and immune function [13]. In fact, social well-being is defined by the Gallup Purdue Index as: having strong and supportive relationships and love in your life. In terms of health, poor social well-being is equivalent to smoking 15 cigarettes a day [14].

The bulk of the research on the importance of loving relationships has focused on romantic love. Marriage, in particular, has been consistently associated with improved physical health, mental health, and longevity. The most striking findings include:

- Marriage is associated with a decreased rate of heart attacks for both men and women [15], and married people are more likely to survive a heart attack.
- Married people are more likely to survive coronary artery bypass grafting in the long term [16].
- Marriage is an independent prognostic factor for survival in pancreatic cancer [17].
- Marriage is associated with lower rates of mental illness [18].
- Married people have lower all-cause mortality [19].

It is tempting to question whether healthy people are more likely to get married, and that this may be the reason behind favorable health outcomes in married couples. However, there is strong evidence that true causal pathways exist in the relationship between marriage and health outcomes [18]:

- Married couples support health-promoting behaviors in their partners, including smoking cessation and decreased alcohol use. There is also evidence that married people tend to keep regular doctor's appointments and follow doctor's recommendations more often than single people.
- The combined incomes of married individuals may lead to improved financial well-being, which is strongly associated with health and longevity.
- Marriage provides an intimate, fulfilling relationship which may directly stimulate biological health, particularly through neuroendocrine and immunological mechanisms. This appears to be largely driven by decreased levels of cortisol [18, 19].

An important caveat in discussing the impact of marriage on wellness is that the benefits disappear in the setting of low marriage quality. In fact, marital strain can predict the onset of anxiety, depression, and substance disorders, each of which has a well-described negative impact on health outcomes [20]. Furthermore, the relationship between marital partnerships and biological changes in cardiovascular, neuroendocrine, and immune functioning is bidirectional, and individuals who report low satisfaction in their marriages have unfavorable effects on these systems [19].

In addition to marriage and romantic love, there is also abundant data to suggest that other meaningful relationships – with friends, family members, or colleagues – have a substantial impact on well-being. In a meta-analysis, those who had strong and satisfying relationships had a 50 percent increase in odds of survival compared to those with insufficient, weak, or inadequate relationships. When multidimensional assessments of social relationships were considered, the odds of mortality increased by 91 percent among the socially isolated [14]. This effect size rivals that of smoking cessation, and far exceeds that of obesity prevention and physical activity. Several studies have explored potential causal pathways for this dramatic effect, and have found that social isolation has been tied to inflammation, hypertension, abdominal obesity, and overall obesity across various stages of life [21]. Furthermore, in a study published by McClintock et al., greater mobility predicted well-being and being alive in the next five years, while poor mental health (loneliness), sensory function (hearing), and social engagement, and having a broken bone any time after age 45, were all strong markers for future health problems and death in the next five years regardless of diagnoses, such as only having obesity as a diagnosis [22].

In the same way that marriage quality impacts the direction of the potential health impact, the quality of non-romantic relationships appears to be more significant than the quantity of relationships. Components of high-quality, unstrained relationships include warmth and intimacy, reliability, mutual understanding, feelings of being cared for and valued, lack of criticism, and ability to have fun shared experiences [21].

Play

Though play is an integral aspect of healthy childhood development, it also has a role in well-being in adulthood. For instance, playing tag provides a positive feedback loop for fleeing and is suggested by neuroscientists to reward the primitive part of the brain located in the limbic system. The study of adult playfulness has not historically been a focus of interest in psychological research, but in the last two decades this has changed, likely due to the rise of positive psychology. There are two major tenets of play. First, it is pursued for the purpose of entertainment and enjoyment; and second, it is intrinsically motivated and voluntary, without any external coercion.

For our purposes, "play" can also be loosely equated with the broader concept of leisure, which has been defined as engagement in pleasurable activities that individuals engage in voluntarily when they are free from the demands of work or other responsibilities [23]. Certain play or leisure activities have been particularly associated with improved health outcomes. For example:

- Leisure-time physical activity has been shown to decrease mortality and reduce risk of chronic diseases [24].
- Spending time in nature may have a positive effect on wellness via multiple pathways, including stress reduction [25].
- Laughter is associated with improved short-term cardiovascular function, decreased cortisol levels, higher tolerance for pain, as well as increased quality of life, well-being, and decreased stress [26].
- Vacation and travel appear to be associated with a broad range of health benefits, and may even be associated with decreased mortality [27, 28].
- Certain games have been tied to improved cognitive function [29].
- Engaging in social activities or social relationships has been tied to longevity [14].

In addition to specific benefits tied to certain leisure activities, there is strong evidence that supports a link between wellness and engagement in leisure activities as a whole. For example, adults who rate themselves highly on subjective measures of playfulness tend to have increased well-being and life satisfaction [30]. In addition, individuals who engage in more frequent leisure activities, of any variety, have better psychological and physical functioning [23]. Specific health benefits associated with play and leisure include:

- increased positive affect, increased life satisfaction and engagement, and more social support;
- less depression and negative affect;

Table 45.2 Types of playfulness

Type of playfulness	Description
Other-directed	• Enjoyment of playing with others • Using playfulness to make social relations more interesting and/or loosen up tense situations
Lighthearted	• Seeing life as a game • Not worrying about future consequences of one's behavior • A propensity to improvise
Intellectual	• Cognitive-oriented play • Problem-solving • Playing with words
Whimsical	• Finding amusement in ordinary events • Making light of grotesque or strange situations

- lower blood pressure, waist circumference, and BMI; and
- better perceived physical function.

Furthermore, engaging in leisure activities also likely plays an important "buffer" role in negative psychological impact of stress, and makes it easier for individuals to cope with negative experiences. It is important to acknowledge that more frequent engagement in leisure activities is associated with higher socioeconomic status, which is in turn associated with improved health metrics and outcomes; however, even after controlling for these factors, the significant correlation between engagement in enjoyable activities and the above health benefits persists [23].

Obviously, play and leisure should be tailored to individual preferences and personality types. An activity that one individual finds exciting and pleasurable may be perceived by another as torture. One model of playfulness proposes that playfulness takes the form of four distinct types, and that one's propensity to engage in certain types of playfulness is related to unique personality traits. These are listed in Table 45.2 [31].

It also possible for individuals to enhance the gratification and enjoyment associated with play and leisure activities. In the well-being model put forward by Deyell Hood and Carruthers, leisure can be enhanced by prioritizing the following [32]:

- *Savoring leisure* refers to paying attention to positive aspects and emotions associated with leisure, and purposefully seeking leisure experiences that lead to those emotions.
- *Authentic leisure* refers to selecting leisure activities that are reflective of essential aspects of self.
- *Leisure gratifications* are defined as experiences that are optimally challenging and engaging, and lead to sustained personal effort and commitment, which in turn results in personal development.
- *Mindful leisure* is an experience that involves attention to the entirety of the current situation and a simultaneous disengagement from other life concerns.
- *Virtuous leisure* refers to the capacity to engage in leisure experiences that develop personal strengths, interests, and abilities in the service of something larger than oneself.

Joie de Vivre

"Joie de vivre" is a French term often used in English to express an overall enjoyment of life. It refers to the joy associated with virtually any human activity.

Findings from the English Longitudinal Study of Ageing found sustained enjoyment of life has been associated with increased longevity [33]. Although greater enjoyment of life is also associated with greater wealth and education, being married, and being in paid employment, all of which have established links with survival, greater enjoyment of life was still associated with a 28 percent lower risk of death even after these factors, as well as depression and health behaviors, were accounted for [34]. Another analysis of the same cohort found older adults with high levels of life enjoyment are relatively resistant to functional decline in terms of activities of daily living and gait speed [35]. In a different study, healthy individuals with higher reported levels of life satisfaction were found to have lower rates of coronary heart disease relative to those with lower life satisfaction [36].

Enjoyment of life is tightly correlated with positive affect, as well as related personality traits such as optimism and cheerfulness. The broader concept that encompasses these related constructs, positive psychological well-being, has also been associated with decreased mortality. A meta-analysis revealed that positive psychological well-being is associated with decreased mortality in both healthy and diseased populations, including those with cardiovascular disease, renal disease, and HIV. Importantly, the effect was independent of negative affect states, indicating that the favorable impact of positive psychological well-being does not merely reflect the absence of negative states, such as depression, which have been repeatedly linked to poor health outcomes [37].

Multiple pathways by which enjoyment of life and related positive psychological states lead to improved subjective and objective measures of health have been proposed. Individuals with positive psychological states tend to engage in more positive health behaviors, such as regular exercise and abstinence from drugs and alcohol. In addition, positive psychological states are inversely correlated with incidence of sleep problems such as insomnia, which has been linked to multiple health problems. Thus, at least part of the beneficial effect is likely indirect. However, there is also evidence to support a direct biological effect, particularly with regard to neuroendocrine, cardiovascular, and immunologic function [38]. Key associations include:

- Individuals with high reported levels of positive affect, happiness, and life satisfaction tend to have lower levels of cortisol throughout the day.
- Positive affect is associated with multiple positive cardiovascular metrics, including decreased blood pressure, high heart rate variability, and rapid recovery of elevated blood pressure and heart rate after a stressful event.
- Positive affect is associated with increased cellular immune competence, including heightened antibody responses.

Many factors contribute to a sense of one's enjoyment of life, and are clearly variable according to individual differences. Still, certain elements appear to be consistently linked to increased life enjoyment and life satisfaction, including [34]:

- self-actualization [39]
- meaningful social relationships
- satisfying sexual activity [40]
- religion and spirituality

- job and career satisfaction
- physical well-being and energy.

The importance of life satisfaction and enjoyment, and their critical role in overall subjective well-being, has become a focus of public health professionals. Recently, multiple countries have designed social policy efforts to promote subjective and psychological well-being [41].

To conclude, here are 10 suggestions on how to promote work, love, play, and joie de vivre:

1. Work: organize your tasks and goals.
2. Love: keep up with friends/family weekly.
3. Play: plan daily, weekly, monthly fun activities.
4. Work: enjoy lunch outside with a friend.
5. Love: spend time with loved ones with no distractions.
6. Play: watch comedy, sports, movies.
7. Work: focus on the positives.
8. Love: express gratitude daily.
9. Play: play cards, music, or make art.
10. Joie de vivre: completely focus on the joy of the moment.

References

1. American Psychological Association. Stress in America: the state of our nation. Stress in America Survey. 2018. www.apa.org/news/press/releases/stress (accessed March 1, 2020).

2. EB Faragher, M Cass, CL Cooper. The relationship between job satisfaction and health: a meta-analysis. *Occup Environ Med* 2005; **62**(2): 105–112.

3. JE Myers, TJ Sweeney, JM Witmer. The Wheel of Wellness counseling for wellness: a holistic model for treatment planning. *J Couns Dev* 2000; **78**(3), 251–266.

4. BA Maslow. A theory of human motivation. *Psychol Rev* 1943; **50**(4), 370–396.

5. M Csikszentmihalyi. *Flow and the Foundations of Positive Psychology.* Basel, Springer Nature Switzerland AG; 2014.

6. TJ Sweeney, JM Witmer. Beyond social interest: striving towards optimum health and wellness. *Individ Psychol* 1991; **47**(4), 527–540.

7. B Hettler. The Six Dimensions of Wellness model. www.nationalwellness.org/pdf/Six DimensionsFactSheet.pdf (accessed March 1, 2020).

8. M Swarbrick. A wellness approach. *Psychiatr Rehabil J* 2006; **29**(4): 311–314.

9. J Dirlam, H Zheng. Job satisfaction developmental trajectories and health: a life course perspective. *Soc Sci Med* 2017; **78**: 95–103.

10. A Sousa-Poza, AA Sousa-Poza. Well-being at work: a cross-national analysis of the levels and determinants of job satisfaction. *J Socio Econ* 2000; **29**(6): 517–538.

11. KM Parks, LA Steelman. Organizational wellness programs: a meta-analysis. *J Occup Health Psychol* 2008; **13**(1): 58–68.

12. The Illinois Workplace Wellness Study [Internet]. 2018. www.nber.org/workplace wellness (accessed March 1, 2020).

13. BN Uchino. Social support and health: a review of physiological processes potentially underlying links to disease outcomes. *J Behav Med* 2006; **29**(4): 377–387.

14. J Holt-Lunstad, TB Smith, JB Layton. Social relationships and mortality risk: a meta-analytic review. *PLoS Medicine* 2010; 7(7): e1000316.

15. A Lammintausta, JK Airaksinen, P Immonen-Räihä, et al. Prognosis of acute coronary events is worse in patients living alone: the FINAMI myocardial infarction register. *Eur J Prev Cardiol* 2014; **21**(8): 989–996.

16. KB King, HT Reis. Marriage and long-term survival after coronary artery bypass grafting. *Heal Psychol* 2012; **31**(1): 55–62.

17. M Baine, F Sahak, C Lin, et al. Marital status and survival in pancreatic cancer patients: a SEER based analysis. *PLoS One* 2011; **6**(6): e21052.

18. RG Wood, B Goesling, S Avellar. *The Effects of Marriage on Health: A Synthesis of Recent Research Evidence*. Princeton, NJ, ASPE; 2007.

19. TF Robles, RB Slatcher, JM Trombello, MM McGinn. Marital quality and health: a meta-analytic review. *Psychol Bull* 2014; **140**(1): 140–187.

20. MA Whisman, DH Baucom. Intimate relationships and psychopathology. *Clin Child Family Psychol Rev* 2012; **15**: 4–13.

21. YC Yang, C Boen, K Gerken, et al. Social relationships and physiological determinants of longevity across the human life span. *Proc Natl Acad Sci* 2016; **113**(3): 578–583.

22. P Zaninotto, J Wardle, A Steptoe. Sustained enjoyment of life and mortality at older ages: analysis of the English Longitudinal Study of Ageing. *BMJ*. 2016; **355**: i6267.

23. SD Pressman, KA Matthews, S Cohen, et al. Association of enjoyable leisure activities with psychological and physical well-being. *Psychosom Med* 2009; **71**(7): 725–732.

24. H Arem, SC Moore, A Patel, et al. Leisure time physical activity and mortality: a detailed pooled analysis of the dose-response relationship. *JAMA Intern Med* 2015; **175**(6): 959–967.

25. DE Bowler, LM Buyung-Ali, TM Knight, AS Pullin. A systematic review of evidence for the added benefits to health of exposure to natural environments. *BMC Public Health* 2010; **10**: 456.

26. R Mora-Ripoll. The therapeutic value of laughter in medicine. *Altern Ther Health Med* 2010; **16**(6): 56–64.

27. BB Gump, KA Matthews. Are vacations good for your health? The 9-year mortality experience after the Multiple Risk Factor Intervention Trial. *Psychosom Med* 2000; **62**(5), 608–612

28. J de Bloom, M Kompier, S Geurts, et al. Do we recover from vacation? Meta-analysis of vacation effects on health and well-being. *J Occup Health* 2009; **51**: 13–25.

29. E Stanmore, B Stubbs, D Vancampfort, ED de Bruin, J Firth. The effect of active video games on cognitive functioning in clinical and non-clinical populations: a meta-analysis of randomized controlled trials. *Neurosci Biobehav Rev* 2017; **8**: 34–43.

30. RT Proyer. The well-being of playful adults: adult playfulness, subjective well-being, physical well-being, and the pursuit of enjoyable activities. *Eur J Humour Res* 2013; **1**(1): 84–98.

31. RT Proyer. A new structural model for the study of adult playfulness: assessment and exploration of an understudied individual differences variable. *Pers Individ Dif* 2017; **108**: 113–122.

32. C Deyell Hood, C Carruthers. Enhancing leisure experience and developing resources: the Leisure and Well-Being Model, part II. *Ther Recreation J* 2007; **41**(4): 298–325.

33. MK McClintock, W Daleb, EO Laumannc, L Waite. Empirical redefinition of comprehensive health and well-being in the older adults of the United States. *Proc Natl Acad Sci* 2016; **113**: E3071–E3080.

34. A Steptoe, J Wardle. Enjoying life and living longer. *Arch Intern Med* 2012; **172**(3): 273–275.

35. A Steptoe, C de Oliveira, P Demakakos, P Zaninotto. Enjoyment of life and declining physical function at older ages: a longitudinal cohort study. *CMAJ* 2014; **186**(4): E150–E156.

36. JK Boehm, C Peterson, M Kivimaki, LD Kubzansky. Heart health when life is

satisfying: evidence from the Whitehall II cohort study. *Eur Heart J* 2011; **70**(7): 741–756.

37. Y Chida, A Steptoe. Positive psychological well-being and mortality: a quantitative review of prospective observational studies. *Psychosom Med* 2008; **77**(6): 1747–1776.

38. A Steptoe, S Dockray, J Wardle. Positive affect and psychobiological processes relevant to health. *J Pers* 2009; **77**(6): 1747–1776.

39. C Rogers. *On Becoming A Person: A Therapist's View of Psychotherapy.* Boston, MA, Houghton Mifflin Company, 1961.

40. L Smith, L Tang, N Veronesse, P Soysal, BJS Tubbs. Sexual activity is associated with greater enjoyment of life in older adults. *Sex Med* 2019; **7**(1): 11–18.

41. C Deeming. Addressing the social determinants of subjective wellbeing: the latest challenge for social policy. *J Soc Policy* 2013; **42**(3): 541–565.

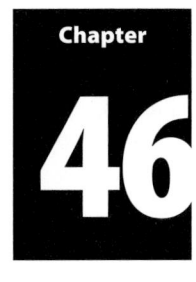

Chapter 46

Well-Being and Work–Life Balance

Cultural, Positive Psychology, and Practical Perspectives

Michael Bolton, Ingrid Lobben, Tom Pruzinsky, and Theodore A. Stern

Introduction

Work–life balance facilitates positive affect, happiness, and satisfaction [1–4]; absence of it contributes to depression and anxiety [1]. However, achieving a "balance" is easier said than done. Strategies to increase positive affect, happiness, and quality of life have often been simplistic.

For example, some suggestions to enhance work–life balance include "learn to say no if you are too busy," "practice self-care," "don't take work home with you," "make time for friends and family outside of work," and "reduce work email and work phone access" [5]. In contrast, our chapter focuses on how to increase well-being. Well-being and positive affect are well described in the positive psychology literature [6, 7].

Culture and Well-Being: The Nordic Way

Before we present a framework for assessing and implementing well-being, we would like to present an illustrative example of a culture in which well-being and happiness are achieved at rates that far outpace other cultures.

Balance is a central aspect of Scandinavian culture. Most Scandinavians believe you should not have to choose between your work and your family life. The Scandinavian countries consistently top the rankings each year in the United Nation's World Happiness Report [8]. By way of contrast, the USA was ranked number 18 last year, despite striving to achieve balance. Nordic countries have a comparable GDP per capita to that of the USA, meaning that economic success does not require spending more time at work; balance does not interfere with productivity [8].

Since both women and men participate in the workforce, and dual-income households are the norm, the focus in Scandinavia on ensuring a good balance between professional and family obligations and well-being has increased [9]. Role conflicts and conflicting expectations still occur. However, creation of new models in which workers can balance work and private life has been particularly important.

For example, for physicians in Norway, the standard schedule is 38–40 hours per week [10]. Decisions to extend working hours beyond this are only permitted by mutual agreement. The national employer's organization and the Norwegian Medical Association set a maximum of 60 hours per week for doctors, and a maximum working period of 19 hours per 24-hour period. A minimum rest period was also established; if a physician's schedule exceeds the limit, it must be compensated for in another week. These policies led to an environment in which physicians in Norway work significantly fewer hours per week than physicians in many European Union countries [10]. Between 1994 and 2012, junior doctors in Norway worked 45–46 hours per week, on average, and senior doctors worked 46–47 hours, compared to 50–90-hour averages in most EU countries [10]. This has also led to generous parental leave (mothers are entitled to one year's leave with full pay after giving birth/adopting, while fathers are entitled to three months).

In the USA, work–life flexibility practices (like flex-time, voluntary telework, and leave for family and personal needs) remain limited by employers. This is very different from Denmark, a country the OECD Better Life Index ranked highest in terms of work–life balance in 2017. According to the report, Denmark ranks above average among OECD countries in many dimensions, including work–life balance, social connections, civic engagement, work–life balance health status, subjective well-being, and personal security. Perhaps the country's progressive work–life policies play a significant role in its population's general satisfaction, with life score of 7.5 (out of 10), which is higher than that of the OECD average of 6.5. Many Danes report that they prioritize life over work, and they enjoy a high degree of flexibility when they are at work. Many can choose when they start their workday and are also able to work from home [11]. Surprisingly, productivity is higher when people spend fewer hours working [12].

PERMA: The Positive Psychology of Well-Being

The PERMA model of well-being (Figure 46.1), with each letter of the mnemonic standing for a specific domain of psychological experience (**p**ositive emotion, **e**ngagement, **r**elationships, **m**eaning, and **a**ccomplishment), was developed by Seligman [13], the acknowledged "father" of the field of positive psychology. It operationalizes a path to well-being and work–life balance. It is based on his multi-decade understanding and synthesis of the empirical and conceptual literature on happiness, satisfaction with life, and well-being, terms that are often used interchangeably [6, 13–16]. PERMA is a highly structured, yet individualizable and concise way of understanding well-being and its components [17, 18].

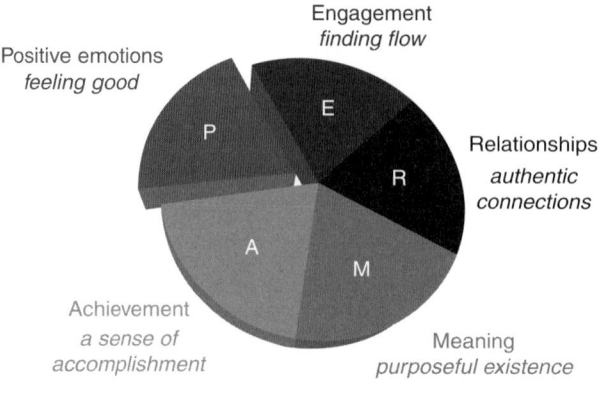

Figure 46.1 Seligman's PERMA model.

As a conceptual and practical organizational structure, PERMA is also best understood in the much broader scholarly context of the nomenclature of character strengths and virtues [17, 18]. That is, PERMA is conceptually embedded in a much broader understanding of human functioning that is separate and distinct from psychopathological models of understanding.

PERMA provides the basis for a practical/clinical intervention that is focused on work/non-work issues. For example, a possible job change could be discussed in terms of the potential emotional, relationships, engagement, and accomplishment variables. Additionally, specific empirically validated, psychometric measures are available for effectively measuring each PERMA component, as well as multiple measures of well-being [19–22].

Positive Emotion

What are the benefits of positive emotions? Lyubomirsky and colleagues [23] provided a persuasive answer after reviewing the literature on the relationship between positive affect and "happiness" (i.e., well-being, success, satisfaction with life). They concluded that there were significant relationships among positive affect and a wide range of positive life outcomes (e.g., physical health, longevity, employment, income, as well as social and intimate relationships).

One of many compelling empirical examples of the benefits of positive emotion was found in the dramatic increase in length of life associated with early life positive affect in the experience of females who entered into the Catholic organization the School Sisters of Notre Dame [24, 25]. If at the time of their entrance into nunhood they described their lives using more positive affect, they were much more likely to live significantly more than six decades compared to their peers who reported less positive affect in their biographical descriptions. Additional similarly compelling empirical findings are those of cognitive psychologist Alice Isen, who consistently found that positive affect enhanced problem-solving, decision-making, and thinking in physicians [26, 27].

Given the abundance of benefits resulting from the experience of positive affect, it logically follows that scientific positive psychology would ask: *Can positive emotions be systematically increased?* The answer is *yes* [28]. Lyubomirsky and colleagues developed the Positive Activity Model. Here, they posed the question: How do simple positive activities increase well-being? [29].

Engagement

The experience of engagement has been most closely tied to the seminal work of Csikszentmihalyi [30, 31] on flow. "Flow is a psychological state of complete absorption," which individuals experience as intrinsically motivating [30]. Such attentional absorption can be associated with a distorted sense of time (time slowing down or speeding up) and/or distorted sense of self (e.g., momentary loss of self-awareness), such as what might occur when deeply engrossed in an activity (e.g., playing chess, performing surgery).

Social flow, an interpersonal experience of absorption that is intrinsically motivated, also occurs in work-related contexts [32–34]. Interestingly, social flow has been associated with high-quality connections at work [33]. Flow has been extensively studied with respect to its influence on the highest levels of human performance in a range of activities [35], and therefore it is directly connected to the PERMA variable of accomplishment.

Relationships

In the literature on work–life balance there is invariably an emphasis on the need to pay close attention to all types of interpersonal relationships (e.g., with children, a spouse, parents, coworkers) [13]. In explicating PERMA, Seligman makes clear that relationships are inextricably related to positive affect, meaning, and accomplishment, even though they are intrinsically important independent of positive affect, engagement, and meaning [13]. Clearly, time and attention need to be given to relationships. For example, Gottman's research on marriage documents the importance of giving persistent attention to specific patterns of marital interaction (e.g., repairs and positive interactions) to ensure long-term marital well-being [36]. Interestingly, there has been some compelling work done on the importance of emotion in work-related relationships, in what Dutton calls high-quality connections, which are defined in terms of "aliveness, vitality, heightened sense of positive regard, and mutuality." Dutton and colleagues have further gone on to systematically articulate the role of compassion at work [37].

Meaning

The literature on meaning in life is voluminous [38]. Meaning is created by the successive choices about how we use our time and energy and where we chose to focus our attention [39–42]. Meaning that goes beyond the pursuit of pleasure and material wealth is argued to give people a greater sense of purpose in life [43], and a meaningful life is thought to be related to attaching oneself to something larger than oneself, and has been known to be an effective barrier against depression [44].

Accomplishment

The variable of "accomplishment" is a relatively recent addition to Seligman's PERMA model of well-being. Seligman and colleagues noted that "accomplishment (or achievement), is often pursued for its own sake, even if it brings no positive emotion, no meaning and no positive relationships. Accomplishment can be defined in terms of achievement, success, or mastery at the highest level possible within a particular domain" [6].

For some individuals, accomplishment may be a driving force in one's pursuit of well-being; for example, if one is fulling a "calling" with respect to a work-related role or another role in life (e.g., parenting) [42]. Accomplishment may be also be dominant if one is motivated to pursue excellence in some endeavor (e.g., sports, scientific inquiry, scholarly activities, service).

PERMA as a Framework for Decision-Making and Intervention

PERMA embodies a practical and conceptual emphasis that is distinct from deficit/pathology-oriented perspectives that focus on "fixing" what is "broken" (e.g., stop abusing alcohol and drugs, being controlling, and yelling at your spouse). It is an empirically based rationale with specific interventions for the cultivation of positive affect to enhance success.

Although using positive psychology concepts in therapy is not new, we know of no known studies using PERMA as a model for work–life balance. The PERMA model allows clinicians to guide patients through each of the five areas of well-being, but it also allows the patient to use the acronym as a standardized, stepwise method for coming to a decision. If a person were about to quit their job, end their relationship or marriage, or decide to move to a different city or country due to a decision made on an impulsive, emotional surge, perhaps the decision would have been different had they systematically applied PERMA to arrive at the decision. What does it mean to say that someone has "bad decision-making"? It could mean that the endpoint (the decision) is worse than what would be expected, but it could also mean that the person is using a method of decision-making that is worse than expected. PERMA imparts a style of questions to guide decision-making.

Consider as an example a father's wish for his daughter to take over the family farm. Without PERMA the daughter may say "No, I don't want to be a farmer." The reasons for this decision may be emotional, transient, or concrete, but if the daughter does not have a standardized method of working through the issue in a manner that can be replicated, important variables that may affect the decision may not always be addressed. However, if the daughter applies PERMA, there is a standard set of questions to be asked, which lead to a systematic, thorough, reproducible method of analysis – namely, the consideration of *p*ositive emotion, *e*ngagement, *r*elationships, *m*eaning, and *a*chievement – PERMA. The dialog in such a case may proceed as follows: "If I take over the farm the positive emotion scores low, my engagement scores low, positive relationships score high, meaning scores very high (because of the father's dying wish), and accomplishment may score moderately." Depending on how highly the daughter values the "meaning" component compared to the other components of PERMA, she might decide to run the farm after all. This demonstrates the issue of "weighting" the individual components of PERMA relative to each other, as not everyone will assign equal or similar value to each part, and high scores on one component of PERMA may compensate for low scores on the remaining components.

One of the limitations of any clinical model is that the treater cannot make all the decisions for a patient once the patient leaves the hospital or office. Being able to use PERMA as a portable coaching strategy can potentially overcome decision-making that is less than thorough, analytical, and thoughtful when a patient has left the treater's office, clinic, or hospital.

Bullet Points

What we hope you take away from this short chapter on an extensive subject are the following bullet points:

- The work–life landscape is changing.
- Research shows it may not be enough to focus on "balance" alone between work and non-work living if the goal is to increase well-being.
- Instead, by having well-being as the primary focus when choosing what to do for work, where to work, who to surround yourself with, and what to do when not working, what has been referred to as "balance" may occur.
- PERMA is a model that is supported in the literature as a way to increase well-being, and may provide a systematic method for value-based decision-making about work and non-work activities.
- The PERMA model may have an application as a tool for intervention in mental healthcare.

Final Thought

If you knew you were to die tomorrow, what would matter most to you today?

References

1. D Antai, DS Anthony, B Braithwaite, A Oke. A "balanced" life: work–life balance and sickness absence in four Nordic countries. *Int J Occup Environ Med* 2015; **6**(4): 205–222.

2. T Lunau, C Bambra, TA Eikemo, KA van der Wel, N Dragano. A balancing act? Work–life balance, health, and well-being in European welfare states. *Eur J Publ Health* 2014; **24**(3): 422–427.

3. K Kvande. Work–life balance for fathers in globalized knowledge work: some insights from the Norwegian context. *Gender Work Org* 2008; **16**. DOI:10.1111/j.1468-0432.2008.00430.x.

4. L Artazcoz, I Cortes, V Puig-Barrachina, et al. Combining employment and family in Europe: the role of family policies in health. *Eur J Publ Health* 2013; **24**(4): 649–655.

5. Mayo Clinic. Work–life balance: tips to reclaim control. www.mayoclinic.org/healthy-lifestyle/adult-health/in-depth/work-life-balance/art-20048134 (accessed March 2, 2019).

6. E Jayawickreme, M Foregard, MEP Seligman. The engine of well-being, *Rev Gen Psychol* 2012; **16**(4): 327–342.

7. G Henriques, K Kleinman. The nested model of well-being: a unified approach. *Rev Gen Psychol* 2014; **18**(1): 7–18.

8. J Helliwell, R Layard, J Sachs. *World Happiness Report 2018*. New York: Sustainable Development Solutions Network; 2018. http://worldhappiness.report/ed/2018 (accessed February 20, 2019).

9. K Knudsen. Striking a different balance: work–family conflict for female and male managers in a Scandinavian context. *Gender Manage* 2009; **24**(4): 252–269.

10. M Limb. Could UK doctors learn from Norwegian doctors' shorter working hours? *BMJ* 2014; **349**: 74–90.

11. OECD. OECD Better Life Index. 2019. www.oecdbetterlifeindex.org/countries/denmark (accessed February 1, 2019).

12. J Pencavel The productivity of working hours. 2019. http://ftp.iza.org/dp8129.pdf (accessed March 1, 2019).

13. M Seligman. *Flourish: A Visionary New Understanding of Happiness and Well-Being*. New York, Free Press; 2011.

14. E Diener, MEP Seligman. Beyond money: progress on an economy of well-being. *Perspect Psychol Sci* 2018; **13**(2): 171–175.

15. JL Duarte. Beyond life satisfaction: a scientific approach to well-being gives us much more to measure. In: AC Parks, SM Schueller, eds., *The Wiley Blackwell Handbook of Positive Psychological Interventions*. Chichester, Wiley-Blackwell; 2014; 433–449.

16. JE Gillham, ed. *The Science of Optimism and Hope: Research Essays in Honor of Martin E P Seligman*. London, Templeton Foundation Press; 2000.

17. C Peterson, N Park. Character strengths and the life of meaning. In PTP Wong, ed., *The Human Quest for Meaning: Theories, Research, and Applications* (2nd ed.). New York, Routledge; 2012; 277–295.

18. C Peterson, MEP Seligman. *Character Strengths and Virtues: A Handbook and Classification*. Washington, DC, American Psychological Association; 2004.

19. M Brandel, F Vescovelli, C Ruini. Beyond Ryff's scale: comprehensive measures of eudaimonic well-being in clinical populations – a systematic review. *Clin Psychol Psychother* 2017; **24**(6): O1524–O1546.

20. E Diener, D Wirtz, W Tov, et al. New well-being measures: short scales to assess flourishing and positive and negative feelings. *Social Indicators Res* 2010; **97**(2): 143–156.

21. J Lindert, PA Bain, LD Kubzansky, C Stein. Well-being measurement and the WHO health policy Health 2010: systematic review of measurement scales. *Eur J Publ Health* 2015; **25**(4): 731–740.

22. Wikimedia. The Perma Model of Well-Being. https://commons.wikimedia.org/wiki/Main_Page (accessed April 15, 2019).

23. S Lybomirsky, L King, E Diener. The benefits of frequent positive affect: does happiness lead to success? *Psychol Bull* 2015; **131**(6): 803–855.

24. DD Danner, WV Friesen, SM Collier. Personal narratives, positive emotions, and long lives: the Nun Study. In: SJ Lopez, ed., *Positive Psychology: Exploring the Best in People, Vol 2: Capitalizing on Emotional Experiences.* Westport, CT, Praeger Publishers/Greenwood Publishing Group; 2008; 21–36.

25. DD Danner, DA Snowdon, WV Friesen. Positive emotions in early life and longevity: findings from the Nun Study. *J Pers Soc Psychol* 2001; **80**(5): 804–813.

26. AM Isen. Some perspectives on positive feelings and emotions: positive affect facilitates thinking and problem solving. In: ASR Manstead, N Frijda, A Fischer, eds., *Feelings and Emotions: The Amsterdam Symposium.* New York, Cambridge University Press; 2004; 263–281.

27. JT Moskowitz, MS Clark, AD Ong, J Gruber. The role of positive affect on thinking and decision-making: a tribute to Alice Isen. In: J Gruber, JT Moskowitz, eds., *Positive Emotion: Integrating the Light Sides and Dark Sides.* New York, Oxford University Press; 2014; 72–77.

28. AC Parks, SM Schueller, eds. *The Wiley Blackwell Handbook of Positive Psychological Interventions.* Chichester, Wiley-Blackwell; 2014.

29. S Lyubomirsky, K Layous. How do simple positive activities increase well-being? *Curr Dir Psychol Sci* 2013; **22**(1): 57–62.

30. M Csikszentmihalyi. *Creativity: Flow and the Psychology of Discovery and Invention.* New York, HarperCollins Publishers; 1997.

31. M Csikszentmihalyi. *Applications of Flow in Human Development and Education: The Collected Works of Mihaly Csikszentmihalyi.* New York, Springer Science + Business Media; 2014.

32. M Boffi, E Riva, N Rainisio, P Inghilleri. Social psychology of flow: a situated framework for optimal experience. In: L Harmat, FØ Andersen, F Ullén, J Wright,

G Sadlo, eds., *Flow Experience: Empirical Research and Applications.* Cham, Springer; 2016; 215–231.

33. HE Lucas. Social Flow: Optimal Experience With Others at Work and Play. In: MA Warren, SI Donaldson, eds., *Toward a Positive Psychology of Relationships: New Directions in Theory and Research.* Santa Barbara, CA, Praeger/ABC-CLIO; 2018; 179–192.

34. R Maeran, F Cangiano. Flow experience and job characteristics: analyzing the role of flow in job satisfaction. *TPM* 2013; **20**(1): 13–26.

35. M Csikszentmihalyi, MN Montijo, AR Mouton. Flow theory: optimizing elite performance in the creative realm. In: SI Pfeiffer, E Shaunessy-Dedrick, M Foley-Nicpon, eds., *APA Handbook of Giftedness and Talent.* Washington, DC, American Psychological Association; 2018; 215–229.

36. J Driver, A Tabares, AF Shapiro, JM Gottman. Couple interaction in happy and unhappy marriages: Gottman Laboratory studies. In: F Walsh, ed., *Normal Family Processes: Growing Diversity and Complexity* (4th ed.). New York, Guilford Press; 2012; 57–77.

37. JE Dutton, KM Workman, AE Hardin. Compassion at work. *Ann Rev Org Psychol Org Behav* 2014; **1**: 277–304.

38. PTP Wong, ed. *The Human Quest for Meaning: Theories, Research, and Applications* (2nd ed.). New York, Routledge; 2012.

39. PTP Wong. Viktor Frankl's meaning-seeking model and positive psychology. In: A Batthyany, P Russo-Netzer, eds., *Meaning in Positive and Existential Psychology.* New York, Springer Science + Business Media; 2014; 149–184.

40. A Eakman. A subjectively-based definition of life balance using personal meaning in occupation. *J Occup Sci* 2014; **23**(1): 108–127.

41. A Gregory, S Milner Editorial. Work–life balance: a matter of choice? *Gender Work Orgn* 2009; **16**(1): 1–13.

42. MF Steger, BJ Dik. If one is looking for meaning in life, does it help to find meaning in work? *Appl Psychol Health Well-Being* 2009; **1**(3): 303–320.

43. M Pascha. The PERMA model: your scientific theory of happiness. 2019. https:// positivepsychologyprogram.com/perma-model (accessed April 1, 2019).

44. P Adler. What is PERMA by Martin Seligman. GoStrengths! 2019 https://gos trengths.com/whatisperma (accessed April 1, 2019).

Family Relations, Friendships, and Love

Shelby Alsup, Elli Weisbaum, Talya Vogel, and Daniel J. Siegel

Introduction

Humans are intrinsically social beings. Over time we are shaped by our lived experiences, particularly through our connections and interactions with others. By examining the profound nature of these social relationships, we can begin to understand how the mind emerges across the lifespan and regulates such experiences. In this chapter, we will explore relationships with family, friends, and romantic partners to develop an understanding of our innate social nature and the direct link this has to well-being and health.

Scientific Perspective: Research Links Well-Being to Social Relationships

Positive Effects of Relationships on the Social Brain

Science has made evident the positive effects of relationships on well-being, including longevity, happiness, and mental health. The World Health Organization defines health as "a state of complete physical, mental and social well-being and not merely the absence of disease or infirmity" [1]. Therefore, the absence of disease alone does not signify well-being. Rather, well-being is a quality of life in which there is the presence of positive affective processes, a sense of satisfaction, purpose, and fulfillment in life, and the absence of enduring negative emotions [2, 3]. Research has shown that it is not single components that contribute to overall well-being, but rather a vast amalgamation of internal and external factors, including relationships, environment, physical health, neurobiology, and cognitive, social, and emotional processes [4]. One of the most critical findings in this large body of research is that the quality of social relationships is among the strongest predictors of well-being over a lifespan [4, 5]. The quality of social relationships influences other domains instrumental to the development of well-being. Individuals who feel a sense of connection with others are happier, have better overall physical health, and live longer than their less socially connected peers. Over two decades of research collected from the World Values Survey found a positive association between time spent engaged in activities with others and individuals' subjective sense of well-being [6]. The 2019 World Happiness Report dedicated an entire chapter to the topic "Happiness and Prosocial Behavior: An Evaluation of the Evidence" [7]. In that chapter, a robust link is shown between generous behaviors – such as volunteering and donating to charity – and greater life satisfaction, positive affect, and reduced depression. The positive benefits of these prosocial behaviors or "giving experiences" on an individual's happiness increased when three specific factors were present: there was (1) a sense of free choice; (2) an opportunity for social connection; and (3) a chance to see how their behavior made a difference. The second two factors provide evidence that a sense of connection can increase happiness beyond the baseline satisfaction of engaging in a prosocial activity.

Research has shown that connection to others impacts not only mental well-being but also physical well-being. A longitudinal study found that the magnitude of effects of social relationships on mortality is comparable to well-established risk factors such as smoking, alcohol consumption, and physical inactivity [8]. Nobel Laureate Elizabeth Blackburn and her colleague Elissa Epel [9] found that telomeres, the protective caps at the ends of our chromosomes, profoundly impact our global functioning. More specifically, the length and health of our telomeres significantly affect our bodies, brains, and minds. The production of the enzyme telomerase actively revitalizes and nourishes telomeres – repairing and maintaining these important ends of our chromosomes that establish the integrity of our genetic material in each cell. Positive relationships, attachments, and social connections help promote an optimal level of telomerase that contributes to the lengthening of our telomeres, which, in turn, promotes youthfulness and overall health and functioning.

Scientific research has built a strong case that overall health promotion and well-being are supported by mental and physical health and that a sense of connection through meaningful relationships is foundational to both of these components. Interestingly, research findings have paralleled the necessity of relationships to that of basic needs for survival, such as sleep or food, recognizing relationships as a public health concern [10]. Overall, the experience of good-quality relationships helps make us happier, increases our sense of well-being, and gives meaning to life [11]. Social behaviors, such as prosociality or acts of kindness toward others, have been identified as a "social feedback loop" which results in increased well-being and future positive social behavior [12]. The reciprocal relationship, characterized by a positive social feedback loop, has shown increased well-being in children [12] and adults [13] across cultures [14]. The considerable impact of the quality of social relationships can be seen on all domains of functioning across the lifespan. As human beings, we can qualitatively reflect on the impact that meaningful relationships have on our lives. Viewing this in relation to the research we have just discussed, we can see how the quality of our relationships shapes our bodies, brains, and minds.

Connecting to the Framework of Interpersonal Neurobiology

Our lens as authors is situated in interpersonal neurobiology (IPNB) [15, 16], a framework that integrates diverse fields of thought and science by noting the consilience or common ground across disparate ways of understanding the world. From a cultural studies perspective, a theoretical lens provides a frame through which to perceive social reality [17]. The IPNB framework proposes that the mind is both a relational and embodied process [18]. The mind is defined as having four facets, each of which may be an emergent property of embodied and relational energy and information flow. These facets include subjective experience, consciousness, information processing, and self-organization. Self-organization is how a complex system regulates itself. For the mind, this would be the embodied and relational regulation of the flow of energy and information.

As clinicians, when we have a patient in front of us, our focus may center on this individual and their health; however, IPNB suggests that the self is not defined by the skin-encased body alone, but also by the relational world in which the individual lives. This relational field of communication not only shapes the mind; the mind in this framework actually emerges from it. Therefore, as a clinician, it is important to consider that when we are treating or caring for another human, the interactive experience is not separate from us, but part of a relational process in which the mind is emerging. For example, a physician who identifies the internal state of a patient with a common cold and makes an empathic comment revealing that the inner life of the patient was seen and understood will help the patient recover from their cold a day sooner and have a more robust immune response to help them recover from the illness [19]. This understanding can also help inform therapeutic relationships, not only by impacting the quality of care provided, but also by supporting awareness of how daily interactions at work impact the clinician's own well-being. This awareness can help to prevent empathy fatigue and encourage compassion toward oneself. Increased self-compassion can lead to increases in positive affect, prosocial feelings, and the decrease of stress response in challenging situations [20, 21]. On the topic of relational well-being, Dan Siegel says that "relationships are not the icing on the cake, they aren't even the cake, they are the main meal." If we accept that the self emerges from beyond simply the skull or skin, and is a relational process arising from both our internal and external experiences, we can easily see that the interconnection between us and others is a crucial aspect for our well-being.

From Interconnection to Integration

Meaningful Connection Leads to Healthy Integration

The reality of interconnection (Figure 47.1) is important to understand when we examine the central role that relationships play in the establishment of well-being. Interconnection implies interdependence and is a term we can use to acknowledge that we do not, and cannot, exist independently. Interconnection does not mean that we do not rely on ourselves. Rather, the IPNB framework states that having healthy relationships with others requires us to have a clear *differentiation* between ourselves and another person – characterized by a healthy relationship and understanding of ourselves – while simultaneously being able to form strong *linkages* with others [16]. This linkage of differentiated parts is simply called *integration*. The concept of interconnection can be seen as the recognition that a global state of health must include an awareness that an entirely separate self is actually a constructed illusion. From a scientific perspective, we can easily see that as human beings, we cannot survive without the sun, rain, or other elements that make up our world. This relational nature of our world is mirrored in the IPNB perspectives as we view the mind as part of a complex system, one facet of which is self-organizing and regulates the flow of energy and information within us, between us, and among us [18]. Interconnection can be seen as the health and reality of any given component of an interconnected system. Within this view is the notion that integration creates optimal self-organization, the basis of well-being. The term *Ubuntu* describes the bond that connects humanity and, essentially, translates to "I am because we are" [22].

Understanding the mind through the lens of IPNB as an emergent property of the complex system of embodied and relational energy flow reveals the ways the mind emerges and shapes us and others through interconnection. If we accept one facet of the mind as an emergent, self-organizing system of energy and information flow within and between individuals, what implications might this have in terms of our own identity and its relation to others? IPNB proposes that to create well-being, we must develop an integrated identity, one that accounts for

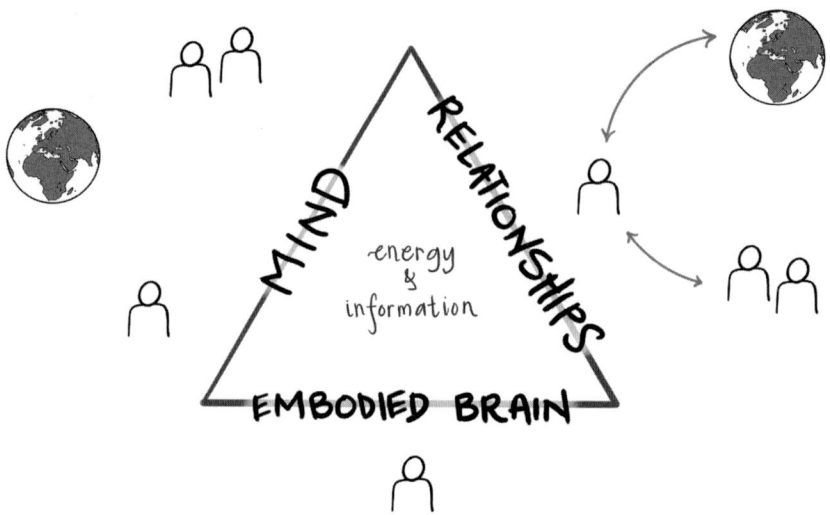

Figure 47.1 The Triangle of Human Experience reveals the connections of the mind, embodied brain, and relationships. Illustration by Madeleine W. Siegel as depicted in DJ Siegel, *Aware: The Science and Practice of Presence*. New York, TarcherPerigee; 2018. © 2018 Mind Your Brain, Inc. Used with permission from the author.

both the individual, embodied self, and the interconnected nature of our relational self. Integration can be seen as the linking of differentiated parts in a complex, nonlinear system. The framework of a complex system, which originates from the field of mathematics, though capable of chaos or rigidity, is seen to naturally move toward integration when self-organization is optimizing its flow toward harmony – away from the banks of chaos on the one hand, and rigidity on the other (see Figure 47.2). However, integration should not be seen as a resolution, but rather as a state that is constantly being cultivated through our lived experiences.

Building Healthy Relationships: Understanding the River of Integration

Integration is the essence of the functioning of healthy relationships, embodied brain, and the mind, where harmony and health emerge through the linking of differentiated parts of a system. When integration is impaired, there is movement toward chaos, rigidity, or a combination of both. Often, this impairment results in difficulties with self-regulation and psychopathology. Impairment becomes evident through our external behaviors, often impacting our interpersonal relationships.

To better conceptualize the idea of healthy integration IPNB uses a metaphor of a river, which we call *the River of Integration* (Figure 47.2). A complex system has emergent properties that arise from the interactions of the elements of the system. As dispersions of energy and information flow move through differentiation and linkage, they are bounded on one side by chaos and on the other by rigidity. Optimal self-organization generates a flexible, adaptive, coherent, energized, and stable (FACES) flow. In IPNB, we call this *integration* [23].

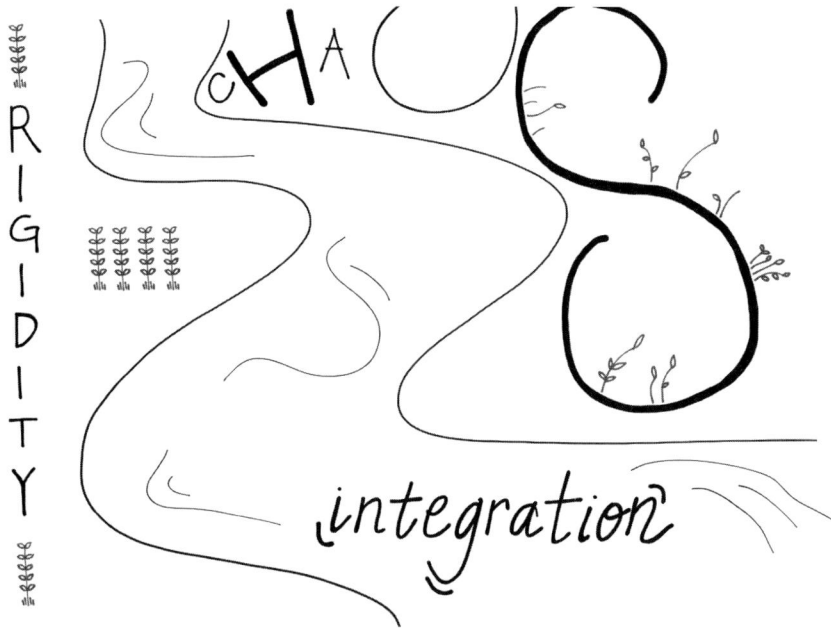

Figure 47.2 The River of Integration represents the movement of systems in which states of integration are harmonious and adaptive, and impairment in integration moves toward chaos, rigidity, or a combination. Illustration by Madeleine W. Siegel as depicted in DJ Siegel, *Aware: The Science and Practice of Presence.* New York, TarcherPerigee; 2018. © 2018 Mind Your Brain, Inc. Used with permission from the author.

To understand how to create a state of healthy integration, we can look to neuroscience to help identify areas of potential disconnection. The area of the brain called the prefrontal cortex is known to link distinct regions of the brain – such as the cortex, limbic system, brainstem, and body proper – and information arising from the social world. As clinicians, we strive to reduce suffering and help others cultivate well-being. Using the integrative functions of the prefrontal cortex, we can identify tools that support the development of well-being. Through the lens of IPNB, we can build a framework of nine integrative functions that encapsulate the components of embodied mental health: bodily regulation, attuned communication, emotional balance, fear extinction, flexibility, insight, empathy, mortality, and intuition [24]. By tuning into these integrative functions, new neural connections and growth can evolve. In addition to these nine functions, our connectome, the map of neural connections among the differentiated and widely distributed regions in the brain and nervous system, when integrated, is a strong predictor of well-being [25]. Internal integration and external integrated relationships – which are based first on differentiation then linkage – influence healthy neural integration. Thus, neural pathways are more likely to activate in the future and contribute to overall health and well-being.

Relational Integration

If we recognize interconnection as a form of integration, we can further come to know the influence of our *inner and inter* self on our relationships. The self is understood through the relational nature that is fundamental to who we are as social beings. Integration across domains of life may be essential to the development of well-being. Earlier we discussed what healthy integration looks like internally. Through interconnection, individuals can also develop healthy integration externally with others through their interpersonal relationships. The process through which two individuals exchange energy and information is termed empathy and compassion and involves regions of the brain that can be called our "resonance circuitry" [15]. When two differentiated individuals link, resonance and integration allow the two separate individual *me* to become an integrated entity. Dan Siegel refers to this relational state as MWe, where the *me* and *we* link together with a sense of integrity, so one's individuality is not lost in the joining with another. Integration is more like a fruit salad than a blended smoothie, wherein individual identities are maintained, and the whole is greater than the sum of its parts. This framing is useful for imagining what a healthy, integrated relationship looks like.

Relational integration is the ultimate expression of integration, where we come to see the demonstration of well-being, awareness, kindness, compassion, and love. We use the term *mindsight* to describe focused attention and awareness of the internal state of the mind of the self as well as the inner world of others [24]. Mindsight builds on the perceptual skills of openness, observation, and objectivity to help us monitor and modify our internal states in the present moment toward integration. When we engage in mindsight conversations with family, friends, romantic partners, and community, we become aware of the inner nature of the mind and move toward states of integration and improved functioning across many domains of life.

Practical Tools: Cultivating Relational Integration

There are many tools and practices that stem from the IPNB lens, which we can use as clinicians and in our relationships across many contexts. Using the acronym ESSENCE [23], we can identify steps to achieve elements that promote well-being across relationships. Emotional spark (ES) is the drive to keep passion alive, which can act as a prominent feature in the fabric of our lives. Social engagement (SE), the core of this chapter, is the understanding that relationships and connection are among the strongest predictors and foundations of well-being. Novelty-seeking (N) is the experience of being open to new things and having the courage to experience change and engage in the unknown. Creative exploration (CE) is how we cultivate the creative mind in the *inner* and *inter* development of the self.

Mindsight conversations can be developed through the application of PART – a helpful acronym that stands for presence, attunement, resonance, and trust [26]. These four functions provide opportunities to cultivate healthy connection and are fundamental components of an integrated relationship in which differences are respected while linking together. Presence involves mindful attention, where there is receptive awareness of both our internal and external states. Attunement is the understanding of, and attention given to, the subjective experiences of others. Resonance, an outcome of presence and attunement, goes beyond simply mirroring another's behavior to actively allowing another to *feel felt* and understood. Trust is an essential condition in relationships that naturally emerges when presence, attunement, and resonance are experienced [27, 28]. The polyvagal theory describes the biology of safety and danger, and the mind–body connection that occurs within ourselves and in our relationships with others [28]. The function of the vagus nerve, the tenth cranial nerve, explains how the autonomic nervous system regulates the *social engagement system*, engendering receptivity, openness, and trust. According to Stephen

Porges, who proposed this theory, the presence of safety and trust helps mobilize and downregulate states of reactivity and allows for transformative change and connection.

A sense of presence promotes positive health for our minds, bodies, and relationships. Presence can act as a gateway through which integration arises. Shari Geller [29] used the term *therapeutic presence* in psychotherapy to describe the foundation for effective therapy and receptive attunement. *Therapeutic presence* is "a way we can receptively attune with our patients, within ourselves, and with the moment-to-moment unfolding of therapy." Through *therapeutic presence,* we can tune into the present moment and help regulate patients through interpersonal connection. Using resonance in the moment, we can guide others to expand and connect both within themselves and between us, creating an integrated relational presence. By way of our own experience of remaining grounded, centered, and in contact with ourselves, we can hold our patients' suffering, while remaining differentiated. This relational process allows us to be truly present without becoming overwhelmed or experiencing empathy fatigue. The four domains that make up PART underscore the movement toward states of integration, in which we maintain a coherent sense of self, both *inner* and *inter*. Mindsight, PART, and our social engagement system help us to understand how we create integrated relationships, allowing us to develop thriving relationships with family, friends, and romantic partners that are an expression of well-being.

Recognizing interconnection as a form of integration and a fundamental foundation of well-being, we should seek to enhance integration both within our inner lives and in our relational world. In IPNB, nine domains of integration are individually distinguished and can be used as a framework for promoting well-being through relational integration [16]. The domains of consciousness and interpersonal integration present opportunities to connect relationships, the embodied brain, and mind with practical tools for integration and well-being.

Integration of consciousness is necessary for change and the development of relational integration. Consciousness is the mental experience of knowing and the awareness of the known. Affective and cognitive processes arise within consciousness and allow us to separate our thoughts and feelings from who we are, thus creating a sense of agency and regulation. Practical applications include mindful awareness practices, such as mind-training [30], in which focused attention, open awareness, and kind intention are a catalyst for the experiences of consciousness [31]. Research has shown that where we focus our attention, new connections and pathways can form, thus, "where attention goes, neural firing flows, and neural connection grows" [23]. Through attention training, we join consciousness and attention, expanding the capacity for neuroplasticity [30]. The Wheel of Awareness (Figure 47.3) brings together several mind-training states and is a practical exercise that actively promotes integration through attention, a sense of connectedness, and the experience of being aware.

Interpersonal integration unfolds when the becoming of *we* does not mean the loss of *me*. When we see the mind as emerging from energy flow through our neural circuits and in our relationships with others, we understand that energy and our sense of self are both embodied and relational. Energy flow can take symbolic forms in which it re-presents – or represents – reality as information. Both embodied and relational energy flow can create symbolic meaning that links information processing across connections. Louis Cozolino [32] coined the term *social synapse* to refer to the neural circuitry reinforced through synaptic connection and communicative linkage. The shared experience at the neural level reveals that joint attention, the joining of minds through the relational focus of

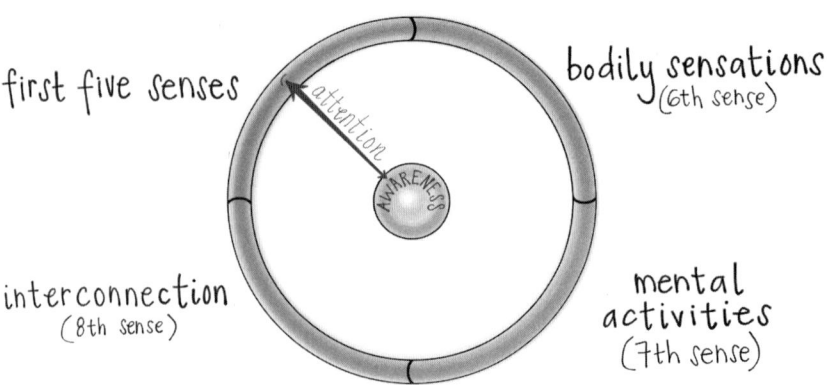

Figure 47.3 The Wheel of Awareness is a time-in mind-training practice that promotes integration through awareness, attention, and connectedness. Illustration by Madeleine W. Siegel as depicted in DJ Siegel, *Aware: The Science and Practice of Presence*. New York, TarcherPerigee; 2018. © 2018 Mind Your Brain, Inc. Used with permission from the author.

attention, can be truly integrative. In psychotherapy and medicine, the patient–clinician relationship may be integrative in the clinician's care for the patient's distress, and the empathic joy found in their progress and accomplishments that promote vitality and well-being [15]. Through this process, we join minds and come to *feel felt*, one of the most rewarding emotional states arising from our interpersonal integration. Some studies explore neural circuits and interpersonal connection focusing on neural coupling, or the communication system between two individuals in the shared environment [33]. The shared experience shapes our interpersonal connection, helping us to infer information about others and communicate successfully. Such findings highlight how relationships and interpersonal communication can connect individuals on a neurological basis. Therefore, the positive and lasting effects of shared experience promote new synaptic connections and open the door for more adaptive capacities to foster well-being in the future.

The Science of Family, Friends, and Love

Family Relations

We have explored how our bodies, brains, and minds respond to interactions with others, building a clear case for the linkage between our connection to others and our own personal well-being. Familial relationships are significant predictors of psychological health and well-being over the lifespan. At an early age, neurobiological processes are active and shaped by our relationships and attachments to help grow the neural networks in the brain [34]. Typically, this early attachment includes the secretion of the neurotransmitter oxytocin, which is known to facilitate social connection and bonding. An attachment figure interacts with the child through the sharing of energy and information flow. In early attachment, the caregiver can position their mind to have presence which, in turn, can facilitate a secure attachment. Secure attachment and parental presence from which it arises promote flexibility, self-regulation, prosocial behavior, empathy, a positive sense of emotional well-being and self-esteem, and a coherent life story – all functions that can be seen as an outcome of integration [35, 36]. Early relationships shape later functioning, as these early attachments provide the foundation for all future relationships. Secure parent–child attachment is associated with better social skills and higher-quality childhood friendships, while non-secure attachments can negatively impact children's social competence and functioning. Research has shown that secure parent–child attachment is predictive of high levels of well-being in adulthood [36, 37]. The National Centre for Social Research found that children and adolescents who have strong social relationships with peers and family endorsed a higher sense of well-being [2]. Research has also shown that a more predictive factor of a child's well-being than family structure is the quality of familial relationships, cohesion, and harmony [3]. Quality family relationships continue to contribute to well-being over the span of a lifetime.

Friendships

Friendships are also important across the lifespan. A large body of research has shown friendships to be central to overall well-being in children and adolescents [3], adults, and older adults [38]. A sense of belonging and connection in relationships tends to be indicative of positive functioning in many different domains. There is also a direct relationship between early secure attachment and social competencies later in life [35, 36]. As a result, in early childhood, children often establish the skills necessary to develop friendships into adulthood. Because science has found that friendships across the lifespan are indicative of well-being, it is crucial, when possible, to develop integrative relationships at an early age. However, neuroplasticity has shown that our brains can form new connections at any stage of our lives [39]. While it is ideal to form secure attachments and healthy connections in childhood, neuroplasticity provides us with the hopeful reality that change and growth are always possible. Thus, neuroplasticity is important when we consider the role of friendships as we and those with whom we work may need to form new relationships as life changes and evolves over time.

Love

Cultivating love in our early attachments and friendships helps prepare us for love in the context of romantic relationships. Healthy romantic love can be viewed as two self-regulating individuals, each with a sense of self, where the *me* or *I* maintain integrity amid the *we* or *us*. As previously discussed, this kind of healthy romantic relationship can be seen as a fruit salad rather than a smoothie. In the fruit salad, we can see all the individual parts that make up the whole, rather than them being blended together, and yet they are part of the single entity of the fruit salad. Thus, the two people in the relationship remain differentiated while linked together as a collective whole. John Gottman [40] suggests that transformation in a couple's relationship happens through emotional attunement, the ability for a couple to process challenging events and painful emotions in such a way that creates trust, resilience, awareness, understanding, and empathy in their relationship. Research has shown that being in a stable relationship is associated with better physical and physiological outcomes, such as lower stress, morbidity, and mortality [41, 42]. Similarly, for older adults, having a romantic relationship and love has been linked to a healthier and happier lifestyle, which, in turn, contributes to longevity [43]. In studying love, Helen Fisher [44] found that the same brain areas active in the use of cocaine were active in the experience of love. This finding showed that when we are in love, our reward system is activated and, in turn, releases oxytocin and vasopressin. Fisher posits that the drive for love is more powerful than the sex drive, and is deeply embedded in our human brain. Ruth Feldman [45], along with Shir Atzil and colleagues [46], reviewed how romantic relationships and our attachment connections involve circuitries of the social brain that go beyond our reward centers to include centers involved in regulating the body. These centers are also involved in sensing the mind of the self and other in what is called mentalizing or theory of mind, and are linked within our relational interconnection. Interpersonal neurobiology proposes that love is *integration made visible*.

Conclusion

The growing body of research on relationships suggests that individuals who feel interconnected to a broader community experience higher levels of well-being through their sense of social identity and connection. From one-on-one to our wider global communities, relational connections help create belonging and cohesion, which arise from a healthy state of integration. As clinicians, we can help create interconnection through our embodied compassionate awareness toward ourselves and others – coming to realize that the terms "self" and "other" can sometimes mislead us to forget our deep interconnected nature. Through our presence, we can skillfully join minds with our children, families, coworkers, friends, romantic partners, and communities.

We hope this chapter will motivate each of us to develop and enhance our connections to ourselves and the broader world of other human beings and nature that is all around us. Relationships with other people and the planet reflect and grow a state of healthy integration that can create well-being within ourselves and in the communities we serve. Through these kinds of interconnected relationships that allow for both linkage and differentiation, we can truly build a foundation for well-being across the lifespan.

To explore further, access www.DrDanSiegel.com.

References

1. World Health Organization. The constitution of the World Health Organization. 2019. www.who.int/about/who-we-are/constitution (accessed April 21, 2020).

2. J Chanfreau, C Lloyd, C Byron, et al. *Predicting Wellbeing*. London, NatCen Social Research; 2013.

3. Children's Society. The good childhood report, 2015. 2015. www.childrenssociety .org.uk/sites/default/files/TheGoodChildho odReport2015.pdf (accessed April 21, 2020).

4. JF Helliwell, R Layard, J Sachs, eds. *World Happiness Report 2015*. New York,

Sustainable Development Solutions Network; 2015.

5. E Diener, EM Suh. National differences in subjective well-being. In: D Kahneman, E Diener, N Schwarz, eds., *Well-Being: The Foundations of Hedonic Psychology*. New York, Russell Sage Foundation Publications; 2003; 434–450.

6. R Inglehart, C Haerpfer, A Moreno, et al. *World Values Survey: Round Six-Country-Pooled Datafile 2010–2014*. Madrid, JD Systems Institute; 2014.

7. J Helliwell, R Layard, J Sachs, eds., *World Happiness Report 2019*. New York, Sustainable Development Solutions Network; 2019.

8. J Holt-Lunstad, TB Smith, JB Layton. Social relationships and mortality risk: a meta-analytic review. *PLoS medicine* 2010; 7(7): e1000316.

9. E Blackburn, E Epel. *The Telomere Effect: A Revolutionary Approach to Living Younger, Healthier, Longer*. London, Hachette UK; 2017.

10. R Meier. Relationships: the missing link in public health. Relationships Alliance, 2013. https://tavistockrelationships.ac.uk/images/uploads/Relationships_-_the_missing_link_in_public_health_-_report_from_the_Relationships_Alliance.pdf (accessed February 29, 2020).

11. M Marmot, J Allen, P Goldblatt, et al. Fair society, healthy lives. The Marmot Review London 2010. www.instituteofhealthequity.org/resources-reports/fair-society-healthy-lives-the-marmot-review (accessed February 29, 2020).

12. LB Aknin, EW Dunn, MI Norton. Happiness runs in a circular motion: evidence for a positive feedback loop between prosocial spending and happiness. *J Happiness Stud* 2011; 13(2): 347–355.

13. W Hofmann, DC Wisneski, MJ Brandt, et al. Morality in everyday life. *Science* 2014; 345(6202): 1340–1343.

14. LB Aknin, CP Barrington-Leigh, EW Dunn, et al. Prosocial spending and well-being: cross-cultural evidence for a psychological universal. *J Pers Soc Psychol* 2013; 104(4): 635.

15. DJ Siegel. *Pocket Guide to Interpersonal Neurobiology: An Integrative Handbook of the Mind*. New York, WW Norton; 2012.

16. DJ Siegel. *The Developing Mind* (3rd ed.) New York, Guilford Press; 2020.

17. P Alasuutari. Theorizing in qualitative research: a cultural studies perspective. *Qualitat Inquiry* 1996; 2(4): 371–384.

18. DJ Siegel. *Mind: A Journey to the Heart of Being Human*. New York, WW Norton; 2016.

19. D Rakel, B Barrett, Z Zhang, et al. Perception of empathy in the therapeutic encounter: effects on the common cold. *Patient Educ Couns* 2011; 85(3): 390–397.

20. G Chierchia, T Singer. The neuroscience of compassion and empathy and their link to prosocial motivation and behavior. In: J-C Dreher, L Tremblay, eds., *Decision Neuroscience*. New York, Academic Press; 2017; 247–257.

21. OM Klimecki, S Leiberg, C Lamm, et al. Functional neural plasticity and associated changes in positive affect after compassion training. *Cerebral Cortex* 2012; 23(7): 1552–1561.

22. D Lama, D Tutu. *The Book of Joy: Lasting Happiness in a Changing World*. New York, Avery, an Imprint of Penguin Random House; 2016.

23. DJ Siegel. *AWARE: The Science and Practice of Presence*. New York, TarcherPerigee; 2018.

24. DJ Siegel. *Mindsight: The New Science of Personal Transformation*. New York, Bantam; 2010.

25. SM Smith, TE Nichols, D Vidaurre, et al. Positive–negative mode of population covariation links brain connectivity, demographics and behavior. *Nature Neurosci* 2015; 18(11): 1565.

26. DJ Siegel. *The Mindful Therapist: A Clinician's Guide to Mindsight and Neural Integration*. New York, WW Norton; 2010.

27. J Panksepp, L Biven. *The Archaeology of Mind: Neuroevolutionary Origins of Human Emotions*. New York, WW Norton; 2012.

28. SW Porges. *The Polyvagal Theory: Neurophysiological Foundations of Emotions, Attachment, Communication, and Self-Regulation*. New York, WW Norton; 2011.

29. SM Geller. *A Practical Guide to Cultivating Therapeutic Presence*. Washington, DC, American Psychological Association; 2017.

30. D Goleman, RJ Davidson. *Altered Traits: Science Reveals How Meditation Changes Your Mind, Brain, and Body.* New York, Penguin; 2017.

31. A Villamil, T Vogel, E Weisbaum, et al. Cultivating well-being through the three pillars of mind training: understanding how training the mind improves physiological and psychological well-being. *OBM Integr Complement Med* 2019; 4(1).

32. L Cozolino. *The Neuroscience of Human Relationships: Attachment and the Developing Social Brain.* New York, WW Norton; 2014.

33. U Hasson, AA Ghazanfar, B Galantucci, et al. Brain-to-brain coupling: a mechanism for creating and sharing a social world. *Trends Cogn Sci* 2012; 16(2): 114–121.

34. AN Schore. *Affect Regulation and the Origin of the Self: The Neurobiology of Emotional Development.* New York, Routledge; 2015.

35. M Main. The organized categories of infant, child, and adult attachment: flexible vs. inflexible attention under attachment-related stress. *J Am Psychoanal Assoc* 2000; 48(4): 1055–1096.

36. LA Sroufe. The coherence of individual development: early care, attachment, and subsequent developmental issues. *Am Psychol* 1979; 34(10): 834.

37. J Bowlby. *A Secure Base: Parent–Child Attachment and Healthy Human Development.* New York, Basic Books; 2008.

38. Mental Health Foundation. *Relationships in the 21st Century.* London, Mental Health Foundation; 2016.

39. N Doidge. *The Brain that Changes Itself: Stories of Personal Triumph from the Frontiers of Brain Science.* New York, Penguin; 2007.

40. JM Gottman. *The Science of Trust: Emotional Attunement for Couples.* New York, WW Norton; 2011.

41. J Holt-Lunstad, W Birmingham, BQ Jones. Is there something unique about marriage? The relative impact of marital status, relationship quality, and network social support on ambulatory blood pressure and mental health. *Ann Behav Med* 2008; 35(2): 239–244.

42. TF Robles, RB Slatcher, JM Trombello, et al. Marital quality and health: a meta-analytic review. *Psychol Bull* 2014; 140(1): 140.

43. BA Bloem, TG Tilburg, F Thomese. Changes in older Dutch adults' role networks after moving. *Pers Relatsh* 2008; 15(4): 465–478.

44. H Fisher. *Why We Love: The Nature and Chemistry of Romantic Love.* Basingstoke, Macmillan; 2004.

45. R Feldman. The neurobiology of human attachments. *Trends Cogn Sci* 2017; 21(2): 80–99.

46. S Atzil, W Gao, I Fradkin, et al. Growing a social brain. *Nat Hum Behav* 2018; 2: 624–636.

Chapter

48

The Role of Leisure, Recreation, and Play in Health and Well-Being

Laura L. Payne and Jaesung An

Introduction

According to a 40-year panel study by Robinson and Godbey [1], most Americans have an average of 40 hours of leisure time per week, outside of work and personal maintenance (e.g., sleeping, eating, bathing). While initially this was encouraging news, it has been disputed, and Robinson and Godbey [1] report that much of that time is spent watching television, which is a vicarious passive activity. The person is being acted upon, instead of being the actor in the experience. As the prevalence of chronic conditions continues to rise (including overweight, obesity, diabetes, and other lifestyle diseases), people are busier than ever, trying to maximize their time through multitasking, which adds to the perception of time famine, or the feeling we never have enough time. Max Weber's axiom "we live to work" still rings true in contemporary society [2]. However, at what cost to our health and well-being? As theologian philosopher Josef Pieper [3] emphasized, we need to strive for a world where we work to live. Or at least to strive for a balance between these two perspectives. In response to technology, however, many people have embraced screen time over coffee socials, and mega-multiplayer online games over vigorous games of tag and other yard games. However, a shift is needed back toward increasing leisure, recreation and play in our lives. Rather than six or more hours per day of television and screen time (e.g., smartphones, social media, Internet browsing), people should increase their engagement in meaningful and enjoyable leisure activities. Thus, the purpose of this chapter is to highlight the role of leisure, recreation, and play in improving and maintaining one's health and well-being.

Because leisure is defined as freely chosen, intrinsically motivated, meaningful, and enjoyable experience, it is the life context in which we have the greatest opportunity to shape our health (Figure 48.1) [4–6]. Leisure activities are those experiences people do for stress relief and attention restoration, social support, joy, and pleasure, among others. In this chapter, the concepts of leisure, recreation, and play are defined and their associations with health and well-being are discussed. Then, we provide evidence from a large body of research that illustrates how leisure, recreation, and play are associated with health in the following contexts: (1) for stress coping and the prevention and management of chronic disease; (2) social and emotional health; (3) life transitions; and (4) how parks and open space can facilitate physical, socioemotional, and cognitive health. These topics only scratch the surface of the many roles that leisure, recreation, and play have in health; for further reading, please see the book *Leisure, Health and Wellness: Making the Connections*, edited by Laura Payne, Geoffrey Godbey, and Barbara Ainsworth [7].

Leisure is often thought of as "free time" or time away from work, in which a person is intrinsically motivated to engage in a personally meaningful activity that is enjoyable [8]. Another hallmark of leisure is that to truly be a leisure experience, which emphasizes one's

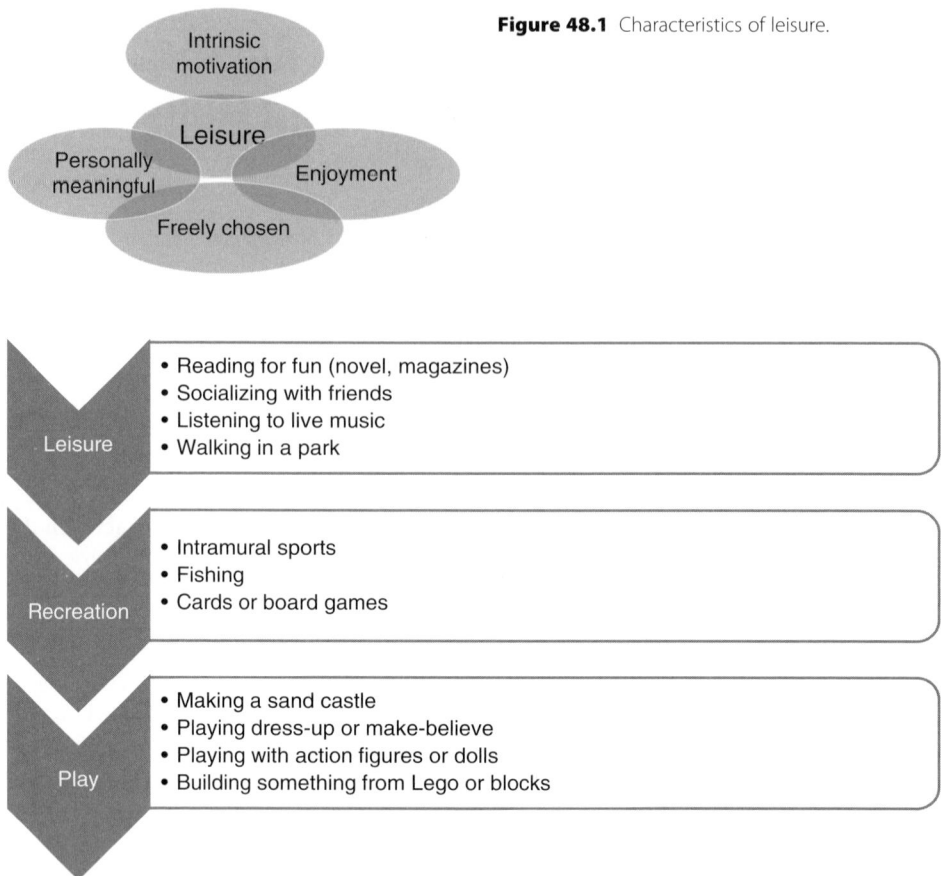

Figure 48.1 Characteristics of leisure.

Figure 48.2 Leisure, recreation, and play examples.

state of mind while engaged in it, the activity should be freely chosen. A number of leisure scholars and philosophers have emphasized the importance of these characteristics of leisure. However, leisure is also subjective, meaning that the person who is doing it can decide if it is leisure or not, given the characteristics mentioned above [9–11]. While there are various definitions of recreation and play, many leisure scholars agree that recreation tends to be organized and have some rules, whereas play is more spontaneous, with rules that are flexible, changing, or absent, and creativity is encouraged [12, 13]. Play is more open-ended, and often begins and ends without respect to a schedule [13]. Enjoyment is a common thread among leisure, recreation, and play. Examples of leisure include walking in a park, reading a book, or having coffee with a friend. Recreation can include an organized bridge club gathering, intramural basketball, or trivia nights at a local restaurant or pub. Play might include building sandcastles and other things at the beach, a jazz jam session highlighted by improvisation, or playing with Lego. More examples of leisure, recreation, and play are described in Figure 48.2. Thus, leisure, recreation and play are important experiences that can enhance individual health and well-being, improve social and emotional health, and be a context for learning, challenge, and a sense of accomplishment [5, 6]. They can also be an important resource and context for building understanding between and among groups from different backgrounds (e.g., socioeconomic, race/ethnicity, gender, age, culture), thereby assisting with social health and well-being [14, 15]. Thus, as aptly asserted by philosophers such as Huizinga [2] and Pieper [3], leisure and play are vitally important to culture and society, all of which have the potential to benefit our health and well-being.

Leisure, Stress Coping, and Chronic Disease Prevention/ Management

Leisure has consistently been identified as a significant resource, facilitating people to positively and effectively cope with the "negatives" in life, including stress [16]. As multiple stress researchers have also emphasized the importance of leisure in stress coping, findings from numerous studies indicate that leisure and recreation (especially outdoor and nature-based) are important to buffer and manage stress. Leisure-generated social support (i.e., companionship/friendship) and self-determination disposition (i.e., autonomy, competence, relatedness), for instance, buffer the adverse effects of stress on physical and mental health problems [17]. In particular, nature-based outdoor recreation has been shown to reduce negative feelings (e.g., anxiety) and promote positive mood, therefore reducing the level of perceived stress [5]. Chronic diseases certainly account for major and common barriers to people's quality of life. The prevalence of chronic health conditions is especially high among older adults, as over 85 percent of the older adult population report having at least one chronic disease [18]. Participating in leisure activities may enable people of all ages to remain physically, socially, and mentally active. For older adults, leisure engagement allows them to express their strengths and enduring interests. It also provides opportunities for older adults to maintain or improve their physical and mental health. For instance, physically active leisure has been associated with enhanced independence, longevity, and improved cognitive and physical functioning for older adults with chronic conditions [19, 20]. Also, leisure engagement may serve as a positive distraction from their ongoing health conditions, thereby improving their affect and fostering hope [16].

The experience of chronic disease is often associated with elevated stress. When these two are mingled together in a vicious cycle, it can have a severe impact on people's quality of life. Participating in valued leisure activities can add purpose and meaning to their lives. Having a greater sense of control and regaining meaning in life provide important benefits in coping with and managing both chronic conditions and stress over the long-term [21].

Social and Emotional Health

The social and emotional benefits of leisure have been studied fairly extensively across the lifespan. An overview of major contributions is presented in this chapter. As early as the late 1800s, the social and emotional well-being of urban working-class citizens was the focus of significant social programs. Jane Addams established a community center in Chicago that strived to improve residents' health, family (e.g., daycare for working mothers), educational, environmental, and recreational opportunities [22]. Working with supporters, Addams carried out programs with a strong social justice focus that improved the socioemotional health and quality of life of hard-working Chicagoans.

Post-World War II was marked by the rapid expansion of community parks and recreation systems across the USA, which made more parks, programs, and facilities available to residents across income levels, ethnicity/race, and life stages. Due to interest by developmental psychologists, more research on the value of play in childhood was conducted. Children's play is vitally important to social and emotional development, as evidenced by the significant body of knowledge created by scholars such as Lynn Barnett [23]. Play was shown to facilitate motor abilities, socioemotional skills (e.g., sharing, empathy, conflict resolution), cognitive development (e.g., logical thinking, problem-solving, executive functioning skills), and more [13, 23]. In adolescence and emerging adulthood, leisure can be seen as an obstacle to development, particularly in the context of risky leisure (e.g., sexual risk-taking, substance-use/abuse), and a facilitator of healthy development [24, 25]. Compounded by high dropout rates in sport among girls, combined with cuts in extracurricular activities, now more than ever adolescents and emerging adults need positive activities and social experiences to further enhance socioemotional learning and development [26]. Researchers largely agree that young people with high self-determination (comprised of perceived competence, relatedness, and autonomy) will navigate malaise or amotivation in free time to engage in meaningful and satisfying leisure [27]. While women's socioemotional health has been well examined [28, 29], the leisure lives of middle-aged people and men have largely been overlooked [30, 31]. However, midlife is a time rife with caregiving (e.g., children, parents), careers, and household and civic responsibilities. A longitudinal study on leisure among adults provided important insights as to how values and identities are maintained and developed through leisure [31]. Carpenter et al.'s findings suggested that many midlife events may lead to structure building or structure changing, thereby affecting leisure values, patterns, and identity. Overall, across the 10-year study, they found more stability than change in leisure values over time, despite life events, and characterized the changes as smaller adjustments [31].

Although many women report feeling constraints to engaging in leisure, research also suggests leisure is important for enhancing social support and coping with midlife challenges (e.g., menopause), empowerment, and improving health [32–35]. For example, in her study of dragon boat racing, Parry found that breast cancer survivors involved in this activity reported more physical activity, improved social support, and a more positive outlook, in addition to having fun [29]. In contrast, Henderson examined women's leisure within a family context and found that their leisure was constrained by daily activities and caregiving, which led to the notion that "a women's work is never done" [33]. Rather than experiencing leisure within the family, these women were more focused on caregiving and family responsibilities, thus compromising their experience of leisure.

Leisure and Managing Life Transitions

People navigate a variety of changes and transitions throughout the lifespan. Whether it is involuntary retirement, caregiving for children and aging parents, or the transition from high school to college or work, transitions can be disruptive, but are also important to identity development and self-concept [36]. Transitions can constrain or change one's leisure or they can facilitate growth and exploration in leisure. For example, Nimrod studied older people's leisure patterns after retirement and found that some people add new activities to their repertoires [37]. However, she found that adding (i.e., innovating) depended on some factors such as health, work history, and whether the retirement decision was voluntary. Nimrod recognized this experience as a form of innovation in later life, which is contrary to past studies that suggest people cease or reduce leisure activities as they age [37]. While ceasing activities is often touted as having negative effects on health and quality of life, Kleiber et al. purported that selective disengagement from activities could be beneficial for people as they age [38]. They asserted that in later life, people's functional abilities change and their social worlds often shrink to meet the changing demands of their abilities within their environments. Thus, achieving more benefits by doing less might be a way to conserve energy and maximize meaning and enjoyment as we age.

Although later life is associated with a number of transitions, other stages of development involve transitions that affect leisure and health. For example, Raymore studied the leisure patterns of adolescents who transitioned to college [39]. Using data from the Michigan Study of Adolescent Life Transitions (MSALT), they found males and females maintained some continuity in their leisure from high school to college, but males were more physically active than females in college. This has important implications for physical health and mental health (e.g., stress coping, social support). In fact, Bland et al. surveyed 900 college students about stress tolerance and activity [40]. They found a significant relationship between engagement in leisure and physical activity and stress tolerance. Moreover, Vankim and Nelson found that individuals who met the US Centers for Disease Control and Prevention (CDC) physical activity guidelines reported better mental health than college students who did not meet CDC physical activity standards [41]. Social activity partially mediated the relationship between physical activity, stress, and perceived mental health, which highlights the value of social engagement on health.

Other transitions that can disrupt leisure and health include the onset of chronic disease and traumatic health events. For example, in a study of older adults with arthritis, Janke et al. found that the participants use a variety of self-regulation strategies to maintain involvement in valued leisure activities [42]. These included conserving energy, seizing the moment, modifying leisure to maintain engagement, and using assistive devices/aids to continue participating.

In their study of life after a traumatic event, Kleiber et al. examined the role of leisure in the experiences of people who lost a loved one unexpectedly, acquired a significant disability, or experienced a major natural disaster [16]. They suggested pleasant events such as leisure are important for helping people cope with these transitions in four ways: (1) Leisure can provide a buffer by being a positive distraction from the situation/event; (2) the distractions can make space for more positive emotions that lead to hope [43], and thus leisure can facilitate transformation and recasting oneself in the wake of the event; (3) this transformation is aided by leisure, which helps a person create a future that continues from one's past; and (4) this positions leisure as a mechanism of transformation. For example, a man with a spinal cord injury from a car accident could find a new way to express himself through painting and adapted sport, rather than doing triathlons.

Parks, Green Space, and Health

Environmental psychologists, landscape architects, planners, and parks and natural resource researchers have long been interested in understanding the health benefits associated with parks and green space. In an early study, Ulrich compared the recovery of people whose hospital rooms had a view of nature with individuals whose rooms had no view [44]. He found that individuals with a view recovered faster than those without a view, controlling for the type of surgery. The need for nearby nature became more urgent as two issues collided: alarmingly low rates of physical activity and the overbuilding of cities, which left residents with little green space or green views [6]. Since the 1990s, many researchers have documented the health outcomes associated with parks and green space. Much of this research suggests having a park within walking distance is important to facilitate park use, that parks provide opportunities for physical activity, and that people are physically active in parks, in addition to important benefits such as stress relief, attention restoration, social interaction, awe, and spiritual contemplation [45]. While parks and nature are important for promoting health and physical activity, many urban and rural communities lack sufficient access to parks, underscoring the need for more equitable distribution of parks and natural areas [6].

The value of green space and parks has been emphasized by studies of urban greenness. For example, Kuo and Sullivan compared people who lived in Chicago Public Housing buildings with adjacent green space to those surrounded by little greenery and mostly concrete [46]. They found that residents with more green space surrounding their building had significantly lower feelings of aggression and better attention restoration than people whose housing lacked nearby nature. These authors suggested that mental fatigue is associated with more aggressive dispositions and behavior, and that nearby nature could help restore attention, thereby reducing aggression.

In order to better understand how restorative natural environments are compared to other settings, Hartig et al. randomly assigned people to three conditions: (1) a walk in the park, (2) a walk in an urban environment, and (3) relaxing in a chair [47]. They induced cognitive fatigue and then led each participant in a 40-minute experience. A comparison of pre- and posttest results indicated that the nature environment group reported significantly higher happiness scores, more positive affect, and lower anger and aggression scores than either the urban walk or chair relaxation. This suggests the park environment was more restorative than the urban or relaxing environments. Further, from a policy standpoint, the importance of parks for health has been underscored by recent initiatives such as healthcare professionals making "park prescriptions," the Walk with a Doc program, the Healthy Parks Healthy People program, and the National Park Service's "Find your Park" campaign.

Conclusion

Leisure, recreation, and play contribute to health and well-being across the lifespan. The variety of ways leisure is associated with health are extensive and too diverse to address in one chapter. Since leisure is intrinsically motivated, freely chosen, and an enjoyable activity, it has great potential as a life context for shaping our health and quality of life. Thus, this chapter focused on ways leisure can be used for stress coping and the prevention and management of chronic diseases. Settings such as parks and natural areas are also important to promote health and can be physically, cognitively, and emotionally restorative. Leisure is also important for social and emotional health and is a key component to effectively manage life transitions. Across the lifespan, leisure is an important context for healthy development and contributes to quality of life.

References

1. JP Robinson, GC Godbey. *Time for Life: The Surprising Ways Americans Use Time.* University Park, PA, Pennsylvania State University Press; 1999.

2. J Huizinga. *Homo Ludens: A Study of the Play Element in Culture.* Boston, MA, Beacon Press; 1950.

3. J Pieper. *Leisure: The Basis of Culture.* New York, Pantheon Books; 1952.

4. L Caldwell. Leisure and health: why is leisure therapeutic? *Br J Guid Counc* 2005; **33**: 7–26.

5. L Caldwell, E Smith. Leisure: an overlooked component of health promotion. *Can J Public Health* 1988; **79**: S44–S48.

6. G Godbey, L Caldwell, M Floyd, L Payne. Implications from leisure studies and recreation and park management research for active living. *Am J Prev Med* 2005; **28**: 150–158.

7. L Payne, G Godbey, B Ainsworth., eds. *Leisure, Health and Wellness: Making the Connections.* State College, PA, Venture Publishing; 2010.

8. S Iso-Ahola. Basic dimensions of definitions of leisure. *J Leis Res* 1979; **11**: 28–39.

9. DM Samdahl. Issues in the measurement of leisure: a comparison of theoretical and connotative meanings. *Leis Sci* 1991; **13**: 33–49.

10. HEA Tinsley, DJ Tinsley. A theory of the attributes, benefits, and causes of leisure experience. *Leis Sci* 1986; **8**: 1–45.

11. DA Kleiber, GJ Walker, RC Mannell. *A Social Psychology of Leisure.* State College, PA, Venture Publishing; 2011.

12. J Piaget. *Play, Dreams and Imitation in Childhood.* Boston, MA, Beacon Publishing; 1962.

13. L Payne, L Barnett. Leisure and recreation across the lifespan. In: T Tapps, MS Wells, eds., *Introduction to Leisure and Recreation.* Champaign, IL, Human Kinetics; 2006; 229–250.

14. JWR Baur, E Gomez, JF Tynan. Urban nature parks and neighborhood social health in Portland, Oregon. *J Park Rec Admin* 2013; **31**: 23–44.

15. TD Glover, DC Parry, KJ Shinew. Building relationships, accessing resources: mobilizing social capital in community garden contexts. *J Leis Res* 2005; **37**: 450–474.

16. DA Kleiber, SL Hutchinson, R Williams. Leisure as a resource in transcending negative life events: self-protection, self-restoration, and personal transformation. *Lei Sci* 2002; **24**: 219–235.

17. SE Iso-Ahola, CJ Park. Leisure-related social support and self-determination as buffers of stress–illness relationship. *J Leis Res* 1996; **28**: 169–187.

18. C Hoffman, D Rice, HY Sung. Persons with chronic conditions: their prevalence and costs. *JAMA* 1996; **276**: 1473–1479.

19. EM Orsega-Smith, LL Payne, AJ Mowen, CH Ho, GC Godbey. The role of social support and self-efficacy in shaping the leisure time physical activity of older adults. *J Leis Res* 2007; **39**: 705–727.

20. P Lampinen, RL Heikkinen, M Kauppinen, E Heikkinen. Activity as a predictor of mental well-being among older adults. *Aging Ment Health* 2006; **10**: 454–466.

21. J McQuoid. Finding joy in poor health: the leisure-scapes of chronic illness. *Soc Sci Med* 2017; **183**: 88–96.

22. CR Edginton, DJ Jordan, DG DeGraaf, SR Edginton. *Leisure and Life Satisfaction: Foundational Perspectives.* New York, McGraw-Hill; 2002.

23. LA Barnett. Developmental benefits of play for children. *J Leis Res* 1990; **22**: 138–153.

24. L Berdychevsky. Antecedents of young women's sexual risk taking in tourist experiences. *J Sex Res* 2016; **53**: 927–941.

25. C Watts, JL Cremeens. Leisure, adolescence and health. In: L Payne, B Ainsworth, G Godbey, eds., *Leisure, Health, and Wellness: Making the Connections.* State College, PA, Venture Publishing; 2010; 213–226.

26. LB Ransdell, DL Schmalz. Healthy sports. In: L Payne, B Ainsworth, G Godbey, eds., *Leisure, Health, and Wellness: Making the Connections.* State College, PA, Venture Publishing; 2010; 425–435.

27. CE Watts, LL Caldwell. Self-determination and free time activity participation as predictors of initiative. *J Leis Res* 2008; **40**: 156–181.

28. KA Henderson, WJ Brown. Leisure, health and leisure: a lot like music making. In: L Payne, B Ainworth, G Godbey, eds., *Leisure, Health, and Wellness: Making the Connections*. State College, PA, Venture Publishing; 2010; 305–312.

29. DC Parry. There is life after breast cancer: nine vignettes exploring dragon boat racing for breast cancer survivors. *Leis Sci* 2007; **29**: 53–69.

30. K Broughton, L Payne, T Liechty. An exploration of older men's social lives and well-being in the context of a coffee group. *Leis Sci* 2017; **39**: 261–276.

31. J Stockton, G Carpenter, LR Kahle. Continuity and change in values in midlife: testing the age stability hypothesis. *Exp Aging Res* 2014; **40**: 224–244.

32. R Deem. *All Work and No Play? The Sociology of Women and Leisure*. Milton Keynes, Open University Press; 1986.

33. KA Henderson. Broadening and understanding of women, gender and leisure. *J Leis Res* 1994; **26**: 1–7.

34. DC Parry, SM Shaw. The role of leisure in women's experience of menopause in mid-life. *Leis Sci* 1999; **21**: 205–218.

35. CM Yarnal, G Chick, DL Kerstetter. "I did not have time to play growing up . . . so this is my play time. It's the best thing I have ever done for myself": what is play to older women? *Leis Sci* 2008; **30**: 235–252.

36. M Janke, A Davey, D Kleiber. Modeling change in older adults' leisure activities. *Leis Sci* 2006; **28**: 285–303.

37. G Nimrod. In support of innovation theory: innovation in activity patterns and life satisfaction among recently retired individuals. *Ageing Soc* 2008; **28**: 831–846.

38. D Kleiber, FA Maguire, B Ayber-Damali, W Norman. Having more by doing less: the paradox of leisure constraints in later life. *J Leis Res* 2008; **40**: 343–359.

39. LA Raymore, BL Barber, JS Eccles, GC Godbey. Leisure behavior pattern stability during the transition from adolescence to young adulthood. *J Youth Adol* 1999; **28**: 79–103.

40. HW Bland, BF Melton, LE Bigham, PD Welle. Quantifying the impact of physical activity on stress tolerance in college students. *Coll Stud J* 2014; **48**: 559–568.

41. NA Vankim, TF Nelson. Vigorous physical activity, mental health, perceived stress and socializing among college students. *Am J Health Promot* 2013; **28**: 7–15.

42. MC Janke, JJ Jones, LL Payne, JS Son. Living with arthritis: using self-management of valued activities to promote health. *Qual Health Res* 2012; **22**: 360–372.

43. RS Lazarus. *Stress and Emotion: A New Synthesis*. New York, Springer; 1999.

44. R Ulrich. View through a window may influence recovery from surgery. *Science* 1984; **224**: 420–421.

45. L Payne, E Orsega-Smith, G Godbey, M Roy. The relationship between personal health and park use among adults 50 and over: results of an exploratory study. *J Park Rec Admin* 2005; **23**: 1–20.

46. FE Kuo, WC Sullivan. Aggression and violence in the innter city: effects of environment via mental fatigue. *Environ Behav* 2011; **33**: 543–571.

47. T Hartig, M Mang, GW Evans. Restorative effects of natural environment experiences. *Environ Behav* 1991; **23**: 3–26.

Chapter 49

Wellness and Whole-Person Care

Tom A. Hutchinson and Nora Hutchinson

Introduction

Whole-person care is medical or other care that includes separating the person from the problem, taking measures to cure or prevent the problem or disease, and facilitating and supporting healing [1]. This is the approach to wellness taken in this chapter. There are three ways to imagine whole-person care interventions that might affect wellness.

The first is the reductionist approach that divides a whole person into their many component parts, identifies the location of the problem that is interfering with wellness, and takes appropriate measures to alleviate or fix the problem. There is a lot to be said for this approach. If I have a toothache that is interfering with my sense of wellness, I want that problem identified and fixed. I would want a physician or other healthcare professional caring for me to be able to deliver this kind of care or to refer me to someone who could deliver this care.

The second approach to wellness interventions is to use preventive measures aimed at the whole body [2]. These would include many of the approaches discussed in this book, such as nutrition, exercise, sleep, meditation, and so on. They are not aimed at fixing a particular problem, but aim to prevent problems and are good for the body as a whole. These are almost always a good idea and are part, but not the most important part, of whole-person care.

The third and most important part of whole-person care is interventions aimed at the whole person. These, we believe, are the most powerful determinants of wellness but surprisingly are sometimes directly opposed to interventions in the first two categories. An example will clarify the difference. In Vienna during World War II the Nazis were invading Austria. Viktor Frankl, a Jewish physician who was living in Vienna, was quite aware of the risks to him and his family. He applied for and was granted a visa to the USA. His family encouraged him to take the visa as this would preserve his life and presumably contribute to his wellness compared to the likely alternative – suffering and possibly death in a concentration camp. Frankl decided to stay in order to do what he could to care for and protect his family. He was unsuccessful. He and all of his family were transported to concentration camps. Frankl was the only one who survived. As illustrated in the film *The Choice Is Yours* [3], we would contend that Frankl made the choice most likely to contribute to his long-term wellness despite the terrible suffering he subsequently experienced. To understand this reasoning, we need to look more closely at what wellness is and how it relates to happiness and quality of life.

Happiness and Wellness

The simplest frame for wellness is to equate wellness with experienced happiness. In this formulation, when we are feeling happy we are well. It does not take much reflection to realize that this formulation does not always work. Ryan and Huta provide illustrative examples of a drug addict with a good supply of drugs or a person with bipolar disorder in the manic phase [4]. In both of these situations an individual may feel very well, but few would accept these as good examples of true wellness.

We need to delve a little deeper to arrive at a better definition of wellness. In their article on subjective well-being in aging, Steptoe et al. outline three types of subjective well-being: (1) hedonic well-being, (2) evaluative well-being – which can be equated with life satisfaction, and (3) eudaimonic well-being [5]. Wellness, in this formulation, involves our feelings and emotions (hedonic), our perceptions and expectations about life (evaluative), and our true longings and purpose in life (eudaimonic). These elements are also reflected in Virginia Satir's iceberg model of the whole person [6].

The Iceberg Model of the Whole Person

Given the complexity of human beings, we have found the iceberg metaphor a very helpful way to understand ourselves as whole persons. The components of the iceberg are shown in Figure 49.1. Above the water is what is visible to an outside observer: a person's appearance, speech, actions, and so on. However, there is a lot going on beneath the surface.

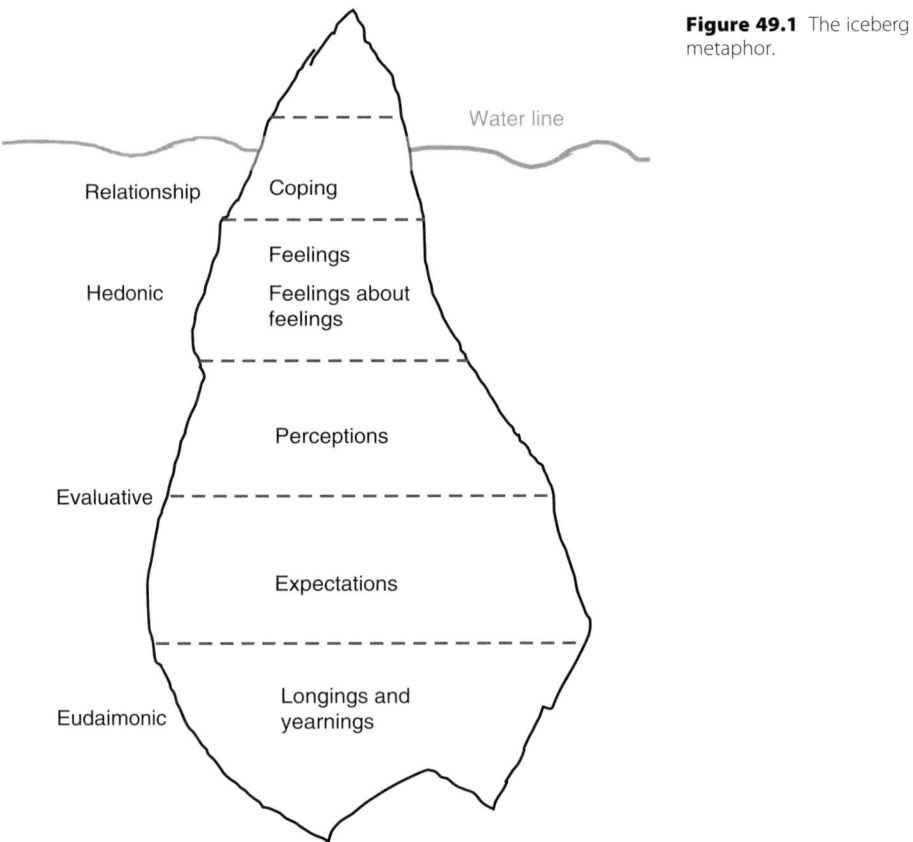

Figure 49.1 The iceberg metaphor.

Coping Stances

The first layer, labeled coping, is the stance that the person has taken toward the world or another person with whom they are relating, and constitutes our relationship well-being. In any such interaction, there are three components: self, other, and context. Satir, the originator of the iceberg metaphor, has pointed out that unconsciously, particularly under stress, we tend to omit one or more of these elements [7], resulting in the stances shown in Figure 49.2. In the placating stance we leave out ourselves; in the blaming stance the other person; in the super-reasonable stance the self as a person and the other person as a person; and in the distracting stance we lose touch with all three elements. The ideal stance according to Satir is congruence, in which we remain in contact with all three elements [8].

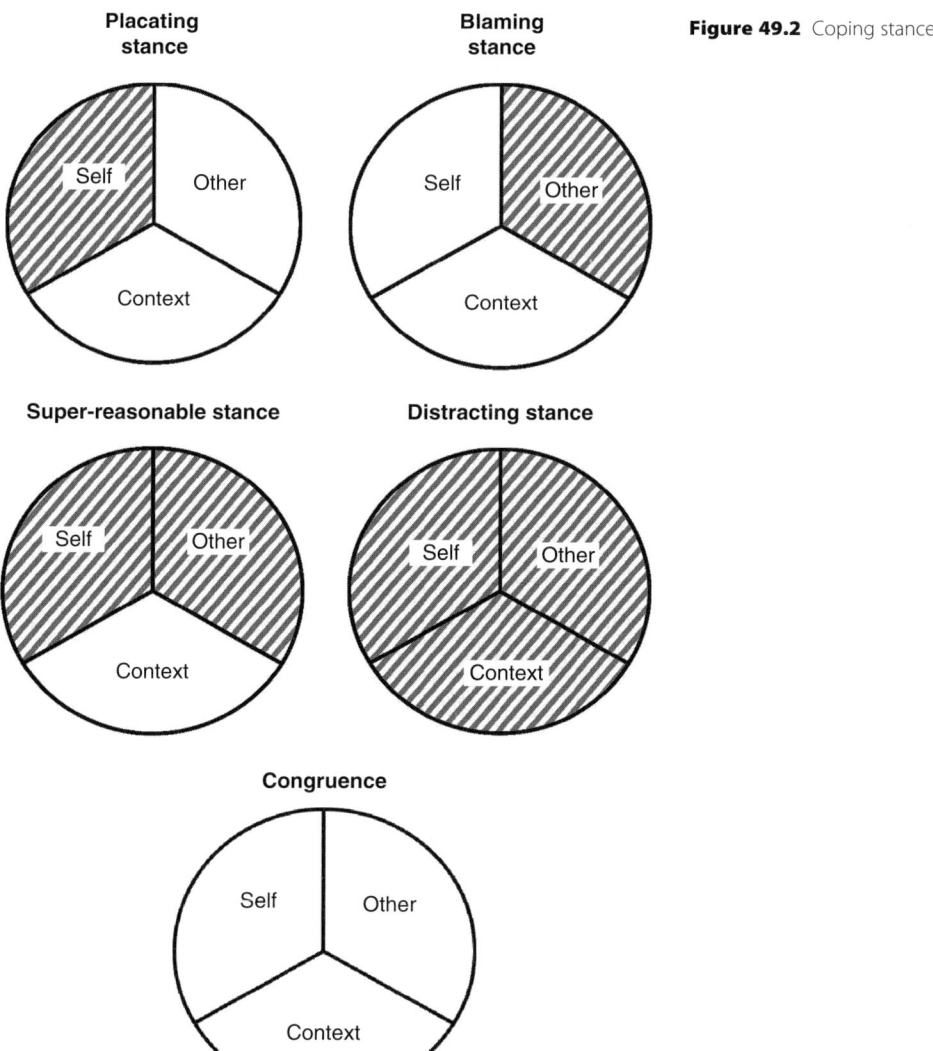

Figure 49.2 Coping stances.

Feelings and Feelings about Feelings

The layer below the coping stances deals with feelings, and feelings about feelings, and this constitutes our hedonic well-being. We all have feelings such as sadness, anger, fear, and so on, and it is probably our feelings about our feelings that primarily determine our coping stance. In placating, we suppress our feelings; in blaming, we project our feelings; in the super-reasonable stance, we deny our feelings; in the distracting stance, we distract ourselves from our feelings. When we are congruent, we are present to and accept our feelings and the feelings about our feelings.

Perceptions and Expectations

The layer below our feelings is our perceptions: the meaning we give to the world and what is happening. Below perceptions are the expectations that we have of the world, ourselves, and other people. Our expectations also help frame our perceptions.

Expectations usually contain a "should" or implied "should." At the simplest level, if something happens or someone does something that we do not think should happen, our perception will likely be that something has gone wrong or a mistake has been made. Another person with different expectations might see it completely differently. Perceptions and expectations correspond to our evaluative well-being, and they are also the primary drivers of our feelings.

Longings and Yearnings

Below our expectations is the deepest layer of the iceberg, our longings and yearnings. These are sometimes difficult to articulate, but are the source of our energy and aliveness. They include such longings as to be loved, to love, to be acknowledged, to make a difference. Our longings and yearnings provide meaning and purpose to life. Our eudaimonic well-being is contingent upon deep presence to our longings and yearnings.

The Iceberg as a Tool in Wellness: An Example

Longings and Yearnings (Eudaimonic Wellness)

To see how the iceberg metaphor might clarify wellness, let us take a medical student who has just begun intense clinical rotations. We will start at the deepest layer of the iceberg, the longings and yearnings. This student, like many medical students, longs to help and to provide care to those in need, to be valued and appreciated, to be part of a team with laudable common goals, probably to be loved. Our student may or may not be in touch with her yearnings. Many students either before entering medical school or in the first few years have learned to shelve or suppress their yearnings as being inappropriate, unrealistic, possibly embarrassing to admit to themselves. The first step toward wellness might be allowing herself to acknowledge and validate her longings, which will provide energy for the rest of the iceberg and is the foundation for eudaimonic wellness.

Expectations and Perceptions (Evaluative Wellness)

This student's expectations are to become part of a medical system that enacts the values of curing and empathy, and to combine these values with the expertise that she has learned in lectures and small groups early in medical school. She may find that the day-to-day experience in the hospital bears very little relationship to what she expected. Physicians are often rushed, don't appear caring and empathetic, sometimes mistreat patients and others, including students, may even at times be completely inappropriate or abusive. This may cause our student to conclude that medicine has no place for the kind of doctor she wants to be. She may decide that she no longer wishes to pursue a medical career, or if she does continue, that she needs to give up the values of empathy and caring and join what appears to be an uncaring and somewhat mechanical medical system. There is obviously a severe risk to wellness here that may take considerable effort to resolve. The risk is that our student may give up the values with which she entered medical school and thus inevitably forgo successfully helping people in need, which is probably the primary satisfaction of a life in medicine. Our student will need to find ways to act on her values, to find parts of the system and mentors who will support that way of being, and take some control of her own trajectory through the medical system in order to experience long-term evaluative wellness.

Feelings and Feelings about Feelings (Hedonic Wellness)

Our student's feelings may be of fear (that she will be crushed by the system), anger (at the system and people within it who have failed to meet her expectations), sadness (at the unaddressed suffering that she sees), guilt and shame (that she is somehow to blame), and possibly other feelings. She will probably have feelings about these feelings. These might include shame for feeling this way, fear that her feelings may become known to others and possibly affect her evaluations and progress in the system. She may decide to suppress her feelings, which may appear to be a good solution but will probably interfere with her hedonic wellness. In the long run the best approach for wellness would be to allow herself to feel her feelings even if they are currently unpleasant, because this will allow space for more positive feelings to emerge as and when they arise in the future.

Coping Stances (Relationship Wellness)

The stance our student is most likely to adopt is the placating stance. By suppressing her own feelings, she will discount herself in interactions with the system and focus primarily on pleasing the system and other people. In our experience, this is a very common stance in medical students. The price to be paid includes losing touch with oneself; making decisions that are not in one's own best interest; and the long-term effects of suppressed emotions, often anger, on personal health and well-being. The step to improve well-being would be to start to include themselves more as persons of value in interactions with others in the system. Given the hierarchical nature of medical care, this must be done judiciously, as most students realize, but it is certainly possible and makes a real difference to wellness.

Reacting, Responding, and Mindfulness

In our work with medical students we have found that the greatest difficulty in promoting our own long-term wellness is our reactivity. Something happens that triggers us and we find ourselves automatically in a defensive coping stance that affects our well-being. The placating student is a good example of this phenomenon. Most often students do not make a conscious choice to be placating. They simply find themselves doing so in reaction to the perceived expectations of the system. However, placating is not the only stance we may take in reaction to an event we experience.

To give a contrasting personal example: I am teaching a course for medical students on mindful medical practice, and 5 out of 20 students are unaccountably missing at the start of the class. Instead of focusing on the 15 students who are present and modeling the mindful presence I am attempting to teach, I am caught in a reactive stance that blames the students for being late and infers various reasons, including their lack of interest in my teaching. If I stay in that stance or attempt to suppress it or deny it, the energy for my teaching will drain away and I will simply be going through the motions. An alternative response, and one which we believe provides an answer in this situation, is a mindful presence defined as "moment to moment nonjudgmental awareness" [9] that allows the reaction to exist and makes space for a chosen response, which in this case would be to refocus on the teaching with some awareness of the longings and yearnings that led to this teaching in the first place. The class and I can then move forward. In any attempt to nurture our own long-term wellness, our reactivity will be a frequently repeated challenge that will be acted out in every conceivable context in our lives. It is for this reason that mindfulness is such an important skill and way of being in the lifelong journey to wellness.

Wellness, Longing, and Yearning

The most important determinant of our wellness is probably our relationship to the deepest layer of the iceberg, our longings and yearnings. It is our longings and yearnings that give life to the rest of the iceberg, but they are the most challenging to bring to awareness. We may long to love, to be loved, to be cared for, but it makes us very vulnerable to admit even to ourselves how powerful these longings are because our longings may not be met, at least in the way we would recognize and anticipate. It is very important to realize that longings and yearnings are not fixed desires or goals, which would be expectations. And it is likely that how our longings will be lived out is not predictable but is completely dependent on the context in which we live and our moment-to-moment response to it. In their examination of wellness from a self-determination perspective, authors DeHaan and Ryan describe wellness as an authentic process that involves a congruent approach to the world, which is appreciative and responsive to both the external environment and internal states [10]. They note that eudaimonic living, which is centered on living an authentic and purposeful life in which you are in touch with your true nature, is a pathway toward wellness [10]. However, we are not, as sometimes suggested by formulations of Aristotle's eudaimonic model, "true natures" for whom there is some prescribed best way to live. We are unformed potentials that could be lived out satisfactorily in myriad possible ways. And perhaps it is not where we arrive at that determines our wellness, but the process that we experience in getting there, which fits well with the healing aspect of whole-person care.

Whole-Person Care, Healing, and Wellness

Whole-person care comprises two complementary approaches: curing or preventing what can be fixed or prevented; and promoting healing [11]. Healing is a subjective improvement in quality of life in response to illness or wounding. This phenomenon has been observed most clearly in the care of people who are dying. Balfour Mount describes the paradigmatic case [12]:

> CD was 30 years old when he presented with a widely disseminated germinal testicular cancer. Radical surgery and chemotherapy initially resulted in his tumor markers reverting to negative

and the hope of cure, but within months his disease progressed with ensuing extreme cachexia. He died slowly over a 12-month period. CD had always stood out from his peers. He had always been a winner. Strong. Outgoing. Gracious. A world-class athlete, he was a member of the national ski team. He was successful in business and engaged to be married. A champion from a family of competitive champions, he was now melting before the raging forces of the embryonal cell. Then, just days before he died he married his fiancée and said goodbye to those he loved, observing, "This last year has been the best year of my life."

This subjective improvement in quality of life with severe and even terminal illness is not an infrequent occurrence and has led Balfour Mount and Michael Kearney to call for healing to be reincorporated into the medical mandate [13]. They point out that subjective quality of life is not determined by objective disease status or measures of physical health. In fact, the two often change in opposite directions, as illustrated by CD. This explains the lack of relationship between different physical states of disease and disability and subjective quality of life [14]. It also explains the sometimes paradoxical effect of disease on wellness – wellness sometimes actually increasing as patients deteriorate [15]. Healing is growth in response to illness [11], and we believe that it is the growth that these patients are experiencing that explains their improved wellness. This fits well with the view of the Irish artist J.B. Yeats: "Happiness is not virtue or pleasure, or this thing or that. It is merely growth. We are happy when we are growing" [16]. This changes the whole way we frame wellness. It is no longer about fixing this or that aspect of our lives, filling this or that deficiency. It is simply a measure of how much we are growing. It also explains the disconnect between external circumstances and wellness, which leads to the relationship between suffering, comfort, and wellness.

Suffering, Comfort, and Wellness

It might at first be assumed that suffering is opposed to wellness and that comfort is an essential ingredient of wellness. This is not the case. Following Eric Cassell's proposal that suffering occurs when there is a threat to our intactness as a person [17], we might suppose that the aim in furthering wellness would be to avoid such threats. But to avoid such threats would be to limit our growth because all growth requires us to step outside of who we currently know ourselves to be. The story of Viktor Frankl at the beginning of the chapter is an example of stepping out [3]. To take a less dramatic example, medical students as they progress through medical school are repeatedly asked to step into new roles that change their perception of themselves, from students listening to lectures to supervised visitors on the wards of the hospital, to ward clerks responsible for the supervised day-to-day care of sick patients.

Each of these transitions involves a change in identity, and growth. Each transition also comes with suffering – a threat to their intactness as a person – as anyone who has supervised medical students will easily recognize. And yet each of these transitions can also contribute to growth and wellness. A medical student who insisted on never stepping outside their comfort zone would not be able to make these transitions and would thereby prevent their development as a physician, their growth, and we believe their wellness. It is true that too rapid and confronting a transition can overwhelm the individual's ability to grow in response to change and can result in damage and decreased wellness, as has been observed in medical students [18]. The answer is not the avoidance of suffering and discomfort, which are an inevitable accompaniment of growth, but a balance between change and stability, and sufficient support as the process unfolds. Our underlying assumption is that human beings are inherently creatures of growth and dynamic change, and that they require such change in order to be well.

Whole-Person Wellness

We believe that the most important factors in long-term wellness are not only specific measures aimed at particular problems or preventive measures aimed at the whole body, both of which are primarily defensive approaches. Wellness and happiness are products of the relationship of the whole person to life, and the important and essential ingredient in that relationship is growth. This is not a simple path but will require increasing self-knowledge and self-acceptance, particularly of our deep longings and yearnings, an ability to be mindful under stress and respond rather than react, a willingness to let go of some defenses, to risk the suffering that comes with change, and to embrace the adventure of life lived as a developing and growing whole person, which we believe is the key to long-term wellness.

References

1. TA Hutchinson, N Hutchinson, A Arnaert. Whole person care: encompassing the two faces of medicine. *CMAJ* 2009; **180**(8): 845–846.

2. TA Hutchinson. Prevention and the whole person. In: *Whole Person Care. Transforming Healthcare.* Cham, Springer; 2017; 115–122.

3. RY Drazen. *The Choice is Yours.* DVD. Drazen Productions; 2001.

4. RM Ryan, V Huta. Wellness as healthy functioning or wellness as happiness: the importance of eudaimonic thinking (response to the Kashdan et al. and Waterman discussion). *J Positive Psych* 2009;**4**(3): 202.

5. A Steptoe, A Deaton, AA Stone. Subjective wellbeing, health, and ageing. *Lancet* 2015; **385**(9968): 640–648.

6. V Satir, J Banmen, J Gerber, M Gomori. The transformation process. In: *The Satir Model. Family Therapy and Beyond.* Palo Alto, CA, Science and Behavior Books; 1991; 147–174.

7. V Satir, J Banmen, J Gerber, M Gomori. The survival stances. In: *The Satir Model: Family Therapy and Beyond.* Palo Alto, CA, Science and Behavior Books; 1991; 31–64.

8. V Satir, J Banmen, J Gerber, M Gomori. Congruence. In: *The Satir Model: Family Therapy and Beyond.* Palo Alto, CA, Science and Behavior Books; 1991; 65–84.

9. J Kabat-Zinn. Introduction: stress, pain, and illness – facing the wisdom of your body and mind to face stress, pain, and illness. In: *Full Catastrophe Living: Using the Wisdom of Your Body and Mind to Face Stress, Pain, and Illness.* New York, Delta; 1990; 1–14.

10. CR DeHaan, RM Ryan. Symptoms of wellness, happiness and eudaimonia from a self-determination perspective. In: KM Sheldon, RE Lucus, eds., *Stability of Happiness: Theories and Evidence on Whether Happiness Can Change.* Amsterdam, Elsevier; 2014; 37–55.

11. TA Hutchinson The focus of medical care. In: *Whole Person Care: Transforming Healthcare.* Cham, Springer; 2017; 29–36.

12. SR Cohen, BM Mount. Quality of life in terminal illness: defining and measuring subjective well-being in the dying. *J Palliat Care* 1992; **8**: 40–45.

13. B Mount, M Kearney. Healing and palliative care: charting our way forward. *Palliat Med* 2003; **17**: 657–658.

14. CJ Gill. Facts about disability and "quality of life." Independent Living Institute. 1999. www.independentliving.org/gill99.html (accessed April 4, 2019).

15. M Kagawa-Singer. Redefining health: living with cancer. *Soc Sci Med* 1993; **37**: 295–304.

16. JB Yeats. *Letters to His Son W. B. Yeats and Others 1869–1922*. New York, E. P. Dutton & Company, Inc.; 1946; 121.

17. EJ Cassell. *The Nature of Suffering and the Goals of Medicine*. New York, Oxford University Press; 2004.

18. LN Dyrbye, MR Thomas, TD Shanafelt. Systematic review of depression, anxiety, and other indicators of psychological distress among U.S. and Canadian medical students. *Acad Med* 2006; **81**(4): 354–373.

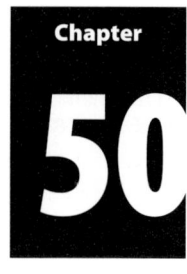

Chapter

50

The Personalized Wellness Life Plan

Waguih William IsHak, Ryan Bart,* Yasmine Gohar, Natalie Lorea, Lidia Eskander, Tiffany Chang, Samantha Cohen, Katerina Furman, Piyush Peter Nayyar, and Katrina DeBonis

Introduction

Wellness is often intimidating. Pursuing it requires significant commitment and carries emotional risk/vulnerability [1]. While fear can be a strong motivator, it can also be the reason one may not try or follow-through with a plan. In most cases, fear prevents us from being able to accomplish what we wish to. In the case of wellness, we found that due to the commitment many were challenged by the fear of not being able to achieve the results and goals they had set for themselves. For example, if one was never taught, or had modeled, how to live a life full of joy, love, and wellness, they will fear a life different than what they were taught, whether by observation or directly. Occasionally it can be more difficult and painful to break a pattern than to live in it [2]. The path to wellness will likely be unique for each and every one of us. If one has experienced any adverse childhood experiences or is a survivor of adult emotional trauma, it may take a lot of support from self and others to adopt wellness practices. Practices of wellness often require us to look at facts of life that many try to outrun or ignore. This can be true even for those who have not faced any trauma. Taking care of oneself means taking care of all of oneself, i.e., emotional, spiritual, and physical body.

Wellness requires a willingness to recognize, feel, and address all of one's feelings, feeding one's soul, and nourishing one's body. This also involves recognizing one's short-comings, which is not comfortable. Because consistent adherence to the plan for wellness is required [3], it may feel at times that it is like taking two steps forward and one step back as people integrate wellness; that is okay! It is a part of the growth process. Adhering to a wellness plan will demand a lot of patience and acceptance to see lasting changes, and it is unlikely to be linear. In order to optimize personalization, each individual has to be viewed as the master and expert of their own experience and empowered to create their own plan for wellness, measuring its effectiveness, and reaping the benefits of creating and adhering to the plan [4]. We may never reach the perfect ideal, but rather be on a constant journey. Every moment is as complete as it can be as we strive toward the ideal. When we recognize and accept our constant drive for progress, this is when growth and inner peace can occur simultaneously, which will consequently promote personal wellness.

---

* Disclaimer: The views expressed in this material are those of the author, and do not reflect the official policy or position of the US Government, the Department of Defense, or the Department of the Air Force.

Personalization

While many of the chapters of this book cover the whole range of wellness interventions, it is paramount that each one of us pick and choose what works best for ourselves. Please bear in mind that we owe it to ourselves to try new ideas at least once. Important parameters to drive personalization and "what works for me" include the following: characterization of interest level (and looking forward to the activity), effects (preferably using measurement), side effects, cost, and sustainability [5]. In working with others to develop a personalized wellness plan, it is important to consider cultural and structural factors that might influence the activities that are available, accessible, and effective in promoting wellness. Although wellness as marketed to the public is not synonymous with wellness as defined by the World Health Organization, people might associate the term with yoga, juice cleanses, expensive supplements, and images of thin Caucasian women [6]. Recommending that someone with limited income who lives in an under-resourced neighborhood eat more fruits and vegetables and join a gym, without consideration of the structural factors that would make this difficult or impossible, is not a helpful intervention. Therefore, it is recommended that you approach conversations about wellness with humility and openness. Actively discussing activities that promote wellness with people from a variety of backgrounds, cultures, and financial means will enable you to broaden your perspective and suggestions when engaging in this work.

Personalization of the wellness plan involves investing time and effort in the activities defined by the World Health Organization (WHO) [7, 8], and highlighted in Figure 50.1.

The process of developing the personalized wellness life plan involves the six steps depicted in Figure 50.2: setting the plan, scheduling the plan, getting support for the plan, tracking the plan, measuring the impact, and updating the plan. The process involves choosing activities from each of the eight dimensions of wellness in order to set the plan: physical, emotional, social, spiritual, intellectual, financial, occupational, and environmental. For the next step, individuals are required to schedule their wellness interventions on a daily, weekly, monthly, and yearly basis. It is crucial for everyone to get support for the plan. Support can be from an intimate partner, significant other, and/or friend(s), in addition to professionals and allocating resources. Tracking the plan and measuring its impact is essential to its success in order for one to be able to gauge which techniques and interventions are working, as opposed to those that need adjustment. Appendix II contains some state-of-the-art self-report measures that are in the public domain, created by the Patient-Reported Outcomes Measurement Information System (PROMIS) supported by the US National Institute of Health [9]. Updating the plan and renewing the commitment to wellness is of utmost importance in integrating and sustaining wellness in our lives [10].

Resources for activities to include in the personalized wellness life plan from the chapters in this volume are depicted in Box 50.1. Websites that contain wellness activities that could be used to create the personalized wellness life plan are displayed in Box 50.2.

We also provide sample personalized wellness life plans in Tables 50.1–50.10.

Conclusion

It is important to accept from the outset that due to the personal nature of wellness, pursuing and achieving it successfully will likely look very different from person to person. There is no one "correct" path. The key is to be intentional and to be consistently moving

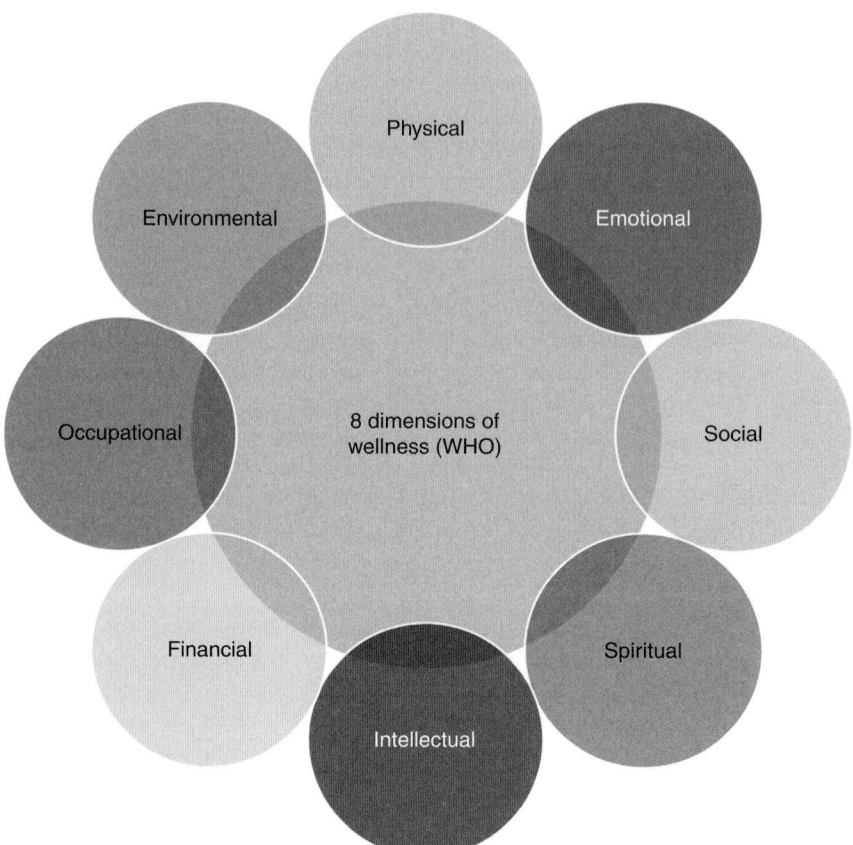

Figure 50.1 Wellness activities along the eight dimensions of wellness defined by the WHO.

toward improved wellness. The methods highlighted in this volume will not apply to every person. There is more or less an agreement in research studies, expert consensus, and anecdotal reports that any personalized effort to achieve wellness will lead to developing a life plan that encompasses the following components:

- Prioritize one's physical health (with adequate nutrition, adequate sleep, avoiding health-destructive habits, and seeking medical care as needed).
- Pursue meaningful and purposeful activities for work, home life, or volunteering.
- Develop and nurture loving relationships and sharing one's gifts with others.
- Organize yourself, conserve your energy, and allow yourself time between activities.
- Approach problems with a solution-oriented positive attitude.
- Have faith in yourself, in others, and in a higher power.
- Fill your day with pleasurable activities that you enjoy and could share with the people you love.
- Contribute to others with whom you might or might not have a connection

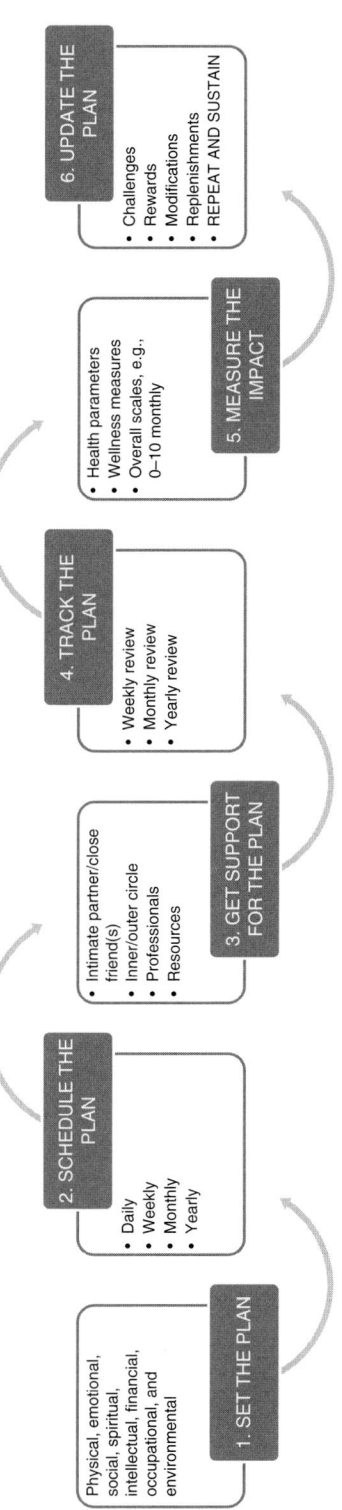

Figure 50.2 The process of developing the personalized wellness life plan.

1. SET THE PLAN
- Physical, emotional, social, spiritual, intellectual, financial, occupational, and environmental

2. SCHEDULE THE PLAN
- Daily
- Weekly
- Monthly
- Yearly

3. GET SUPPORT FOR THE PLAN
- Intimate partner/close friend(s)
- Inner/outer circle
- Professionals
- Resources

4. TRACK THE PLAN
- Weekly review
- Monthly review
- Yearly review

5. MEASURE THE IMPACT
- Health parameters
- Wellness measures
- Overall scales, e.g., 0–10 monthly

6. UPDATE THE PLAN
- Challenges
- Rewards
- Modifications
- Replenishments
- REPEAT AND SUSTAIN

Box 50.1 Wellness Activities from this Book

Chapter 22: Nutrition
Chapter 23: Nutraceuticals and Wellness
Chapter 24: Pharmaceuticals and Alternatives for Wellness
Chapter 25: Exercise, Dance, Tai Chi, Pilates, and Alexander Technique
Chapter 26: Sleep, Rest, and Relaxation
Chapter 27: Sex, Intimacy, and Well-Being
Chapter 28: Mindfulness, Meditation, and Yoga
Chapter 29: Gratitude, Forgiveness, and Spirituality
Chapter 30: Positive Neuropsychology, Cognitive Rehabilitation, Neuroenhancement
Chapter 31: Acupuncture, Herbs, and Ayurvedic Medicine
Chapter 32: The Role of Aesthetics in Wellness
Chapter 33: Massage, Humor, and Music
Chapter 34: Nature and Pets
Chapter 35: Circadian Rhythm in the Digital Age
Chapter 36: The Arts in Health Settings
Chapter 37: Engaging the Five Senses: Taste, Smell, See, Listen, and Touch
Chapter 38: Emotional Intelligence and its Role in Sustaining Fulfillment in Life
Chapter 39: Psychotherapy and Positive Psychology
Chapter 40: Resilience and Wellness
Chapter 41: Developing Purpose, Meaning, and Achievements
Chapter 42: Healing and Wellness
Chapter 43: Connection, Compassion, and Community

Box 50.2 Websites for Wellness Activities

SAMHSA: https://store.samhsa.gov/product/Creating-a-Healthier-Life-/SMA16-4958

Dimensions of wellness: change your habits, change your life: www.ncbi.nlm.nih.gov/pmc/articles/PMC5508938

Pleasurable activities: http://elishagoldstein.com/assets/183-pleasurable-activities-to-choose-from.pdf

Pleasant activities: http://uwaims.org/files/behavioral-activation/pleasantactivitieslist.pdf

University of Central Arkansas: https://uca.edu/wellness/dimensions-of-wellness

Jake Behrens, MD: www.wikihow.com/Create-a-Wellness-Plan

If you are reading this, you are likely already engaging in some/most of the above recommendations. The goal of this chapter is to equip you with a means of implementing the above facets into your daily life. Doing so will help you to hold yourself accountable to continue to build upon your personal wellness. We hope you find it useful and practical.

Table 50.1 Sample personalized wellness life plan #1

Dimension	Daily	Weekly	Monthly	Yearly
Physical	Walk 30 minutes Eat low-carb Drink plenty of water	Shop for fresh and wholesome foods	Monitor my weight and medication intake	Get a physical check-up and labs
Emotional	Stay positive	Meditation	Learn/practice one stress management skill	Take a two-week vacation solid
Social	Meal with intimate partner/family	Lunch with a friend	Get together with family	Call and speak to friends on their birthdays
Spiritual	Say grace before meal	Count my blessings	Go to service 2x per month	Attend a spiritual retreat
Intellectual	Read before bed	Watch a TED talk weekly	Attend an event or lecture	Read two best-sellers
Financial	Cut on wasteful spending	Review expenses and income	Pay yourself 1 percent of each paycheck and save	Unsubscribe to services not used for six months
Occupational	Acknowledge and greet my colleagues	Mentorship availability: two office hours	Advocate for system-based wellness ideas	Promote/execute idea that is mission-relevant
Environmental	Cut down on waste	Take a walk/hike in the fresh air by water/greenery once a week	Organize and cut down on clutter	Plant a new tree

Table 50.2 Sample personalized wellness life plan #2

Dimension	Daily	Weekly	Monthly	Yearly
Physical	Eat plant-centric wholefoods Moderate–high intensity activity ×30 min Avoid sitting >40 min at a time	Outdoor half-day activity	Outdoor full-day or multiday adventure	Learn a new sport/ physical activity
Emotional	Be patient amid stress	Express gratitude to others	Self-reflection of interpersonal interactions	Spend extended period of time in nature
Social	Be approachable Uninterrupted check-in with significant other	Call my parents	Go to a social gathering/ group outing	Handwritten thank you cards
Spiritual	Daily gratitude list	Meditate	Spend quiet time in nature	Volunteer at a homeless shelter or with disadvantaged youth
Intellectual	Read primary literature	Focused teaching for junior residents	Complete 100 board review questions	Contribute to academic literature
Financial	Pack a lunch	Listen to white coat investor podcast	50 percent income toward financial independence Track bills and spending	Give to a credible charity Reassess asset allocation and investment plan
Occupational	Expand knowledge and skills Be kind	Seek and provide feedback to team members	Go the extra mile for a patient in need	Reassess long-term career goals and necessary steps toward them
Environmental	Recycle Eat sustainable foods	Support local businesses	Pay fees/give donations at parks	Neighborhood trash clean up

Table 50.3 Sample personalized wellness life plan #3

Dimension	Daily	Weekly	Monthly	Yearly
Physical	Engage in one hour of exercise while maintaining a healthy and balanced diet	Weigh yourself and adjust diet as necessary	Grocery shopping and meal preparations 2x a month	Visit the doctor for a full-body check-up
Emotional	Morning positive affirmations and daily journaling	Therapy sessions and meditation (hot yoga)	Self-care day or weekend	Take a 1–2- week electronics-free vacation
Social	Spend quality time (in person/on the phone) with a significant other/family member	Go out for a meal/coffee with a friend	Have a family gathering	Take a trip with family/ best friends
Spiritual	Gratitude journal	Incense cleanse throughout the house	Volunteer to help the less fortunate	Spiritual retreat
Intellectual	Catch up on world news	Spend 1–2 hours practicing a new language	Read or listen to a new book	Attend a conference
Financial	Create and stay within a daily budget	Make coffee/ breakfast at home 1–2 times per week	Place 50 percent of income into savings (after bills)	Reassess all subscriptions (Dish/Amazon) and cancel extra unneeded expenses
Occupational	Greet coworkers	Update weekly to- do lists and organize work files	Engage in a new project	Evaluate performance of self and employees
Environmental	Recycle, reuse, and reduce	Spend a day in nature (hike/beach/picnic)	Turn off all electricity for two hours	Volunteer with a clean the beaches group

Table 50.4 Sample personalized wellness life plan #4

Dimension	Daily	Weekly	Monthly	Yearly
Physical	20 min yoga at home, or walking	Buy pasture-raised organic meats and small-farm veggies from local farmers markets	Walking/hiking in nature 2x a month	Visit the doctor for a full-body check-up
Emotional	Write myself 2–3 sentence love letters before bed	Schedule 2 hours of doing something I love for myself every week	Meet with a friend 2x a month for co-counseling and intentional space	Go on mini vacations 6x a year
Social	Call one I love a day for 15–30 minutes	Go see one friend a week	Have a game night once a month	Go on a camping trip with friends
Spiritual	Participate in activities to engage with my inner-most being	Meet with friends to read from spiritual text	Attend intuitive dance session 1x a month	Take an inventory of my life, dreams, and aspirations
Intellectual	Learn something new every day	Allow myself to investigate an interest	Listen to a new audio book 1x a month	Take 1 class of something I am interested in
Financial	Track my spending and where it is being spent	Put money into different envelopes such as "camping," "my loving home," and "scuba"	Place 5 percent of income into prudent reserve	Take inventory of financial goals, reassess spending every 3 months
Occupational	Set intentions to be of service and not take things personally	Meet with supervisor and discuss progress	Assess career goals, make changes in next steps as necessary	Attend non-violent communication workshop
Environmental	Buy pasture-raised meats (carbon sequestration) and repair products	Tend to compost pile	Attend environmental activism group 1x a month	Research and build sawdust toilet

Table 50.5 Sample personalized wellness life plan #5

Dimension	Daily	Weekly	Monthly	Yearly
Physical	Do 20 min cardio on the elliptical machine along with light stretching	Cook and meal prep for the week	Take a hike with a friend	Do a fitness assessment at the gym to monitor progress
Emotional	Five-minute body scan meditation	Write down two things you are grateful for in a journal	Plan a mid-month activity to look forward to (e.g., massage)	Plan a summer road trip with closest friends
Social	Phone call with my sister	Friday night dinner with family	Go to the beach with friends	Celebrate my birthday with friends and family
Spiritual	Say prayers before bed	Go to temple every Saturday for morning services	Participate in a fundraising event for my temple	Attend services at temple for every religious holiday
Intellectual	Listen to one chapter of an audio book before bed	Watch a documentary weekly	Attend a university or work lecture/presentation	Subscribe to an interesting journal or newsletter
Financial	Cut down on eating out at restaurants	Review expenses of the week using a budgeting app	Limit monthly subscriptions to a gym membership	Meet with financial advisor to review expenses, loans, and budgeting
Occupational	Make a to-do list for the day	Weekly meeting with mentor to discuss work concerns and ideas	Participate in a work wellness activity (e.g., team yoga or meditation class)	Attend a national work conference for networking opportunities
Environmental	Use reusable cups and containers	Purchase groceries in bulk to reduce packaging waste	Attend an environmental health organization event (e.g., lecture on toxin-free beauty products)	Switch to energy-conserving appliances

Table 50.6 Sample personalized wellness life plan #6

Dimension	Daily	Weekly	Monthly	Yearly
Physical	Use stand-up desk and take stairs at work	Nature hike	Reflect on nutritional/physical state and make plan to adjust as needed	Assess and set new goals
Emotional	Ask myself "how am I feeling today?"	Plan an enjoyable weekend activity	Monitor screen time	Spend one week of vacation completely disconnected from email, phone, and internet use
Social	Be as present as possible when with my family	Have a meaningful conversation with a friend	Reflect on which relationships might need more of my time/energy	Weekend trip with closest friends
Spiritual	Practice mindful awareness	Express gratitude	Celebrate meaningful traditions and connection with family	Commit to community service activities
Intellectual	Read an article related to field	Read the *New Yorker*	Go to a museum or play	Attend a work-related conference
Financial	Try to keep budget	Track spending	Save portion of income for children's college fund	Maximize retirement savings
Occupational	Focus on one activity at a time	Reflect on patients from the week and process difficult cases with colleagues	Take one full weekend away from work emails	Adjust work commitments to best align with values
Environmental	Walk my children to school	Work to reduce waste	Track water use and work toward reducing	Assess energy use and identify areas for improvement

Table 50.7 Sample personalized wellness life plan #7

Dimension	Daily	Weekly	Monthly	Yearly
Physical	Engage in one hour of exercise (weight training, outdoor run, cycling, etc.)	Compete in a recreational league soccer game	Try a new fitness class	Undergo a comprehensive health evaluation with my primary care doctor
Emotional	Listen to music during my commute	Meditate in a yoga class	Spend a day in nature with friends	Take a vacation to somewhere I have not been yet
Social	Eat lunch with coworkers	Spend time with friends after work	Speak on the phone to long-distance friends	Remove individuals from my social media who do not positively contribute to my well-being
Spiritual	Practice mindfulness	Set intentions for my meditation practice and life in general	Engage in a reflection of gratitude	Attend services at synagogue for the High Holidays and reflect on resolutions for the Jewish New Year
Intellectual	Spend 5–10 min learning about current world affairs	Read for pleasure	Engage in a discussion with a friend about their work in a different field	Write and edit academic literature
Financial	Take public transportation to and from work	Cook food at home instead of eating out	Move a percentage of my income to a savings account	Pay off a percentage of loans
Occupational	Block off 30 min on my calendar for lunch and set working hours for client calls	Make a to-do list	Participate in a team wellness walk	Meet with manager to discuss career development and compensation
Environmental	Maintain a pescatarian diet	Recycle at home	Pick up trash in a park or at the beach	Volunteer at an environmental advocacy event

Table 50.8 Sample personalized wellness life plan #8

Dimension	Daily	Weekly	Monthly	Yearly
Physical	Deep breathing (pranayama) for 5 min	Practice yoga (three to four times per week for 30 min)	Play in a recreational competitive league (prefer soccer)	Take a formalized one-week yoga course
Emotional	Note three instances of positive interactions with others	Meditate on what makes me happy	Communicate to maintain loving relationships with close friends and family	Take a week vacation with my significant other (no phones)
Social	Ask open-ended questions and allow people to open up	Attend at least one organized event for a cause	Network with one person working on a stimulating idea or project	Host a dinner with friends/ family
Spiritual	Be consciously aware of diverse viewpoints	Listen to spiritual podcast (such as Waking up with Sam Harris)	Read one book/essay on the evolving nature of consciousness	24-hour retreat disconnected from all technology and luxuries
Intellectual	Listen more and talk less	Research case reports for unique current patients	Read newly released research topics in medicine (What's New section of Uptodate)	Learn and fulfill continued medical education requirements
Financial	Link income and expenses to a budget-tracking app	Monitor budget application and compare expenses over time	Identify large expenses and assess utility of purchases	Balance contributions to retirement, savings and student loan repayment
Occupational	Provide supportive listening to patients to enhance work satisfaction	Be aware of possible burnout and its effect on professional interactions	Get 360-degree feedback from coworkers and staff around me	Evaluate career trajectory and meet with mentors
Environmental	Reduce use of single-use plastic	Limit car use when walking is appropriate	Track utility bills and monitor usage	Consider a more eco-friendly vehicle

Table 50.9 Sample personalized wellness life plan #9

Dimension	Daily	Weekly	Monthly	Yearly
Physical	30 min walk daily	Go to the gym for one hour	Go for a long hike	Schedule my annual physical exam
Emotional	Jot down three things I am grateful for	Write a thank-you note to someone who helped	Spend a day in nature with friends	Attend a positive thinking retreat
Social	Call or see one close friend	Never miss birthdays on my social media network	Play soccer with friends	Make new friends
Spiritual	Practice the rules of my faith	Make time for the Friday prayer	Attend a Holy Koran study group	Fast in Ramadan and donate to the less fortunate
Intellectual	Catch up with current events	Download and read my favorite magazine	Attend the book club	Watch the movies on my must-see list
Financial	Save loose change for donations	Plan my meals	Save to buy a house	Update my investment plan
Occupational	Organize my desk before I leave	Return all phone calls before the week ends	Clean my email inbox and address all pending issues	Update my career goals
Environmental	Moderate my use of electricity and water	Water my plants	Organize my drawers and closets	Participate in a neighborhood clean-up

Table 50.10 Sample personalized wellness life plan #10

Dimension	Daily	Weekly	Monthly	Yearly
Physical	Park far from the entrance	Play tennis	Check and update my fitness plan	Meet with my doctor
Emotional	Practice deep breathing	Weekly meditation class	Go to the comedy club	Plan my vacation with family or friends
Social	Speak with family or friends	Go to happy hour with my friends	Plan a dinner party	Plan a Christmas party
Spiritual	Pray before bedtime	Attend mass in my church	Attend Bible study	Go the annual church retreat
Intellectual	Read before bed	Read the articles I saved	Attend a cultural event	Write a short story
Financial	Keep track of my expenses	Have my latte on the weekend (not on weekdays)	Donate to my favorite charity	Meet with my financial planner
Occupational	Start with challenging tasks first	Review and complete my to-do list	Start and maintain a newsletter at work	Meet with my manager for feedback
Environmental	Use washable utensils (not disposable)	Use and maintain my water bottle	Donate items that I no longer use	Support an advocacy organization

References

1. CB Brown. *The Power of Vulnerability.* Louisville, Sounds True; 2012.

2. A Levine, R Heller. *Attached: The New Science of Adult Attachment and How It Can Help You Find – and Keep – Love.* New York, Penguin Random House; 2012.

3. SA Miller. Easier said than done: practicing self-care and health and wellness in higher education and student affairs. *Vermont Connection* 2016; 37(13). https://scholar works.uvm.edu/tvc/vol37/iss1/13 (accessed September 1, 2019).

4. SM Bhanji. Respect and unconditional positive regard as mental health promotion practice. *J Clin Res Bioeth* 2013; 4: 147.

5. R Bart, WW IsHak, S Ganjian, et al. The assessment and measurement of wellness in the clinical medical setting: a systematic review. *Innov Clin Neurosci* 2018; 15: 14–23.

6. J Hamblin. The art of woke wellness. *The Atlantic.* 2018. www.theatlantic.com/health/ archive/2018/11/wellspring-festival-woke-wellness/576103 (accessed September 12, 2019).

7. World Health Organization (WHO). Constitution. 1949. www.loc.gov/law/help/ us-treaties/bevans/m-ust000004-0119.pdf (accessed September 1, 2019).

8. B Smith, K Tang, D Nutbeam. WHO health promotion glossary: new terms. *Health Promot Int* 2006; 21: 340–345.

9. Health Measures. Patient-Reported Outcomes Measurement Information System (PROMIS). www.healthmea sures.net/explore-measurement-systems/ promis/obtain-administer-measures/pre senting-results (accessed September 1, 2019).

10. J Myers, T Sweeney, J Witmer. The wheel of wellness counseling for wellness: a holistic model for treatment planning. *J Couns Dev* 2000; 78: 251–266.

Appendix I Wellness Measures

Waguih William IsHak

This appendix contains wellness measures created by the Patient Reported Outcomes Measurement Information System (PROMIS®). Funding for PROMIS was provided by the United States National Institutes of Health (NIH). Scoring information is available at www.hea lthmeasures.net/explore-measurement-systems/promis/obtain-administer-measures/present ing-results.

PROMIS Global Health Scale

		Excellent	Very good	Good	Fair	Poor
Global01	In general, would you say your health is:	☐ 5	☐ 4	☐ 3	☐ 2	☐ 1
Global02	In general, would you say your quality of life is:..	☐ 5	☐ 4	☐ 3	☐ 2	☐ 1
Global03	In general, how would you rate your physical health?	☐ 5	☐ 4	☐ 3	☐ 2	☐ 1
Global04	In general, how would you rate your mental health, including your mood and your ability to think?	☐ 5	☐ 4	☐ 3	☐ 2	☐ 1
Global05	In general, how would you rate your satisfaction with your social activities and relationships?	☐ 5	☐ 4	☐ 3	☐ 2	☐ 1
Global09r	In general, please rate how well you carry out your usual social activities and roles. (This includes activities at home, at work and in your community, and responsibilities as a parent, child, spouse, employee, friend, etc.)......	☐ 5	☐ 4	☐ 3	☐ 2	☐ 1
		Completely	Mostly	Moderately	A little	Not at all
Global06	To what extent are you able to carry out your everyday physical activities such as walking, climbing stairs, carrying groceries, or moving a chair?	☐ 5	☐ 4	☐ 3	☐ 2	☐ 1

Figure A1.1 Global health scale. © 2008–2016 PROMIS Health Organization and PROMIS Cooperative Group. Reprinted with permission.

In the past 7 days...

		Never	Rarely	Sometimes	Often	Always
Global10r	How often have you been bothered by emotional problems such as feeling anxious, depressed or irritable?	☐ 5	☐ 4	☐ 3	☐ 2	☐ 1

		None	Mild	Moderate	Severe	Very severe
Global08r	How would you rate your fatigue on average?	☐ 5	☐ 4	☐ 3	☐ 2	☐ 1

Global07r	How would you rate your pain on average?	☐ 0 No pain	☐ 1	☐ 2	☐ 3	☐ 4	☐ 5	☐ 6	☐ 7	☐ 8	☐ 9	☐ 10 Worst pain imaginable

Figure A1.1 (cont.)

PROMIS Positive Affect and Well-Being

Lately...

		Never	Rarely	Sometimes	Often	Always
NQPPF14	I had a sense of well-being...................	☐ 1	☐ 2	☐ 3	☐ 4	☐ 5
NQPPF12	I felt hopeful....................................	☐ 1	☐ 2	☐ 3	☐ 4	☐ 5
NQPPF15	My life was satisfying........................	☐ 1	☐ 2	☐ 3	☐ 4	☐ 5
NQPPF20	My life had purpose...........................	☐ 1	☐ 2	☐ 3	☐ 4	☐ 5
NQPPF17	My life had meaning..........................	☐ 1	☐ 2	☐ 3	☐ 4	☐ 5
NQPPF22	I felt cheerful..................................	☐ 1	☐ 2	☐ 3	☐ 4	☐ 5
NQPPF19	My life was worth living....................	☐ 1	☐ 2	☐ 3	☐ 4	☐ 5
NQPPF16	I had a sense of balance in my life.........	☐ 1	☐ 2	☐ 3	☐ 4	☐ 5
NQPPF07	Many areas of my life were interesting to me..	☐ 1	☐ 2	☐ 3	☐ 4	☐ 5
NQPPF02	I was able to enjoy life.......................	☐ 1	☐ 2	☐ 3	☐ 4	☐ 5
NQPPF03	I felt a sense of purpose in my life.........	☐ 1	☐ 2	☐ 3	☐ 4	☐ 5
NQPPF04	I could laugh and see the humor in situations......................................	☐ 1	☐ 2	☐ 3	☐ 4	☐ 5
NQPPF05	I was able to be at ease and feel relaxed...	☐ 1	☐ 2	☐ 3	☐ 4	☐ 5
NQPPF06	I looked forward with enjoyment to upcoming events...............................	☐ 1	☐ 2	☐ 3	☐ 4	☐ 5
NQPPF08	I felt emotionally stable......................	☐ 1	☐ 2	☐ 3	☐ 4	☐ 5
NQPPF10	I felt lovable...................................	☐ 1	☐ 2	☐ 3	☐ 4	☐ 5

Figure A1.2 Positive affect and well-being. © 2008–2016 PROMIS Health Organization and PROMIS Cooperative Group. Reprinted with permission.

Lately…

		Never	Rarely	Sometimes	Often	Always
NQPPF11	I felt confident………………………	☐ 1	☐ 2	☐ 3	☐ 4	☐ 5
NQPPF13	I had a good life……………………..	☐ 1	☐ 2	☐ 3	☐ 4	☐ 5
NQPPF18	My life was peaceful………………..	☐ 1	☐ 2	☐ 3	☐ 4	☐ 5
NQPPF21	I was living life to the fullest……………	☐ 1	☐ 2	☐ 3	☐ 4	☐ 5
NQPPF23	In most ways my life was close to my ideal………………………………….	☐ 1	☐ 2	☐ 3	☐ 4	☐ 5
NQPPF24	I had good control of my thoughts……….	☐ 1	☐ 2	☐ 3	☐ 4	☐ 5
NQPPF26	Even when things were going badly, I still had hope………………………….	☐ 1	☐ 2	☐ 3	☐ 4	☐ 5

Figure A1.2 (cont.)

PROMIS General Life Satisfaction

		Strongly disagree	Disagree	Slightly disagree	Neither agree nor disagree	Slightly agree	Agree	Strongly agree
PA045m	In most ways, my life is close to perfect ….	☐ 1	☐ 2	☐ 3	☐ 4	☐ 5	☐ 6	☐ 7
PA046	If I could live my life over, I would change almost nothing……………………	☐ 1	☐ 2	☐ 3	☐ 4	☐ 5	☐ 6	☐ 7
PA047	I am satisfied with my life ………………	☐ 1	☐ 2	☐ 3	☐ 4	☐ 5	☐ 6	☐ 7
PA048	So far I have gotten the important things I want in life ……………………………	☐ 1	☐ 2	☐ 3	☐ 4	☐ 5	☐ 6	☐ 7
PA049m	My life situation is excellent……………….	☐ 1	☐ 2	☐ 3	☐ 4	☐ 5	☐ 6	☐ 7

Figure A1.3 General life satisfaction. © 2008–2016 PROMIS Health Organization and PROMIS Cooperative Group. Reprinted with permission.

	Indicate how much you agree or disagree...	Not at all	A little bit	Somewhat	Quite a bit	Very much
PA077	I am satisfied with my education..............	☐ 1	☐ 2	☐ 3	☐ 4	☐ 5
PA078	I am satisfied with my present job or work...	☐ 1	☐ 2	☐ 3	☐ 4	☐ 5
PA079	I am satisfied with my well-being from spiritual, religious or philosophical beliefs	☐ 1	☐ 2	☐ 3	☐ 4	☐ 5
PA080	I am satisfied with my housing.	☐ 1	☐ 2	☐ 3	☐ 4	☐ 5
PA081	I am satisfied with my family life	☐ 1	☐ 2	☐ 3	☐ 4	☐ 5
PA082	I am satisfied with my health	☐ 1	☐ 2	☐ 3	☐ 4	☐ 5
PA083	I am satisfied with my friends and social life...	☐ 1	☐ 2	☐ 3	☐ 4	☐ 5
PA084	I am satisfied with my neighborhood overall...	☐ 1	☐ 2	☐ 3	☐ 4	☐ 5
PA085	I am satisfied with my ability to help others	☐ 1	☐ 2	☐ 3	☐ 4	☐ 5
PA086	I am satisfied with my achievement of my goals	☐ 1	☐ 2	☐ 3	☐ 4	☐ 5
PA087	I am satisfied with my leisure	☐ 1	☐ 2	☐ 3	☐ 4	☐ 5

Figure A1.3 (cont.)

PROMIS Domain-Specific Life Satisfaction

	Indicate how much you agree or disagree...	Not at all	A little bit	Somewhat	Quite a bit	Very much
PA088	I am satisfied with my physical safety	☐ 1	☐ 2	☐ 3	☐ 4	☐ 5
PA089	I am satisfied with my energy level	☐ 1	☐ 2	☐ 3	☐ 4	☐ 5

Figure A1.4 Domain-specific life satisfaction. © 2008–2016 PROMIS Health Organization and PROMIS Cooperative Group. Reprinted with permission.

PROMIS 29+2 Profile

	Physical Function	Without any difficulty	With a little difficulty	With some difficulty	With much difficulty	Unable to do
PFA11	Are you able to do chores such as vacuuming or yard work?........................	☐ 5	☐ 4	☐ 3	☐ 2	☐ 1
PFA21	Are you able to go up and down stairs at a normal pace?....................................	☐ 5	☐ 4	☐ 3	☐ 2	☐ 1
PFA23	Are you able to go for a walk of at least 15 minutes?..............................	☐ 5	☐ 4	☐ 3	☐ 2	☐ 1
PFA53	Are you able to run errands and shop?.....	☐ 5	☐ 4	☐ 3	☐ 2	☐ 1

	Anxiety In the past 7 days...	Never	Rarely	Sometimes	Often	Always
EDANX01	I felt fearful..	☐ 1	☐ 2	☐ 3	☐ 4	☐ 5
EDANX40	I found it hard to focus on anything other than my anxiety	☐ 1	☐ 2	☐ 3	☐ 4	☐ 5
EDANX41	My worries overwhelmed me..................	☐ 1	☐ 2	☐ 3	☐ 4	☐ 5
EDANX53	I felt uneasy	☐ 1	☐ 2	☐ 3	☐ 4	☐ 5

	Depression In the past 7 days...	Never	Rarely	Sometimes	Often	Always
EDDEP04	I felt worthless	☐ 1	☐ 2	☐ 3	☐ 4	☐ 5
EDDEP06	I felt helpless..	☐ 1	☐ 2	☐ 3	☐ 4	☐ 5
EDDEP29	I felt depressed...	☐ 1	☐ 2	☐ 3	☐ 4	☐ 5
EDDEP41	I felt hopeless..	☐ 1	☐ 2	☐ 3	☐ 4	☐ 5

	Fatigue During the past 7 days...	Not at all	A little bit	Somewhat	Quite a bit	Very much
HI7	I feel fatigued..	☐ 1	☐ 2	☐ 3	☐ 4	☐ 5
AN3	I have trouble starting things because I am tired..	☐ 1	☐ 2	☐ 3	☐ 4	☐ 5

Figure A1.5 PROMIS 29+2 Profile. © 2008–2016 PROMIS Health Organization and PROMIS Cooperative Group. Reprinted with permission.

PROMIS 29+2 Profile v2.1 (PROPr)

	Fatigue In the past 7 days...	Not at all	A little bit	Somewhat	Quite a bit	Very much
FATEXP41	How run-down did you feel on average?	☐ 1	☐ 2	☐ 3	☐ 4	☐ 5
FATEXP40	How fatigued were you on average?	☐ 1	☐ 2	☐ 3	☐ 4	☐ 5
	Sleep Disturbance In the past 7 days...	Very poor	Poor	Fair	Good	Very good
Sleep109	My sleep quality was	☐ 5	☐ 4	☐ 3	☐ 2	☐ 1
	In the past 7 days...	Not at all	A little bit	Somewhat	Quite a bit	Very much
Sleep116	My sleep was refreshing.	☐ 5	☐ 4	☐ 3	☐ 2	☐ 1
Sleep20	I had a problem with my sleep	☐ 1	☐ 2	☐ 3	☐ 4	☐ 5
Sleep44	I had difficulty falling asleep	☐ 1	☐ 2	☐ 3	☐ 4	☐ 5
	Ability to Participate in Social Roles and Activities	Never	Rarely	Sometimes	Usually	Always
SRPPER11 _CaPS	I have trouble doing all of my regular leisure activities with others	☐ 5	☐ 4	☐ 3	☐ 2	☐ 1
SRPPER18 _CaPS	I have trouble doing all of the family activities that I want to do	☐ 5	☐ 4	☐ 3	☐ 2	☐ 1
SRPPER23 _CaPS	I have trouble doing all of my usual work (include work at home)	☐ 5	☐ 4	☐ 3	☐ 2	☐ 1
SRPPER46 _CaPS	I have trouble doing all of the activities with friends that I want to do	☐ 5	☐ 4	☐ 3	☐ 2	☐ 1
	Pain Interference In the past 7 days...	Not at all	A little bit	Somewhat	Quite a bit	Very much
PAININ9	How much did pain interfere with your day to day activities?	☐ 1	☐ 2	☐ 3	☐ 4	☐ 5
PAININ22	How much did pain interfere with work around the home?	☐ 1	☐ 2	☐ 3	☐ 4	☐ 5
PAININ31	How much did pain interfere with your ability to participate in social activities?	☐ 1	☐ 2	☐ 3	☐ 4	☐ 5

Figure A1.5 (cont.)

Pain Interference

In the past 7 days...	Not at all	A little bit	Somewhat	Quite a bit	Very much
PAININ34 How much did pain interfere with your household chores?	☐ 1	☐ 2	☐ 3	☐ 4	☐ 5

Cognitive Function Abilities

In the past 7 days...	Not at all	A little bit	Somewhat	Quite a bit	Very much
PC6r I have been able to concentrate	☐ 1	☐ 2	☐ 3	☐ 4	☐ 5
PC27r I have been able to remember to do things, like take medicine or buy something I needed	☐ 1	☐ 2	☐ 3	☐ 4	☐ 5

Pain Intensity

In the past 7 days...

Global07 How would you rate your pain on average?	☐ 0 No pain	☐ 1	☐ 2	☐ 3	☐ 4	☐ 5	☐ 6	☐ 7	☐ 8	☐ 9	☐ 10 Worst pain imaginable

Figure A1.5 (cont.)

Appendix II Wellness Apps and Devices

Brennan Spiegel, Jonathan A. Almendárez, Samuel Korouri, Angela Liu, and Waguih William IsHak

Introduction

Mobile health applications have become a common method for supporting efforts to lead a healthier life. Since the introduction of the smartphone, the app has become a common software tool for users, as shown in Figure A2.1.

Mobile phone users are spending significant amounts of time reading, listening, and watching on their devices, especially using apps specifically designed for optimal functioning on smartphones. One popular application involves mobile health apps (Figure A2.2).

Some of the health apps are introduced by healthcare organizations to intervene and support treatment plans, while others are designed by private businesses to help the consumer lead a healthy lifestyle. Representative examples include Headspace, which is an app designed to support daily meditation practices, and wearables, which are typically devices that track physical activity, such as a Fitbit. Research by Liewel et al. in 2019 examined the success of health and wellness mobile apps. Using a consumer survey, the findings of the research indicated that mobile apps can help to keep consumers

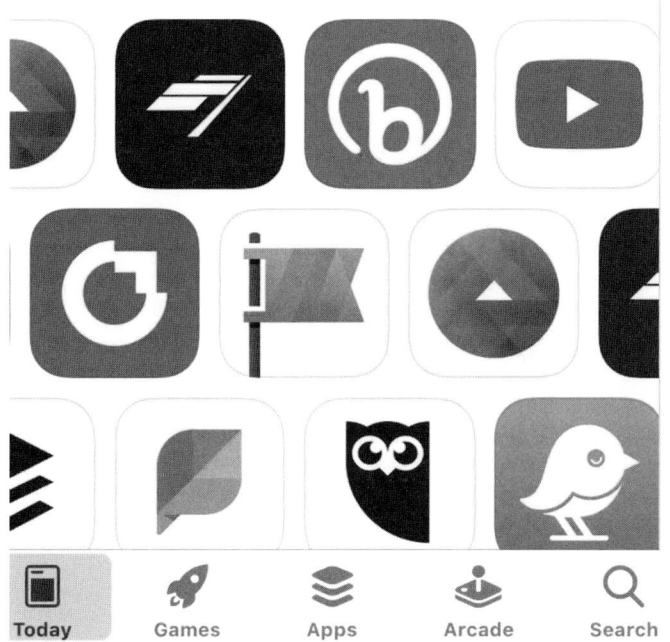

Figure A2.1 Apps.

8:14

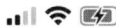

Figure A2.2 Health apps.

Q Health apps ⊗   Cancel

⚲ STORY

Beginner's Guide to Health Track...

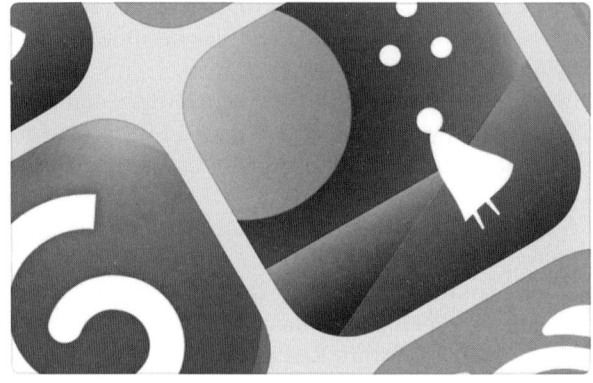

 **Motivation - Dail...**
Positive reminders o...
★★★★★ 165K   GET
In-App Purchases

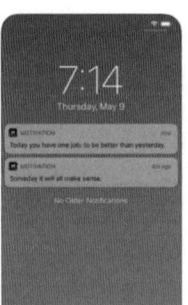 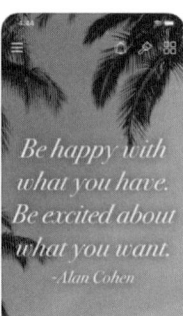 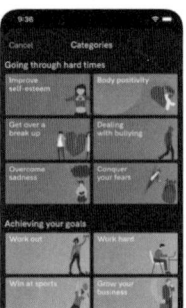

 Today   Games   Apps   Arcade   Search

accountable and the apps are easy to use [1]. One concern was the additional costs for add-ons and advertisements [1]. Users report an overall positive experience. Han and Lee investigated in 2018 the effectiveness of mobile apps in "changing health-related behaviors and improving clinical health outcomes" [2]. When used as intended, health apps can have a positive influence on the user's health and can change health-related behaviors. The following review lists some of the commonly used wellness apps and devices.

Example Wellness App

Research examining the use of the mindfulness-based smartphone apps examined whether the app can enhance the user's psychosocial well-being [3]. In a cohort study, a sample of 38 were given a self-reported satisfaction survey after using the app for 30 days [3]. The results indicated the app benefited the user's psychosocial well-being.

Headspace

The Headspace app is a guided meditation and mindfulness app that is considered one of the most downloaded apps for this purpose (Figure A2.3) [3]. The app helps users develop a plan and track meditation time through graphical tracking, and provides a journal for taking notes [4]. Randomized trials (small sample) showed that the use of Headspace improved well-being [4–6]. Dropout rates from using the app are not atypical of apps in general [3].

Example Wellness Device

Wearable devices are increasingly popular for monitoring activity, exercise, sleep, and weight (Figure A2.4).

Fitbit is an example of such a device, dedicated to measuring change in health behavior over time and during different activities. Fitbit includes an app paired with a device designed to track the activity of the user (Figure A2.5). The goal of the Fitbit is to motivate users to take more steps. Feehan et al. in 2018 measured Fitbit accuracy in monitoring the activity of users. According to the findings of the research, Fitbit was found to be an accurate tool for measuring activity [7].

Nazari et al. conducted research on the reliability of Fitbit in 2019 in a sample of 30 women examined while wearing a Fitbit device [8]. Measurements were taken of heart rate and physical activity to measure the reliability of the app. According to the findings of the research, the Fitbit app can reliably measure heart rate at rest and during fitness activities [8]. Tracking of steps also motivated the user to take more steps to improve overall health. The device can also track food intake and sleep patterns.

Partial Listing of Commonly Used Wellness Apps
Relax Melodies

Research examining the effects of different types of relaxing music on heart rate variability show that autonomic responses to musical stimuli were correlated with users' subjective preferences with respect to relaxing musical styles (Figures A2.6 and A2.7) [9]. This suggests that an application that would allow users to personalize their own relaxing musical experiences could better put them at ease.

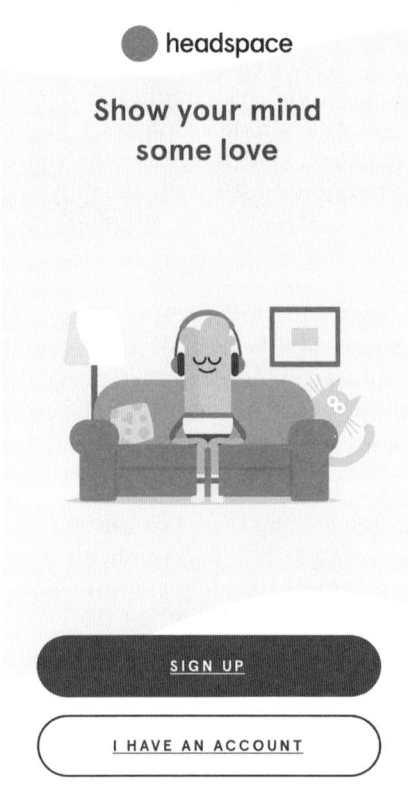

Figure A2.3 Headspace.

Relax Melodies is an application that helps users fall asleep in minutes by combining soothing sounds, bedtime stories, and sleep meditations. Relax Melodies offers innovative music and sounds designed to relieve tension, and the app gives the user the opportunity to use these features to craft a personalized bedtime experience.

Daylio Journal

Research examining the effects of positive affect journaling shows that this type of behavior has positive health benefits (Figure A2.7). In a study on 70 adults with elevated anxiety symptoms randomly assigned to a web-based positive affect journaling group or a usual care group, those who took part in the web-based positive affect journaling showed decreased mental distress and increased well-being relative to baseline, as well as fewer depressive symptoms and less anxiety relative to the usual care group [10]. These results suggest that a web-based application in which users take part in positive affect journaling can be effective in producing positive health benefits.

Daylio Journal is an app that enables users to create daily personalized journals based on their mood and the activities they take part in throughout the day.

Belly Bio

BellyBio is a wellness app that focuses on deep abdominal breathing, biofeedback, and music (Figure A2.8).

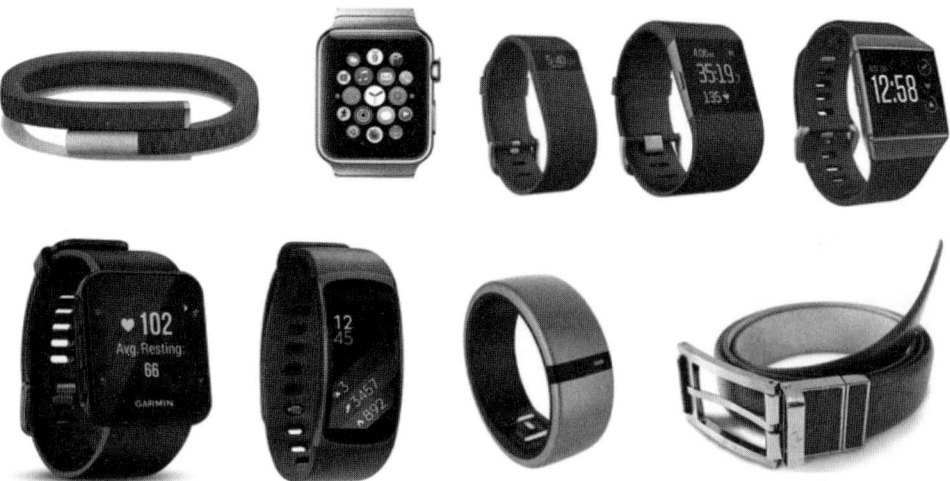

Figure A2.4 Examples of wearable devices.

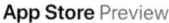

App Store Preview

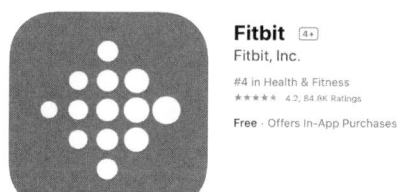

iPhone Screenshots

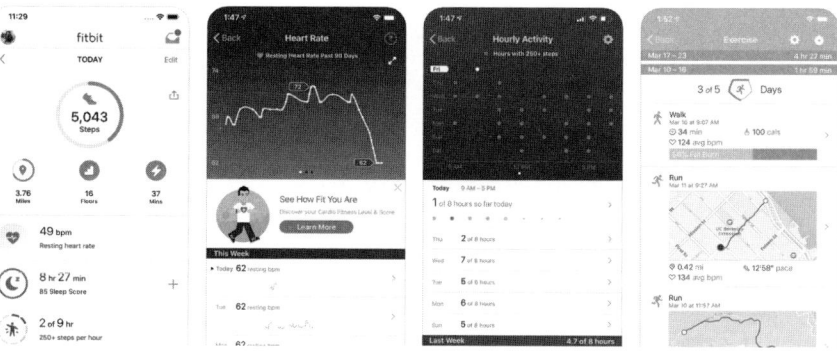

Figure A2.5 Fitbit app.

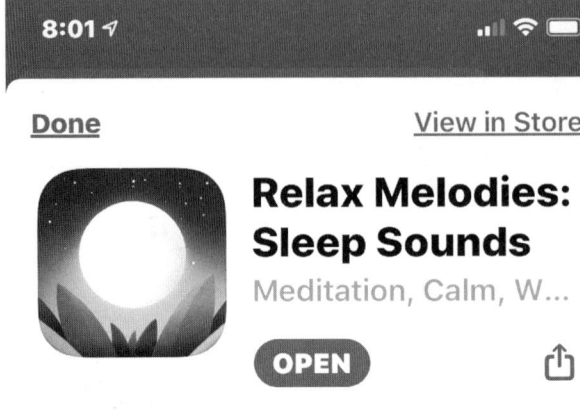

Figure A2.6 Relax Melodies app.

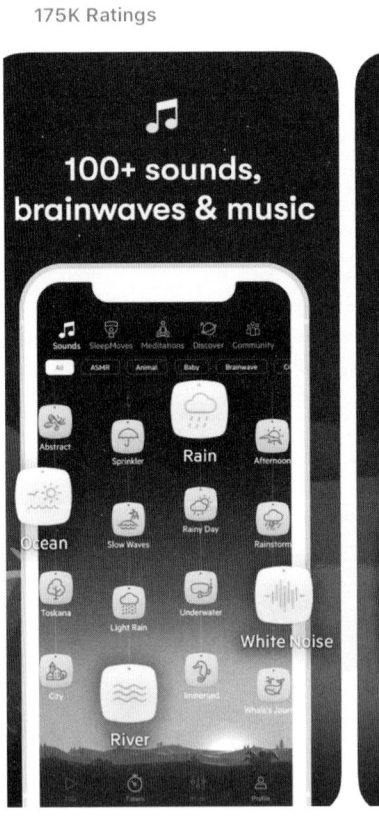

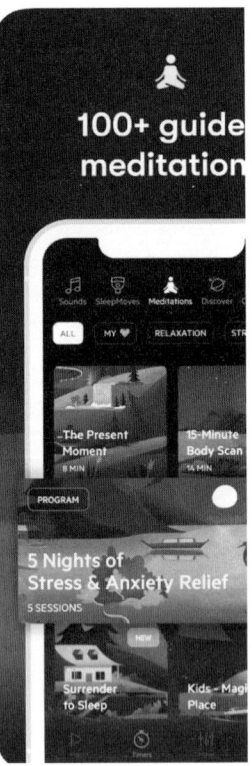

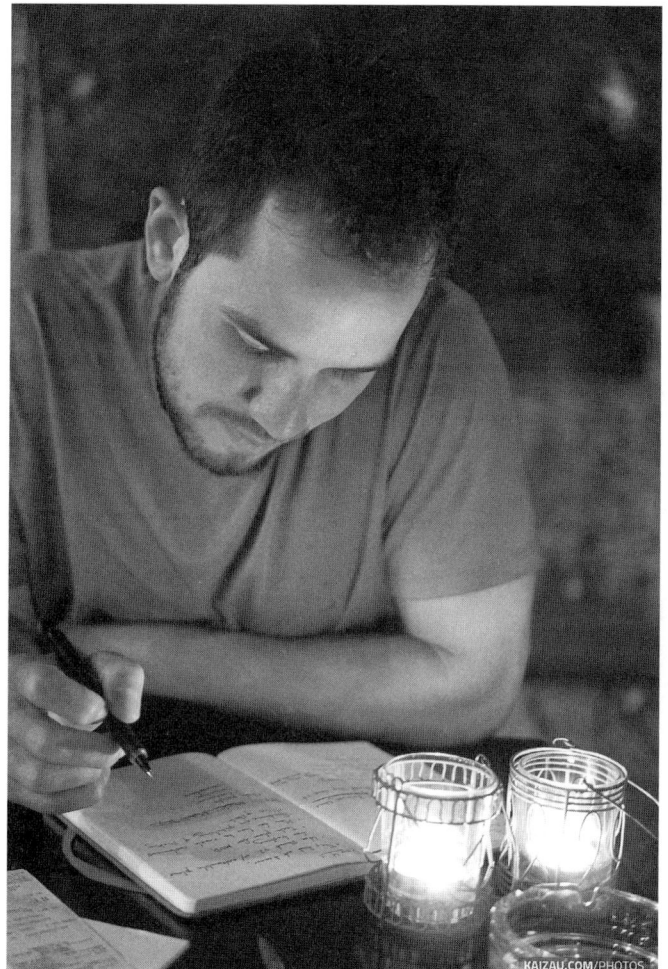

KAIZAU.COM/PHOTOS

Figure A2.7 Journaling. Reprinted from https://commons.w ikimedia.org/wiki/File:Journaling_(7 5048673).jpeg with permission from Creative Commons.

MindBody

The MindBody app allows users to explore millions of different local gym, yoga, fitness, wellness, and beauty classes (Figure A2.9). The app provides all the information about the local studio, as well as categorizing the types of treatments the user is looking for with regards to wellness services.

BodySpace

The BodySpace app combines www.bodybuilding.com, the largest website for health and fitness on the planet, with a complete system of innovative workout tools, cutting-edge trackers, and advice from qualified physicians, nutritionists, athletes, and trainers (Figure A2.10). The app also contains integrated social features to meet like-minded individuals that help users achieve the best version of themselves.

App Store Preview

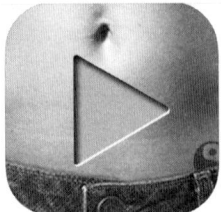

BellyBio Interactive Breathing 4+
RelaxLine

★★★★★ 3.5, 20 Ratings

Free · Offers In-App Purchases

iPhone Screenshots

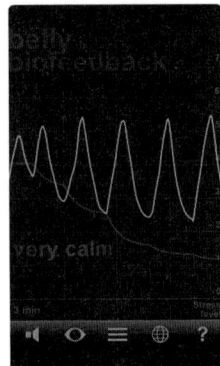 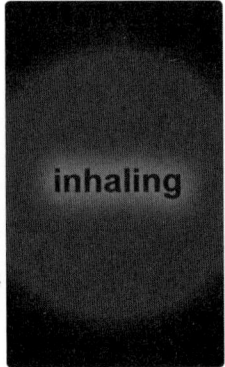 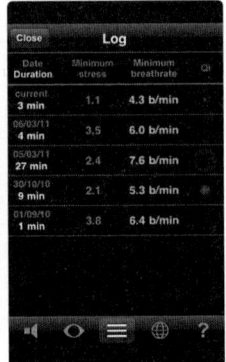 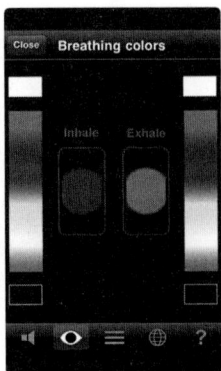

Figure A2.8 BellyBio app.

Achievement

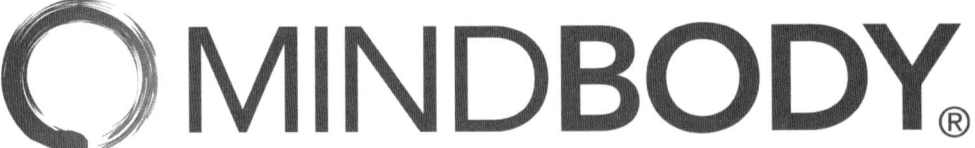

Figure A2.9 MindBody app. Reprinted from https://commons.wikimedia.org/wiki/File:MINDBODY_Logo.png with permission from Creative Commons.

The Achievement app offers users the chance to get paid for tracking steps as well as participating in health research aimed at engaging in health behaviors such as walking, eating well, and sleeping (Figure A2.11). The app also integrates information from other health behavior applications such as Fitbit.

Insight Timer

Insight Timer provides users with thousands of guided meditations and talks led by expert meditation and mindfulness experts, as well as music tracks from world-renowned artists

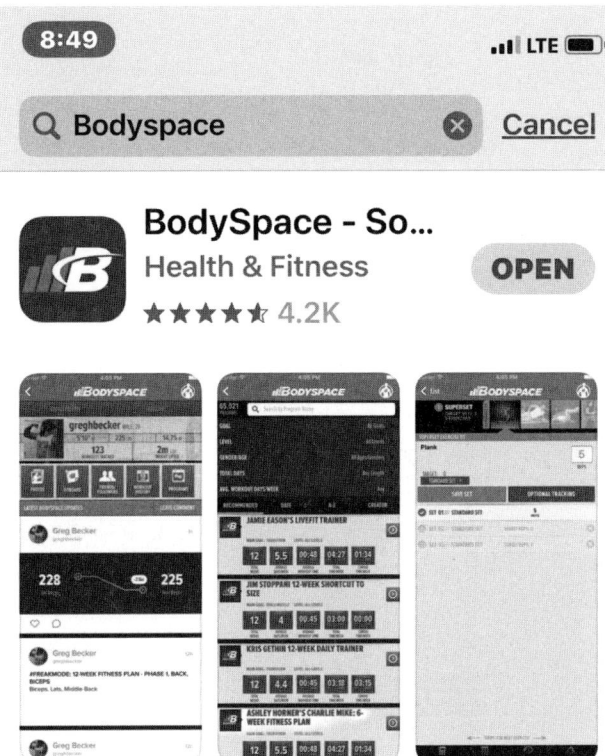

Figure A2.10 BodySpace app.

(Figure A2.12). The app lets users select the duration of their meditation sessions, which is useful for creating simple daily habits.

Breethe

Breethe offers guided meditations, soothing music, nature sounds, and different classes to allow users to destress and become happier and healthier (Figure A2.13).

Virgin Pulse

The Virgin Pulse app is designed to enhance daily healthy living habits (Figure A2.14). Virgin Pulse allows users to track their steps, their active minutes, calories burned, and sleep time, as well as to track program rewards and connect to other devices and apps for automatic tracking.

Sanvello

Sanvello is designed to help users deal with stress, anxiety, and depression (Figure A2.15). The app teaches users cognitive-behavioral therapy, an approach focused on changing negative behavior and thought patterns through immersive activities that integrate videos, audio exercises, mood and health habit tracking, and different activities.

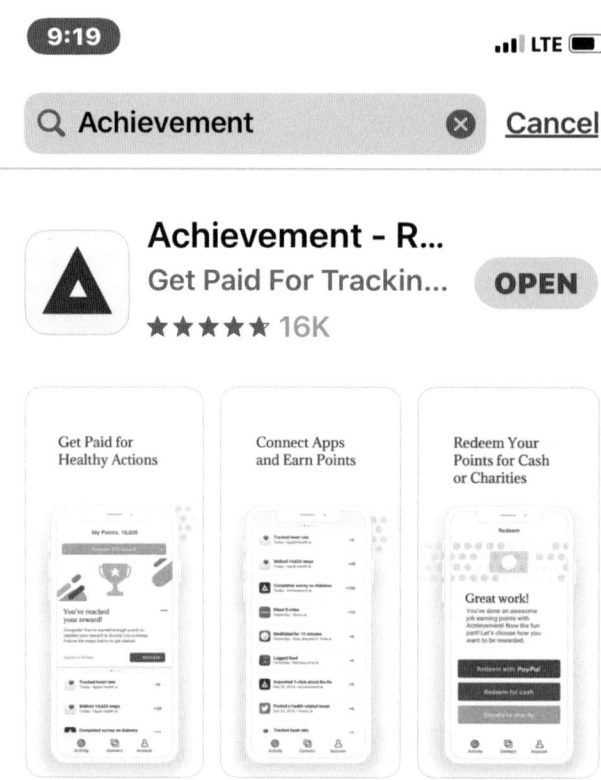

Figure A2.11 Achievement app.

Mantra

Mantra is an application that uses daily unique positive affirmations to help users reduce stress, make healthier choices, and improve performance during daily activities (Figure A2.16).

Calm

Calm, the #1-rated app in health and fitness, is designed to improve sleep, lower stress, and lessen anxiety with guided meditations, sleep stories, breathing exercises, stretching exercises, and relaxing music (Figure A2.17). Meditation sessions are offered in different time blocks, which makes it easy for users to craft sessions that fit best with their schedule.

Partial Listing of Commonly Used Wellness Devices
Example Virtual Reality Device: Mobile Phone Goggles

Virtual reality (VR) has been studied in several medical applications, including pain and behavioral and neurological conditions. Cedars-Sinai Medical Center investigators used a Samsung Gear VR goggle set, fitted with a Samsung Galaxy Note mobile phone (Figure A2.18) to deliver VR images and sound. Patients used VR applications such as the paint brush, underwater ocean exploration, aerial acrobatics, and aerial tour of scenic

4:30 ⌐ ..ll LTE 🔋

🔍 insight timer ⊗ Cancel

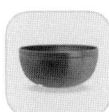

Insight Timer - M...
Meditation for Sleep... OPEN
★★★★★ 173K

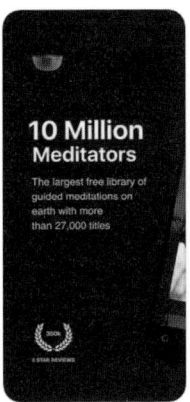
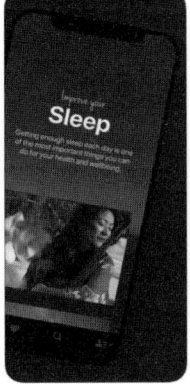
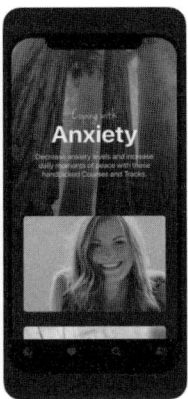

🅰 **FEATURED APP**
Insight Timer - Meditation App

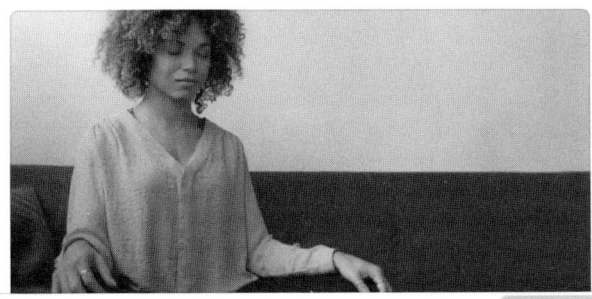

Today | Games | Apps | Arcade | Search

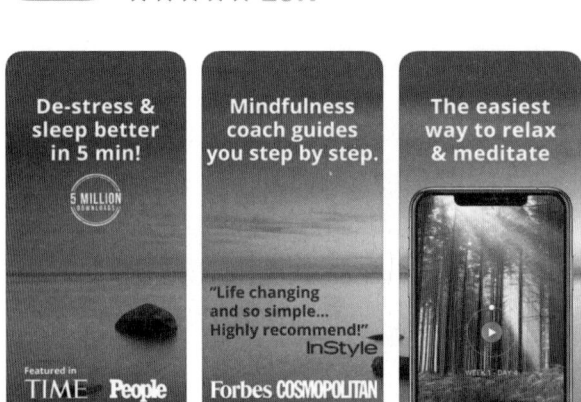

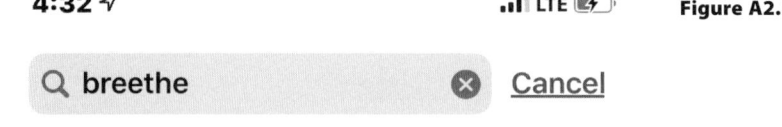

Figure A2.13 Breethe app.

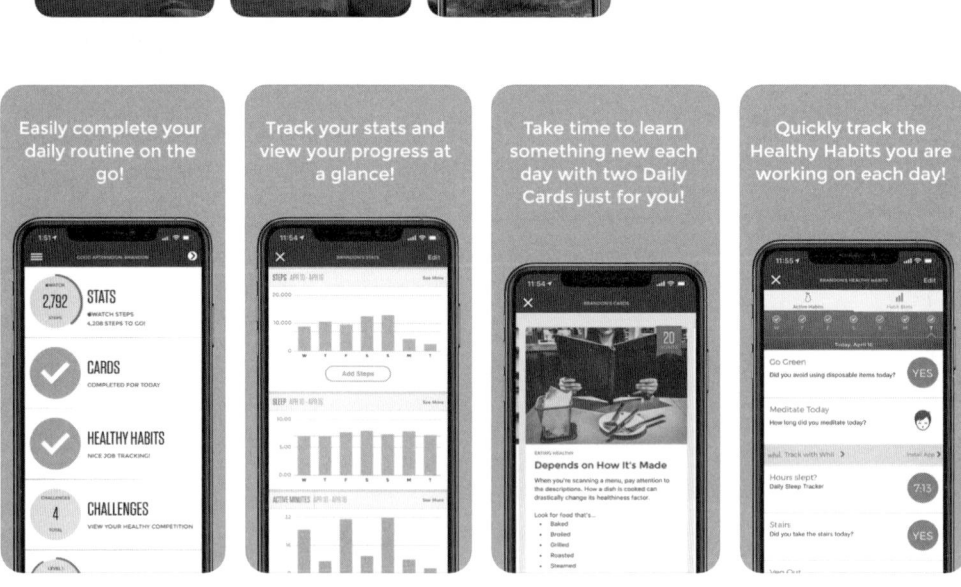

Figure A2.14 Virgin Pulse app.

Sanvello:Stress & Anxiety Help [12+]
Relieve symptoms feel happier
Sanvello Health Inc.

★★★★★ 4.8, 4.2K Ratings

Free · Offers In-App Purchases

Screenshots iPhone   iPad

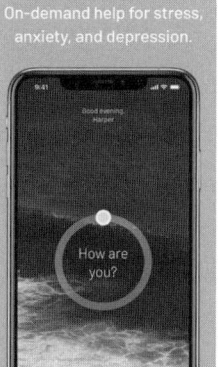 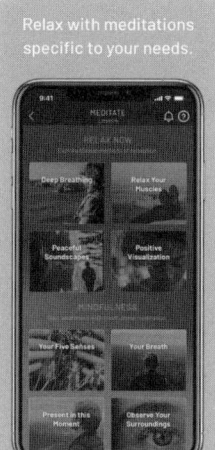 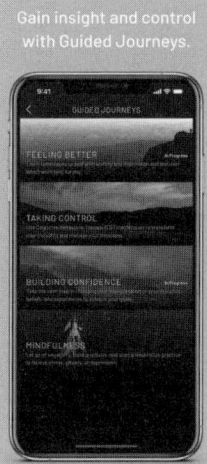 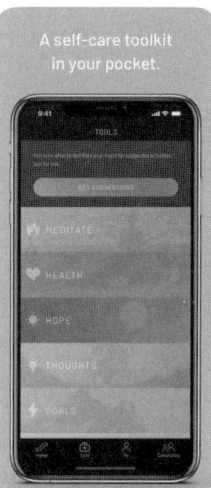

Figure A2.15 Sanvello.

topographies [11]. Research shows effectiveness of this VR method in pain management in hospitalized patients [12]. Future studies are being planned to examine impact on wellness.

Example Stress Measurement Device: PIP

The PIP is a biofeedback device that measures electrodermal activity, i.e., galvanic skin response and skin conductance from fingertips, at a frequency of eight times per second and connects to the PIP mobile phone app (Figure A2.19). Other apps work with PIP, such as Stress Tracker, Steps to Mindfulness, Clarity, and Loom. Controlled studies showed that biofeedback using PIP reduced stress significantly [13].

Example Brain Sensing Device: MUSE

Muse is a headband that detects electrical activity of the brain (Figures A2.20–A2.22) in the form of an electroencephalogram (EEG), with the feedback delivered to the user through a smartphone app such as Calm. This neurofeedback method, which rewards decreasing theta wave activity and increasing alpha wave activity, is thought to enhance attention, concentration, and well-being [14].

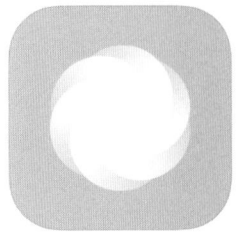

Mantra - Daily Affirmations ⁴⁺
Self Motivation & Be Positive
Efe Helvaci

★★★★★ 4.7, 2.1K Ratings

Free · Offers In-App Purchases

Screenshots   iPhone   iPad

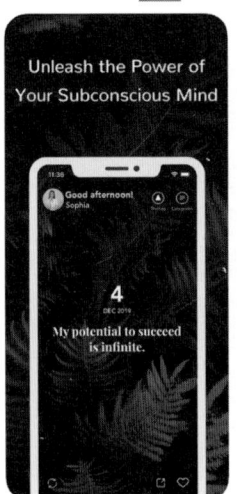
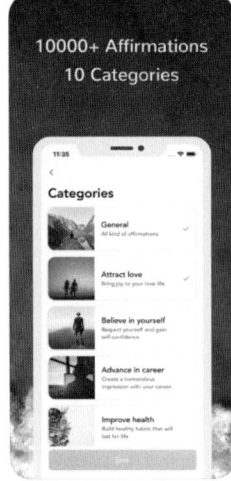
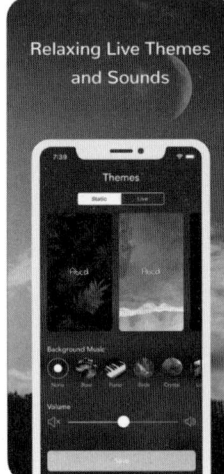
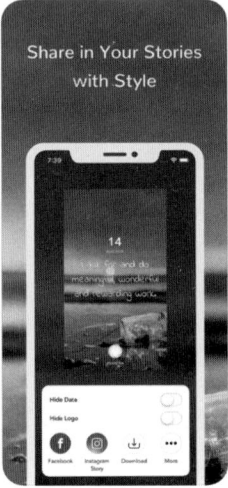

Figure A2.16 Mantra app.

References

1. M Liew, H Zhang, S See, Y Ong. Usability challenges for health and wellness mobile apps: mixed-methods study among health experts and consumers. *JMIR Mhealth Uhealth* 2019; **7**: e12160.

2. M Han, E Lee. Effectiveness of mobile health application use to improve health behavior changes: a systematic review of randomized controlled trials. *Healthc Informat Res* 2018; **24**: 207–226.

3. NA Haug. Headspace: an Expert Review. https://psyberguide.org/expert-review/head space-expert-review (accessed September 15, 2019).

4. L Champion, M Economides, C Chandler. The efficacy of a brief app-based mindfulness intervention on psychosocial outcomes in healthy adults: a pilot randomized controlled trial. *PLoS One* 2018; **13**: e0209482.

5. A Howells, I Ivtzan, FJ Eiroa-Orosa. Putting the "app" in happiness: a randomized controlled trial of a smartphone-based mindfulness intervention to enhance wellbeing. *J Happiness Stud* 2016; **17**: 163–185.

6. D Lim, P Condon, D DeSteno. Mindfulness and compassion: an examination of mechanism and scalability. *PLoS One* 2015; **10**: e0118221.

7. L Feehan, J Geldman, L Li. Accuracy of Fitbit devices: systematic review

Calm 4+
Meditation and Sleep Stories
Calm.com

#1 in Health & Fitness
★★★★★ 4.8, 632.9K Ratings

Free · Offers In-App Purchases

Screenshots   iPhone   iPad   Apple Watch   Apple TV

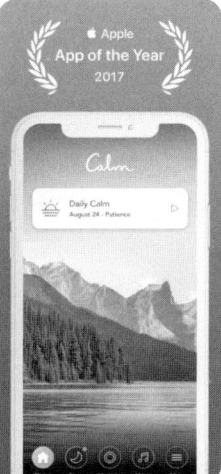 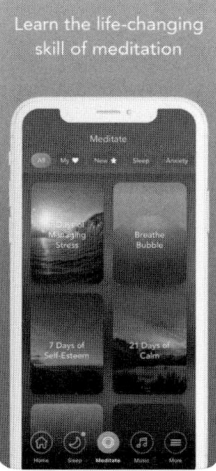 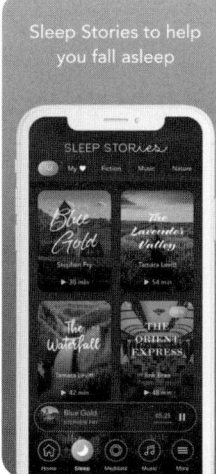 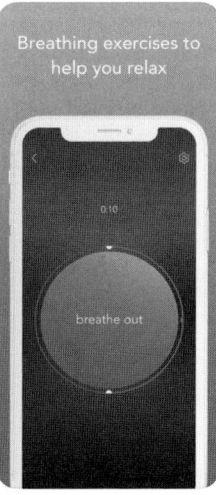

Figure A2.17 Calm app.

and narrative syntheses of quantitative data. *JMIR Mhealth Uhealth* 2018; **6**: e10527.

8. G Nazari, J MacDermid, K Sinden, et al. Reliability of Zephyr Bioharness and Fitbit charge measures of heart rate and activity at rest, during the modified Canadian aerobic fitness test, and recovery. *Strength Cond Res* 2019; **3**: 559–571.

9. S Perez-Lloret, J Diez, MN Dome, et al. Effects of different "relaxing" music styles on the autonomic nervous system. *Noise Health* 2014; **72**: 279–284.

10. J Smyth, J Johnson, B Auer, et al. Online positive affect journaling in the improvement of mental distress and well-being in general medical patients with elevated anxiety patients: a preliminary randomized control trial. *JMIR Ment Health* 2018; **5**: e11290.

11. S Mosadeghi, MW Reid, B Martinez, BT Rosen, BM Spiegel. Feasibility of an immersive virtual reality intervention for hospitalized patients: an observational cohort study. *JMIR Ment Health* 2016; **27**: e28.

12. Tashjian VC, Mosadeghi S, Howard AR, et al. Virtual reality for management of pain in hospitalized patients: results of a controlled trial. *JMIR Ment Health* 2017; **4**: e9.

13. A Dillon, M Kelly, IH Robertson, et al. Smartphone applications utilizing

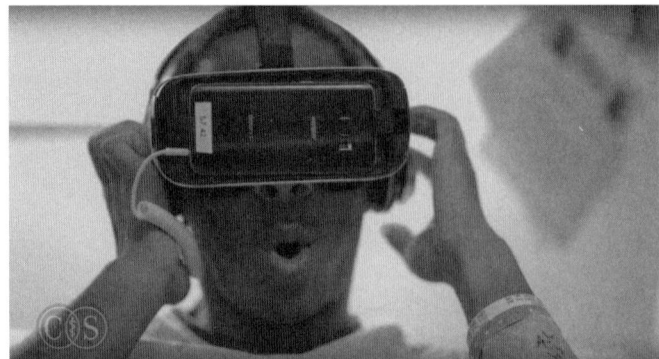

Figure A2.18 Virtual reality using a Samsung Gear VR goggle set, fitted with a Samsung Galaxy Note mobile phone at Cedars-Sinai Medical Center.

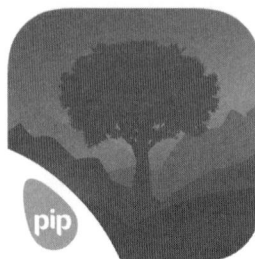

PIP: The Loom

Galvanic Ltd   **Health & Fitness**

E Everyone

★ ★ ★ ★ ⋆ 19 ▲

🔖 Add to Wishlist

Install

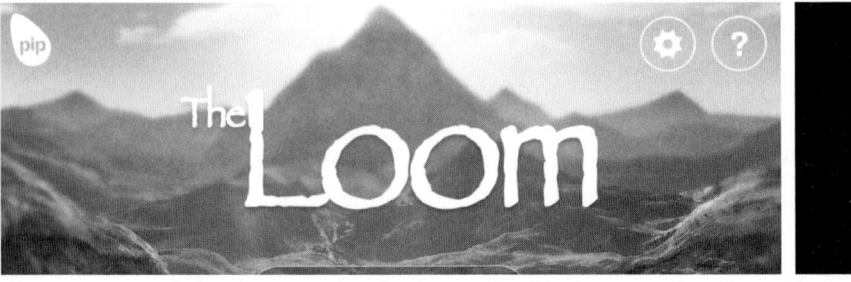

Use your powers of relaxation to transform landscapes. Soothing imagery and music combine to dissolve tension and ease stress away. As you de-stress, the landscape responds to reflect your inner calmness – cold, snowy winter turns into bright, sunny summer; starry night skies transform into radiant dawn.

Figure A2.19 PIP.

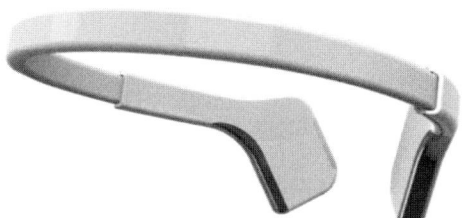

Figure A2.20 Muse app.

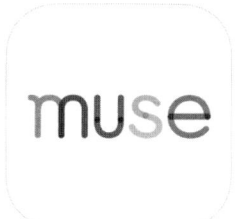

Figure A2.21 Muse headband.

Muse: Meditation Assistant 4+

Brain Sensing Headband
InteraXon

★★★★★ 4.6, 880 Ratings

Free · Offers In-App Purchases

Screenshots iPhone iPad

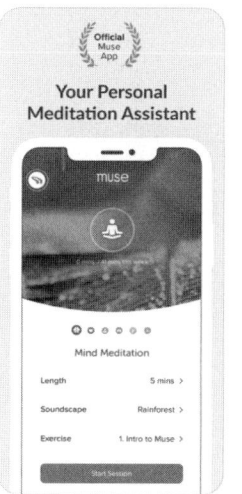

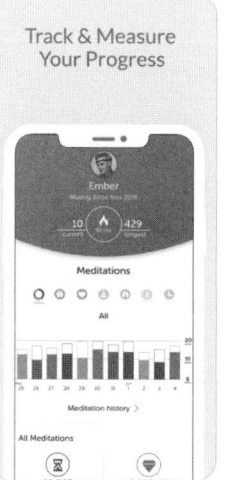

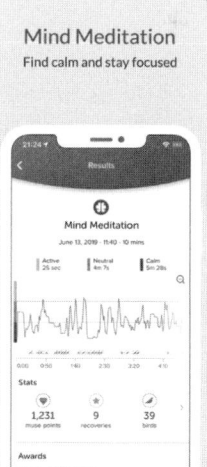

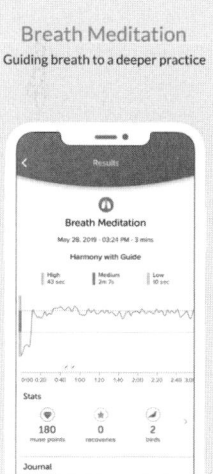

Figure A2.22 Muse results.

biofeedback can aid stress reduction. *Front Psychol* 2016; 7: 832.

14. YJ Lee, HG Kim, EJ Cheon, et al. The analysis of electroencephalography changes before and after a single neurofeedback alpha/theta training session in university students. *Appl Psychophysiol Biofeedback* 2019; 44: 173–184.

Index

5 A's of physical activity,
191–192
5-hydroxtryptophan (5-HTP),
305–306
360-degree evaluation,
469–470

acceptance and commitment
therapy (ACT), 184, 220
accommodating conflict
resolution style, 469
accomplishment, work–life
balance, 548
Accreditation Council for
Graduate Medical
Education (ACGME),
259, 267, 440
achievement
defined, 498
future-directed therapy,
499–502
hope therapy, 498–499
Achievement (computer
application), 612
Acromegaly Quality of Life
Questionnaire, 164
Action Collaborative (NAM),
259–260
Active Australia
Questionnaire, 19–20
active constructive
response, 465
active destructive response, 465
acts of kindness, 204
acupressure, 121
acupuncture
cancer, 381
chronic pain, 219
defined, 75, 90–91
gastroesophageal reflux
disorder (GERD), 89
hypertension and, 380–381
labor pain management, 121
low back pain, 380
and moxibustion, 91–92
multiple sclerosis, 380
traditional Chinese
medicine, 378
UTIs and, 104

acute medical conditions,
178–179
Adams, H. (Patch), 404
Adams, J., 567
Adams, T., 6
adaptogens, 297–298. see also
herbal therapies
Addison's disease, 161–162
adiponectin, 165–166
Adler, R., 388
adrenal deficiency, 161–162
adverse childhood experiences
(ACEs), 29, 151
advocacy, women's
wellness, 118
aesthetics and wellness
cosmetic procedures,
394–396
as form of recovery, 397–399
styling, 399–400
Affordable Care Act, 248
Aggarwàl, B., 389
Aisen, A., 474
alcohol
fertility and, 123
OAB and, 100
Alderman, A.K., 396
Alexander technique, 321
allergic process, 143–149
Alliance for Innovation on
Maternal Health
(AIM), 117
allopathic medicine, 379–380
Alzheimer's disease
MIND diet, 277–278
sleep and, 326–327
American Association of
Fitness Directors, 249
American Cancer Society,
189
American Public Health
Association, 414
American Sleep
Association, 425
amino acids, 222–223
analysis of variance, 61
anger, 10
anterior fornix erogenous zone
stimulation, 341

anticonvulsants, 213
antidepressants, 213
anti-inflammatory diet,
221–222
Antoni, M.H., 141
anxiety
cancer, 231
CBD for, 307
essential oils for, 308
etiology of, 306
kava for, 307
massage therapy and, 403
meditation and, 349
mindfulness and, 346, 347
music therapy, 408
neuroenhancement, 374
pharmaceuticals for,
306–307
sensory therapy, 459
terminal illness, 241
valerian root for, 307–308
aromatherapy, 453
arousal (sexual), 332–334
art therapy
child and adolescent
health, 205
and expression, 70
history of, 435–438
arthritis
neuropathic
medications, 212
NSAIDs, 212
statistics, 310
arts in health, 436, 438–440
asana yoga, 353
assessment instruments
cancer, 227–232
chronic pain, 209
PERMA-Profiler, 18
PROMIS, 19
SF-, 3617
SWLS, 17–18
WHO-, 5, 15–17
Association of American
Medical Colleges
(AAMC), 440
Astor, M.C., 167
Atkins diet. see modified
Atkins diet

atopic dermatitis (AD),
144, 148
audio-visual entrainment
(AVE), 365
autoimmune disease, 149–157
automatic negative thoughts
(ANTs), 367
avoiding conflict resolution
style, 468
Ayurvedic medicine
effectiveness of, 387–389
herbal therapies, 389–390
lifestyle factors and, 390–391
meditation, 389
philosophy, 385–386
practice, 386–387
Azizzadeh, B., 398

Baiker, K., 521
Balasubramaniam, M., 354
Bansal, A., 169
Banz, W.J., 165
Barnett, L., 568
Barsky, A.J., 9
Bart, R., 11
Bates, W., 456
Beauvais, A.M., 466
Bell's palsy, 398
Belly Bio (computer
application), 608
benign prostatic hyperplasia,
108–109
Bennis, W.G., 467
Benson, H., 389
Bensoussan, J.C., 394
best-self visualization method
(BSM), 530
biofeedback
circadian rhythm, 432
PIP (wellness device), 617
positive
neuropsychology, 368
biologically based therapies
chronic medical conditions,
183–184
dietary supplements, 71–72
herbal therapies, 72–73
specialized diet, 73–74
biopsychosocial assessment
chronic medical conditions,
180–181
measurement, 38
medical assessment, 23–24
psychiatric symptoms, 24–25
psychological assessment,
24

psychosocial factors, 25–33
resources, 33–34
biopsychosocial health, 1
Blackburn, E., 554
bladder health
defined, 98
nutrition and, 99
physical activity and, 99
risk factors for bladder
cancer, 99
training/urge
suppression, 100
voiding habits, 98
Bland, H.W., 569
Body–Mind Spirit Wellness
Behaviour and
Characteristics
Inventory, 61
BodySpace (computer
application), 611
Boiler, L., 477
boron, 124
botanicals. see herbal therapies
Botox injections, 398
botulinum toxin (Botox),
306
Brain Smart, 365
brain stimulation, 372–373
breast cancer aesthetics,
397–398
breast cancer screening,
189–190
Breethe (computer
application), 613
brief resilience scale, 490
Brinkworth, G.D., 166
broaden-and-build theory of
positive emotions, 474
buprenorphine, 212
burnout and stress prevention,
258–259

Cáceres-Muñoz, V.S., 328
caffeine
fertility and, 124
OAB and, 100
CAGE-AID, 25
Calm (computer
application), 614
calories in/calories out model,
280–281
cancer
defined, 225
occurrence of, 225
risk factors for, 225–226
in women, 127–128

cancer wellness
anxiety and depression, 231
assessment methods,
227–232
cancer-related fatigue, 231
geriatric, 189–190
methodology, 232
quality of life, 231
sleep patterns, 231–232
survivorship, 226
treatment symptoms and
long-term effects, 226–227
variables affecting, 227
cancer wellness interventions
acupuncture, 381
art therapy, 439
Ayurvedic medicine, 389
exercise and yoga, 233
hormone replacement
therapy and, 162–163
humor therapy, 406–407
massage therapy, 404–405
psychosocial, 234
published articles, 232–233
survivorship care plans, 233
traditional Chinese
medicine, 383–384
cancer-related fatigue, 231
cannabinoid treatment, 72, 307
Cannon, W., 387
carbamazepine, 213
cardiovascular and pulmonary
disorders
definitions and
symptoms, 79
dietary supplements, 83
humor therapy, 82
massage, 80
meaningful social
relationships, 83
meditation, 80
music therapy, 82–83
Ornish diet for, 278
positive thinking, 83
specialized diet therapy,
79–80
yoga, 80
Carlson, L.E., 161
Carpenter, G., 568
Caruthers, C., 540
CASIO model, 477
celecoxib, 212
cell phones
computer applications,
605–607
fertility and, 124

Centers for Disease Control, 251
cervical cancer screening, 190
cesarean-section pain management, 120
Chainanu-Wu, N., 390
Chapman, C.R., 242
character strengths and virtues model, 475
Charmaz, K., 526
Charon, R., 440
Chawla, L., 414
Check Up GP (computer app), 20
Chen, E., 149
Chew, B.H., 466
child and adolescent health
  acts of kindness, 204
  adverse childhood experiences (ACEs), 203–204
  clown therapy, 404
  cognitive-behavioral therapy, 205
  early-life stress, 466
  exercise therapies, 201
  family and, 199–200, 560–561
  gratitude, 204
  humor therapy, 406–407
  massage therapy, 404–405
  mindfulness, 204–205
  music and art, 205
  nutraceuticals, 206
  nutrition, 200–201
  pharmaceuticals, 206
  positive psychology, 204
  positive relationships and, 200
  sleep, 202–203
  social connection, 517
  social media use, 202
  spirituality and religion, 205–206
  yoga, 201–202
Chochinov, H.M., 532
Choi, J., 383
chronic care model, 180
chronic diseases, 1, 110
chronic illness
  demoralization, 530–532
  fostering wellness, 527–530
  occurrence of, 525
  psychology of, 525–527
  stress and, 567
chronic medical conditions

barriers to treatment, 183
clinical issues, 185
defined, 178–179
evidence-based approach, 182, 183–185
psychosocial factors, 185
psychotherapy, 184–185
self-care, 182–183
suboptimal wellness in, 179
wellness theory in, 179–180
chronic pain
  acupuncture, 219
  assessment, 209
  botanicals, 222–223
  curcumin for, 311
  defined, 209
  dietary supplements, 222
  epidural blocks, 217
  etiology of, 309–310
  inflammation and, 367
  low back, 380
  manual therapy, 220
  massage therapy, 219–220, 404–405
  massage therapy and, 403–404
  meditation and, 349
  mind–body therapies, 220–221
  music therapy, 223, 408
  neuromodulation, 218–219
  neuropathic medications, 212–217
  nutrition, 221–222
  pet therapy, 223
  pharmaceuticals for, 209–217, 310–311
  psychotherapy, 220
  radiofrequency ablation, 217
  sympathetic blocks, 218
chronotype, 430–431
Cicerone, K., 369–372
circadian rhythm. see also neuromodulation
  body systems, 429–430
  defined, 423–425
  individual chronotype, 430–431
  influencers, 426–428
  metabolism, 428
  sleep and, 425–426
  stress and, 428–429
  tips for, 431–433
Circle of Wellness in Psychiatric Disorders, 60

clinical issues
  affecting cancer, 227
  psychiatric and substance-use disorders, 63
  senses and diagnosing, 450–451
clinician wellness
  burnout and stress prevention, 258–259
  emotional intelligence, 467
  evaluation, 576–577
  healing practices, 507
  individual interventions, 262–263
  medical school arts education, 440–442
  Norwegian culture, 545–546
  organizational interventions, 265–266
  practice interventions, 263–264
  sleep patterns, 325–326
  strategies, 259–262
  systems interventions, 267
Cloninger, R., 361
clothing and wellness, 400
cocaine, 123
coffee. see caffeine
cognitive disorders
  etiology of, 308
  gingko biloba for, 309
  pharmaceuticals for, 308
cognitive rehabilitation, 369–372
cognitive-behavioral therapy (CBT)
  art, 69–70
  cancer wellness, 234
  child and adolescent health, 205
  insomnia, 119, 366
  irritable bowel syndrome, 92, 94
  perinatal depression, 119
  as psychological-based therapy, 220, 475
  sexual wellness, 340–341
  social relationships, 516
Cohen, M.H., 506
Cohen, N., 388
Cohen, S., 139, 388
coital alignment technique, 341
collaboration conflict resolution style, 469
colon cancer screening, 190

community. *see also* social
relationships
defined, 521
virtual, 522–523
work, 521–522
compassion
defined, 518
interventions, 519
self, 518–519
compassion-focused therapy
(CFT), 520
compassion meditation
(CM), 520
competitive conflict resolution
style, 469
complementary and alternative
medical practices (CAM).
see also
psychoneuroimmunology
biologically based therapies,
71–74
exercise therapies, 74
gynecological wellness,
126–128
labor pain management,
120–121
manual body therapies,
74–75
mind–body therapies,
67–69
prostate health, 109–110
psychosocial therapies,
69–71
usage of, 66–67
complex regional pain
syndrome, 218
comprehensive geriatric
assessment, 190–191
compromising conflict
resolution style, 469
CONCORD program, 226
conflict resolution styles,
468–469
connectors, 464
Connor–Davidson resilience
scale, 490
consciousness of
integration, 559
continuous labor support,
120
cosmetic procedures
as form of recovery, 397–399
minimally invasive
procedures, 395
popularity of, 394
surgical procedures, 396

Cousins, N., 404
Covey, S., 5
Covinsky, K.E., 189
Cozolin, L., 559
cranberry consumption,
103–104, 295–297
creative arts therapies, 436,
437, 442–443
Cretney, R., 485
Crohn's disease. *see*
inflammatory bowel
diseases therapies
Csikszentmihalyi, M., 38,
547
culture
circadian rhythm, 433
healing practices, 505–507
terminal illness, 244
and well-being
measurement, 43
and wellness treatment
plan, 51
work–life balance, 545–546
Cunningham, J., 167
curcumin, 91, 222, 311. *see also*
turmeric
Cusano, N.E., 166
Cushing syndrome, 160–161
cyclooxygenase (COX),
212

dance therapy, 317–319
Daniel Patterson, P., 328
Davis, D.L., 2
Daylio Journal (computer
application), 608
DeHaan, C.R., 578
delayed ejaculation, 107–108
demographics (patient)
cancer, 227
geriatric, 188
humor therapy, 406–407
massage therapy, 404–405
demoralization, 530–532. *see
also* depression
Depken, D., 6
depression. *see also*
demoralization
5-HTP for, 305–306
Botox for, 306
cancer, 231
chronic medical
conditions, 179
DHEA for, 305
etiology of, 304
meditation and, 349

mindfulness and, 346, 347
pharmaceuticals for, 304
during pregnancy, 119
S-adenosyl-L-methionine
for, 305
screening for, 24–25
St. John's wort for,
304–305
terminal illness, 241
yoga and, 353–354
DeSantana, J.M., 367
diabetes, 164–166, 354
Diabetes Prevention
Program, 164
diabetic neuropathy, 212
diathesis-stress model, 485
diclofenac, 310–311
Diener, E., 17–18, 41
diet therapy. *see also* nutrition
bladder health and, 99
comparison between,
279–281
diet commonalities,
278–279
Dietary Approaches to Stop
Hypertension (DASH)
diet, 275–276
exercise therapies and,
73–74, 79–80
FODMAP diet, 93, 276–277
immune system, 92
ketogenic diet, 275
Mediterranean diet,
273–274
MIND diet, 277–278
modified Atkins diet,
277
Ornish diet, 278
Paleolithic diet, 274
practical guidelines,
281–282
search for perfect, 272–273
sexual wellness, 340
vegetarian, 276
weight loss, 278
wellness and health through,
271–272
Dietary Approaches to Stop
Hypertension (DASH)
diet, 275–276
dietary fiber, 93, 293
Dietary Supplement Health
and Education Act,
303
dietary supplements. *see also*
nutraceuticals

cardiovascular and
   pulmonary disorders,
   83
chronic pain, 222
herbal and plant based,
   71–72
obesity, 166
sexual wellness, 339
urinary tract infections
   (UTIs), 104
usage of, 303
dignity therapy, 532
dihydroepiandrosterone
   (DHEA), 305
Dillard, A., 9
disability, 526–527
disgust, 10
Dissanayake, E., 435
D-mannose, 104
Donabedian, A., 191
doula, 120
Dube, S.R., 151
Duckworth, A.L., 467,
Dutton, J.E., 548

early-life stress, 466
Eckman, P., 8–10
Edwards, M.E., 167
eight dimensions of wellness
   model, 536
electronic medical records,
   264, 266
Elliot, A., 438
emotional intelligence (EQ)
   biology of, 465–466
   clinical applications,
      467
   importance of, 463
   scope of, 463–465
   tips to improve, 467–471
   wellness and, 8–10
employee assistance program
   (EAP), 254
end-of-life care, 238–239,
   406–407, 578–579. see also
   terminal illness
endocrine model, 281
endocrine system disorders
   adrenal, 160–162
   diabetes, 164–166
   estrogen and progesterone,
      162–163
   parathyroid hormone,
      166–167
   testosterone, 168–169
   thyroid hormone, 169–170

energy healers, 508
engagement, 547
Engle, G., 1, 23
ensemble empowerment, 400
Epel, E., 554
epidural blocks, 217
EPOCH Measure of
   Adolescent Well-being, 18
erectile disorder, 107
Eriksonian stages of terminal
   illness, 243
essential oils, 308
estrogen
   endocrine system disorders,
      162–163
   UTIs and, 102–103
eudaimonia, 40–41
eudaimonic principle of well-
   being, 6, 576
evaluative wellness, 576–577
exclusive enteral nutrition, 92
exercise screening, 19–20
exercise therapies
   benefits of, 315–316
   cancer, 233
   childhood, 201
   chronic medical
      conditions, 184
   elements of, 316
   fertility and, 122
   geriatric, 191–193
   irritable bowel syndrome,
      92, 94
   neuroenhancement, 373
   neurological disorders, 74
   obesity, 165–166
   positive
      neuropsychology, 368
   workplace wellness
      programs, 252–254
expression therapy, 70

family relationships, 199–200,
   560–561
fashion. see styling
fatty acids. see polyunsaturated
   fatty acids
Fava, G.A., 478–480
fear, 9–10
Feldman, R., 562
female sexual dysfunction
   genito-pelvic pain/
      penetration disorder,
      106–107
   interest/arousal disorder,
      105–106

orgasmic disorder, 106
   testosterone therapy, 168
Ferro-Luzzi, A., 273
fertility treatments
   alcohol and, 123
   caffeine and, 124
   cocaine and, 123
   exercise, 122
   heavy metals and, 124–125
   low-resource settings, 126
   marijuana and, 123
   nutrition, 121
   opiates and, 123
   psychological, 122
   reproductive clock, 121
   resilience training, 125–126
   tobacco use, 122–123
   weight, 121–122
fiber. see dietary fiber
fibromyalgia, 213, 354
fight-or-flight response, 9–10
Fisher, H., 562
Fiskum, A., 415
Fitbit (wellness device), 607
Five Factor Wellness, 61
Flachenecker, P., 156
flibanserin, 106
flu vaccine, 189
fluid intake, OAB and, 100
focused breathing, 67
FODMAP diet, 276–277
food allergies, 145, 147
Food and Drug Administration
   (FDA), 303
Forbes, H., 329
forgiveness, 357–359
Foster, G.D., 166
Fox, R., 417
Frank, J., 531
Frankl, V., 496–497
Fredrickson, B., 474
Frendl, D.M., 17
friendship relationships, 561
Frisch, M.B., 475, 477–478
Fullen, M.C., 491
functional dyspepsia therapies
   acupuncture, 90–91
   peppermint/caraway oil, 90
   STW5, 90
functional magnetic resonance
   (fMRI), 465–466
future-directed therapy,
   499–502

gabapentin, 213
Gallup Purdue Index, 541

gastroesophageal reflux
disorder (GERD)
acupuncture, 89
lifestyle modifications for,
87–89
gastrointestinal system
disorders
functional dyspepsia
therapies, 90–91
GERD therapies, 87–89
inflammatory bowel diseases
therapies, 91–93
irritable bowel syndrome,
93–94
symptoms, 87–88
Gavrin, J., 242
Geller, S., 559
gender identity, 30–31
generalized anxiety
disorder, 25
genito-pelvic pain/penetration
disorder, 106–107
Geriatric Depression Scale,
24
geriatric wellness
breast cancer screening,
189–190
cervical cancer
screening, 190
colon cancer screening,
190
comprehensive geriatric
assessment, 190–191
demographics, 188
exercise therapies, 191–193
flu vaccine, 189
humor therapy, 406–407
joie de vivre, 541–542
massage therapy, 404–405
mobility and, 541
nutrition, 193–195
osteoporosis screening, 190
pneumonia vaccine, 189
prostate cancer
screening, 190
purpose and, 495
resilience and, 491
shingles vaccine, 189
social relationships, 193
TDAP vaccine, 189
three types of well-being
in, 574
Gignac, M.A., 527
Gilbert, P., 520
ginger, 222
gingko biloba, 309

ginseng, 383
Gladwell, M., 464
Godbey, G.C., 565
goji berry, 383
Goleman, D., 463
Goodkin, K., 140, 142
Gottman, J., 548, 561
gratitude, 204, 345, 359–361
Graves' disease, 151, 169
grit, 464, 467
growth hormone, 164–166
Gupta, N., 170
Gurin Global Likert Scale, 61

Hanh, T.N., 345
happiness, 9, 573–574
Hartig, T., 570
Hasani-Ranjbar, S., 166
Haskins, E.C., 369–372
Hassanpour-Dehkordi, A., 329
hatha yoga, 353
headaches, meditation and, 349
Headspace (computer
application), 607
healed state, 505
healing, defined, 504–506
healing practices
cultural, 505–507
effects of, 508–509
energy, 508
holism, 578–579
medical clinicians, 507
healing process
inside influences, 510
outside influences, 509
phenomenology of, 512
reciprocity of, 511–512
speed of, 510–511
health
defined, 2, 45, 303
equity, 117
traditional definition, 5
healthcare professionals. see
clinician wellness
health-related quality of
life, 231
Healthy People, 2010, 251
Healthy People, 2020, 117
hearing, 456–457
heart disease, 1
heavy metals, fertility and,
124–125
hedonic wellness, 6, 577
Heintzelman, S.J., 40, 41
Helvig, A., 327
Henderson, K.A., 568

Henning, R.A., 328
herbal therapies. see also
adaptogens
Ayurvedic medicine, 386,
389–390
cancer, 383–384
cannabinoid treatment,
72–73
chronic pain, 222–223
curcumin, 91
essential oils, 308
peppermint/caraway oil,
90, 94
sexual wellness, 339–340
STW5, 90
traditional Chinese
medicine, 381–383
UTIs and, 105
Herbert, T.B., 388
Heymsfield, S.B., 165
hierarchy of needs, 7–8,
179
HIV, aesthetics and, 397
HIV infection, 140–143
Hojjat, H., 394
holism
Ayurvedic medicine, 384
happiness and, 573–574
healing and, 578–579
iceberg model, 574–577
longing and yearning, 578
nature therapy, 414
reacting, responding, and
mindfulness, 577–578
suffering and, 579–580
wellness approaches to,
573
honesty, intimacy and, 335
Hood, D., 540
hope therapy, 9, 498–499
hormone replacement therapy
(HRT), 162–163
hormones
DHEA, 305
stress response, 487
UTIs and, 102–103
hospice, 239
HowsYourHealth.org
(website), 20–21
Hudziak, J., 206
humor therapy
cardiovascular and
pulmonary disorders, 82
defined, 404–406
demographics, 406–407
effects of, 406

Huntington's chorea, 326–327
Huta, V., 574
hyperparathyroidism, 167
hypertension, 380–381
hyperthyroidism, 169–170
hypoactive sexual desire
    disorder, 105–106, 107
hypoparathyroidism,
    166–167
hypothalamic–pituitary–
    adrenal axis (HPA axis),
    9–10, 160
hypothalamic–pituitary–
    adrenocortical axis, 136
hypothyroidism, 169

iceberg model, 574–577
Iio, M., 145
Ikeda, H., 328
illness uncertainty, 152
immune system
    circadian rhythm, 430
    massage therapy and, 404
Indivisible Self: An Evidence
    Based Model of Wellness,
    46, 54
inflammation, 367
inflammatory bowel diseases
    therapies
    acupuncture and
        moxibustion, 91–92
    cognitive-behavioral therapy
        and mindfulness, 92
    curcumin, 91
    exercise, 92
    probiotics, 93
    specialized diet, 92
Insight Timer (computer
    application), 612–613
insomnia. see also sleep
    CBT for, 119, 366
    etiology of, 309
    meditation and, 349
    melatonin for, 309
    mindfulness and, 346
    pharmaceuticals for, 309
Institute for Health Care
    Improvement, 265–266
Institute of Medicine, 425
Institute of Medicine
    Education and Spirituality
    at Ochsner, 511
integration, 555–557
interactive voice response
    technology (IVR), 14, 20
interconnection, 555–557

interest/arousal disorder,
    105–106
interventional management
    strategies (chronic pain),
    217–219
interventions
    clinician individual,
        262–263
    clinician organizations,
        265–266
    clinician practice, 263–264
    clinician system, 267
    compassion, 519
    forgiveness, 358–359
    gratitude, 360
    meaning therapy, 497–498
    social connection, 516–518
intimacy, 334–336
irritable bowel syndrome
    therapies
    exercise, 94
    fiber, 93
    FODMAP diet, 93, 276–277
    peppermint oil, 94
    probiotics, 94
    psychological, 94
IsHak, W., 140, 142

Jacobsen, K., 415
Jacobsen, P., 233
Jahoda, M., 479
job satisfaction elements,
    537
Johnson & Johnson, 249–250
joie de vivre, 541–542

Kabat-Zinn, J., 204–205,
    346
Kalia, A., 292
Kaptchuk, T.J., 506
Karpatkin, H.I., 380
kava, 307
Kearney, M., 579
Kececi, Y., 396
Kegel exercises, 100
Kerndt, P.R., 164
ketamine, 213
ketogenic diet, 73, 275
Keys, A., 273
Khan, s., 390
kidney health
    chronic kidney disease,
        110
    kidney stones, 110–111
Kim, J.H., 325
kindness, acts of, 204

King, L.A., 40, 41
Kirby, J.N., 519
Kissane, D.W., 531
Klainin-Yobas, P., 329
Kleiber, D., 569,
Klempner, D., 438
Kok, B.E., 83
Kreifelts, B., 465
Kroenke, C.H., 163
Kuo, F.E., 570

labor dance, 120
labor pain management. see
    also pregnancy
    acupressure and
        acupuncture, 121
    cesarean section, 120
    continuous labor
        support, 120
    delivery positions, 120
    labor dance, 120
    water immersion, 120–121
language, 30
Lanzi, R., 163
lead, 124
Lee, N.-H., 383
Lee, S., 165
Lee, T.H., 467,
leisure. see also play
    coping with stress and, 567
    importance of, 565–566
    managing life transitions,
        568–569
    nature and, 569–570
    social and emotional health,
        567–568
leptin, 165–166
Lewis, E.T., 238
Li, X., 152, 154
licorice, 383
Liew, M., 605
life review, 243–244
life summary intervention, 71
Lind, N., 146
Liston, C., 465
Live for Life program, 249–250
Lockwood, N.L., 82
logotherapy, 496–497
loneliness, 39
Loprinzi, P.D., 324
love relationships, 541,
    561–562
loving-kindness meditation
    (LKM), 520
low back pain, 212
low FOPMAP diet, 93

low glycemic index treatment diet, 74
Luxembourg Declaration on Workplace Health Promotion in the European Union, 250
Lyubomirsky, S., 547

Ma, T.T., 91
magnesium deficiency, 222
magnesium oxide, 72
Mahoney, A., 361
make-up, 399
maladaptive thinking reduction, 367
male sexual dysfunction
  delayed ejaculation, 107–108
  erectile disorder, 107
  hypoactive sexual desire disorder, 107
  premature ejaculation, 107
Manderscheid, R.W., 2
Mansukhani, M.P., 325
Mantra (computer application), 614
manual body therapies
  acupuncture, 75
  back pain, 220
  massage, 75
  spinal manipulation, 75
marijuana, 123
Martinson, C., 191
Maslow, A., 7–8, 179
Mason, S., 387
massage therapy
  cardiovascular and pulmonary disorders, 80
  defined, 403
  effects of, 403–404
  low back pain, 219–220
  multiple sclerosis, 75
  osteopathic manipulation, 219–220
  patient demographics of, 404–405
maternal care disparities, 118
maternal mortality and morbidity, 117–118
May, B., 90
Mayer–Salovey–Caruso Emotional Intelligence Test (MSCEIT), 466, 467–468
McChrystal, S., 467
meaning in life

defined, 495–496
logotherapy, 496–497
meaning therapy, 497–498
work–life balance, 548
Meaning in Life Questionnaire, 41
meaning therapy, 497–498
measurement-based care, 42, 227–230
mechanisms of action
  allopathic medicine, 379–380
  traditional Chinese medicine, 378–379
medical humanities, 436, 440–442
meditation
  Ayurvedic medicine, 389
  cardiovascular and pulmonary disorders, 80
  circadian rhythm, 432
  defined, 348
  instructions, 350–351
  loving-kindness and compassion, 520
  mastery of, 348–349
  mindfulness, 67–68
  neuroenhancement, 373–374
  research, 221, 349–350
  role of breathing in, 348
Mediterranean diet, 273–274
medium-chain triglyceride diet, 74
melatonin, 309
menopause, 127
Menopause-Specific Quality of Life Questionnaire, 162
mental health, defined, 57
mental wellness
  humor therapy, 406–407
  rest and, 327–328
  women's, 118–119
mercury, 124
meta-honesty, 335
methadone, 212
methenamine, 104
methylphenidate, 308
migraines, 213, 219
MIND diet, 277–278
MindBody (computer application), 611
Mind–Body Skills Group, 349
mind–body therapies
  chronic pain, 220–221
  meditation, 67–68

neurofeedback, 68
progressive relaxation, 67
usage of, 67
yoga, 69
mindful self-compassion (MSC), 519–520
Mindfulness-Based Stress Reduction, 204–205, 346
mindfulness
  cancer wellness, 234
  Cushing syndrome, 161
  defined, 345
  diabetes, 165
  forgiveness and, 358
  incorporation of, 347
  indications for, 347
  meditation and, 67–68
  overactive bladder (OAB), 100–101
  positive neuropsychology, 368
  during pregnancy, 119
  psychosocial factors, 92
  research, 346–347
  sexual wellness, 341
  social connection, 517–518
  stress reduction, 220
  at work, 254–255, 522
mindsight, 558
Mizokami, T., 151, 153
modified Atkins diet, 74, 277
modular treatment, 369–370
mommy makeover procedure, 396
Mooney, K.A., 475
motivational enhancement therapy with CBT (MET-CBT), 119
Mount, B., 579
movement-based meditation therapies, 221
moxibustion, 91–92
multiple sclerosis, 156, 380
Muse (wellness device), 617
music therapy
  cardiovascular and pulmonary disorders, 82–83
  child and adolescent health, 205
  chronic pain, 223
  effects of, 407–408
  neuroenhancement, 374
Myers, J., 46, 414

nadi suddhi, 348
National Academy of
    Medicine, 259–260
National Wellness Institute,
    4
nature deficit disorder, 432
nature therapy, 413–416,
    419–420, 567, 569–570
nature versus nurture,
    465–466
Nazari, G., 607
Neff, K.D., 471, 518
Neighborhood Asthma
    Coalition, 146
Nelson, T.F., 569
neoplastic disease, 225
neuroenhancement
    brain stimulation,
        372–373
    cognitive enhancement
        and, 372
    exercise therapies, 373
    meditation and yoga,
        373–374
    music therapy, 374
    social relationships,
        554–555
neurofeedback, 68, 365
neurological disorders
    CAM healthcare practices
        usage, 66–67
    complexity of, 66
neuromodulation, 218–219,
    408. *see also* circadian
    rhythm
neuropathic medications,
    212–217
neuroplasticity, 486, 561
Ng, L.K., 2
Nimrod G., 568
Nisbet, E.K., 414
non-steroidal anti-
    inflammatory drugs
    (NSAIDs), 212–213,
    310–311
nutraceuticals. *see also* dietary
    supplements
    adaptogens, 297–298
    clinician tips, 300
    defined, 206, 292
    dietary fiber, 293
    polyphenols, 295–297
    polyunsaturated fatty acids,
        293–294
    prebiotics and
        probiotics, 293

spices, 296
    toxicity potential of, 298–299
    vitamins, 294–296
nutrition. *see also* diet therapy
    child and adolescent health,
        200–201
    chronic pain, 221–222
    fertility, 121
    geriatric wellness, 193–195
    obesity and, 165–166
    positive
        neuropsychology, 367
    testosterone deficiency, 168
    workplace wellness
        programs, 252–254

obesity
    childhood, 200–201
    and fertility, 121–122
    hormones and, 165–166
    OAB and, 100
    sleep and, 327
objective/subjective well-being
    perspectives, 38–39
Occupational Safety and
    Health Act (OSHA), 249
omega-3 fatty acids, 222,
    293–294
operant-behavioral
    therapy, 220
opiates, 123
opioids, 209–212
Optimal Living Profile, 61
optimal sleep, 324–325
Organization for Economic
    Cooperation and
    Development (OECD),
    40
orgasm synchronization, 341
orgasmic disorder
    (female), 106
Ornish diet, 278
Osaki, T.H., 397
osteopathic manipulation, 220
osteoporosis
    screening, 190
    statistics, 310
overactive bladder (OAB)
    behavioral modification for,
        99–101
    symptoms of, 99
oxcarbazepine, 213

Padesky, C.A., 475
pain. *see* chronic pain
Paleolithic diet, 274

palliative care. *see* end-of-life
    care
Palmer, M., 407
pancreas, 427–428
Panda, S., 428
Parás-Bravo, P., 330
parathyroid hormone, 166–167
Pargament, K., 361
Parkinson's disease, 326–327
parks. *see* nature therapy
Parry, C., 568
passive constructive
    response, 465
passive destructive
    response, 465
Patient Checklist-, 5, 25
Patient Health Questionnaire
    (PHQ), 24
Patient Reported Outcomes
    Measurement
    Information System
    (PROMIS), 13, 19, 598
pelvic floor muscle therapy,
    100
Pennebaker, J.W., 440
peppermint/caraway oil, 90, 94
Perceived Wellness Survey, 61
PERMA model, 18, 546–547,
    548–549
PERMA-Profiler, 18
Personal and Social
    Performance Scale, 61
personalized wellness plan,
    311, 583–596
Pert, C., 388
pet therapy, 223, 416–417,
    419–420
Peterson, C., 475
pharmaceuticals
    anxiety, 306–307
    child and adolescent
        health, 206
    chronic medical conditions,
        183–184
    chronic pain, 209–217,
        310–311
    cognitive disorders, 308
    depression, 304
    usage of, 303
phosphodiesterase inhibitor
    (PDE-5), 336
physical activity. *see* exercise
    therapies
physiological relaxation,
    329–330
Pilates, 320

Pimental, P.A., 365–366, 368–369
Pinto, S.L., 165
PIP (wellness device), 617
plant-based diet, 276
play, 539–540. *see also* leisure
pneumonia vaccine, 189
polyphenols, 72–73, 295–297
polyunsaturated fatty acids, 293–294
polyvagal theory, 558
Porges, S., 559
positive neuropsychology
  biofeedback, 368
  defined, 365–366
  exercise therapies, 368
  inflammation and pain, 367
  maladaptive thinking reduction, 367
  nutrition and diet, 367
  restorative techniques, 366
  role of, 474–475
  social relationships, 368
  spirituality and mindfulness, 368
  stimulating activities, 365–366
  trauma healing, 368–369
positive psychology, 38, 528–529, 547
positive psychotherapy (PPT), 475–477
positive savoring, 70
positive thinking, 83
postherpetic neuralgia, 212, 218
posttraumatic growth, 43
posttraumatic stress disorder (PTSD), 350
Pott, P., 248
Potter, D.J., 428
prebiotics, 293
pregabalin, 213
pregnancy. *see also* labor pain management
  anxiety and depression during, 119
  insomnia, 119
  labor pain management, 119–121
  lifestyle changes and, 125
  low-resource settings, 126
  massage therapy, 404–405
  stress and, 118
premature ejaculation, 107

premenstrual syndrome, 126–127
President's Council on Physical Fitness and Sports, 249
Primary Care PTSD Screen for DSM-, 5, 25
primary dysmenorrhea, 128
probiotics
  irritable bowel syndrome therapies, 93, 94
  nutraceuticals, 293
  UTIs and, 103
progesterone, 162–163
progressive muscular relaxation, 329
progressive relaxation, 67
prostate cancer, 109
  screening, 190
prostate health
  alternative treatments, 109–110
  benign prostatic hyperplasia, 108–109
  cancer, 109
  prostatitis, 109
prostatitis, 109
psychiatric and substance-use disorders
  enhancing wellness, 62–63
  history of wellness in, 57–58
  validation of wellness concept, 58–62
psychiatric wellness models, 59–61
psychological health
  chronic illness, 525–527
  fertility, 122
  OAB and, 101
  relaxation, 329
psychoneuroimmunology (PNI). *see also* complementary and alternative medical practices
  allergic process, 143–149
  allergy resilience, 149
  autoimmune disease, 149–157
  Ayurvedic medicine, 387
  defined, 135
  infectious process, 139–143
  integrative approach of, 135–137
psychosocial therapies
  art therapy, 70

cancer wellness, 234
child and adolescent health, 204
chronic medical conditions, 185
cognitive-behavioral therapy, 69–70
gender identity/sexual orientation, 30–31
language, 30
life summary, 71
positive savoring, 70
psychosocial history, 26–29, 32
race/ethnicity, 29–30
religion/spiritual beliefs, 30
senses, 449–450
workplace wellness programs, 254–255
psychotherapy
  autoimmune disease, 156–157
  chronic illness, 528
  chronic medical conditions, 184–185
  chronic pain, 220
  positive, 475–477
  therapeutic presence, 559
pulmonary disorders. *see* cardiovascular and pulmonary disorders
purpose
  defined, 494
  development, 495
Purpose in Life Test, 41

Quality of Care Model, 191
quality of life
  cancer, 231
  mindfulness and, 346
  Short-Form Health Survey (SF-36), 40
  terminal illness, 237–238
  wellness and, 2–3, 178
quality of life therapy, 475
quality of life therapy and coaching, 477–478

race/ethnicity, 29–30
Rachele, J., 5–6, 7
radiation, 124
radiculopathy, 212
Radin, D., 512
radiofrequency ablation, 217

radiofrequency electromagnetic waves (RFEMV), 124
Ramazzini, B., 248
RAND Corporation, 251–252, 255, 256
Rashid, T., 475–477
Raymore, L.A., 569
Recine, A.C., 358
Reece, R.F., 414
rehabilitation, 156
Reig-Ferrer, A., 329
relational integration, 557–560
relationship management, 464–465, 471
relationship wellness, 577
Relax Melodies (computer application), 607–608
relaxation training
  benefits of, 329
  chronic pain, 220–221
  defined, 324
  irritable bowel syndrome therapies, 94
  physiological, 329–330
  psychological, 329
reliability (measurement), 41, 61–62
religion/spiritual beliefs
  cancer wellness, 234
  child and adolescent health, 205–206
  patient, 30
  terminal illness, 244–245
  wellness theory, 47–50
Renger, R., 6
Renz, M., 244
reproductive clock, 121
resilience
  building, 487–490
  defined, 484–485
  genetics, 485
  measurement, 490
  physiology of, 486–487
  training, 125–126, 149, 203–204, 464
  wellness and, 490–491
resilience scale for adults, 490
response bias, 42
rest
  as base of support for physical health, 328–329
  defined, 324, 327
  mental health and, 327–328
Rhatz, E., 511

rheumatoid arthritis, 151, 156
riboflavin, 72
Rich, G., 90
river of integration, 556–557
Robinson, J.P., 565
Roche, A., 395, 397
Rojas, M., 156
Romano, J., 23
Ronzio, R.A., 162
Roscoe, L.J., 4–5
Rose, G.L., 20
Rowles, S.V., 164
Russell, R., 414
Ryan, R.M., 574, 578
Ryff, C., 479

S-adenosyl-L-methionine (SAMe), 305
sadness, 9
Saeed, S., 491
Sanders, C.R., 416
Sandseter, E.B.H., 415
Sanvello (computer application), 613
Satisfaction with Life Scale (SWLS), 17–18, 41
saw palmetto, 108
Schussel, L., 529–530
Scott, J.G., 509
screening and assessment methods
  biopsychosocial, 23–34
  cancer, 227
  goals of, 13–15
  instruments, 15–19
  lifestyle factors, 19–21
  scribes, 264
selective serotonin reuptake inhibitors (SSRIs), 213
self-actualization, 7–8
self-awareness, 463–464, 470, 518–519, 525–526
self-compassion, 518–519
self-esteem, 471
self-management, 471
self-reflection, 33
self-regulation, 464
self-reporting, 61–62
Seligman, M., 18, 38, 204, 465, 474, 475–477, 548,
Seligman's Authentic Happiness Inventory, 70
sensate focus, 341–342
senses and wellness
  blending multiple, 459

clinical diagnosing, 450–451
functions of, 449
hearing, 456–457
historical importance of, 448–449
psychosocial factors, 449–450
sight, 454–456
smell, 452–454
taste, 451–452
touch, 457–459
sensory overstimulation, 450
serotonin–norepinephrine reuptake inhibitors (SNRIs), 213
sertraline, 304
sexual dysfunction
  defined, 105
  female, 105–107
  male, 107–108
sexual health, defined, 105
sexual orientation, 30–31
sexual wellness
  anterior fornix erogenous zone stimulation, 341
  arousal and, 332–334
  CBT for, 340–341
  coital alignment technique, 341
  defined, 332–333
  diet therapy, 340
  dietary supplements for, 339
  herbal therapies, 339–340
  intimacy and, 334–336
  mindfulness for, 341
  orgasm synchronization, 341
  pharmaceuticals for, 335–338
  sensate focus, 341–342
  tips for, 343
shingles vaccine, 189
Short-Form Health Survey (SF-36), 17
Sickness Impact Profile, 60–61
Siegel, D., 555, 558
sight, 454–456
Six Dimensions of Wellness model, 4, 45–46, 53, 536
Skov, A.R., 166
sleep. see also insomnia
  need for, 324
  neurodegenerative diseases, 326–327
  obesity and, 327
  optimal, 324–325

sleep apnea, 327
sleep deprivation, 325–326, 327
sleep patterns
  cancer, 231–232
  child and adolescent health, 202–203
  circadian rhythm, 425–426, 430
  clinician wellness, 325–326
  long and short term, 325–327
smell, 452–454
smoking cessation. see tobacco use
Snyder, C.R., 498–499
social awareness, 464, 471
social connection. see also social relationships
  benefits of, 515–516
  defined, 515
  health risk of isolation, 516
  interventions, 516–518
  love relationships, 541
social flow, 547
social isolation, 516
social jet lag, 431, 433
social media use, 202. see also virtual community
social relationships. see also community; social connection
  allergic process, 146–147
  autoimmune disease, 152–154
  cardiovascular and pulmonary disorders, 83
  child and adolescent health, 200
  chronic illness, 529–530
  emotional intelligence, 464–465
  family and, 560–561
  friendships, 561
  geriatric wellness, 193
  healthy integration, 555–557
  HIV and, 140
  humor therapy and, 406
  love, 561–562
  neuroenhancement, 554–555
  positive effects of, 553–554
  positive neuropsychology, 368
  relational integration, 557–560

social network
  interventions, 126
  terminal illness, 245
  work–life balance, 548
social synapse, 559
social–emotional learning (SEL), 203–204
Solomon, G., 387
somatosensory amplification, 9
Song, Z., 521
spices, 296
spinal cord stimulation, 218
spinal manipulation, 75, 220
spirituality and religion
  chronic illness, 530
  healing practices, 506
  patient, 361–363
  positive neuropsychology, 368
SSC Nodel Outcomes Cascade, 149, 157
St. John's wort, 304–305
Stanford WellMD Center, 259
Stanton, C., 466
Steptoe, A., 574
Stojanovic, L., 150
Stone, A.A., 139
stress
  allergies and, 144–146
  anatomical structures in, 486–487
  autoimmune disease, 150–152
  Ayurvedic medicine, 388–389
  circadian rhythm, 428–429
  clinician, 258–259
  early-life, 466
  HIV and, 140
  and the HPA axis, 9–10
  humor therapy and, 406
  infectious process, 139–143
  intimacy and, 334
  leisure and, 567
  massage therapy and, 403
  mindfulness and, 346
  neurotransmitters in, 487
  and psychoneuroimmunology, 136
  women's wellness, 118
  workplace, 254, 535
  yoga and, 354

Stressor–Support–Coping model (SSC), 135, 136–139
STW5, 85
styling
  clothing, 400
  make-up, 399
suboptimal wellness (chronic medical conditions), 179
substance-use disorders. see psychiatric and substance-use disorders
suffering, 579–580
Suido, S., 204
Sullivan, W.C., 570
superchiasmatic nucleus, 423–425
supplements. see dietary supplements
surprise, 10
survivorship care plans, 233
Suwalska, A., 169
Sweeney, T., 46, 536
sympathetic blocks, 218

tai chi, 221, 319–320
taste, 451–452
TDAP vaccine, 189
teamwork, clinician practice, 264
telomere length, 346, 554
terminal illness. see also end of life care
  versus chronic, 178–179
  defined, 237
  Eriksonian stages, 243
  life review, 243–244
  loss of control adjustments, 242–243
  physiologic well-being, 239–241
  psychological well-being, 241–242
  quality of life, 237–238
  religion/spiritual beliefs, 244–245
  social relationships, 245
testosterone, 168–169, 429
therapeutic presence, 559
Thomas, R.J., 467
Thomas Kilmann Conflict Mode Instrument (TKI), 468–469
Thrash, T., 438
thyroid hormone, 169–170
tissue repair, massage therapy, 404

tobacco use
 fertility and, 122–123
 meditation and, 349
 workplace wellness
  programs, 252–254
total worker health model, 536
touch, 457–459
Toumpanakis, A., 164
Toussaint, L., 358
toxicity potential,
 nutraceutical, 298–299
traditional Chinese medicine
 acupuncture, 378
 cancer, 383–384
 defined, 378
 herbal therapies, 381–383
 mechanisms of action,
  378–379
 taste pathology, 452
transcranial direct current
 stimulation, 372, 373
transcranial magnetic
 stimulation, 218, 373
transcutaneous electrical
 nerve stimulation
 (TENS), 367
trauma healing
 coping mechanisms for,
  487–490
 positive neuropsychology,
  368–369
trazodone, 309
Trichopoulou, A., 273
tricyclic antidepressants, 213
trigeminal neuralgia, 212, 213
turmeric, 222, 383. see also
 curcumin

Ufferman, R.C., 161
ulcerative colitis. see
 inflammatory bowel
 diseases therapies
Ulrich, R., 570
United Nations Sustainable
 Development Goals, 414
urinary symptoms not caused
 by bacteria, 105
urinary tract infections
 (UTIs)
 alternative treatments for
  prevention of, 102–105
 definition and occurrence of,
  101–102
US Preventative Services
 Task Force (USPSTF),
 116, 189

vaccine therapy
 geriatric wellness, 189
 UTIs and, 104

vagus nerve stimulation, 219
Vaidya, G.C., 167
valerian root, 307–308
validity (measurement), 41
Vankim, N.A., 569
Vayalil, P.K., 390
vegetarian diet, 276
Vermont Family Based
 Approach, 206
Villar, H.C., 169
Virgin Pulse (computer
 application), 613
virtual community, 522–523.
  see also social media use
virtual reality, 221, 617
vision. see sight
vitamin B2, 72
vitamin B12, 222
vitamin C, 104
vitamin D, 71–72, 163, 168, 222
vitamins, risks and benefits,
 294–296

Walsh, A.P., 169, 476
Ware, J.E., 17
water consumption, 102–103
water immersion, 120–121
websites for wellness
 activities, 586
weight-loss diets, 278
well-being
 assessment instruments,
  15–19
 defined, 2, 6–7
 eudaimonia, 40–41
 lifestyle factors and, 19–21
 objective/subjective
  perspectives, 38–39
 OECD questionnaire, 40
 principles, 6
 quality of life, 40
 therapy, 478–480
Well-Being Promotion
 Program, 204
wellness
 categories, 302
 chronic diseases and, 1
 chronic illness, 527–530
 defined, 2–3, 11, 58–59, 178,
  226, 448
 emotions and, 8–10
 evaluative, 576–577

hedonic, 577
 operational understanding,
  5–6, 7
 resilience and, 490–491
 self-actualization and, 7–8
wellness computer
 applications, 605–614
wellness devices, 607, 614–617
wellness dimensions
 five core dimensions, 4–5
 National Wellness
  Institute, 4
 six core, 6
 WHO, 3
Wellness Evaluation of
 Lifestyle, 61
wellness measurement
 accuracy, 41
 administration issues,
  42–43
 evolving nature of, 43–44
 PROMIS, 598
 psychiatric and substance-
  use disorders, 61
 what to measure, 37–41
wellness principles, 6
wellness treatment plan
 background
  considerations, 582
 defined, 45
 establishment, 50–51
 Indivisible Self model, 46, 54
 multicultural variables, 51
 personalized, 583–596
 research, 46–50
 Six Dimensions of Wellness,
  4, 45–46, 53
 steps, 51–53
 Wheel of Wellness, 3–4
well-woman chart, 116
What Matters Index, 20–21
Wheel of Wellness model, 3–4,
 536, 560
White, J., 489
whole-person care. see holism
Williams, R.E., 162
Witmer, J.M., 536
women's empowerment, 126
Women's Preventative Services
 Initiative (WPSI),
 116–117, 162
women's wellness
 advocacy, 118
 fertility, 121–125
 gynecological, 126–128
 health equity, 117

women's wellness (cont.)
  labor pain management,
    119–121
  lifestyle changes, 125
  maternal care disparities, 118
  maternal mortality and
    morbidity, 117–118
  mental, 118–119
  prevention care to improve,
    116–117
Wong, P., 497–498
work–life balance
  accomplishment, 548
  engagement, 547
  meaning in life, 548
  Norwegian culture, 545–546
  PERMA model, 546–547,
    548–549
  positive psychology, 547
  social relationships, 548
workplace wellness program
    types
  effectiveness of, 255–256
  physical health, 252–254

  psychological health, 254–255
workplace wellness programs
  history of, 248–250
  individual/organization
    interaction, 250
  job satisfaction, 537
  mindfulness, 522
  occurrence of, 248
  overview of, 535–537
  quality metrics, 251–252
  serious health problem
    prevention, 250–251
  success measurement, 252
World Happiness Report, 553
World Health Organization
    (WHO), 2, 3, 38, 40, 45,
    57, 303, 380, 427, 525, 584
World Health Organization
    Well-Being Index (WHO-
    5), 15–17

Yamauchi, T., 165
yoga
  8 limbs of, 352

asana, 353
cancer, 233
cardiovascular and
    pulmonary disorders, 80
child and adolescent health,
    201–202
chronic pain, 221
clinician tips, 354
Cushing syndrome, 161
defined, 351–352
devotion and, 353
hyperthyroidism, 170
importance of, 69
irritable bowel syndrome
    therapies, 94
laughter, 406
many meanings of, 352–353
neuroenhancement, 373–374
research, 353–354
Yoshimura, S.M., 82

Zhao, X., 380
Zorilla, E.P., 388
Zumrutdal, E., 170